Diabetes: Causes, Diagnosis and Treatment

Diabetes: Causes, Diagnosis and Treatment

Editor: Carlos Rickman

FOSTER ACADEMICS

www.fosteracademics.com

www.fosteracademics.com

FOSTER ACADEMICS

Cataloging-in-Publication Data

Diabetes : causes, diagnosis and treatment / edited by Carlos Rickman.
p. cm.
Includes bibliographical references and index.
ISBN 978-1-63242-539-3
1. Diabetes. 2. Diabetes--Diagnosis. 3. Diabetes--Treatment. I. Rickman, Carlos.
RC660 .D53 2018
616.462--dc23

Foster Academics,
118-35 Queens Blvd., Suite 400,
Forest Hills, NY 11375, USA

ISBN 978-1-63242-539-3 (Hardback)

Printed and bound in China.

Contents

Preface

Diabetes is a medical condition in which the body is either unable to create insulin or rejects insulin leading to the development of serious disorders. This book on diabetes covers all the latest advances that are found in this field. It elucidates the symptoms and conditions of diabetes as well as the long-term risks that develop because of this disorder have been included. It also mentions new diagnostic techniques to detect diabetes. The book will act as a resource guide for both students and researchers. It will provide crucial information that will contribute to the growth of the discipline.

This book is a comprehensive compilation of works of different researchers from varied parts of the world. It includes valuable experiences of the researchers with the sole objective of providing the readers (learners) with a proper knowledge of the concerned field. This book will be beneficial in evoking inspiration and enhancing the knowledge of the interested readers.

In the end, I would like to extend my heartiest thanks to the authors who worked with great determination on their chapters. I also appreciate the publisher's support in the course of the book. I would also like to deeply acknowledge my family who stood by me as a source of inspiration during the project.

Editor

Association between Tissue Characteristics of Coronary Plaque and Distal Embolization after Coronary Intervention in Acute Coronary Syndrome Patients: Insights from a Meta-Analysis of Virtual Histology-Intravascular Ultrasound Studies

Song Ding[a], Longwei Xu[a], Fan Yang, Lingcong Kong, Yichao Zhao, Lingchen Gao, Wei Wang, Rende Xu, Heng Ge, Meng Jiang, Jun Pu*, Ben He*

From Department of Cardiology, Ren Ji Hospital, School of Medicine, Shanghai Jiao Tong University, Shanghai, China

Abstract

Background and Objectives: The predictive value of plaque characteristics assessed by virtual histology-intravascular ultrasound (VH-IVUS) including fibrous tissue (FT), fibrofatty (FF), necrotic core (NC) and dense calcium (DC) in identifying distal embolization after percutaneous coronary intervention (PCI) is still controversial. We performed a systematic review and meta-analysis to summarize the association of pre-PCI plaque composition and post-PCI distal embolization in acute coronary syndrome patients.

Methods: Studies were identified in PubMed, OVID, EMBASE, the Cochrane Library, the Current Controlled Trials Register, reviews, and reference lists of relevant articles. A meta-analysis using both fixed and random effects models with assessment of study heterogeneity and publication bias was performed.

Results: Of the 388 articles screened, 10 studies with a total of 872 subjects (199 with distal embolization and 673 with normal flow) met the eligibility of our study. Compared with normal flow groups, significant higher absolute volume of NC [weighted mean differences (WMD): 5.79 mm^3, 95% CI: 3.02 to 8.55 mm^3; $p<0.001$] and DC (WMD: 2.55 mm^3, 95% CI: 0.22 to 4.88 mm^3; $p=0.03$) were found in acute coronary syndrome patients with distal embolization. Further subgroup analysis demonstrated that the predictive value of tissue characteristics in determining distal embolization was correlated to clinical scenario of the patients, definition of distal embolization, and whether the percutaneous aspiration thrombectomy was applied.

Conclusion: Our study that pooled current evidence showed that plaque components were closely related to the distal embolization after PCI, especially the absolute volume of NC and DC, supporting further studies with larger sample size and high-methodological quality.

Editor: Claudio Moretti, S.G.Battista Hospital, Italy

Funding: This work was supported by the National Natural Science Foundation of China (81330006, 81170192, 81270282, 81070176, and 81400261), International Cooperation Program of Shanghai Committee of Science and Technology (12410708300), Shanghai Leading Medical Talents Program and Shanghai Leading Talents Program (LJ10007), Program for New Century Excellent Talents in University from Ministry of Education of China (NCET-12-0352), Shanghai Shuguang Program (12SG22), Key Basic Research Program of Shanghai Committee of Science and Technology (14JC1404500), and Shanghai Jiao Tong University Science and Technology Foundation (Grant No. YZ1005). The funders had no role in study design, data collection and analysis, decision to publish, or preparation of the manuscript.

Competing Interests: The authors have declared that no competing interests exist.

* Email: pujun310@hotmail.com (JP); heben1025@hotmail.com (BH)

[a] These authors contributed equally to this work.

Introduction

Rationale

Distal embolization (DE) is a common complication after percutaneous coronary intervention (PCI), particularly in the setting of acute coronary syndrome (ACS) or vein graft intervention, which may result in microvascular obstruction and no-reflow phenomenon [1,2]. This undesirable side effect of PCI has been confirmed to be associated with increased post-procedural myocardial infarction, in-hospital mortality, and long-term adverse events [3–5]. However, there is no effective strategy for prediction and prevention of DE, which is an important issue for interventional cardiology.

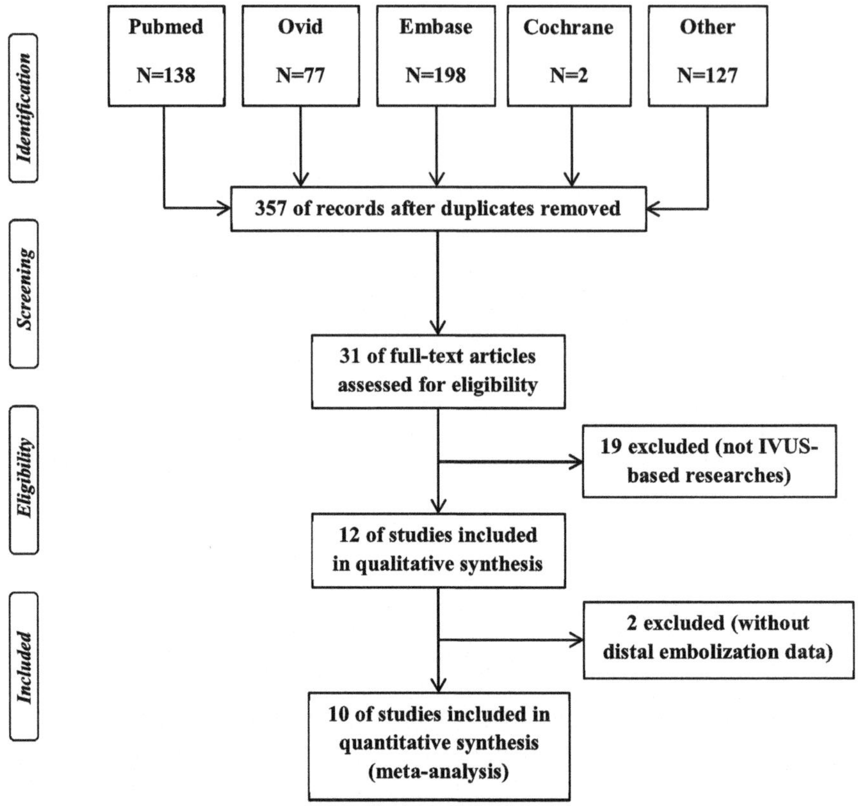

Figure 1. Process of study selection.

Although several studies using grayscale intravascular ultrasound (IVUS) have indicated that plaque characteristics identified by pre-interventional IVUS (i.e., a large plaque burden, a lipid-pool-like image, and positive remodeling) maybe associated with the angiographic no-reflow phenomenon in ACS patients [6–10], gray-scale IVUS is dependent on the simple interpretation of acoustic reflections and of limited value for identifying specific plaque components [11]. Recently, some new methods able to assess both plaque morphology and tissue characteristics, such as virtual histology-IVUS (VH-IVUS), have become clinically available. VH-IVUS is based on spectral and amplitude analysis of IVUS backscattered radiofrequency that allows for characterization of in-vivo atherosclerotic plaque into four types: fibrous (FT), fibrofatty (FF), necrotic core (NC), and dense calcium (DC) [12–23]. However, whether pre-PCI plaque characteristics of culprit lesion assessed by VH-IVUS could predict post-PCI angiographic DE, and which plaque components are associated with no-reflow phenomenon remain debated. We therefore performed a systematic review that pooled current evidence to investigate the relationship between pre-PCI plaque composition characteristics assessed by VH-IVUS and post-PCI DE phenomenon in ACS patients.

Methods

Search strategy

PubMed, Ovid, EMBASE, and the Cochrane Library databases were searched in their entirety from January 2002 to April 2013. Complex search strategies were formulated using the following MESH terms and text words: intravascular ultrasound, virtual histology, IVUS, VH-IVUS, plaque component, plaque composition, plaque characteristic, no reflow, DE, microembolization, and obstruction. In order to identify any studies missed by the literature searches, we had searched reference lists of all eligible studies and relevant review articles. In addition, we searched from published and ongoing trials in clinical trial registries (ClinicalTrials.gov, Controlled-trials.com and the WHO International Clinical Trials Registry Platform). Searches were not restricted by language, time published, or publication status. Duplicate reports were eliminated (Appendix S1).

Study selection

We included studies when the following criteria were met:(1) Plaque characteristics were assessed by VH-IVUS; (2) VH-IVUS was performed before coronary intervention in ACS patients; and (3) DE was defined according to angiographic evidence or clinical relevancy. Studies without normal flow (NF) group were excluded from our analysis.

Data extraction

Two reviewers (D. S. and P. J.) assessed the eligibility of studies using a standardized form developed for this purpose in duplicate and independently. Disagreements were adjudicated by resolved by consensus. Data extraction was completed by the same observers using a standardized data extraction form developed for this study. The following information was extracted from each study: sample size, mean age, gender distribution, risk factors, clinical scenario, definition of DE, and the volume (mm^3)and percentage of each tissue component of plaque (including FT, FF, NC, and DC). Several studies met our inclusion criteria but were

Table 1. Basical characteristics of studies included in meta-analysis (Normal flow vs. distal embolization).

Study	Study interval	Location	Sample size (n)	Design	Clinical scenario	PAT	Definition of distal embolization
Bae 2008	NR	Daejeon, South Korea	45/12	RSC	AMI	Yes	TIMI flow grade ≤2
Higashikuni 2008	2005.6–2006.4	Tokyo, Japan	40/9	RSC	ACS (AMI and UA)	Yes	Decrease of at least 1 grade in TIMI
Hong 2009	NR	Washington DC, United States	42/38	RSC	UA	No	cTnI elevation >3X the ULN
Hong 2011	2006.2–2008.1	Gwangju, South Korea	166/24	RSC	ACS (STEMI, NSTEMI and UA)	No	TIMI flow grade ≤2
Kawaguchi 2007	2005.8–2006.12	Gunma, Japan	60/11	PSC	AMI (STEMI)	Yes	ST-segment re-elevation
Nakamura 2007	2006.1–2006.3	Saitama, Japan	42/8	PSC	AMI (STEMI)	Yes	Decrease in TIMI flow grade
Ohshima 2009	2007.1–2007.12	Ehime, Japan	24/20	PSC	AMI (STEMI)	Yes	TIMI flow grade ≤2
Ohshima 2011	NR	Ehime, Japan	19/34	RSC	AMI (STEMI)	Yes	TIMI flow grade ≤2
Shin 2011	NR	Ulsan, South Korea	90/22	RSC	UA	No	CK-MB elevation >1X the ULN
Zhao 2013	2010.9–2011.11	Zhengzhou, China	145/21	RSC	UA	Yes	TIMI flow grade ≤2

ACS, acute coronary injury; AMI, acute myocardial infarction; NR, not reported; NSTEMI, non ST-segment elevation myocardial infarction; PAT, percutaneous aspiration thrombectomy; PSC, prospective single center; RSC, retrospective single center; STEMI, ST-segment elevation myocardial infarction; ULN, upper limit of normal.

Table 2. Clinical characteristics of studies included in meta-analysis (Normal flow vs. distal embolization).

Study	Mean age (years)	Males (%)	Comorbidities			Pre-PCI use of Aspirin (%)	Use of Statins	Use of GP IIb/IIIa inhibitor	Use of Statins	Use of distal protectiondevices
			HT (%)	DM (%)	HL (%)					
Bae 2008	56.2/67.5	82.2/66.7	40.0/33.3	13.3/33.3	31.1/25.0	100/100	NR	0/0	NR	No
Higashikuni 2008	66.6/60.6	92.5/77.8	70.0/55.6	30.0/55.6	65.0/8	30.0/44.4	22.5/22.2	0/0	22.5/22.2	No
Hong 2009	65/63	47.6/76.3	64.3/73.7	23.8/31.6	NR	92.9/86.8	NR	14.3/10.5	NR	No
Hong 2011	60.5/60.1	65.7/58.3	52.4/70.8	19.3/25	NR	NR	NR	23.5/29.2	NR	NR
Kawaguchi 2007	NR	NR	68.3/81.8	41.7/9.1	45.0/81.8	NR	NR	0/0	NR	No
Nakamura 2007	65.3/58.5	85.7/87.5	42.9/25.0	23.8/37.5	61.9/62.5	100/100	NR	0/0	NR	No
Ohshima 2009	66.0/74.0	83.3/65.0	58.3/75.0	54.2/60.0	62.5/45.0	100/100	NR	NR	NR	No
Ohshima 2011	73/67	68.4/85.3	78.9/70.6	26.3/38.2	47.4/61.8	100/100	NR	NR	NR	No
Shin 2011	61.4/65.5	61.1/50.0	51.1/72.7	32.2/22.7	53.3/63.6	100/100	21.1/27.3	0/0	21.1/27.3	No
Zhao 2013	51/49	66.2/66.6	59.3/61.9	26.9/47.6	NR	100/100	98.6/95.2	NR	98.6/95.2	No

DM, diabetes mellitus; HT, hypertension; HL, hyperlipidaemia; NR, not reported;

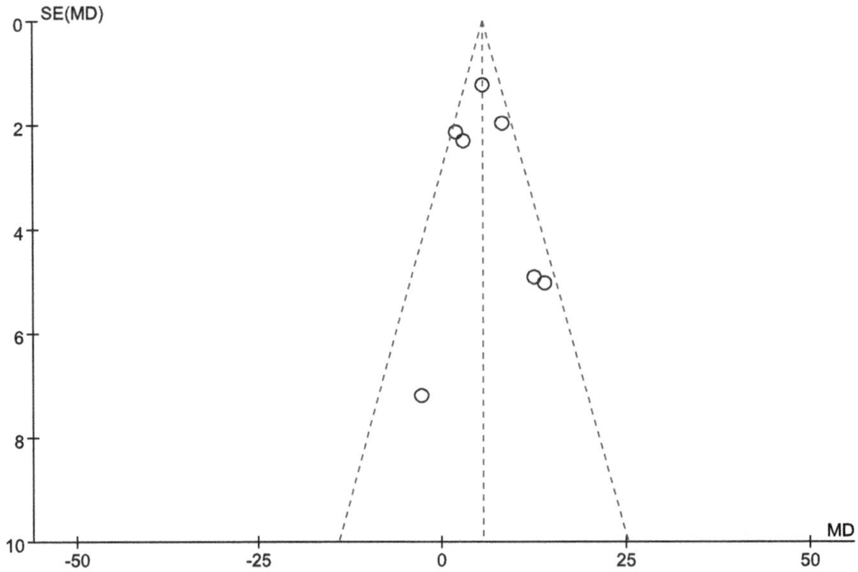

Figure 2. Funnel plot for necrotic core volume outcome data of involved studies.

missing data vital to our analysis; in these cases, we contacted the authors to obtain raw data whenever possible.

Statistical analysis

Statistical analysis in this study was carried out using RevMan software version 5.2 (The Cochrane Collaboration). Results were summarized as weighted mean differences (WMD) with their associated 95% confidence intervals (CI) using both fixed and random effects models, the latter was more conservative where heterogeneity beyond that expected by chance alone was encountered. In addition, the odds ratio (OR) was calculated for baseline comorbidities. Heterogeneity between studies was analyzed by the Q statistic and the I^2 statistic. A p value of the Q statistic <0.1 was defined as an indicator of heterogeneity, and an $I^2 <50\%$ indicated that the magnitude of the heterogeneity might not be significant. Funnel plots were plotted to investigate possible small study effects/publication bias by using Revman 5.2. Planned subgroup analyses were conducted based on the clinical scenario, definition of DE, and whether percutaneous aspiration thrombectomy was applied.

Quality assessment

Methodological quality was assessed independently by 2 reviewers (D. S. and P. J.) using the Newcastle-Ottawa Scale.

Results

Search result

After initial literature search, we identified 388 potential studies, of which 357 studies were excluded based on the title and abstracts, because they were unrelated papers, reviews, editorials, letters, case reports or animal studies. The remaining 31 articles were considered of interest and examined in full-text. Of these, 19 studies those were not IVUS-based were excluded. Of the remainder, 2 studies without DE data were excluded [12,13]. Therefore, 10 observational studies were included in our final meta-analysis [14–23]. Figure 1 shows the study selection process.

Characteristics of included studies

Table 1 and 2 summarize the main features of the included studies. A total of 872 patients (199 patients in DE group and 673 patients in NF group) were enrolled in the 10 studies, and the sample sizes were 44–190 in each study. Among the included studies, 5 studies involved AMI patients [14,18–21] (4 of them only involved STEMI patients), 3 studies enrolled unstable angina (UA) patients [16,22,23], and the remaining 2 studies involved ACS (including both AMI and UA) patients [15,17]. Percutaneous aspiration thrombectomy was performed before IVUS examinations in 7 studies [14,15,18–21,23]. There were no significant differences between DE and NF groups in age and gender of patients. Moreover, there was no significant difference in the incidence of hypertension (OR: 1.36, 95% CI: 0.95 to 1.95, $p=0.10$), diabetes (OR: 1.36, 95% CI: 0.94 to 1.96, $p=0.10$) and hyperlipidaemia (OR: 1.44, 95% CI: 0.89 to 2.31, $p=0.13$) between the two groups. A Funnel plot for NC volume outcome data was used to assess any potential small study effects or publication bias (Figure 2). The Funnel plot was roughly symmetrical as to the mean-effect size line.

Moreover, we evaluated the quality of primary studies using the Newcastle–Ottawa Scale, a validated technique for assessing the quality of observational and non randomized studies. As shown in Table 3, all observational studies were intermediate to low intermediate bias risk as assessed by the Newcastle-Ottawa Scale for quality assessment risk evaluation of adequacy of selection, comparability of study groups, and assessment of outcome or exposure.

Relationship between coronary plaque characteristics and DE

As shown in Table 4, Figure 3 and 4, the absolute volume and percentage of four different plaque compositions through the entire culprit lesion were assessed. Compared with NF group, the overall pooled results with random-effects analysis showed DE group had significant higher absolute volume of NC (WMD: 5.79 mm^3, 95% CI: 3.02 to 8.55 mm^3; $p<0.001$) and DC (WMD:

Table 3. Newcastle-Ottawa Scale of bias risk for the involved studies.

Study	Adequacy of selection			Comparability	Outcomes assessment		
	Representativeness of the exposed cohort	Selection of the non-exposed cohort	Ascertainment of exposure		Assessment of Outcomes	Follow-up period long enough for outcome to occur	Adequacy of follow-up period among cohorts
Bae 2008	**	**	***	***	**	**	**
Higashikuni 2008	**	**	***	***	***	**	**
Hong 2009	**	**	**	***	**	**	**
Hong 2011	**	**	***	***	**	**	**
Kawaguchi 2007	**	**	**	**	**	**	**
Nakamura 2007	**	**	***	***	***	**	**
Ohshima 2009	**	**	***	***	**	**	**
Ohshima 2011	**	**	***	***	***	**	**
Shin 2011	**	**	**	**	***	**	**
Zhao 2013	**	**	***	**	**	**	**

Asterisks are the star rating as per the Newcastle-Ottawa Scale; ** and *** indicate highest rating for these categories.

2.55 mm^3, 95% CI: 0.22 to 4.88 mm^3; $p = 0.03$). The difference between the two groups was not statistically significant with respect to percentage of NC (WMD: 4.35%, 95% CI: −1.44% to 10.15%; $p = 0.14$) and DC (WMD: 0.81%, 95% CI: −1.20% to 2.82%; $p = 0.43$). In addition, there were no significant differences in absolute volume and percentage of FT and FF at the entire culprit lesions between the two groups. Substantial statistical heterogeneity was detected in all of the comparisons among these trials, except for the absolute volume of FT ($I^2 = 0\%$).

Subgroup analysis

Planned subgroup analyses were conducted based on the different clinical scenario, definition of DE, and whether percutaneous aspiration thrombectomy was applied (Table 5 and 6). Subgroup analysis by different clinical scenario showed that patients with DE had significantly higher absolute volume and percentage of NC (WMD: 6.61 mm^3, 95% CI: 4.11 to 9.12 mm^3; $p<0.001$ and WMD: 8.64%, 95% CI: 5.29% to 11.99%; $p< 0.001$) in subgroup of UA patients.

In order to assess the impact of the definition of DE in determining DE on our analyses, subgroup analysis by angiographic or clinical relevance definition was performed. The results showed that there was significantly higher absolute volume of NC (WMD: 7.13 mm3, 95% CI: 4.40 to 9.87 mm3; $p = 0.04$) in subgroup of DE in clinical relevance definition.

In order to investigate whether percutaneous aspiration thrombectomy would affect the outcomes, trials were divided into two subgroups according to whether thrombectomy was applied. The results showed that in the subgroup without thrombectomy, patients with DE had significantly higher absolute volume and percentage of NC (WMD: 7.47 mm3, 95% CI: 4.25 to 10.69 mm3; $p<0.001$ and WMD: −7.45%, 95% CI: 4.38% to 10.53%; $p<0.001$), and significantly lower absolute volume of FF (WMD: −7.38 mm3, 95% CI: −9.86 to −4.90 mm3; $p<0.001$).

Discussion

The present meta-analysis that pooled all currently available published data indicated that, among four phenotypes of coronary plaque composition assessed by VH-IVUS, absolute volume of NC components was closely related to the DE after PCI in ACS patients. Besides, absolute volume of DC component might also be related to the DE after PCI. Further subgroup analysis revealed that the predictive value of VH-IVUS plaque characteristics in determining DE was correlated to the clinical scenario of the patients, the definition of DE, and whether percutaneous aspiration thrombectomy was applied.

Two recent review/meta-analyses [24,25] that investigated the relationship between plaque characteristics and DE after PCI have also reported that the extent of NC was larger in patients with DE. The meta-analysis by Jang et al. [24] evaluated the effect of plaque characteristics on embolization after PCI by grayscale-IVUS and VH-IVUS, and found that the morphologic characteristics of plaque derived from grayscale-IVUS (i.e.,eccentric plaque, ruptured plaque, and attenuated plaque) and the NC component derived from VH-IVUS are closely related to the DE phenomenon after PCI. The systematic review by Claessen et al. [25] summarized the published data on the use of plaque composition assessment by VH-IVUS to predict the occurrence of DE, and found that the NC component was associated with DE in all but 2 of the 11 reviewed studies. In the present study, we performed a systematic review that pooled all the currently available published data investigating the relationship between pre-PCI plaque composition characteristics assessed by VH-IVUS and post-PCI

Table 4. Composition of plaque by VH-IVUS.

Study		Absolute volume (mm³)				Percentage (%)			
		FT	FF	DC	NC	FT	FF	DC	NC
Bae 2008	Reflow	83.8 (66.8)	18.0 (18.6)	12.7 (13.9)	28.8 (26.0)	NR	NR	NR	NR
	No reflow	119.6 (61.7)	36.7 (25.5)	9.3 (8.9)	26.1 (21.0)	NR	NR	NR	NR
Higashikuni 2008	Reflow	NR	NR	NR	NR	68.3 (10.2)	15.5 (7.1)	4.8 (3.6)	11.7 (7.9)
	No reflow	NR	NR	NR	NR	59.6 (11.2)	12.0 (9.7)	4.7 (3.3)	22.1 (9.3)
Hong 2009	Reflow	33.9(14.2)	16.9(11.6)	3.2(3.0)	7.9(4.4)	55.0(11.6)	27.5(13.0)	4.8(3.4)	12.8(8.4)
	No reflow	38.4(19.0)	13.1(9.9)	3.8(3.0)	13.6(6.4)	55.7(13.1)	19.0(9.3)	5.5(3.9)	19.8(10.4)
Hong 2011	Reflow	77 (75.4)	20 (25.4)	10 (11.5)	16 (16.9)	61 (9.9)	16 (9.9)	9 (6.8)	14 (8.0)
	No reflow	76 (50.0)	15 (18.5)	19 (20.0)	30 (23.8)	55 (14.0)	9 (6.1)	14 (8.0)	22 (11.0)
Kawaguchi 2007	Reflow	68.2 (35.3)	13.2 (11.4)	9.6 (13.9)	20.4 (19.2)	NR	NR	NR	NR
	No reflow	67.1 (30.7)	9.8 (10.4)	12.2 (8.6)	32.9 (14.1)	NR	NR	NR	NR
Nakamura 2007	Reflow	NR	NR	NR	NR	67.0 (1.5)	17.0 (1.1)	4.8 (0.6)	11.2 (1.2)
	No reflow	NR	NR	NR	NR	68.3 (2.1)	23.1 (3.5)	2.6 (0.6)	6.3 (1.0)
Ohshima 2009	Reflow	56.6 (21.8)	8.6 (5.2)	6.5 (5.3)	12.0 (7.4)	67.8 (10.2)	10.1 (3.9)	7.8 (5.2)	14.3 (6.7)
	No reflow	56.2 (32.6)	14.2 (11.4)	10.3 (7.6)	14.1 (6.7)	57.5 (10.7)	14.5 (9.6)	11.8 (8.9)	15.8 (7.4)
Ohshima 2011	Reflow	57.0 (33.3)	14.7 (11.5)	9.3 (6.0)	13.7 (6.7)	57.5 (11.0)	14.8 (9.7)	11.3 (9.0)	15.8 (7.6)
	No reflow	67.5 (29.7)	15.0 (11.7)	11.0 (8.8)	16.8 (10.0)	61.2 (10.8)	13.4 (8.1)	10.2 (7.2)	15.3 (6.0)
Shin 2011	Reflow	NR	NR	3.9 (3.7)	8.8 (5.8)	NR	NR	NR	NR
	No reflow	NR	NR	9.1 (5.8)	17.2 (8.8)	NR	NR	NR	NR
Zhao 2013	Reflow	NR	NR	NR	NR	59.24 (6.72)	17.90 (3.21)	8.36 (3.13)	14.50 (5.48)
	No reflow	NR	NR	NR	NR	50.26 (8.72)	15.29 (2.83)	9.53 (2.99)	24.92 (10.04)

Data are presented as mean (SD)
FT, fibrous tissue; FF, fibrofatty; NC, necrotic core; DC, dense calcium.

A

Study or Subgroup	No-reflow Mean	No-reflow SD	No-reflow Total	Reflow Mean	Reflow SD	Reflow Total	Weight	Mean Difference IV, Fixed, 95% CI
Bae 2008	119.6	61.7	12	83.8	66.8	45	2.1%	35.80 [-4.19, 75.79]
Hong 2009	38.4	19	38	33.9	14.2	42	61.1%	4.50 [-2.91, 11.91]
Hong 2011	76	50	24	77	75.4	166	6.3%	-1.00 [-24.06, 22.06]
Kawaguchi 2007	67.1	30.7	11	68.2	35.3	60	8.2%	-1.10 [-21.32, 19.12]
Ohshima 2009	56.2	32.6	20	56.6	21.8	24	12.0%	-0.40 [-17.14, 16.34]
Ohshima 2011	67.5	29.7	34	57	33.3	19	10.4%	10.50 [-7.50, 28.50]
Total (95% CI)			**139**			**356**	**100.0%**	**4.38 [-1.41, 10.18]**

Heterogeneity: Chi² = 3.62, df = 5 (P = 0.61); I² = 0%
Test for overall effect: Z = 1.48 (P = 0.14)

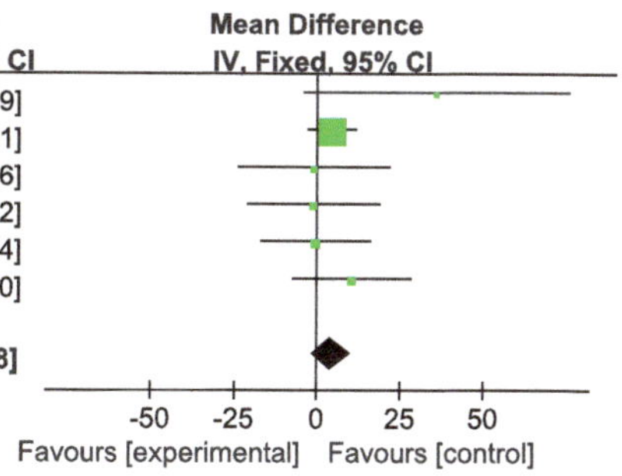

B

Study or Subgroup	No-reflow Mean	No-reflow SD	No-reflow Total	Reflow Mean	Reflow SD	Reflow Total	Weight	Mean Difference IV, Random, 95% CI
Bae 2008	36.7	25.5	12	18	18.6	45	7.2%	18.70 [3.28, 34.12]
Hong 2009	13.1	9.9	38	16.9	11.6	42	21.6%	-3.80 [-8.51, 0.91]
Hong 2011	15	18.5	24	20	25.4	166	15.0%	-5.00 [-13.35, 3.35]
Kawaguchi 2007	9.8	10.4	11	13.2	11.4	60	17.7%	-3.40 [-10.19, 3.39]
Ohshima 2009	14.2	11.4	20	8.6	5.2	24	20.3%	5.60 [0.19, 11.01]
Ohshima 2011	15	11.7	34	14.7	11.5	19	18.2%	0.30 [-6.20, 6.80]
Total (95% CI)			**139**			**356**	**100.0%**	**0.36 [-4.46, 5.19]**

Heterogeneity: Tau² = 22.24; Chi² = 14.57, df = 5 (P = 0.01); I² = 66%
Test for overall effect: Z = 0.15 (P = 0.88)

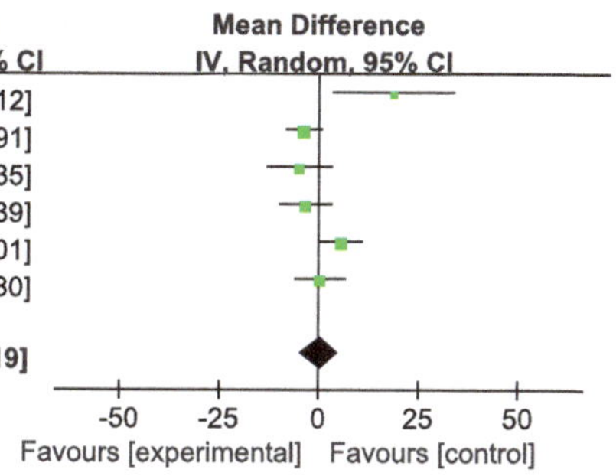

C

Study or Subgroup	No-reflow Mean	No-reflow SD	No-reflow Total	Reflow Mean	Reflow SD	Reflow Total	Weight	Mean Difference IV, Random, 95% CI
Bae 2008	9.3	8.9	12	12.7	13.9	45	8.8%	-3.40 [-9.87, 3.07]
Hong 2009	3.8	3	38	3.2	3	42	24.9%	0.60 [-0.72, 1.92]
Hong 2011	19	20	24	10	11.5	166	6.2%	9.00 [0.81, 17.19]
Kawaguchi 2007	12.2	8.6	11	9.6	13.9	60	9.3%	2.60 [-3.58, 8.78]
Ohshima 2009	10.3	7.6	20	6.5	5.3	24	15.2%	3.80 [-0.15, 7.75]
Ohshima 2011	11	8.8	34	9.3	6	19	15.0%	1.70 [-2.30, 5.70]
Shin 2011	9.1	5.8	22	3.9	3.7	90	20.5%	5.20 [2.66, 7.74]
Total (95% CI)			**161**			**446**	**100.0%**	**2.55 [0.22, 4.88]**

Heterogeneity: Tau² = 5.22; Chi² = 16.56, df = 6 (P = 0.01); I² = 64%
Test for overall effect: Z = 2.15 (P = 0.03)

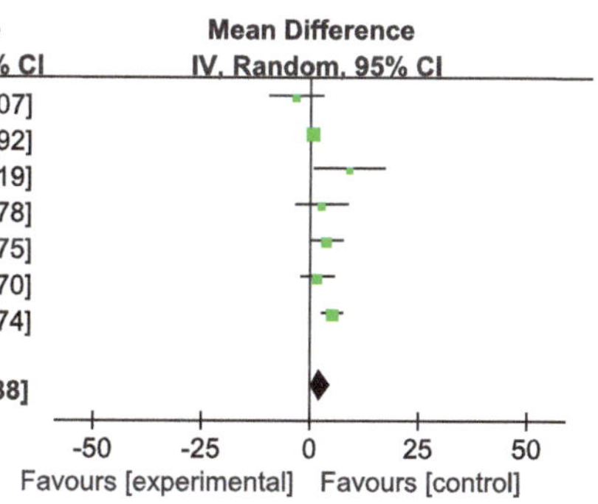

D

Study or Subgroup	No-reflow Mean	No-reflow SD	No-reflow Total	Reflow Mean	Reflow SD	Reflow Total	Weight	Mean Difference IV, Random, 95% CI
Bae 2008	26.1	21	12	28.8	26	45	3.4%	-2.70 [-16.80, 11.40]
Hong 2009	13.6	6.4	38	7.9	4.4	42	26.6%	5.70 [3.27, 8.13]
Hong 2011	30	23.8	24	16	16.9	166	6.4%	14.00 [4.14, 23.86]
Kawaguchi 2007	32.9	14.1	11	20.4	19.2	60	6.6%	12.50 [2.85, 22.15]
Ohshima 2009	14.1	6.7	20	12	7.4	24	19.0%	2.10 [-2.07, 6.27]
Ohshima 2011	16.8	10	34	13.7	6.7	19	17.7%	3.10 [-1.41, 7.61]
Shin 2011	17.2	8.8	22	8.8	5.8	90	20.2%	8.40 [4.53, 12.27]
Total (95% CI)			**161**			**446**	**100.0%**	**5.79 [3.02, 8.55]**

Heterogeneity: Tau² = 5.93; Chi² = 11.99, df = 6 (P = 0.06); I² = 50%
Test for overall effect: Z = 4.10 (P < 0.0001)

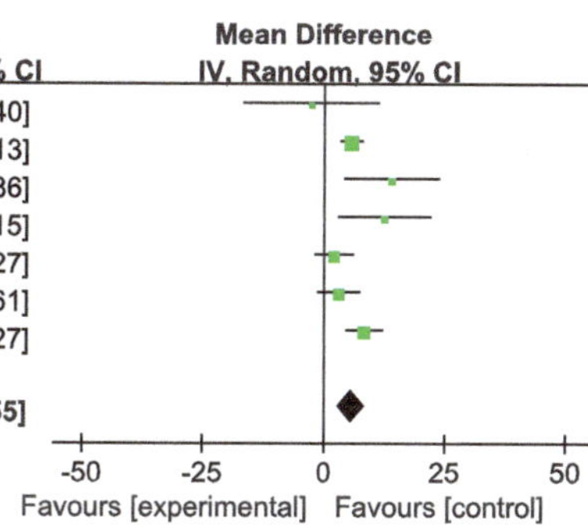

Figure 3. Absolute volume comparison of four different plaque compositions through the entire culprit lesion between the normal flow group and the distal embolization group. (A) Absolute fibrous volume comparison; (B) Absolute fibrofatty volume comparison; (C) Absolute dense calcium volume comparison; (D) Absolute necrotic core volume comparison;

DE phenomenon in ACS patients, and we updated the meta-analysis by adding two VH-IVUS studies [22,23] that did not include in the previous meta-analysis by Jang et al. [24]. We found that absolute volume of NC component, but not percentage of NC component, was closely related to the DE after PCI in ACS patients, confirming the findings of previous review/meta-analyses. In addition, our analysis that pooled all current evidence found that besides NC volume, absolute DC volume was also closely related to the DE phenomenon after PCI. There is some evidence which indicated that DC might be related to DE. For example, pathologic studies revealed that coronary calcification is related to the total plaque burden, NC component, plaque erosion or rupture that is responsible for coronary thrombosis [26–29]. In addition, some studies have also reported that coronary calcium

A

Study or Subgroup	No-reflow Mean	No-reflow SD	No-reflow Total	Reflow Mean	Reflow SD	Reflow Total	Weight	Mean Difference IV, Random, 95% CI
Higashikuni 2008	59.6	11.2	9	68.3	10.2	40	13.8%	-8.70 [-16.67, -0.73]
Hong 2009	55.7	13.1	0	55	11.6	42		Not estimable
Hong 2011	55	14	24	61	9.9	166	16.3%	-6.00 [-11.80, -0.20]
Nakamura 2007	68.3	2.1	8	67	1.5	42	19.9%	1.30 [-0.22, 2.82]
Ohshima 2009	57.5	10.7	20	67.8	10.2	24	15.8%	-10.30 [-16.52, -4.08]
Ohshima 2011	61.2	10.8	34	57.5	11	19	15.9%	3.70 [-2.44, 9.84]
Zhao 2013	50.26	8.72	21	59.24	6.72	145	18.3%	-8.98 [-12.87, -5.09]
Total (95% CI)			**116**			**478**	**100.0%**	**-4.60 [-9.87, 0.67]**

Heterogeneity: Tau² = 35.69; Chi² = 42.20, df = 5 (P < 0.00001); I² = 88%
Test for overall effect: Z = 1.71 (P = 0.09)

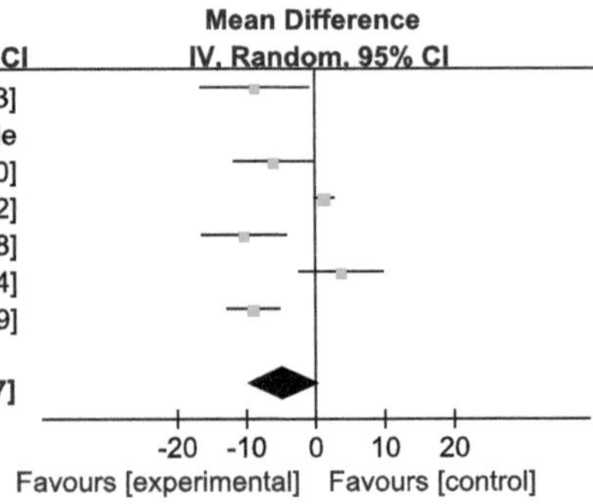

B

Study or Subgroup	No-reflow Mean	No-reflow SD	No-reflow Total	Reflow Mean	Reflow SD	Reflow Total	Weight	Mean Difference IV, Random, 95% CI
Higashikuni 2008	12	9.7	9	15.5	7.1	40	11.5%	-3.50 [-10.21, 3.21]
Hong 2009	19	9.3	38	27.5	13	42	13.5%	-8.50 [-13.42, -3.58]
Hong 2011	9	6.1	24	16	9.9	166	15.5%	-7.00 [-9.87, -4.13]
Nakamura 2007	23.1	3.5	8	17	1.1	42	15.8%	6.10 [3.65, 8.55]
Ohshima 2009	14.5	9.6	20	10.1	3.9	24	13.9%	4.40 [-0.09, 8.89]
Ohshima 2011	13.4	8.1	34	14.8	9.7	19	13.2%	-1.40 [-6.54, 3.74]
Zhao 2013	15.29	2.83	21	17.9	3.21	145	16.5%	-2.61 [-3.93, -1.29]
Total (95% CI)			**154**			**478**	**100.0%**	**-1.67 [-5.72, 2.38]**

Heterogeneity: Tau² = 25.44; Chi² = 68.62, df = 6 (P < 0.00001); I² = 91%
Test for overall effect: Z = 0.81 (P = 0.42)

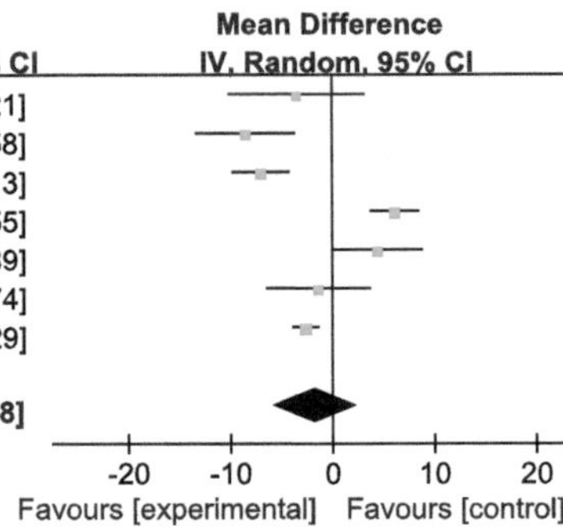

C

Study or Subgroup	No-reflow Mean	No-reflow SD	No-reflow Total	Reflow Mean	Reflow SD	Reflow Total	Weight	Mean Difference IV, Random, 95% CI
Higashikuni 2008	4.7	3.3	9	4.8	3.6	40	14.9%	-0.10 [-2.53, 2.33]
Hong 2009	5.5	3.9	38	4.8	3.4	42	17.0%	0.70 [-0.91, 2.31]
Hong 2011	14	8	24	9	6.8	166	12.4%	5.00 [1.64, 8.36]
Nakamura 2007	2.6	0.6	8	4.8	0.6	42	18.9%	-2.20 [-2.65, -1.75]
Ohshima 2009	11.8	8.9	20	7.8	5.2	24	9.9%	4.00 [-0.42, 8.42]
Ohshima 2011	10.2	7.2	34	11.3	9	19	9.3%	-1.10 [-5.82, 3.62]
Zhao 2013	9.53	2.99	21	8.36	3.13	145	17.5%	1.17 [-0.21, 2.55]
Total (95% CI)			**154**			**478**	**100.0%**	**0.81 [-1.20, 2.82]**

Heterogeneity: Tau² = 5.50; Chi² = 52.36, df = 6 (P < 0.00001); I² = 89%
Test for overall effect: Z = 0.79 (P = 0.43)

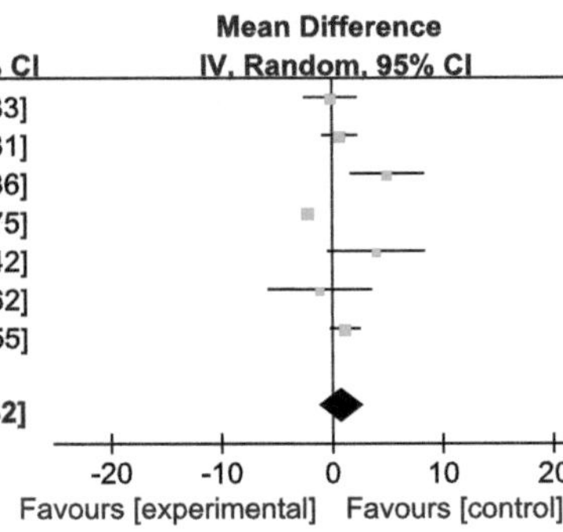

D

Study or Subgroup	No-reflow Mean	No-reflow SD	No-reflow Total	Reflow Mean	Reflow SD	Reflow Total	Weight	Mean Difference IV, Random, 95% CI
Higashikuni 2008	22.1	9.3	9	11.7	7.9	40	13.0%	10.40 [3.85, 16.95]
Hong 2009	19.8	10.4	38	12.8	8.4	42	14.4%	7.00 [2.83, 11.17]
Hong 2011	22	11	24	14	8	166	14.2%	8.00 [3.43, 12.57]
Nakamura 2007	6.3	1	8	11.2	1.2	42	15.5%	-4.90 [-5.68, -4.12]
Ohshima 2009	15.8	7.4	20	14.3	6.7	24	14.3%	1.50 [-2.71, 5.71]
Ohshima 2011	15.3	6	34	15.8	7.6	19	14.5%	-0.50 [-4.47, 3.47]
Zhao 2013	24.92	10.04	21	14.5	5.48	145	14.3%	10.42 [6.03, 14.81]
Total (95% CI)			**154**			**478**	**100.0%**	**4.35 [-1.44, 10.15]**

Heterogeneity: Tau² = 56.37; Chi² = 124.35, df = 6 (P < 0.00001); I² = 95%
Test for overall effect: Z = 1.47 (P = 0.14)

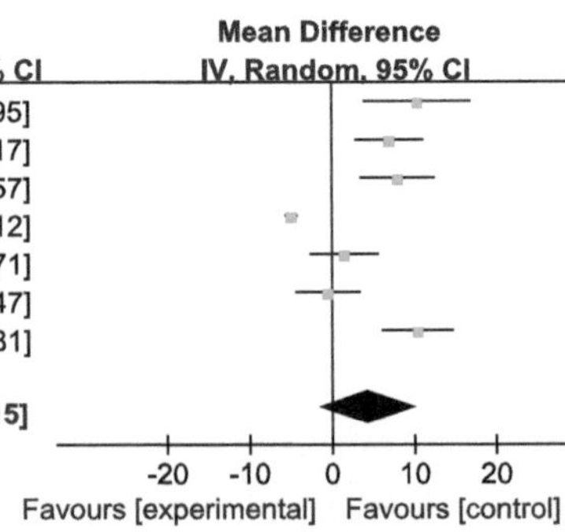

Figure 4. Percentage comparison of four different plaque compositions through the entire culprit lesion between the normal flow group and the distal embolization group. (A) Fibrous percentage comparison; (B) Fibrofatty percentage comparison; (C) Dense calcium percentage comparison; (D) Necrotic core percentage comparison.

was associated with coronary event including myocardial infarction or death in symptomatic/asymptomatic persons [30–33].

In our analysis, we noted a considerable degree of heterogeneity among the included trials. Thus, we performed further subgroup analyses and tried to appraise the possible sources of differences and heterogeneity among trials. Our results suggested that the clinical scenario of the patients, the definition of DE and the use of thrombectomy may influence the correlation between tissue characteristics of coronary plaque and DE. When analyzed in the context of clinical scenario, increased absolute volume of NC was found in DE group in studies including UA patients, but not in those including AMI patients. This phenomenon might be

Table 5. Subgroup analyses of the association of the absolute volume of plaque components with the onset of distal embolization.

	FT		FF		DC		NC	
Subgroup	**WMD (95% CI, mm^3)**	*p*	**WMD (95% CI, mm^3)**	*p*	**WMD (95% CI, mm^3)**	*p*	**WMD (95% CI, mm^3)**	*p*
Clinical scenario								
AMI	5.21 (−4.93, 15.35)	0.31	3.17 (−3.25, 9.59)	0.33	1.81 (−0.81, 4.44)	0.18	3.56 (−0.37, 7.50)	0.08
Unstable angina	4.50 (−2.91, 11.91)	0.23	−3.80 (−8.51, 0.91)	0.11	2.77 (−1.73, 7.27)	0.23	6.61 (4.11, 9.12)	<0.001
Definition of distal embolization								
Angiographic evidence	5.62 (−4.83, 16.07)	0.29	3.11 (−3.77, 10.00)	0.38	2.44 (−1.34, 6.22)	0.21	3.88 (−0.62, 8.38)	0.09
Clinical relevancy	3.84 (−3.12, 10.80)	0.28	−3.67 (−7.54, 0.20)	0.06	2.71 (−0.88, 6.29)	0.14	7.13 (4.40, 9.87)	<0.001
Thrombectomy								
With thrombectomy	−4.36 (−10.42, 1.71)	0.16	0.80 (−3.89, 5.49)	0.74	0.06 (−2.17, 2.30)	0.96	3.56 (−0.37, 7.50)	0.08
Without thrombectomy	−2.57 (−9.14, 3.99)	0.44	−7.38 (−9.86, −4.90)	<0.001	2.59 (−1.60, 6.77)	0.23	7.47 (4.25, 10.69)	<0.001

FT, fibrous tissue; FF, fibrofatty; NC, necrotic core; DC, dense calcium; WMD, weighted mean differences; AMI, acute myocardial infarction.

Table 6. Subgroup analyses of the association of the percentage of plaque components with the onset of distal embolization.

	FT		FF		DC		NC	
Subgroup	**WMD (95% CI, %)**	*p*	**WMD (95% CI, %)**	*p*	**WMD (95% CI, %)**	*p*	**WMD (95% CI, %)**	*p*
Clinical scenario								
AMI	−1.48 (−8.40, 5.44)	0.68	3.49 (−0.68, 7.66)	0.10	−0.18 (−3.89, 3.53)	0.92	−1.67 (−6.04, 2.70)	0.45
Unstable angina	−4.34 (−13.81, 5.14)	0.37	−5.06 (−10.75, 0.63)	0.08	0.97 (−0.07, 2.02)	0.07	8.64 (5.29, 11.99)	<0.001
Definition of distal embolization								
Angiographic evidence	−4.60 (−9.87, 0.67)	0.09	−0.61 (−4.91, 3.70)	0.78	0.87 (−1.49, 3.24)	0.47	3.91 (−2.30, 10.11)	0.22
Clinical relevancy	0.70 (−4.75, 6.15)	0.80	−8.50 (−13.42, −3.58)	<0.001	0.70 (−0.91, 2.31)	0.39	7.00 (2.83,11.17)	0.001
Thrombectomy								
With thrombectomy	5.21 (−4.93, 15.35)	0.31	3.17 (−3.25, 9.59)	0.33	1.81 (−0.81, 4.44)	0.18	3.07 (−3.45,9.59)	0.36
Without thrombectomy	3.98 (−3.07, 11.04)	0.27	−4.09 (−8.19, 0.01)	0.05	3.85 (−0.46, 8.17)	0.08	7.45 (4.38, 10.53)	<0.001

FT, fibrous tissue; FF, fibrofatty; NC, necrotic core; DC, dense calcium; WMD, weighted mean differences; AMI, acute myocardial infarction.

explained by the rupture and migration of NC plaque in AMI patients. In addition, VH-IVUS is limited to detecting thrombus (in fact, thrombus appears as either fibrotic or fibrofatty plaque depending on the age of the thrombus) [34]. Moreover, large amount of NC may have migrated into the distal coronary bed before or during primary PCI in AMI patients [14]. An unexpected finding in our analysis was that no association was found between plaque components and DE in the subgroup of angiographically defined DE. Although angiography has been commonly used as a gold standard for assessing DE, TIMI flow grade is a subjective method to assess epicardial blood flow. As suggested by published literatures, the qualitative nature of TIMI grade renders it somewhat dependent on the technical skill of the observer, and significant differences were found in inter-observer variabilities among different reports, particularly for TIMI 2 grade (Kappa value was 0.4963 for inter-observer variability), which may introduce selection bias in the enrollment of the participants [35,36].

In addition, our results indicated that pre-stent percutaneous aspiration thrombectomy may also be a important factor in determining the predictive value of VH-IVUS-derived plaque characteristics.

Study limitations

Several important limitations of our study should be taken into account, in order to place our findings in the proper context. Firstly, as mentioned above, there was considerable heterogeneity in patient characteristics, use of pre-stent thrombectomy, and definitions of DE among the included trials. Secondly, although the consensus document recommends measurement of the absolute and relative components of each plaque at the minimum lumen site and over the whole lesion, these measurements were not usually reported uniformly in the individual studies involved in our study. Thirdly, although our pooled analysis found that besides NC volume, absolute DC volume was also closely related to the DE phenomenon after PCI, more evidence should be obtained to confirm this finding because only two of the studies included in our meta-analysis reported statistically significant association between DC component and post-PCI DE. Finally, all of the involved trials were non-randomized studies and of small sample sizes, which might have brought some bias. Therefore further studies with larger sample size and high-methodological quality are needed.

Supporting Information

Appendix S1 Search strategy.

Checklist S1 Meta-Analysis on Genetic Association Studies Checklist.

Acknowledgments

The authors gratefully acknowledge the authors of the original studies.

Author Contributions

Conceived and designed the experiments: SD LX RX JP BH. Performed the experiments: SD LX RX JP BH. Analyzed the data: SD LX FY LK YZ LG WW RX. Contributed reagents/materials/analysis tools: SD LX HG MJ JP BH. Wrote the paper: SD LX RX LK JP BH.

References

1. Morishima I, Sone T, Okumura K, Tsuboi H, Kondo J, et al. (2000) Angiographic no-reflow phenomenon as a predictor of adverse long-term outcome in patients treated with percutaneous transluminal coronary angioplasty for first acute myocardial infarction. J Am Coll Cardiol 36: 1202–1209.
2. Grines CL, Cox DA, Stone GW, Garcia E, Mattos LA, et al. (1999) Coronary angioplasty with or without stent implantation for acute myocardial infarction. Stent Primary Angioplasty in Myocardial Infarction Study Group. N Engl J Med 341: 1949–1956.
3. Pu J, Shan P, Ding S, Qiao Z, Jiang L, et al. (2011) Gender differences in epicardial and tissue-level reperfusion in patients undergoing primary angioplasty for acute myocardial infarction. Atherosclerosis 215: 203–208.
4. Cura FA, L'Allier PL, Kapadia SR, Houghtaling PL, Dipaola LM, et al. (2001) Predictors and prognosis of suboptimal coronary blood flow after primary coronary angioplasty in patients with acute myocardial infarction. Am J Cardiol 88: 124–128.
5. Ding S, Pu J, Qiao ZQ, Shan P, Song W, et al. (2010) TIMI myocardial perfusion frame count: a new method to assess myocardial perfusion and its predictive value for short-term prognosis. Catheter Cardiovasc Interv 75: 722–732.
6. Iijima R, Shinji H, Ikeda N, Itaya H, Makino K, et al. (2006) Comparison of coronary arterial finding by intravascular ultrasound in patients with "transient no-reflow" versus "reflow" during percutaneous coronary intervention in acute coronary syndrome. Am J Cardiol 97: 29–33.
7. Ohshima K, Ikeda S, Kadota H, Yamane K, Izumi N, et al. (2013) Impact of culprit plaque volume and composition on myocardial microcirculation following primary angioplasty in patients with ST-segment elevation myocardial infarction: virtual histology intravascular ultrasound analysis. Int J Cardiol 167: 1000–1005.
8. Kusama I, Hibi K, Kosuge M, Nozawa N, Ozaki H, et al. (2007) Impact of plaque rupture on infarct size in ST-segment elevation anterior acute myocardial infarction. J Am Coll Cardiol 50: 1230–1237.
9. Tanaka A, Kawarabayashi T, Nishibori Y, Sano T, Nishida Y, et al. (2002) No-reflow phenomenon and lesion morphology in patients with acute myocardial infarction. Circulation 105: 2148–2152.
10. Katayama T, Kubo N, Takagi Y, Funayama H, Ikeda N, et al. (2006) Relation of atherothrombosis burden and volume detected by intravascular ultrasound to angiographic no-reflow phenomenon during stent implantation in patients with acute myocardial infarction. Am J Cardiol 97: 301–304.
11. Pu J, Mintz GS, Brilakis ES, Banerjee S, Abdel-Karim AR, et al. (2012) In vivo characterization of coronary plaques: novel findings from comparing greyscale and virtual histology intravascular ultrasound and near-infrared spectroscopy. Eur Heart J 33: 372–383.
12. Bose D, von Birgelen C, Zhou XY, Schmermund A, Philipp S, et al. (2008) Impact of atherosclerotic plaque composition on coronary microembolization during percutaneous coronary interventions. Basic Res Cardiol 103: 587–597.
13. Yamada R, Okura H, Kume T, Neishi Y, Kawamoto T, et al. (2010) Target lesion thin-cap fibroatheroma defined by virtual histology intravascular ultrasound affects microvascular injury during percutaneous coronary intervention in patients with angina pectoris. Circ J 74: 1658–1662.
14. Bae JH, Kwon TG, Hyun DW, Rihal CS, Lerman A (2008) Predictors of slow flow during primary percutaneous coronary intervention: an intravascular ultrasound-virtual histology study. Heart 94: 1559–1564.
15. Higashikuni Y, Tanabe K, Tanimoto S, Aoki J, Yamamoto H, et al. (2008) Impact of culprit plaque composition on the no-reflow phenomenon in patients with acute coronary syndrome: an intravascular ultrasound radiofrequency analysis. Circ J 72: 1235–1241.
16. Hong YJ, Mintz GS, Kim SW, Lee SY, Okabe T, et al. (2009) Impact of plaque composition on cardiac troponin elevation after percutaneous coronary intervention: an ultrasound analysis. JACC Cardiovasc Imaging 2: 458–468.
17. Hong YJ, Jeong MH, Choi YH, Ko JS, Lee MG, et al. (2011) Impact of plaque components on no-reflow phenomenon after stent deployment in patients with acute coronary syndrome: a virtual histology-intravascular ultrasound analysis. Eur Heart J 32: 2059–2066.
18. Kawaguchi R, Oshima S, Jingu M, Tsurugaya H, Toyama T, et al. (2007) Usefulness of virtual histology intravascular ultrasound to predict distal embolization for ST-segment elevation myocardial infarction. J Am Coll Cardiol 50: 1641–1646.
19. Nakamura T, Kubo N, Ako J, Momomura S (2007) Angiographic no-reflow phenomenon and plaque characteristics by virtual histology intravascular ultrasound in patients with acute myocardial infarction. J Interv Cardiol 20: 335–339.
20. Ohshima K, Ikeda S, Watanabe K, Yamane K, Izumi N, et al. (2009) Relationship between plaque composition and no-reflow phenomenon following primary angioplasty in patients with ST-segment elevation myocardial infarction—analysis with virtual histology intravascular ultrasound. J Cardiol 54: 205–213.
21. Ohshima K, Ikeda S, Kadota H, Yamane K, Izumi N, et al. (2011) Cavity volume of ruptured plaque is an independent predictor for angiographic no-reflow phenomenon during primary angioplasty in patients with ST-segment elevation myocardial infarction. J Cardiol 57: 36–43.

22. Shin ES, Garcia-Garcia HM, Garg S, Park J, Kim SJ, et al. (2011) The assessment of Shin's method for the prediction of creatinine kinase-MB elevation after percutaneous coronary intervention: an intravascular ultrasound study. Int J Cardiovasc Imaging 27: 883–892.
23. Zhao XY, Wang XF, Li L, Zhang JY, Du YY, et al. (2013) Plaque characteristics and serum pregnancy-associated plasma protein A levels predict the no-reflow phenomenon after percutaneous coronary intervention. J Int Med Res 41: 307–316.
24. Jang JS, Jin HY, Seo JS, Yang TH, Kim DK, et al. (2013) Meta-analysis of plaque composition by intravascular ultrasound and its relation to distal embolization after percutaneous coronary intervention. Am J Cardiol 111: 968–972.
25. Claessen BE, Maehara A, Fahy M, Xu K, Stone GW, et al. (2012) Plaque composition by intravascular ultrasound and distal embolization after percutaneous coronary intervention. JACC Cardiovasc Imaging 5: S111–118.
26. Taylor AJ, Burke AP, O'Malley PG, Farb A, Malcom GT, et al. (2000) A comparison of the Framingham risk index, coronary artery calcification, and culprit plaque morphology in sudden cardiac death. Circulation 101: 1243–1248.
27. Pu J, Mintz GS, Biro S, Lee JB, Sum ST, et al. (2014) Insights into echo-attenuated plaques, echolucent plaques, and plaques with spotty calcification: novel findings from comparisons among intravascular ultrasound, near-infrared spectroscopy, and pathological histology in 2,294 human coronary artery segments. J Am Coll Cardiol 63: 2220–2233.
28. Schmermund A, Schwartz RS, Adamzik M, Sangiorgi G, Pfeifer EA, et al. (2001) Coronary atherosclerosis in unheralded sudden coronary death under age 50: histo-pathologic comparison with 'healthy' subjects dying out of hospital. Atherosclerosis 155: 499–508.
29. Virmani R, Kolodgie FD, Burke AP, Farb A, Schwartz SM (2000) Lessons from sudden coronary death: a comprehensive morphological classification scheme for atherosclerotic lesions. Arterioscler Thromb Vasc Biol 20: 1262–1275.
30. Keelan PC, Bielak LF, Ashai K, Jamjoum LS, Denktas AE, et al. (2001) Long-term prognostic value of coronary calcification detected by electron-beam computed tomography in patients undergoing coronary angiography. Circulation 104: 412–417.
31. Shaw LJ, Raggi P, Schisterman E, Berman DS, Callister TQ (2003) Prognostic value of cardiac risk factors and coronary artery calcium screening for all-cause mortality. Radiology 228: 826–833.
32. Detrano R, Hsiai T, Wang S, Puentes G, Fallavollita J, et al. (1996) Prognostic value of coronary calcification and angiographic stenoses in patients undergoing coronary angiography. J Am Coll Cardiol 27: 285–290.
33. Raggi P, Cooil B, Shaw LJ, Aboulhson J, Takasu J, et al. (2003) Progression of coronary calcium on serial electron beam tomographic scanning is greater in patients with future myocardial infarction. Am J Cardiol 92: 827–829.
34. Maehara A, Mintz GS, Weissman NJ. (2009) Advances in intravascular imaging. Circ Cardiovasc Interv 2: 482–490.
35. Steigen TK, Claudio C, Abbott D, Schulzer M, Burton J, et al. (2008) Angiographic core laboratory reproducibility analyses: implications for planning clinical trials using coronary angiography and left ventriculography end-points. Int J Cardiovasc Imaging 24: 453–462.
36. Gibson CM, Cannon CP, Daley WL, Dodge JT, Jr., Alexander B, Jr., et al. (1996) TIMI frame count: a quantitative method of assessing coronary artery flow. Circulation 93: 879–888.

2

Effects of the Use of Assisted Reproductive Technologies and an Obesogenic Environment on Resistance Artery Function and Diabetes Biomarkers in Mice Offspring

Francisco I. Ramirez-Perez[1,2], Angela L. Schenewerk[3], Katy L. Coffman[4], Christopher Foote[1], Tieming Ji[4], Rocio M. Rivera[3]*, Luis A. Martinez-Lemus[1,2,5]*

1 Dalton Cardiovascular Research Center, University of Missouri, Columbia, Missouri, 65211, United States of America, **2** Department of Biological Engineering, University of Missouri, Columbia, Missouri, 65211, United States of America, **3** Division of Animal Sciences, University of Missouri, Columbia, Missouri, 65211, United States of America, **4** Department of Statistics, University of Missouri, Columbia, Missouri, 65211, United States of America, **5** Department of Medical Pharmacology and Physiology, University of Missouri, Columbia, Missouri, 65211, United States of America

Abstract

Maternal obesity affects the incidence of cardiovascular disease and diabetes in offspring. Also the use of assisted reproductive technologies (ART) has been associated with cardiovascular deficiencies in offspring. Obese women often suffer from infertility and use ART to achieve a pregnancy, but the combined effects of maternal obesity and ART on cardiovascular health and incidence of diabetes in the offspring is not known. Here, we report the effects of the use of ART within an obesogenic environment, consisting of feeding a western diet (WD) to dams and offspring, on resistance artery function and presence of diabetes biomarkers in juvenile mice offspring. Our results indicate that WD and ART interacted to induce endothelial dysfunction in mesenteric resistance arteries isolated from 7-week-old mice offspring. This was determined by presence of a reduced acetylcholine-induced dilation compared to controls. The arteries from these WD-ART mice also had greater wall cross-sectional areas and wall to lumen ratios indicative of vascular hypertrophic remodeling. Of the diabetes biomarkers measured, only resistin was affected by a WD×ART interaction. Serum resistin was significantly greater in WD-ART offspring compared to controls. Diet and sex effects were observed in other diabetes biomarkers. Our conclusion is that in mice the use of ART within an obesogenic environment interacts to favor the development of endothelial dysfunction in the resistance arteries of juvenile offspring, while having marginal effects on diabetes biomarkers.

Editor: Michael Bader, Max-Delbrück Center for Molecular Medicine (MDC), Germany

Funding: This work was supported by the National Institutes of Health (RO1 HL088105 to LAM), and Animal Reproductive Biology Cluster (F21C to RMR). The funders had no role in study design, data collection and analysis, decision to publish, or preparation of the manuscript.

Competing Interests: The authors have declared that no competing interests exist.

* Email: martinezlemusl@missouri.edu (LAM); riverarm@missouri.edu (RMR)

Introduction

Obesity has become a major health problem worldwide [1,2]. Excessive body weight in the form of accumulated adipose tissue is accompanied by adverse pathophysiological conditions. Of these conditions, hypertension and type 2 diabetes mellitus (T2DM) are particularly important for their association with cardiovascular disease and the incidence of life threatening cardiovascular events such as myocardial infarction and stroke [1]. The epidemic proportions at which obesity is increasing are associated with an increased consumption of hypercaloric diets rich in fats and carbohydrates, as well as with more sedentary lifestyles [3,4,5]. In addition to these factors, evidence is increasing that indicates exposure to an obesogenic environment during embryonic and fetal development programs individuals for obesity, hypertension and T2DM later in life [6,7,8,9,10,11,12,13]. This developmental programming of adult diseases is hypothesized to participate in perpetuating the incidence of obesity and cardiovascular disease across generations [5].

An additional consequence of the obesity epidemic is that many women of reproductive age are overweight and have difficulties getting pregnant [14]. Many of these women pursue the use of assisted reproductive technologies (ART) to address their infertility. The use of ART has been associated with an increased incidence of developmental abnormalities including cardiovascular malformations that is further increased when mothers are obese [15,16,17]. This suggests that ART has the potential of influencing the developmental programming of adult diseases. However, little is known about the interactions that ART and maternal obesity may have on the development of adult diseases in offspring.

In order to emulate the increasing association between the use of ART and obesity in women with the incidence of obesity, hypertension and T2DM in the offspring, we recently developed a mouse model of this condition [18]. We have already reported that, in this model, consumption of a western diet (WD) high in fat and carbohydrates by both mother and offspring resulted in augmented mean arterial pressure at seven weeks of age. We also reported that the use of ART resulted in increased body weight at weaning, as well as in the presence of an increased production of reactive oxygen species (ROS) by the resistance arteries of the juvenile offspring [18].

Presence of an increased production of ROS or an imbalance in the redox status of tissues can cause oxidative stress, which in turn has been associated with vascular dysfunction and the development of T2DM [19,20]. In particular, ROS can cause vascular endothelial dysfunction, which is associated with decreased vasodilation efficiency, a hallmark of both hypertension and diabetes. An increased production of ROS, in conjunction with obesity, is indicative of a pro-inflammatory state that has been associated with changes in biomarkers related to orexia, glucose metabolism and the development of T2DM. In the present study we investigated the effects of the use of ART in the context of an obesogenic environment from embryonic development to early life on the vasoconstriction and vasodilation properties of mesenteric resistance arteries, as well as on the presence of T2DM associated biomarkers in juvenile mice. We report that a significant interaction exists between an obesogenic environment and the use of ART that affects the endothelial function and structure of mesenteric resistance arteries, while having only a small effect on T2DM associated biomarkers in juvenile mice offspring.

Methods

Ethics Statement

All animal procedures were performed in accordance to the Guide for the Care and Use of Laboratory Animals published by the U.S. National Institutes of Health. The Institutional Animal Care and Use Committee at the University of Missouri approved all animal procedures used in the study. Animal use protocol was 7501.

Mice and ART

Female mice used for reproductive purposes were of the NSA strain (CF1; Harlan Laboratories, Indianapolis, IN, USA). Males used for reproductive purposes were B6D2F1/J mice (The Jackson Laboratory, Bar Harbor, ME, USA). Dams were split in two groups to receive different diets beginning three weeks before mating with males. The control diet (CD) group of dams was fed chow containing 6.5% fat (LabDiet 5008). The western diet (WD) group received feed containing 24% fat and 17% high fructose corn syrup (TestDiet 58Y1, St. Louis, MO, USA) as previously described [18]. Each group of dams was divided into two subgroups. In the No ART subgroup, dams were mated naturally and allowed to carry their pregnancies from beginning to end. In the ART subgroup, female mice 6–10 weeks old were superovulated with an intraperitoneal injection of equine chorionic gonadotropin (5 IU) followed by human chorionic gonadotropin (5 IU) 45 hours later. Embryo donors were mated with intact males, while embryo recipient dams (surrogates) were mated with vasectomized males. Two-cell embryos were collected 46 hours following superovulation from the embryo donors and cultured in Whitten's medium for three days. Cultured embryos where then transferred to 2.5 days pseudopregnant recipients that received ten embryos per uterine horn. Pseudopregnant surrogate dams were fed the same diet as the embryo donors. We purposely chose to use Whitten's medium for embryo culture because this medium is known to provide suboptimal conditions that affect the molecular structure of the embryo [21,22], but supports full development to term [18,23,24]. In order to equalize litter sizes, pups were culled to constitute litters of four males and four females whenever possible. After weaning, mice were fed the same diet as their mothers and were euthanized at 7 weeks of age. We developed this protocol to emulate, as much as possible, those conditions found in human subjects, in that a woman undergoing ART is usually the recipient of her own embryos and children remain in the same environment after birth [25,26]. Thus, our experimental design created eight groups of offspring, namely, CD-No ART-males, CD-No ART-females, CD-ART-males, CD-ART-females, WD-No ART-males, WD-No ART-females, WD-ART-males and WD-ART-females (Figure 1). The distribution of offspring per surrogate dam is shown in Table S1. As we are particularly interested in the mechanisms that program offspring exposed to ART and/or an obesogenic environment to hypertension and T2DM early in life, we euthanized mice at an age comparable to human puberty.

Vessel Isolation

Mesenteric arteries were collected immediately after euthanasia at 7 weeks of age. Two arteries were isolated from each mouse. The arteries were cannulated onto glass micropipettes, pressurized at 70 mmHg without flow, and warmed to 37°C in commercial myograph chambers (Living Systems Instrumentation, Burlington, VT, USA) as previously described [27]. The chambers contained physiological saline solution (PSS) with (in mM) 145.0 NaCl, 4.7 KCL, 2.0 $CaCl_2$, 1.2 $MgSO_4$, 1.0 NaH_2PO_4, 5.0 dextrose, 3.0 3-(N-morpholino) propanesulfonic acid (MOPS), 2.0 pyruvate, and 0.02 EDTA at a pH of 7.4. The micropipettes were filled with PSS that contained 0.15 mM bovine serum albumin. To test for viability, cannulated arteries were allowed to stabilize for 40 min and then exposed to PSS in which NaCl was equimolarly substituted with 80 mM KCl. Only arteries that constricted more than 20% to this 80 mM K^+ solution were used in the analyses.

After the exposure to high K^+, the arteries were washed three times with fresh PSS and exposed to increasing concentrations of phenylephrine (10^{-8} to 10^{-4} M) to examine adrenergic-dependent vasoconstriction. Subsequently, arteries were washed and pre-constricted with 10^{-6} M phenylephrine. The arteries were then exposed to increasing concentrations of acetylcholine (10^{-9} to 10^{-5} M). After washing these agents from the arteries, they were again pre-constricted with 10^{-6} M phenylephrine and exposed to increasing concentrations of sodium nitroprusside (SNP, 10^{-8} to 10^{-4} M). All vasoactive agents were added in a cumulative fashion to the bath solution at increments of 0.5 M. Each concentration was maintained in the bath for 2 minutes. At the end of each experiment arteries were exposed to Ca^{2+}-free PSS with 2 mM EGTA and 10^{-4} M adenosine to obtain maximal passive diameter. Throughout the experiment, chambers were mounted on inverted microscopes with CCD cameras. Luminal diameter and wall thicknesses were recorded using a video caliper (Living Systems Instrumentation, Burlington, VT, USA) and a Powerlab data acquisition system (ADInstruments Inc, Colorado Springs, CO, USA).

The elastic characteristics of the arteries were determined at the end of each experiment. Vessels were exposed to consecutive changes in intraluminal pressure from 70 mmHg to 5, 10, 20, 30, 40, 60, 80, 100, 120, and back 70 mmHg while under passive conditions (Ca^{2+}-free PSS). Each pressure was maintained for 2 minutes while luminal diameter and wall thicknesses were recorded.

Plasma measurement of diabetes associated biomarkers

At euthanasia, blood from non-fasted mice was collected by cardiac puncture. Blood was allowed to clot and the plasma was collected and centrifuged at 3,000×g for 15 minutes at 4°C to separate any cellular debris from the plasma. Plasma samples were frozen and kept at −70°C for subsequent analyses.

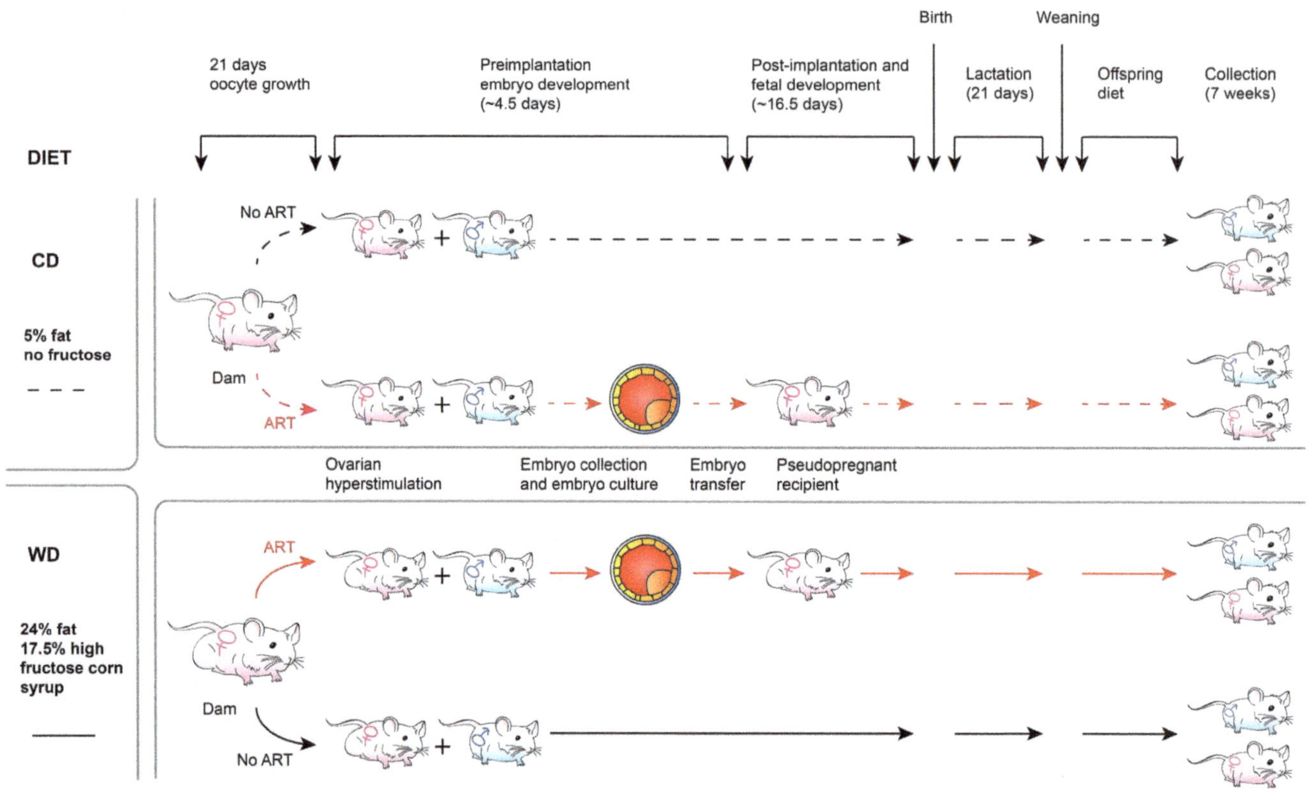

Figure 1. Diagrammatic representation of the experimental design. The design consisted of a factorial arrangement of diet effects (CD = Control Diet; WD = Western Diet), the effects of the use of assisted reproductive technologies (ART; No ART), and sex (males; females) on juvenile mice offspring.

A volume of 50 µl of plasma from each mouse was used to measure the concentration of ghrelin, glucose-dependent insulinotropic polypeptide (GIP), glucagon-like peptide-1 (GLP-1), glucagon, insulin, leptin, plasminogen activator inhibitor-1 (PAI-1), and resistin. The concentration of these biomarkers was measured using the Bio-Plex Pro Mouse Diabetes 8-Plex Assay Kit from Bio-Rad. Plasma samples were analyzed in a BioPlex 200 following instructions from the manufacturer.

Data Analysis

Luminal diameters of arteries were normalized to maximal passive diameter or the level of initial vasoconstriction (phenylephrine-induced pre-constriction). The normalized data were then regressed to ART, diet, sex, intraluminal pressure, and their interactions. Important fixed factors were selected by controlling the statistical significance at level 0.10. According to experimental design, the offspring effect and mother effect were also included as random effects to incorporate covariances among observations. Correlated repeated measurements on the same experimental unit (each artery) were modeled by several different variance-covariance structures, and the best was chosen based on AIC (Akaike information criterion) and BIC (Bayesian information criterion) as well as biological interpretation. Models were implemented in SAS (version 9.4). Residual plots were carefully examined to check model assumptions. Proper Box-Cox transformations were applied to data to maintain normality and constant variance assumptions. Tukey-Kramer HSD (Honestly Significant Difference) test was applied to adjust multiple tests in pair wise comparisons. Statistical significance was considered at $P \leq 0.05$. All data are presented as means ± SEM. An extended version of the statistical analysis is included in Methods S1.

Results

Vasoconstriction to phenylephrine was greater in males than in females

No significant effects were found for diet, ART or their interaction with regard to maximal phenylephrine contraction or the half maximal concentration (EC50) of this vasoconstrictor. The only significant effect found for the vasoconstriction induced by increasing concentrations of phenylephrine was that of sex. Maximal constriction was achieved at a concentration of 10^{-5} M phenylephrine and was significantly ($P \leq 0.05$) greater in males than in females (Figure 2A). Exposure of vessels to concentrations of phenylephrine greater than 10^{-5} M was associated with paradoxical reductions in maximal constriction. In comparison, no significant differences were observed between arteries from males or females on the constriction caused by KCl-induced depolarization (Figure 2B).

Acetylcholine-induced vasodilation was significantly affected by sex and diet x ART interaction

Acetylcholine-induced vasodilation was significantly ($P \leq 0.05$) greater in mesenteric arteries isolated from females than in those isolated from males (Figure 3A). This was particularly noticeable at an acetylcholine concentration of $10^{-6.5}$ M. Acetylcholine-induced dilation was also significantly affected ($P \leq 0.05$) by the interaction between diet and ART (Figure 3C). Mesenteric

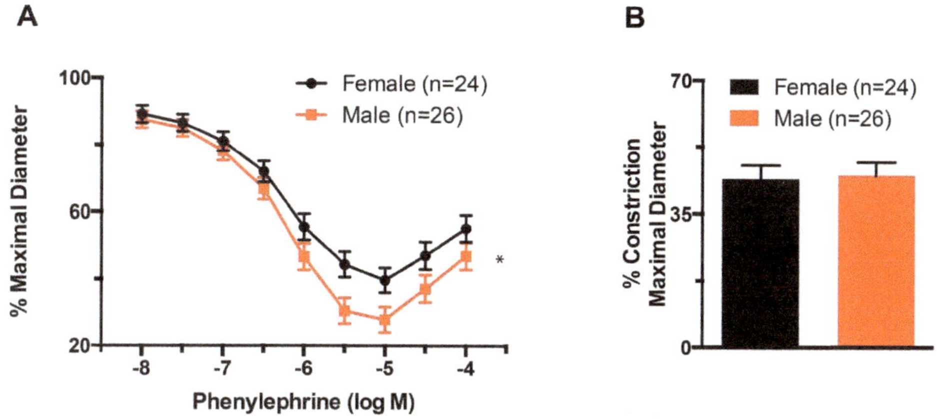

Figure 2. Phenylephrine-induced vasoconstriction is greater in male than in female mice. (A) Percent maximal diameter of mesenteric resistance arteries isolated from male and female mice, and exposed to incremental concentrations of phenylephrine. The maximal constriction to phenylephrine was significantly greater (*P≤0.05) in males than females. (B) Percent constriction after exposure to 80 mM KCl of mesenteric resistance arteries isolated from male and female mice. Data are means ± SEM.

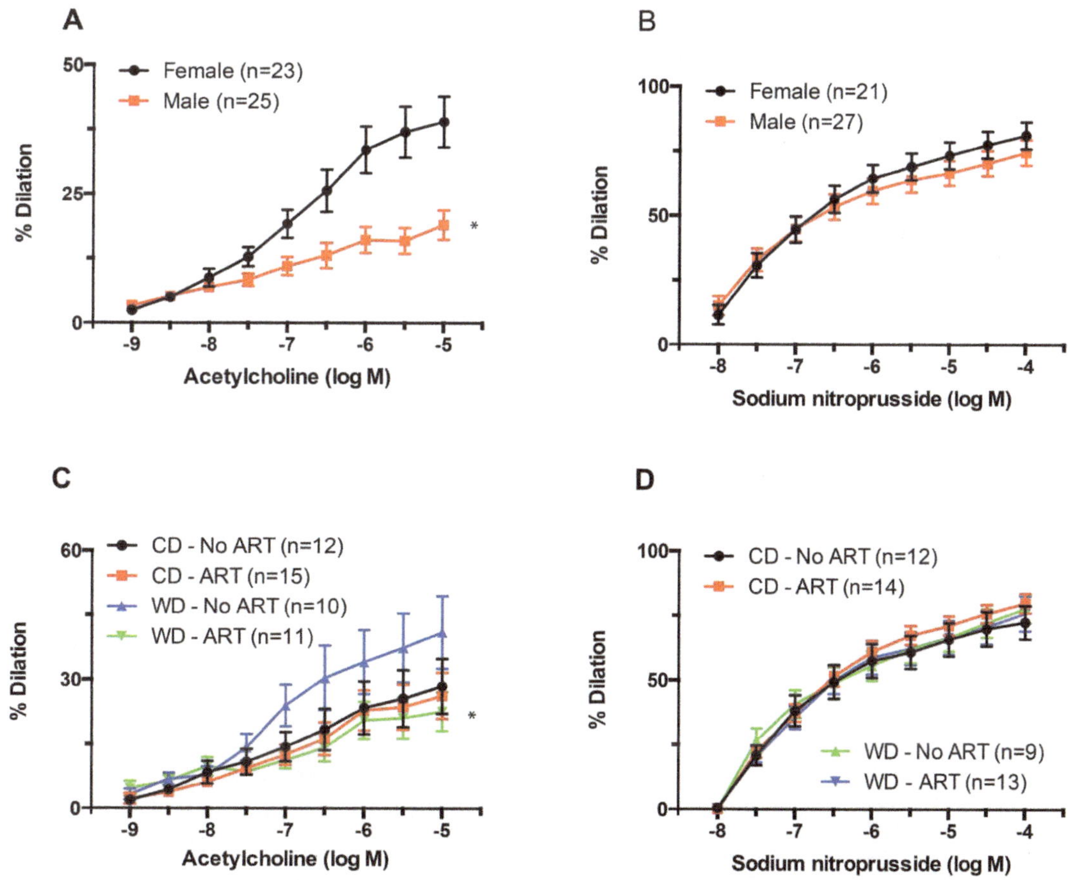

Figure 3. Effects of sex and diet x ART interaction on relaxation responses of mesenteric resistance arteries. (A) Percent dilation of mesenteric resistance arteries isolated from male and female mice, and exposed to incremental concentrations of acetylcholine. Maximal dilations to acetylcholine were significantly greater (*P≤0.05) in females than in males. (B) Percent dilation of mesenteric resistance arteries isolated from male and female mice, and exposed to incremental concentrations of SNP. (C) Percent dilation of mesenteric resistance arteries isolated from mice fed a WD or CD and obtained by natural birth (No ART) or the use of ART, and exposed to incremental concentrations of acetylcholine. Maximal dilations to acetylcholine were significantly smaller (*P≤0.05) in arteries from WD-ART mice than in those from WD-No ART mice. (D) Percent dilation of mesenteric resistance arteries isolated from mice fed a WD or CD and obtained by natural birth (No ART) or the use of ART, and exposed to incremental concentrations of SNP. Data are means ± SEM.

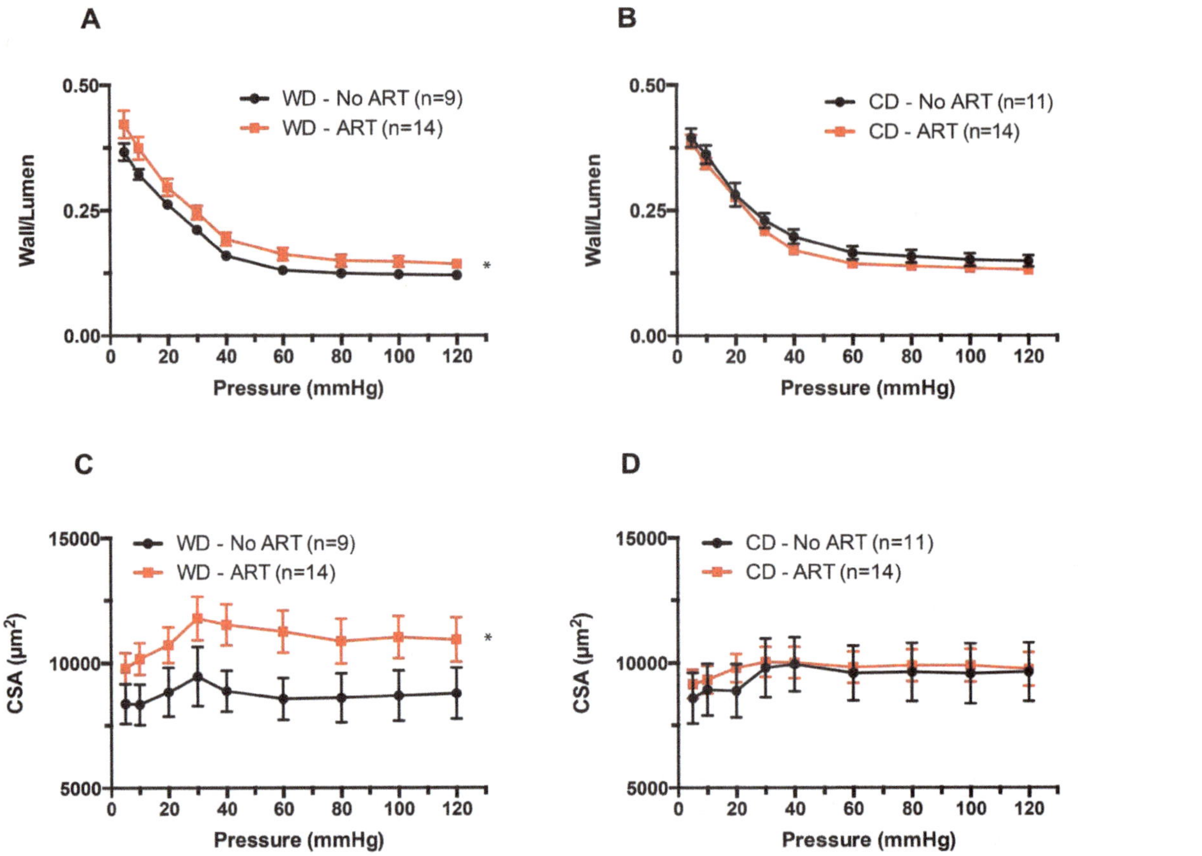

Figure 4. Effects of diet x ART interaction on arterial wall-to-lumen ratios and wall cross-sectional areas. (A) Wall to lumen ratios obtained under passive conditions (Calcium-free) and at different intravascular pressures in mesenteric resistance arteries isolated from mice fed a WD or CD and obtained by natural birth (No ART) or the use of ART. Wall to lumen ratios were significantly greater (*P≤0.05) in ART-WD vs. No ART-WD arteries. (B) Wall cross-sectional areas (CSA) obtained under passive conditions (Calcium-free) and at different intravascular pressures in mesenteric resistance arteries isolated from mice fed a WD or CD and obtained by natural birth (No ART) or the use of ART. CSA were significantly greater (*P≤0.05) in ART-WD vs. No ART-WD arteries. Data are means ± SEM.

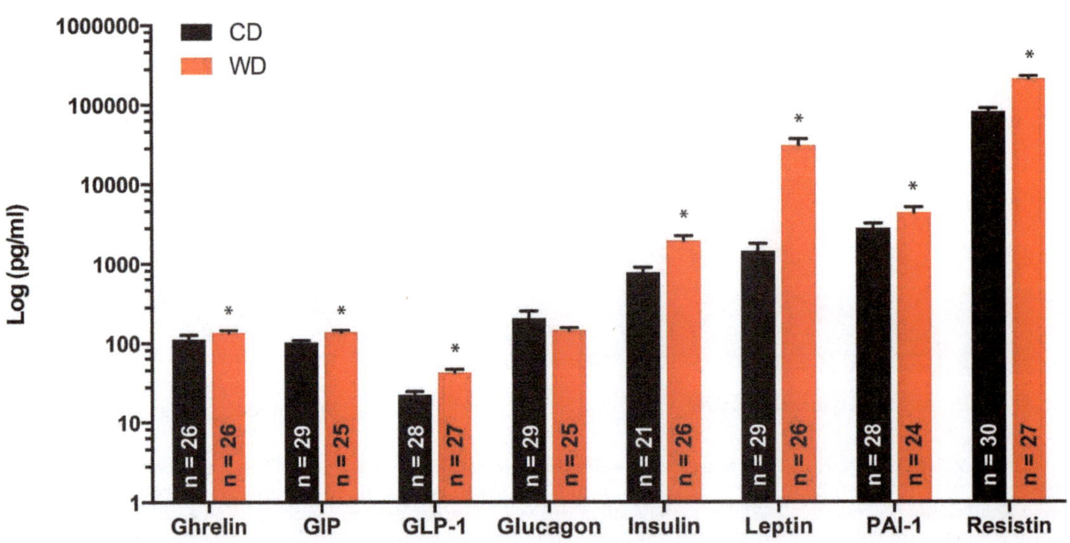

Figure 5. Effect of diet on the serum concentrations of diabetes biomarkers. Serum concentrations of ghrelin, GIP, GLP-1, glucagon, insulin, leptin, PAI-1 and resistin in mice fed a WD or CD. Serum concentrations of ghrelin, GIP, GLP-1, insulin, leptin, PAI-1 and resistin were significantly greater (*P≤0.05) in WD vs. CD fed mice. Data are means ± SEM.

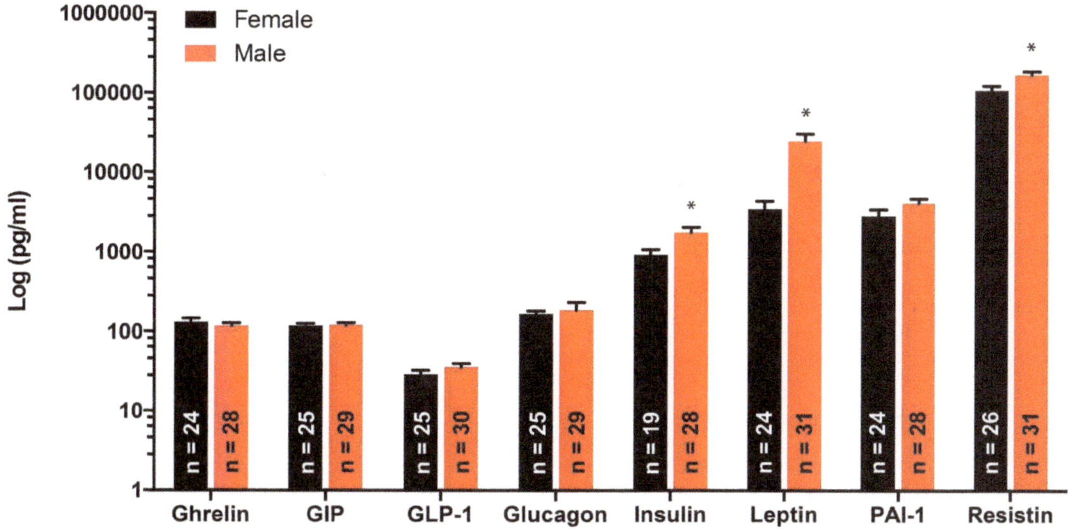

Figure 6. Effects of sex on the serum concentrations of diabetes biomarkers. Serum concentrations of ghrelin, GIP, GLP-1, glucagon, insulin, leptin, PAI-1 and resistin in male and female mice. Serum concentrations of insulin, leptin, and resistin were significantly greater (*P≤0.05) in male vs. female mice. Data are means ± SEM.

resistance arteries from both males and females in the WD-No ART group had greater maximal vasodilations to acetylcholine than those in the WD-ART group. In comparison, no differences in maximal acetylcholine-induced vasodilation were observed between the CD-ART and CD-No ART groups. Vasodilatory responses to SNP were not significantly different between any of the groups (Figure 3B,D)

Effects of diet and ART on vascular structure

A significant effect (P≤0.05) was found for the interaction between diet and ART on the media to lumen ratios (Figure 4A), and vascular wall cross-sectional areas (Figure 4C) of mouse mesenteric resistance arteries maintained under passive conditions. Arteries obtained from ART mice had greater wall to lumen ratios and wall cross-sectional areas than those obtained from No ART mice only when the animals were fed a WD. No differences between ART and No ART were observed in arteries from mice fed CD (Figure 4B,D). Not significant differences were observed either for the internal passive diameter of the arteries or their elastic characteristics, including stress-strain relationships and Young's modulus of elasticity between any of the groups (Figure S1).

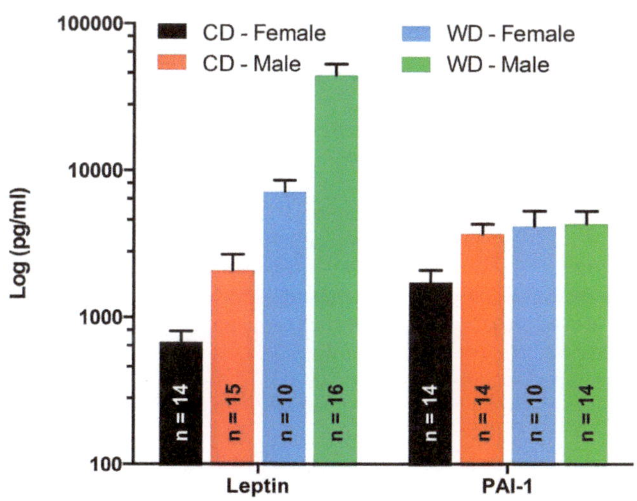

Figure 7. Effects of diet x sex interaction on the serum concentrations of diabetes biomarkers. Serum concentrations of leptin and PAI-1 in male or female mice fed a WD or CD. The increase in serum concentrations of leptin associated with consumption of WD was greater (P≤0.05) in male than female mice, while WD increased (P≤ 0.05) PAI-1 concentrations in females, but not in male mice. Data are means ± SEM.

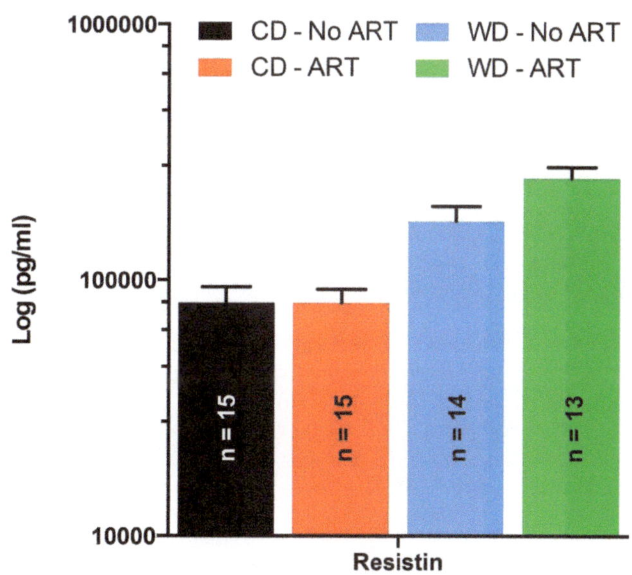

Figure 8. Effects of the diet x ART interaction on the serum concentrations of diabetes biomarkers. Serum concentrations of resistin in mice fed a WD or CD and obtained by natural birth (No ART) or the use of ART. The increase in serum concentrations of resistin associated with consumption of WD was greater (P≤0.05) in ART than in No ART mice. Data are means ± SEM.

Diet had a significant effect on most of the diabetes related biomarkers measured

The concentrations of ghrelin, GIP, GLP-1, insulin, leptin, and resistin were all significantly greater ($P \leq 0.05$) in serum collected from mice in the WD group vs. the CD group irrespective of sex or ART status (Figure 5). Glucagon was the only biomarker measured that was not significantly affected by diet.

Effects of sex on the diabetes related biomarkers measured

Sex had a significant effect ($P \leq 0.05$) on the concentrations of insulin, leptin, and resistin, with males having consistently greater levels of these biomarkers in serum (Figure 6).

Leptin and PAI-1 were significantly affected by a diet x sex interaction

The interaction of diet x sex on leptin serum concentrations was manifested as a significantly greater difference between males and females when mice were fed the WD (Figure 7). In comparison, PAI-1 levels in serum were significantly lower in females than in males only in mice fed CD (Figure 7). No significant differences in PAI-1 serum levels were observed between sexes of mice fed WD. Consequently, WD increased serum levels of PAI-1 only in female mice.

Resistin was significantly affected by a diet x ART interaction

As mentioned above, WD increased overall resistin levels, but the increase was significantly greater in ART mice than in No ART mice, resulting in a significant ($P \leq 0.05$) diet x ART interaction (Figure 8). A trend interaction ($P = 0.06$) in PAI-1 serum levels was also observed between diet and ART. PAI-1 tended to be increased in ART mice only when fed a WD. No effect of diet on PAI-1 was observed in mice of the No ART group (Figure S2).

Discussion

The primary finding of the present study is that the use of ART in an obesogenic environment is associated with a reduced acetylcholine-induce dilation of mesenteric resistance arteries in juvenile mice offspring. We previously reported that the mesenteric resistance arteries of these same mice had an increased level of reactive oxygen species (ROS) in the vascular wall, independent of diet or sex effects [18]. Our present results suggest that exposure to an obesogenic environment tends to increase the ability of mesenteric resistance arteries to dilate more in response to endothelium-dependent acetylcholine stimulation, and that the use of ART under these obesogenic conditions causes endothelial dysfunction. Because ROS reacts with nitric oxide (NO) and reduces its bioavailability, it is likely that the endothelial dysfunction we observed is associated with the well-known scavenging of NO by ROS [12,28]. We observed a numerical reduction in the transcription level of superoxide dismutase 1 (*Sod1*) in the blood vessels of ART mice (Figure S3). Therefore, it is possible that in the resistance arteries of No ART mice there are sufficient antioxidant mediators to prevent the manifestation of endothelial dysfunction, while in the ART mice even a marginal reduction in oxidant defenses allow ROS to reduce the bioavailability of NO, but this remains to be experimentally corroborated.

Our current results also indicate that the interaction of ART with an obesogenic environment was associated with hypertrophic remodeling of the mesenteric resistance vasculature in juvenile mice offspring. This was manifested as an increased media to lumen ratio of the arteries and an augmented cross sectional area of the vascular wall. Although we observed no significant changes in passive luminal diameter in association with the obesogenic environment, overnutrition in mice has been previously associated with outward hypertrophic remodeling in db/db mice [29]. In the latter study, outward remodeling was deemed to have occurred as a consequence of persistent increased flow-induced vasodilation, which is NO dependent. Therefore, it is plausible that the increased vascular oxidative stress we found in the arteries of ART mice prevented the development of outward remodeling associated with the WD in our current study. The observation that endothelium-independent vasodilatory responses to SNP were not affected by WD or ART suggests that both the functional and structural changes we found in mesenteric resistance arteries are likely associated to vascular endothelial dysfunction.

The literature consistently indicates that, early in life, males are more susceptible than females to develop endothelial dysfunction and hypertension [30]. Accordingly we found that male mice had increased vasoconstrictor responses to phenylephrine and reduced vasodilator responses to acetylcholine compared to females. These results are consistent with our previous report in which we showed that these same male mice had greater mean arterial pressures than females at seven weeks of age [18].

Developmental programming of diseases such as hypertension and diabetes has been associated with oxidative stress. Our current finding that ART reduced the vasodilatory capacity of resistance arteries from mice in the WD group suggests that an interaction exists between an obesogenic environment and the use of ART to induce endothelial dysfunction. Our previous finding that the use of ART is associated with an increased level of ROS in the wall of resistance vessels further suggests that the mechanism responsible for this interaction may very well be oxidative stress. At this time there is no clear evidence on which mechanism(s) may be responsible for increasing ROS in the resistance vessels of ART mice and why only ART mice in the WD group showed functional endothelial dysfunction. We previously showed that the expression of the NADPH oxidase, NOX2, in the resistance arteries of these mice is not affected by ART or diet [18]. Our current results indicating that there is a marginal reduction of SOD1 in ART mice suggest that ART may cause a reduction in vascular antioxidant capacity. Whether this reduction in SOD1 expression is sufficient to functionally increase vascular oxidation remains to be determined.

As we observed that the use of ART increased vascular ROS, and as obesity and diabetes are commonly accompanied by oxidative stress [31], we probed the plasma of mice for a number of biomarkers commonly associated with glucose metabolism, diabetes or diabetes development. Not surprisingly, the obesogenic environment caused by feeding dams and offspring a WD resulted in increased plasma concentrations of GIP, GLP-1, insulin, leptin, and resistin. GIP and GLP-1 are incretins, gastrointestinal peptide hormones that increase insulin secretion in response to meal intake. Consistent with our findings, previous reports have indicated that both GIP and GLP-1 levels are increased in response to high-fat obesogenic diets [32,33]. An overwhelming body of literature also associates obesogenic WDs with hyperinsulinemia, hyperleptinemia, and insulin resistance [31,34,35]. As leptin is an anorexic cytokine produced by adipose tissue, it is considered that the hyperleptinemia observed in obese subjects is associated with reduced leptin sensitivity [36,37]. Contrary to our expectations, no significant interactions between diet and ART were observed to affect these biomarkers.

Reports on the levels of circulating resistin found in individuals with obesity and T2DM is controversial [38], but it is clear that resistin is associated with reduced insulin sensitivity [39,40]. Consequently, our finding that resistin levels were increased in WD fed mice is consistent with our observation that these mice were also hyperinsulinemic. We also found a significant diet x ART interaction indicating that the increased levels of resistin found in the WD fed mice were greater in animals obtained by ART than in those obtained via natural conception, gestation, and birth. It remains to be determined whether the association between ART and an obesogenic environment had any mechanistic relation with the increased levels of oxidative stress we found in the resistance vessels of ART mice.

Significant diet x sex interactions were observed for leptin and PAI-1. Leptin was significantly greater in males vs. female only in mice fed a WD. As mentioned above WD was associated with greater leptin levels in both sexes. In comparison, PAI-1 levels were significantly greater in males vs. females only in mice fed CD. Consumption of a WD increased PAI-1 serum concentrations only in females. Male offspring have been shown to be more severely programmed for obesity and cardiovascular disease than females when exposed to a maternal obesogenic environment [41,42]. Our observation that leptin levels increased more in males than in females when fed a WD is in accord with those reports. As for the differential effect of a WD on PAI-1 levels in male and females, our results suggest that a WD increased PAI-1 concentrations only in females. Previously, PAI-1 concentrations have been found to be correlated with body mass index, which is an indirect measure of adiposity in humans [43,44]. We did not measure adiposity in our current study, but we have previously reported that both male and female mice fed the WD were significantly heavier than those fed the CD [18]. Whether this increase in PAI-1 concentration in female mice fed a WD translates into a more prothrombotic phenotype remains to be determined. Additional studies are also needed to determine if the trend for an ART x diet interaction ($P = 0.06$) we observed for PAI-1 affects thrombosis. That trend suggests that the use of ART may increase PAI-1 concentrations only in mice exposed to an obesogenic environment.

Our observation that plasma ghrelin was increased in mice fed a WD is contradictory to previous results indicating diet-induced obesity in mice is associated with low plasma levels of ghrelin [45,46], but consistent with the enlarged body weight of these mice. Increased serum levels of ghrelin are also contrary to the increased levels of insulin, leptin and resistin we found, as previous reports indicate ghrelin reduces insulin secretion and is negatively correlated with leptin and resistin [47,48,49,50]. However, it is important to consider that the assay we used in this study measured total ghrelin and not only the active acylated form of this gastric peptide hormone [51]. Additional experiments will be needed to investigate the level of the acylated form of ghrelin, as well as the other measured biomarkers in fasted animals and at different times during feed intake and the development of obesity.

An important limitation of our study resides in the fact that our experimental design was not developed to interrogate the differential effects of exposure to an obesogenic environment during fetal development vs. exposure after birth. This study was designed to investigate the interaction between the use of ART and an obesogenic environment as it occurs in obese women using ART. An additional limitation of our study is that our experimental design does not allow for identification of the independent contributions of each of the components of our ART protocol in mice to specific effects attributed to ART on the measurements obtained in the offspring [52]. We have used the term ART in this study in reference to all three procedures combined in our protocol namely, superovulation, embryo culture and embryo transfer. Future experiments will be developed to determine the specific effects of each of these procedures on the offspring. Our major conclusion is that ART, as defined in this study, interacts with the presence of an obesogenic environment to reduce the capacity of mesenteric resistance arteries to vasodilate in response to acetylcholine stimulation and to become remodeled. Further studies will be required to determine whether these interactions will influence the development of cardiovascular disease later in life.

Supporting Information

Figure S1 Effect of diet and ART on the passive properties of resistance arteries.

Figure S2 Effect of diet and ART on serum PAI-1 concentrations.

Figure S3 Effect of ART on arterial SOD-1 expression.

Table S1 Offspring distribution per surrogate dam.

Methods S1 Extended version of the statistical analysis.

Acknowledgments

The authors thank Guiling Zhao for her excellent technical support, Laura Moon for technical assistance with the *Sod-1* qRT-PCR assay, and Summer Foote for editorial assistance.

Author Contributions

Conceived and designed the experiments: FIR TJ RMR LAM. Performed the experiments: FIR ALS CF. Analyzed the data: FIR ALS KLC CF TJ LAM. Contributed reagents/materials/analysis tools: TJ RMR LAM. Wrote the paper: FIR ALS KLC CF TJ RMR LAM.

References

1. Bibiloni MD, Pons A, Tur JA (2013) Prevalence of Overweight and Obesity in Adolescents: A Systematic Review. ISRN Obes 2013: 392747.
2. Sturm R (2007) Increases in morbid obesity in the USA: 2000–2005. Public Health 121: 492–496.
3. Church TS, Thomas DM, Tudor-Locke C, Katzmarzyk PT, Earnest CP, et al. (2011) Trends over 5 decades in U.S. occupation-related physical activity and their associations with obesity. PLoS ONE 6: e19657.
4. Katan MB, Ludwig DS (2010) Extra calories cause weight gain–but how much? Jama 303: 65–66.
5. McAllister EJ, Dhurandhar NV, Keith SW, Aronne LJ, Barger J, et al. (2009) Ten putative contributors to the obesity epidemic. Crit Rev Food Sci Nutr 49: 868–913.
6. Samuelsson AM, Matthews PA, Argenton M, Christie MR, McConnell JM, et al. (2008) Diet-induced obesity in female mice leads to offspring hyperphagia, adiposity, hypertension, and insulin resistance: a novel murine model of developmental programming. Hypertension 51: 383–392.
7. Samuelsson AM, Morris A, Igosheva N, Kirk SL, Pombo JM, et al. (2010) Evidence for sympathetic origins of hypertension in juvenile offspring of obese rats. Hypertension 55: 76–82.
8. Gillman MW, Rifas-Shiman S, Berkey CS, Field AE, Colditz GA (2003) Maternal gestational diabetes, birth weight, and adolescent obesity. Pediatrics 111: e221–226.

9. Reynolds RM, Osmond C, Phillips DI, Godfrey KM (2010) Maternal BMI, parity, and pregnancy weight gain: influences on offspring adiposity in young adulthood. J Clin Endocrinol Metab 95: 5365–5369.
10. Petitt DJ, Bennett PH, Knowler WC, Baird HR, Aleck KA (1985) Gestational diabetes mellitus and impaired glucose tolerance during pregnancy. Long-term effects on obesity and glucose tolerance in the offspring. Diabetes 34 Suppl 2: 119–122.
11. Barbero A, Astiz S, Lopez-Bote CJ, Perez-Solana ML, Ayuso M, et al. (2013) Maternal malnutrition and offspring sex determine juvenile obesity and metabolic disorders in a swine model of leptin resistance. PLoS ONE 8: e78424.
12. Torrens C, Ethirajan P, Bruce KD, Cagampang FR, Siow RC, et al. (2012) Interaction between maternal and offspring diet to impair vascular function and oxidative balance in high fat fed male mice. PLoS ONE 7: e50671.
13. Kelsall CJ, Hoile SP, Irvine NA, Masoodi M, Torrens C, et al. (2012) Vascular dysfunction induced in offspring by maternal dietary fat involves altered arterial polyunsaturated fatty acid biosynthesis. PLoS ONE 7: e34492.
14. Jungheim ES, Travieso JL, Hopeman MM (2013) Weighing the impact of obesity on female reproductive function and fertility. Nutr Rev 71 Suppl 1: S3–8.
15. Olson CK, Keppler-Noreuil KM, Romitti PA, Budelier WT, Ryan G, et al. (2005) In vitro fertilization is associated with an increase in major birth defects. Fertil Steril 84: 1308–1315.
16. Reefhuis J, Honein MA, Schieve LA, Correa A, Hobbs CA, et al. (2009) Assisted reproductive technology and major structural birth defects in the United States. Hum Reprod 24: 360–366.
17. Kallen B, Finnstrom O, Lindam A, Nilsson E, Nygren KG, et al. (2010) Congenital malformations in infants born after in vitro fertilization in Sweden. Birth Defects Res A Clin Mol Teratol 88: 137–143.
18. Schenewerk AL, Ramirez FI, Foote C, Ji T, Martinez-Lemus LA, et al. (2014) Effects of the use of assisted reproduction and high-caloric diet consumption on body weight and cardiovascular health of juvenile mouse offspring. Reproduction 147: 111–123.
19. Rochette L, Zeller M, Cottin Y, Vergely C (2014) Diabetes, oxidative stress and therapeutic strategies. Biochim Biophys Acta 1840: 2709–2729.
20. Cai H, Griendling KK, Harrison DG (2003) The vascular NAD(P)H oxidases as therapeutic targets in cardiovascular diseases. Trends Pharmacol Sci 24: 471–478.
21. Rinaudo P, Schultz RM (2004) Effects of embryo culture on global pattern of gene expression in preimplantation mouse embryos. Reproduction 128: 301–311.
22. Doherty AS, Mann MR, Tremblay KD, Bartolomei MS, Schultz RM (2000) Differential effects of culture on imprinted H19 expression in the preimplantation mouse embryo. Biol Reprod 62: 1526–1535.
23. Ecker DJ, Stein P, Xu Z, Williams CJ, Kopf GS, et al. (2004) Long-term effects of culture of preimplantation mouse embryos on behavior. Proc Natl Acad Sci U S A 101: 1595–1600.
24. Sommovilla J, Bilker WB, Abel T, Schultz RM (2005) Embryo culture does not affect the longevity of offspring in mice. Reproduction 130: 599–601.
25. Katz P, Showstack J, Smith JF, Nachtigall RD, Millstein SG, et al. (2011) Costs of infertility treatment: results from an 18-month prospective cohort study. Fertil Steril 95: 915–921.
26. Wang J, Sauer MV (2006) In vitro fertilization (IVF): a review of 3 decades of clinical innovation and technological advancement. Ther Clin Risk Manag 2: 355–364.
27. Martinez-Lemus LA (2008) Persistent Agonist-Induced Vasoconstriction Is Not Required for Angiotensin II to Mediate Inward Remodeling of Isolated Arterioles with Myogenic Tone. J Vasc Res 45: 211–221.
28. Chrissobolis S, Miller AA, Drummond GR, Kemp-Harper BK, Sobey CG (2011) Oxidative stress and endothelial dysfunction in cerebrovascular disease. Front Biosci (Landmark Ed) 16: 1733–1745.
29. Souza-Smith FM, Katz PS, Trask AJ, Stewart JA Jr, Lord KC, et al. (2011) Mesenteric resistance arteries in type 2 diabetic db/db mice undergo outward remodeling. PLoS ONE 6: e23337.
30. Lopez-Ruiz A, Sartori-Valinotti J, Yanes LL, Iliescu R, Reckelhoff JF (2008) Sex differences in control of blood pressure: role of oxidative stress in hypertension in females. Am J Physiol Heart Circ Physiol 295: H466–474.
31. Rindler PM, Crewe CL, Fernandes J, Kinter M, Szweda LI (2013) Redox regulation of insulin sensitivity due to enhanced fatty acid utilization in the mitochondria. Am J Physiol Heart Circ Physiol 305: H634–643.
32. Lodefalk M, Carlsson-Skwirut C, Holst JJ, Aman J, Bang P (2010) Effects of fat supplementation on postprandial GIP, GLP-1, ghrelin and IGFBP-1 levels: a pilot study on adolescents with type 1 diabetes. Horm Res Paediatr 73: 355–362.
33. Suzuki K, Harada N, Yamane S, Nakamura Y, Sasaki K, et al. (2013) Transcriptional regulatory factor X6 (Rfx6) increases gastric inhibitory polypeptide (GIP) expression in enteroendocrine K-cells and is involved in GIP hypersecretion in high fat diet-induced obesity. J Biol Chem 288: 1929–1938.
34. Ferezou-Viala J, Roy AF, Serougne C, Gripois D, Parquet M, et al. (2007) Long-term consequences of maternal high-fat feeding on hypothalamic leptin sensitivity and diet-induced obesity in the offspring. Am J Physiol Regul Integr Comp Physiol 293: R1056–1062.
35. Birk RZ, Rubio-Aliaga I, Boekschoten MV, Danino H, Muller M, et al. (2014) Differential regulation of pancreatic digestive enzymes during chronic high-fat diet-induced obesity in C57BL/6J mice. Br J Nutr 112: 154–161.
36. McGillicuddy FC, Reynolds CM, Finucane O, Coleman E, Harford KA, et al. (2013) Long-term exposure to a high-fat diet results in the development of glucose intolerance and insulin resistance in interleukin-1 receptor I-deficient mice. Am J Physiol Endocrinol Metab 305: E834–844.
37. Jayaram B, Pan W, Wang Y, Hsuchou H, Mace A, et al. (2013) Astrocytic leptin-receptor knockout mice show partial rescue of leptin resistance in diet-induced obesity. J Appl Physiol (1985) 114: 734–741.
38. Lobo TF, Torloni MR, Gueuvoghlanian-Silva BY, Mattar R, Daher S (2013) Resistin concentration and gestational diabetes: a systematic review of the literature. J Reprod Immunol 97: 120–127.
39. Kusminski CM, McTernan PG, Kumar S (2005) Role of resistin in obesity, insulin resistance and Type II diabetes. Clin Sci (Lond) 109: 243–256.
40. McTernan PG, Kusminski CM, Kumar S (2006) Resistin. Curr Opin Lipidol 17: 170–175.
41. Dahlhoff M, Pfister S, Blutke A, Rozman J, Klingenspor M, et al. (2014) Periconceptional obesogenic exposure induces sex-specific programming of disease susceptibilities in adult mouse offspring. Biochim Biophys Acta 1842: 304–317.
42. Calvert JW, Lefer DJ, Gundewar S, Poston L, Coetzee WA (2009) Developmental programming resulting from maternal obesity in mice: effects on myocardial ischaemia-reperfusion injury. Exp Physiol 94: 805–814.
43. Landin K, Stigendal L, Eriksson E, Krotkiewski M, Risberg B, et al. (1990) Abdominal obesity is associated with an impaired fibrinolytic activity and elevated plasminogen activator inhibitor-1. Metabolism: clinical and experimental 39: 1044–1048.
44. Verschuur M, Jellema A, Bladbjerg EM, EJ MF, Mensink RP, et al. (2005) The plasminogen activator inhibitor-1 (PAI-1) promoter haplotype is related to PAI-1 plasma concentrations in lean individuals. Atherosclerosis 181: 275–284.
45. Lacerda-Miranda G, Soares VM, Vieira AK, Lessa JG, Rodrigues-Cunha AC, et al. (2012) Ghrelin signaling in heart remodeling of adult obese mice. Peptides 35: 65–73.
46. Briggs DI, Enriori PJ, Lemus MB, Cowley MA, Andrews ZB (2010) Diet-induced obesity causes ghrelin resistance in arcuate NPY/AgRP neurons. Endocrinology 151: 4745–4755.
47. Broglio F, Arvat E, Benso A, Gottero C, Muccioli G, et al. (2001) Ghrelin, a natural GH secretagogue produced by the stomach, induces hyperglycemia and reduces insulin secretion in humans. J Clin Endocrinol Metab 86: 5083–5086.
48. El Gawad SS, El Kenawy F, Mousa AA, Omar AA (2012) Plasma levels of resistin and ghrelin before and after treatment in patients with hyperthyroidism. Endocr Pract 18: 376–381.
49. Palik E, Baranyi E, Melczer Z, Audikovszky M, Szocs A, et al. (2007) Elevated serum acylated (biologically active) ghrelin and resistin levels associate with pregnancy-induced weight gain and insulin resistance. Diabetes Res Clin Pract 76: 351–357.
50. Zhang S, Zhang Q, Zhang L, Li C, Jiang H (2013) Expression of ghrelin and leptin during the development of type 2 diabetes mellitus in a rat model. Mol Med Rep 7: 223–228.
51. Delporte C (2013) Structure and Physiological Actions of Ghrelin. Scientifica (Cairo) 2013: 518909.
52. Tran M, Gallo LA, Hanvey AN, Jefferies AJ, Westcott KT, et al. (2014) Embryo transfer cannot delineate between the maternal pregnancy environment and germ line effects in the transgenerational transmission of disease in rats. Am J Physiol Regul Integr Comp Physiol 306: R607–618.

Adiponectin Gene Polymorphism rs2241766 T/G Is Associated with Response to Pioglitazone Treatment in Type 2 Diabetic Patients from Southern China

Hong Yang[1,2]☯, Enling Ye[1,2]☯, Guangxin Si[3], Liangmiao Chen[1,2], Lingqiao Cai[1,2], Chengfu Ye[1,2], Chi Zhang[2], Xuemian Lu[1,2]*

1 Department of Endocrinology, the Third Hospital Affiliate to Wenzhou Medical University, Ruian, Zhejiang, China, **2** Ruian Center of the Chinese-American Research Institute for Diabetic Complications, the Third Affiliated Hospital of the Wenzhou Medical University, Wenzhou, China, **3** Department of Endocrinology, Shangdong Jining No. 1 People's Hospital, Jining, Shangdong, China

Abstract

Introduction: Insulin sensitizing drugs such as pioglitazone are not uniformly treatment effective among individual type 2 diabetic patients. Here, the relationship of pioglitazone efficacy to single nucleotide polymorphisms (SNP) of the adiponectin gene, a critical gene directly regulated by the drug, was examined in a cohort of Chinese Han type 2 diabetic patients.

Methods: Eighty type 2 diabetic patients were treated with pioglitazone (15 mg/day) for 12 weeks without interruption of their current therapeutic regimen. Fasting plasma glucose, fasting insulin, homeostasis model assessment for insulin resistance (HOMA-IR), and glycated hemoglobin (HbA1c%) were collected both prior to and following pioglitazone treatment. Response to pioglitazone was defined as a decrease of at least 15% in HbA1c% levels. Three regions of the adiponectin gene containing SNPs (promoter, intron 2 and exon 2, and exon 3) were amplified and sequenced to determine genotype.

Results: Serum adiponectin levels were significantly increased ($p<0.001$) whereas fasting plasma glucose, fasting insulin, HOMA-IR, and HbA1c% values were significantly decreased relative to baseline measurements ($p<0.001$). Response of patients with TG and TT genotypes at rs2241766 (exon2; 52.9% vs. 12.7%, respectively $p=0.001$) was statistically significant relative to all other patients. Amongst rs2241766 TG and TT patients, the mean decrease in HbA1c% levels was greater where the genotype was TG (1.15 ± 0.80 vs. 0.52 ± 0.64, $p=0.001$).

Conclusions: The adiponectin gene polymorphism rs2241766 T/G is associated with pioglitazone efficacy in type 2 diabetic patients, and status of the polymorphism may be an important clinical factor to consider prior to pioglitazone treatment.

Editor: Harpal Singh Randeva, University of Warwick – Medical School, United Kingdom

Funding: This study was supported by a research grant from the Wenzhou Science and Technology Plan (Y20080007, to XL). The funders had no role in study design, data collection and analysis, decision to publish, or preparation of the manuscript.

Competing Interests: The authors have declared that no competing interests exist.

* Email: lu89118@medmail.com.cn

☯ These authors contributed equally to this work.

Introduction

Type 2 diabetes mellitus (T2DM) is on the rise in current populations worldwide due to changes in weight, for example. Alternative therapeutic strategies are necessary, as patients are known to develop resistance to treatment with insulin. A breakthrough in strategies for these patients occurred when it was discovered that adipocytes secrete a protein, adiponectin (ADIPOQ), which plays a role in in the regulation of glucose and lipid metabolism [1]. ADIPOQ is encoded by one of the most abundant adipose gene transcripts [2]. Regulation of the gene is known to occur at least in part through the nuclear receptor transcription factor, peroxisome proliferator activated receptor γ (PPARγ) [3]. Pharmacological compounds, such as the thiazolidinediones (TDZ), that target PPARγ activity have thus been exploited as insulin sensitizers, and are now widely used for the treatment of insulin resistance in T2DM patients.

Pioglitazone is a TZD compound that is currently used as an insulin-sensitizing drug. However, many clinical trials have shown that the therapeutic efficacy of pioglitazone is inconsistentamong individual T2DM patients [4,5]. One explanation is underlying genetic variationas genetic mutation has been shown to be the basis for some metabolic syndromes. A number of studies have demonstrated that subtle changes in DNA sequence, single nucleotide polymorphisms (SNP), are often associated with differences in drug efficacy and toxicity among patients [6]. In recent years, many SNPs in ADIPOQ have been linked to body mass index (BMI), insulin sensitivity, and T2DM in some cross-sectional studies [4,7–9]. However, relatively few studies have addressed whether *ADIPOQ* gene polymorphisms are associated with pioglitazone therapeutic efficacy. The results so far have not been consistent. In a study with 113 T2DM Chinese patients, the rs266729 polymorphism was associated with response to pioglitazone, whereas in an Iranian population, the rs2241766 and rs16928751 polymorphisms were not related to response [10,11]. In the current study, the association of *ADIPOQ* gene polymorphisms with pioglitazone therapeutic efficacy was investigated in Chinese Han patients with T2DM.

Materials and Methods

Ethics statement

The study protocol was approved by the ethics committee of the Third Affiliated Hospital of Wenzhou Medical University. The 80 unrelated individuals were long-term residents in the Wenzhou area of China, and all patients signed the informed consent prior to the study.

Patients

Data were collected from a total of 80 outpatients with T2DM. All patients were derived from the Chinese Han population treated at the Department of Endocrinology of the Third Affiliated Hospital of Wenzhou Medical University between the years 2010 to 2012. Patients included 32 men and 48 women whose ages ranged from 34 to 80 yr (mean 57.05±10.48 yr). T2DM was diagnosed according to the World Health Organization criteria from 1999: (1) random plasma glucose≥11.1 mmol/L, fasting plasma glucose (FPG) ≥7.0 mmol/L, or 2-hour oral glucose tolerance test result was ≥11.1 mmol/L; (2) symptomless: repeat the test a second time on a different day to confirm the diagnosis; (3) any stress (due to infection, trauma, or condition) that causes the level of blood glucose to temporarily rise was excluded. The inclusion criteria were as follows: (1) FPG between 7.0 and 14.0 mmol/L and glycated hemoglobin (HbA1c%) between 7.0 and 11.5%; (2) no change in antidiabetic agents in the last three months; (3) no TZD medications of any type in the past year; and (4) no pregnancy within the past year. Patients were excluded on the basis of the following criteria: (1) type 1 diabetes; (2) a history of diabetic ketoacidosis or acute complications of diabetes, such as hyperosmolar hyperglycemic state; (3) ischemic heart disease or heart failure class II to IV (New York Heart Association; NYHA); (4) insulin treatment; and (5) pregnancy or nursing.

Clinical measurements

Patients took 15 mg/day pioglitazone orally for 12 weeks without interruption of their current therapeutic regimen for T2DM. Venous blood samples were collected from patients after fasting overnight. Clinical and biochemical data, including age, height, weight, waist circumference (WC), blood pressure, fasting plasma glucose (FPG), fasting insulin, HbA1c%, total cholesterol (TC), triglycerides (TG), high-density lipoprotein cholesterol (HDL-C), low-density lipoprotein cholesterol (LDL-C), and ADIPOQ were collected from all 80 patients. FPG, TC, HDL-C, LDL-C, and TG were determined with the Olympus AU 5400 Automatic Biochemical Analyzer (Olympus Corporation, Mishama, Japan). Serum insulin levels were determined with the Beckman Unicel DxI 800 Chemiluminescence Analyzer (Beckman-Coulter, Fullerton, CA). Serum ADIPOQ levels were detected by a double antibody sandwich ELISA (Shanghai Westang Bio-tech Co., Ltd.; Shanghai, China). The insulin resistance (IR) index was assessed by homeostasis model assessment (HOMA). The following formula was used to calculate the IR index: HOMA-IR = (FPI×FPG)/22.5 where 22.5 is a constant.

Efficacy evaluation

Clinical samples were analyzed, and "effectiveness" was defined as a decrease in the HbA1c% level by more than 15% relative to the baseline measurement (prior to piaglitazone treatment) in individual patients.

Genotyping analyses

Genomic DNA was isolated from patient blood with a DNA extraction kit according to the manufacturer's protocol (Shanghai Generay Biotech Co., Ltd.; Shanghai, China). Adiponectin gene SNPs were amplified by polymerase chain reaction (PCR). Primer pairs (Shanghai Generay Biotech Co., Ltd.) were designed using Primer Premier 5 and Oligo 6.0 software to amplify three regions of the adiponectin gene containing 13 polymorphisms (rs266729, rs16861194, rs1501299, rs2241767, rs3821799, rs145335235, rs3774261, rs2241766, rs17846872, rs35469083, rs1063537, rs2082940, rs1063538): promoter, upstream of exon 2 and intron 2, and upstream of intron 3 (Table 1). The reactions were performed in a total volume of 25 µl containing 0.1-1ug DNA, 0.8 µl of each primer (10 µmol/L), and 12.5 µl 2 × PCR Master Mix (Thermo Scientific; Pittsburgh, PA, USA). The cycling parameters for PCR were the following: denaturation 94°C 4 min, followed by 30 cycles of denaturation 94°C 40 s, annealing 56°C 35 s, and extension 72°C 40 s. Specificity of PCR was confirmed by 5% polyacrylamide gel electrophoresis, and products were commercially sequenced (Shanghai Sangon Biological Engineering Technology & Services Co., Ltd.; Shanghai, China).

Statistical analysis

Statistical analyses were performed with SPSS software Version 16.0 for Windows (SPSS Inc.; Chicago, IL, USA). Data showing a normal distribution were summarized as the mean ± standard deviation (SD), and data showing a non-normal distribution were summarized as medians (P25%–P75%). Data with a normal distribution were compared with a Student's t-test; data with non-normal distributions were compared with the Wilcoxon rank-sum test. Numeration data were presented as a frequency and compared using the chi-square test. The relationship between the therapeutic efficacy of pioglitazone and individual polymorphic variants of the adiponectin gene was analyzed using the chi-square test. Logistic regression analysis of relevant variables was performed to identify predictors for therapeutic efficacy of pioglitazone. A value of $p<0.05$ was considered to be statistically significant.

Results

Clinical characteristics are regulated by pioglitazone

The clinical characteristics, and anthropometric and metabolic findings in the patients prior to and following 12 weeks of pioiglitazone treatment are presented in Table 2. Based on critical clinical parameters, pioglitazone appeared to have an overall effect on this cohort of Chinese Han patients. The primary measure of pioglitazone efficacy was that the change in serum ADIPOQ concentration significantly increased from 3.42 mg/l to 5.67 mg/l ($p<0.001$). Other critical clinical correlates (FPG, fasting insulin, HbA1c% levels and HOMA-IR) of the 80 patients significantly decreased with treatment (8.73±1.55 mmol/l, 6.85±3.86 mg/ml, 7.65% and 2.29 respectively vs. 7.25±1.36 mmol/l, 5.38±2.59 mg/ml, 7.10% and 1.51 respec-

Table 1. Polymerase chain reaction primers and the amplified products for adiponectin gene polymorphisms.

Region	Primer sequence	Fragment
Promoter	F:5′-TGGTGGACTTGACTTTACTGGT-3′	563 bp
	R:5′-GCTTGTGGCCTCGAATCGTA-3′	
Intron 2 and exon 2	F:5′-TGCTGTTGCTGGGAGCTGTTCT-3′	738 bp
	R:5′-CATTCTTCATCAGGTCCACGGT-3′	
Exon 3	F:5′-TGAATCCCATATCTACCC-3′	609 bp
	R:5′-TCATGCCACTGCACTCTA-3′	

F: Forward primer; R: Reverse primer.

tively; $p<0.001$). Lower levels of FPG, fasting insulin, HOMA-IR, and HbA1c%, in combination with higher serum ADIPOQ concentration indicated that pioglitazone had beneficial effects on the patients. Other clinical indicators (TC, TG, LDL-C and HDL-C) did not change significantly when examined as a group; neither did weight, BMI, WC, and systolic or diastolic blood pressures.

Genotyping

Thirteen SNPs of the *ADIPOQ* gene were genotyped in this study. The distribution of all genotypes (homozygous and heterozygous polymorphic variants) and allelic frequencies are shown in Table 3. All SNPs were found to be in Hardy-Weinberg equilibrium ($p>0.05$). However, three SNPs (rs35469083, rs17846872 and rs145335235) were eliminated from further analysis due to a low frequency in the target patient population.

Effectiveness of pioglitazone treatment

In general, HbA1c concentrations are used as the definitive measure for whether a drug has any health benefits for patients. Any decrease by greater than 15% is defined as a response to pioglitazone. After 12 weeks of pioglitazone treatment, 21.25% of the 80 patients achieved a decrease in HbA1c% of ≥15%.

rs2241766 is independently associated with response to pioglitazone

In general, pioglitazone appeared to be beneficial to patients. However, the major objective was to determine whether the overall efficacy of pioglitazone could be attributed to any specific subgroups of patients. Patients were, thus, grouped according to their genotype, and the change in HbA1c% levels was determined. The patients exhibiting the greatest response to 12 weeks of treatment with pioglitazone were in the group with the rs2241766 (exon 2) TG genotype (52.9%). A second rs2241766 genotype, TT, was also associated with an increased response to pioglitazone within this timeframe (12.7%). The difference in the response of patients between rs2241766 genotype TG and TT was statistically significant ($p=0.001$). No other associations between individual *ADIPOQ* gene polymorphisms and response to pioglitazone treatment were found (Table 4). Finally, logistic regression analysis revealed that rs2241766 was independently associated with response to pioglitazone. Patients carrying the TG genotype responded significantly better in general to pioglitazone compared to the patients carrying the TT genotype (OR = 11.483, 95% CI = 2.637–50.002, $p=0.001$; Table 5).

Table 2. Clinical characteristics of subjects before and after pioglitazone treatment.

	Before	After	p-value
Fasting plasma glucose (mmol/L)	8.73±1.55	7.25±1.36	<0.001*
Adiponectin (mg/L)	3.42 [2.19,7.21]	5.67 [2.83,10.14]	<0.001*
Fasting insulin(mg/ml)	6.85±3.86	5.38±2.59	<0.001*
HOMA-IR	2.29 [1.61,3.28]	1.51 [1.08,2.16]	<0.001*
HbA1c(%)	7.65 [7.30,8.40]	7.10 [6.70,7.95]	<0.001*
TG(mmol/L)	1.70 [1.20,2.37]	1.52 [1.19,2.00]	0.478
TC(mmol/L)	4.73±0.87	4.72±0.96	0.955
LDL-C(mmol/L)	2.87±0.80	2.81±0.84	0.460
HDL-C(mmol/L)	1.28±0.29	1.33±0.32	0.052
Weight (Kg)	66.13±9.88	66.43±9.81	0.184
BMI(Kg/m2)	25.49±3.05	25.61±3.09	0.163
Waist circumference(cm)	90.65±8.83	90.19±8.60	0.229
Systolic blood pressure(mmHg)	133.98±20.74	132.34±17.93	0.386
Diastolic blood pressure (mmHg)	80.00 75.25,90.00]	80.00 [70.00,89.00]	0.254

HOMA-IR, homeostasis model assessment for insulin resistance; HbA1c, glycated hemoglobin; TG, triglyceride; TC, total cholesterol; LDL-C, low-density lipoprotein cholesterol; HDL-C, high-density lipoprotein cholesterol; BMI, body mass index.

Table 3. SNP genotypes of the adiponectin gene and allele frequencies in the Chinese cohort.

db SNP number	Gene region	Alleles (1/2)	Genotype distribution		
			11	12	22
rs266729	Promoter	C/G	70%	26.25%	3.75%
rs16861194	Promoter	A/G	85%	15%	0.00%
rs1501299	Intron 2	G/T	45%	46.25%	8.75%
rs2241767	Intron 2	A/G	55%	41.25%	3.75%
rs3821799	Intron 2	T/C	38.75%	53.75%	7.50%
rs145335235	Intron 2	C/T	97.50%	2.50%	0.00%
rs3774261	Intron 2	A/G	37.50%	50%	12.50%
rs2241766	Exon 2	T/G	78.75%	21.25%	0.00%
rs17846872	Exon 3	G/T	91.25%	8.75%	0.00%
rs35469083	Exon 3	C/T	97.50%	0.00%	2.50%
rs1063537	Exon 3	C/T	57.50%	30%	12.50%
rs2082940	Exon 3	C/T	47.50%	33.75%	18.75%
rs1063538	Exon 3	T/C	30%	51.25%	18.75%

Mean changes in clinical characteristics before and after pioglitazone treatment are statistically significant between genotypes

The previous analysis was based on the number of patients, out of 80 total or within genotype subgroups, with ≥15% change in HbA1c%. In order to gain further insight into the physiological benefits of pioglitazone to patients, genotype was examined with regard to each clinical parameter in terms of mean change between the measurements made prior to and following treatment. Polymorphisms at rs2241766 exhibited statistically significant changes within clinical correlates in response to treatment that were not apparent in the previous analysis. The mean decrease in HbA1c% levels after pioglitazone treatment was greater in patients with the rs2241766 genotype TG than the patients with genotype TT (TG: 1.15±0.80% vs. TT: 0.52±0.64%, $p = 0.001$), indicating a synergy of the G allele (rs2241766) with efficacy of pioglitazone in these patients. There were no other significant differences of mean change in FPG, fasting insulin, HOMA-IR, ADIPOQ, TG, TC, LDL-C, HDL-C, BMI, and WC between rs2241766 TG and TT genotypes (Table 6).

The second clinical correlate to emerge as a potential predictor of pioglitazone efficacy was WC. Genotypes of two SNPs within the intron 2 region of the *ADIPOQ* gene (rs3774261 and rs3821799) were associated with significant differences in WC. Patients of the rs3774261 genotypes AA and AG + GG experienced a significant mean decrease of WC (AA: 1.00 [−0.63, 3.00] vs. AG + GG; 0.00 [−1.00, 1.00]; $p = 0.019$). The mean decrease in the insulin value, however, was less for genotype AA than for genotypes AG + GG

Table 4. Association of adiponectin gene SNP with response to pioglitazone.

SNP	Response rate	P-value (χ^2)	SNP	Response rate	P-value (χ^2)
Rs1501299G/T			Rs2241767A/G		
GG	16.67%		AA	27.27%	
GT+TT	25%	0.365	AG+GG	13.89%	0.145
Rs2241766T/G			Rs2082940C/T		
TG	52.94%		CC	26.32%	
TT	12.70%	0.001*	CT+TT	16.67%	0.292
Rs266729C/G			Rs1063538T/C		
CC	21.43%		TT	20.83%	
CG+GG	20.83%	0.952	TC+CC	21.43%	0.952
Rs16861194A/G			Rs1063537C/T		
AA	20.59%		CC	26.09%	
AG	25%	0.711	CT+TT	14.71%	0.219
Rs3821799T/C			Rs3774261A/G		
TT	19.35%		AA	16.67%	
TC+CC	22.45%	0.742	AG+GG	24%	0.438

Table 5. Logistic regression analysis for the influence of clinical and genetic factors on the response to pioglitazone treatment.

Variable	Odds ratio	95% CI	P-value
Rs1501299 (GT+TT vs. GG)	1.718	0.408–7.230	0.461
Rs2241767 (AA vs. AG+GG)	1.201	0.236–6.120	0.826
Rs3821799 (TC+CC vs. TT)	1.131	0.139–9.204	0.908
Rs3774261 (AG+GG vs. AA)	1.209	0.156–9.352	0.856
Rs266729 (CC vs. CG+GG)	1.219	0.307–4.836	0.778
Rs16861194 (AG vs. AA)	1.274	0.231–7.019	0.781
Rs1063537 (CC vs. CT+TT)	2.972	0.492–17.947	0.235
Rs2082940 (CC vs. CT+TT)	1.303	0.308–5.515	0.719
Rs1063538 (TC+CC vs. TT)	1.255	0.283–5.562	0.765
Rs2241766 (TG vs. TT)	11.483	2.637–50.002	0.001*

(AA: 0.45 [−0.24, 1.67]; AG + GG: 1.44 [0.33, 2.52]; $p = 0.030$). For the second intron 2 polymorphism (rs3821799), the mean decrease in WC was significantly greater in those patients with genotype TT than in those with the other genotypes (TT: 1.23±2.59 cm; TC+CC: −0.03±2.39 cm; $p = 0.033$; Table 7). No significant differences in the mean change of FPG, fasting insulin, HbA1c%, HOMA-IR, ADIPOQ, TG, TC, LDL-C, HDL-C, BMI, or WC after pioglitazone treatment were found when rs2241767 and rs1501299 genotypes within the intron 2 region of *ADIPOQ* gene were examined (Table 8).

Interestingly, in light of the fact that pioglitazone influences transcription of *ADIPOQ*, the two SNPs within the promoter region of the *ADIPOQ* gene (rs266729 and rs16861194), were not associated with a significant difference in the mean change of FPG, fasting insulin, HbA1c%, HOMA-IR, ADIPOQ, TG, TC, LDL-C, HDL-C, BMI, or WC between patients with rs266729 genotypes CC and CG + GG or between patients with rs16861194 genotypes AA and AG (data not shown).

Likewise, the mean changes in FPG, fasting insulin, HbA1c%, HOMA-IR, ADIPOQ, TG, TC, LDL-C, HDL-C, BMI, and WC after the pioglitazone treatment were not significantly different among the three SNPs within the exon 3 region of the *ADIPOQ* gene (rs2082940, rs1063538 and rs1063537; data not shown).

Discussion

Individual differences in patient response to pioglitazone do exist, and many studies have focused on underlying genetic diversity at the *ADIPOQ* locus as the fundamental cause. Although there is agreement among studies performed by various investigators that *ADIPOQ* gene polymorphisms do influence the response to pioglitazone in T2DM patients, the results of individual studies are inconsistent [11,12,13]. The primary objective of this prospective intervention study was to determine whether genetic variation in the *ADIPOQ* gene might be the basis for the inconsistencies reported in response to pioglitazone treatment. The results revealed two major points. Firstly, the decrease in HbA1c% levels after the pioglitazone treatment was greater in those patients with the rs2241766 TG genotype than in patients with other genotypes. Secondly, where response was not evident by the HbA1c% criteria, significant changes in individual clinical correlates were associated with genotypes of individual polymorphisms. For example, the mean change in the FPG levels between the rs3774261 AA and AG + GG genotypes was significantly different. These findings may be clinically relevant to predict patients who will benefit most from pioglitazone treatment.

The most straightforward scenario for differences in pioglitazone response would be that the transcriptional activity of PPARγ, and thus plasma ADIPOQ levels, may differ based on sequence variability in the promoter region of the gene. Although pioglitazone has been shown to directly regulate transcription of the *ADIPOQ* gene through PPARγ, our data indicate ironically that there is no association between polymorphisms in the promoter region of the *ADIPOQ* gene (rs266729 and rs16861194) and response to the drug. The present findings confirm some of the previous findings reported on 80 northern Chinese Han patients with T2DM [10]. This study also revealed that there was no association between the promoter polymorphism rs16861194 and pioglitazone response. However, a weak association between a polymorphism in the second promoter region (rs266729) and HbA1c% values was found [10]. Specifically, rs266729 CG + GG versus CC was associated with a greater decrease in the HbA1c% value after the pioglitazone treatment (0.13% vs. 0.08%). Treatment protocols between the two studies differed slightly and may account for the association in their results: 10 weeks of treatment pioglitazone at a dose of 30 mg/day study [10] versus 12 weeks at a dose of 15 mg/day in this study.

The synonymous *ADIPOQ* SNP, rs2241766 (+45 T>G, glycine-to-glycine change), is one of the most common polymorphisms of the gene. Rs2241766 is in close proximity to the splice junction of intron 1 and exon 2 and may affect the splicing of the mRNA. Differences in response to pioglitazone may, thus, be the result of subsequent changes in ADIPOQ protein levels and activity. One of the interesting findings from our study is that the rs2241766 polymorphism was significantly associated with the response to pioglitazone in patients. Furthermore, response amongst these patients alone differed based on genotype. The response rate and mean decrease in HbA1c% values with pioglitazone treatment for patients with genotype TG was 52.94% and 1.15%, respectively. A response and mean decrease was also evident in HbA1c% values for patients with the TT genotype but to a lesser degree, 12.70% and 0.52%, respectively. These differences between the genotypes were statistically significant ($p < 0.001$), indicating that a base pair difference of G to T may influence the efficacy of pioglitazone.

As one of the most common polymorphisms of the *ADIPOQ* gene, rs2241766 has been examined for association to treatment response by other investigators. In Iranian patients with T2DM, the rs2241766 polymorphism was not found to be associated with

Table 6. Clinical characteristics of patients with various genotypes for the rs2241766 before and after the administration of pioglitazone.

		rs2241766		P-value
		TT	TG	
FPG (mmol/L)	Before treatment	8.62±1.52	9.17±1.61	0.195
	After treatment	7.22±1.43	7.40±1.07	0.637
	Mean change	1.40±1.88	1.77±1.21	0.440
Fasting insulin (mg/ml)	Before treatment	6.87±4.14	6.81±2.67	0.959
	After treatment	5.24±2.62	5.89±2.51	0.362
	Mean change	1.14 [−0.02,2.51]	0.71 [0.07,1.35]	0.473
HbA1c (%)	Before treatment	7.60 [7.20,8.20]	7.90 [7.30,8.95]	0.256
	After treatment	7.41±0.94	7.12±1.05	0.286
	Mean change	0.52±0.64	1.15±0.80	0.001*
HOMA-IR	Before treatment	2.16 [1.46,3.26]	2.45 [1.94,3.39]	0.298
	After treatment	1.47 [1.06,2.02]	1.83 [1.22,2.39]	0.137
	Mean change	0.66 [0.11,1.23]	0.77 [0.34,1.16]	0.663
Adiponectin (mg/L)	Before treatment	4.51±3.92	6.07±3.64	0.145
	After treatment	6.63±5.07	8.48±5.03	0.185
	Mean change	−2.11±3.95	−2.41±5.19	0.800
TG (mmol/l)	Before treatment	1.84±0.95	2.14±0.90	0.249
	After treatment	1.46 [1.16,2.19]	1.62 [1.31,1.86]	0.394
	Mean change	0.01±0.78	0.28±0.106	0.245
TC (mmol/l)	Before treatment	4.65±0.85	5.02±0.91	0.120
	After treatment	4.72±1.00	4.74±0.87	0.955
	Mean change	−0.07±0.90	0.28±0.90	0.153
LDL-C (mmol/l)	Before treatment	2.84±0.83	2.99±0.69	0.479
	After treatment	2.81±0.87	2.81±0.70	0.998
	Mean change	0.03±0.75	0.18±0.70	0.447
HDL-C (mmol/l)	Before treatment	1.29±0.29	1.26±0.31	0.667
	After treatment	1.35±0.34	1.26±0.23	0.261
	Mean change	−0.06±0.22	0.00±0.23	0.297
BMI (kg/m2)	Before treatment	25.63±3.28	24.94±1.96	0.276
	After treatment	25.76±3.34	25.05±1.86	0.253
	Mean change	−0.13±0.83	−0.11±0.65	0.930
Waist circumference (cm)	Before treatment	91.41±9.43	87.82±5.43	0.049*
	After treatment	90.91±9.04	87.53±6.20	0.151
	Mean change	0.00 [−1.00,2.00]	0.00 [−2.00,1.25]	0.609

FPG, fasting plasma glucose; HOMA-IR, homeostasis model assessment for insulin resistance; HbA1c, glycated hemoglobin; TG, triglyceride; TC, total cholesterol; LDL-C, low-density lipoprotein cholesterol; HDL-C, high-density lipoprotein cholesterol; BMI, body mass index.

the response to pioglitazone [11], although overall Iranian patients did respond better to pioglitazone, 31.7% versus 21.25% in our study. The basis for the difference in response in Iranian patients is unknown and may be due to ethnic differences in the populations analyzed [14,15]. One other possibility is that pioglitazone has physiological effects in addition to transcription mediated by PPARγ[16].

Rs2082940, rs1063538 and rs1063537, polymorphisms in exon 3 regions of the *ADIPOQ* gene, were also examined for associations with therapeutic efficacy of pioglitazone was investigated. However, there was no evidence of an association between response to pioglitazone and these polymorphisms. Additional studies including larger cohorts, as well as other common polymorphisms in *ADIPOQ* gene, will be helpful to further confirm our results.

A final analysis was performed to identify associations between polymorphisms and specific clinical phenotypes that might be obscured simply because of our definition of response to treatment. In this analysis, a unique, previously undescribed relationship of respone to pioglitazone with intron 2 SNPs, rs3774261, rs3821799, rs2241767, and rs1501299, emerged. Two clinical parameters, WC and insulin resistance, exhibited significant changes in patients with specific SNPs. The mean change in WC was significantly greater in treated patients with the rs3821799 genotype AA compared to those carrying genotypes AG + GG (P = 0.019). In contrast, the reduction in the insulin

Table 7. Clinical characteristics of patients with various genotypes for the rs3821799 and rs3774261 before and after the administration of pioglitazone.

		rs3821799		p-value	rs3774261		p-value
		TT	TC+CC		AA	AG+GG	
FPG (mmol/L)	Before treatment	8.63±1.48	8.81±1.60	0.622	8.57±1.49	8.83±1.59	0.469
	After treatment	7.09±1.43	7.36±1.32	0.383	6.88±1.27	7.49±1.37	0.052
	Mean change	1.54±1.88	1.44±1.69	0.810	1.70±1.78	1.35±1.75	0.396
Fasting insulin (mg/ml)	Before treatment	6.02±2.95	7.38±4.29	0.125	6.11±2.95	7.30±4.29	0.183
	After treatment	5.10±2.01	5.56±2.91	0.408	5.31±2.29	5.42±2.78	0.847
	Mean change	0.59 [−0.21,1.64]	1.25 [0.32,2.54]	0.076	0.45 [−0.24,1.67]	1.44 [0.33,2.52]	0.030*
HbA1c (%)	Before treatment	8.20±1.34	7.88±0.82	0.227	8.17±1.30	7.90±0.88	0.322
	After treatment	7.47±1.12	7.27±0.86	0.374	7.49±1.15	7.26±0.83	0.345
	Mean change	0.74±0.68	0.61±0.74	0.435	0.68±0.74	0.64±0.71	0.820
HOMA-IR	Before treatment	2.16 [1.46,3.02]	2.43 [1.71,3.43]	0.187	2.06 [1.44,3.07]	2.44[1.68,3.37]	0.229
	After treatment	1.47 [1.06,1.86]	1.69 [1.09,2.33]	0.477	1.63±0.87	1.77 ±0.87	0.491
	Mean change	0.41 [0.21,0.82]	0.80 [0.30,1.27]	0.142	0.45 [0.19,0.92]	0.79[0.29,1.24]	0.178
Adiponectin (mg/L)	Before treatment	3.15 [2.68,5.53]	4.14 [1.80,7.43]	0.726	3.06 [2.67,5.75]	4.29 [1.87,7.41]	0.773
	After treatment	6.96±4.82	7.06±5.29	0.935	7.12±5.59	6.96 ±4.81	0.897
	Mean change	−2.48±4.47	−1.99±4.07	0.615	−2.49±4.93	−1.99±3.75	0.604
TG (mmol/l)	Before treatment	1.84±0.93	1.94±0.96	0.642	1.85±0.95	1.94±0.95	0.685
	After treatment	1.46 [1.05,1.90]	1.55 [1.27,2.29]	0.186	1.61 [1.18,2.07]	1.48[1.22,2.06]	0.917
	Mean change	0.20±0.79	−0.01±0.88	0.286	0.10±0.73	0.05±0.92	0.778
TC (mmol/l)	Before treatment	4.79±0.83	4.69±0.89	0.595	4.89±0.73	4.63±0.93	0.199
	After treatment	4.60±1.01	4.80±0.93	0.365	4.66±1.01	4.76±0.95	0.649
	Mean change	0.19±0.86	−0.11±0.92	0.138	0.23±0.77	−0.13±0.96	0.084
LDL-C (mmol/l)	Before treatment	2.96±0.86	2.82±0.76	0.425	3.01±0.81	2.79±0.79	0.220
	After treatment	2.84±1.04	2.79±0.69	0.807	2.87±1.03	2.78±0.71	0.636
	Mean change	0.12±0.73	0.02±0.75	0.561	0.15±0.67	0.01±0.78	0.434
HDL-C (mmol/l)	Before treatment	1.24±0.31	1.31±0.28	0.310	1.29±0.29	1.28±0.30	0.870
	After treatment	1.30±0.30	1.35±0.33	0.460	1.32±0.31	1.34±0.33	0.830
	Mean change	−0.06±0.16	−0.04±0.25	0.749	−0.03±0.13	−0.06±0.26	0.540
BMI (kg/m^2)	Before treatment	25.30±2.83	25.60±3.20	0.666	25.64±3.40	25.40±2.85	0.734
	After treatment	25.34±2.84	25.78±3.25	0.536	25.59±3.24	25.62±3.03	0.957
	Mean change	−0.04±0.90	−0.18±0.71	0.446	0.05±0.92	−0.23±0.69	0.126
Waist circumference(cm)	Before treatment	89.71±7.96	91.24±9.37	0.452	91.38±9.62	90.21±8.39	0.568
	After treatment	88.48±8.30	91.28±8.69	0.158	90.18±9.65	90.20±8.00	0.993
	Mean change	1.23±2.59	−0.03±2.39	0.033*	1.00 [−0.63,3.00]	0.00 [−1.00,1.00]	0.019*

FPG, fasting plasma glucose; HOMA-IR, homeostasis model assessment for insulin resistance; HbA1c, glycated hemoglobin; TG, triglyceride; TC, total cholesterol; LDL-C, low-density lipoprotein cholesterol; HDL-C, high-density lipoprotein cholesterol; BMI, body mass index.

Table 8. Clinical characteristics of patients with various genotypes for the rs1501299 and rs2241767 before and after the administration of pioglitazone.

		rs1501299		p-value	rs2241767		p-value
		GG	GT+TT		TT	TG	
FPG (mmol/L)	Before treatment	8.35±1.11	9.05±1.78	0.034*	8.74±1.3	8.74±1.81	0.993
	After treatment	7.10±1.29	7.39±1.42	0.342	7.30±1.37	7.21±1.36	0.779
	Mean change	1.25±1.43	1.67±1.98	0.283	1.44±1.70	1.53±1.85	0.834
Fasting insulin (mg/ml)	Before treatment	6.44±2.94	7.20±4.49	0.366	7.10±3.92	6.55±3.83	0.534
	After treatment	5.33 3.69,7.00]	4.46 [3.16,6.92]	0.498	5.65±2.57	5.05±2.63	0.302
	Mean change	0.67 [−0.03,1.89]	1.11 [0.04,2.87]	0.442	0.88 [−0.04,1.89]	1.23 [0.31,2.37]	0.505
HbA1c (%)	Before treatment	7.40 [7.10,7.80]	8.10 [7.4,8.90]	0.001*	8.19±1.12	7.77±0.94	0.073
	After treatment	7.07±0.76	7.57±1.06	0.016*	7.41±1.00	7.27±0.93	0.508
	Mean change	0.58±0.60	0.72±0.80	0.348	0.78±0.78	0.51±0.60	0.081
HOMA-IR	Before treatment	2.36±1.05	2.98±2.33	0.115	2.55 [1.63,3.38]	1.98 [1.57,3.17]	0.333
	After treatment	1.68±0.75	1.74±0.96	0.764	1.66 [1.15,2.22]	1.18 [1.05,2.04]	0.138
	Mean change	0.69 [0.24,0.93]	0.67 [0.14,2.02]	0.395	0.65 [0.24,0.98]	0.77 [0.15,1.25]	0.653
Adiponectin (mg/L)	Before treatment	3.05 [1.54,5.29]	3.83[2.65,7.91]	0.042*	4.78±3.97	4.92±3.86	0.871
	After treatment	5.93 [2.46,9.28	5.6 [2.94,11.81]	0.471	7.40±4.76	6.56±5.48	0.464
	Mean change	−2.35±4.29	−2.03±4.18	0.737	−2.62±3.98	−1.63±4.46	0.299
TG (mmol/l)	Before treatment	1.89±0.86	1.92±1.02	0.913	1.96±0.85	1.83±1.05	0.542
	After treatment	1.46 [1.19,1.91]	1.61 [1.20,2.59]	0.431	1.62 [1.25,2.13]	1.38 [1.13,1.97]	0.216
	Mean change	0.25±0.76	−0.08±0.90	0.080	0.03±0.92	0.11±0.77	0.659
TC (mmol/l)	Before treatment	4.57±0.86	4.86±0.86	0.143	4.79±0.84	4.66±0.91	0.514
	After treatment	4.43±0.79	4.96±1.03	0.013*	4.82±1.03	4.61±0.88	0.343
	Mean change	0.14±0.92	−0.11±0.88	0.227	−0.03±0.97	0.05±0.82	0.700
LDL-C (mmol/l)	Before treatment	2.71 [2.30,3.24]	2.80 [2.40,3.32]	0.562	2.88±0.74	2.87±0.87	0.965
	After treatment	2.78 [2.30,3.11]	2.70 [2.33,3.34]	0.681	2.83±0.87	2.79±0.81	0.845
	Mean change	0.12±0.82	0.01±0.68	0.508	0.05±0.87	0.08±0.56	0.862
HDL-C (mmol/l)	Before treatment	1.24±0.30	1.32±0.29	0.198	1.26±0.28	1.32±0.31	0.358
	After treatment	1.27±0.26	1.38±0.35	0.118	1.31±0.35	1.37±0.28	0.383
	Mean change	−0.03±0.22	−0.06±0.23	0.599	−0.05±0.20	−0.05±0.25	0.976
BMI (kg/m^2)	Before treatment	25.47±2.83	25.50±3.25	0.976	25.63±3.34	25.31±2.68	0.635
	After treatment	25.51±2.90	25.69±3.27	0.804	25.74±3.27	25.45±2.89	0.681
	Mean change	−0.04±0.91	−0.19±0.68	0.398	−0.11±0.84	−0.15±0.74	0.827
Waist circumference(cm)	Before treatment	90.54±7.19	90.74±10.05	0.919	91.00±9.34	90.22±8.27	0.698
	After treatment	89.57±7.34	90.70±9.55	0.550	90.38±9.21	89.97±7.91	0.836
	Mean change	1.00 −1.00,2.38]	0.00 −1.00,0.38]	0.149	0.00 [−1.00,2.00]	0.00 [−1.00,1.00]	0.506

FPG, fasting plasma glucose; HOMA-IR, homeostasis model assessment for insulin resistance; HbA1c, glycated hemoglobin; TG, triglyceride; TC, total cholesterol; LDL-C, low-density lipoprotein cholesterol; HDL-C, high-density lipoprotein cholesterol; BMI, body mass index.

value of the rs3774261 genotype AG + GG patients was greater than for genotype AA ($p = 0.030$). Our results corroborate analysis performed on a cohort of Italian patients [17]. In the Iranian population, however, the putative relationship of the exon 2polymorphisms with WC was obscured. Only a non-significant association between the rs3821799 polymorphism and WC was observed [18].

The main trend of the future of medicine is personalized medicine, based in part on individual genotypes, in order to provide appropriate, safe, and economic use of a drug [19,20]. This study provides novel data on the relationship between SNP in the *ADIPOQ* gene and the response to pioglitazone. Several caveats however still exist regarding the results. The major limitation of this study is the small sample size. Secondly, the study does not illuminate the molecular mechanisms by which genotype variants may influence the response to pioglitazone. Finally, the efficacy of pioglitazone is to a degree is dependent on environmental factors such as diet and exercise, and these factors were not addressed in this study. However, the results should stimulate further studies with a much larger sample size, perhaps encompassing more than simply the Chinese Han population, along with more strictly designed clinical and mechanistic studies.

Author Contributions

Conceived and designed the experiments: XL. Performed the experiments: GS EY. Analyzed the data: XL HY EY GS. Contributed reagents/materials/analysis tools: L. Chen L. Cai CY CZ. Wrote the paper: XL HY EY GS.

References

1. Berg AH, Combs TP, Scherer PE (2002) ACRP30/adiponectin: an adipokine regulating glucose and lipid metabolism. Trends Endocrinol Metab 13: 84–89.
2. Takahashi M, Arita Y, Yamagata K, Matsukawa Y, Okutomi K, et al. (2000) Genomic structure and mutations in adipose-specific gene, adiponectin. Int J Obes Relat Metab Disord 24: 861–868.
3. Iwaki M, Matsuda M, Maeda N, Funahashi T, Matsuzawa Y, et al. (2003) Induction of adiponectin, a fat-derived antidiabetic and antiatherogenic factor, by nuclear receptors. Diabetes 52: 1655–1663.
4. Perez A, Zhao Z, Jacks R, Spanheimer R (2009) Efficacy and safety of pioglitazone/metformin fixed-dose combination therapy compared with pioglitazone and metformin monotherapy in treating patients with T2DM. Curr Med Res Opin 25: 2915–2923.
5. Derosa G, Sibilla S (2007) Optimizing combination treatment in the management of type 2 diabetes. Vasc Health Risk Manag 3: 665–671.
6. Alwi ZB (2005) The Use of SNPs in Pharmacogenomics Studies. Malays J Med Sci 12: 4–12.
7. Bouatia-Naji N, Meyre D, Lobbens S, Seron K, Fumeron F, et al. (2006) ACDC/adiponectin polymorphisms are associated with severe childhood and adult obesity. Diabetes 55: 545–550.
8. Yang WS, Yang YC, Chen CL, Wu IL, Lu JY, et al. (2007) Adiponectin SNP276 is associated with obesity, the metabolic syndrome, and diabetes in the elderly. Am J Clin Nutr 86: 509–513.
9. Ye E, Yang H, Chen L, Chen Q, Sun M, et al. (2014) Adiponectin and peroxisome proliferator-activated receptor-γ gene polymorphisms and gene-gene interactions with type 2 diabetes. Life Sci 98: 55–59.
10. Li Z, Peng X, Wu Y, Xia Y, Liu X, et al. (2008) The influence of adiponectin gene polymorphism on the pioglitazone response in the Chinese with type 2 diabetes. Diabetes Obes Metab 10: 794–802.
11. Namvaran F, Rahimi-Moghaddam P, Azarpira N, Dabbaghmanesh MH (2012) Polymorphism of adiponectin (45T/G) and adiponectin receptor-2 (795G/A) in an Iranian population: relation with insulin resistance and response to treatment with pioglitazone in patients with type 2 diabetes mellitus. Mol Biol Rep 39: 5511–5518.
12. Namvaran F, Azarpira N, Rahimi-Moghaddam P, Dabbaghmanesh MH (2011) Polymorphism of peroxisome proliferator-activated receptor gamma (PPAR-gamma) Pro12Ala in the Iranian population: relation with insulin resistance and response to treatment with pioglitazone in type 2 diabetes. Eur J Pharmacol 671: 1–6.
13. Balaji V (2013) Efficacy and safety of pioglitazone in type 2 diabetes in the Indian patients: Results of an observational study. Indian J Endocrinol Metab 17: 709–715.
14. Gu HF, Abulaiti A, Ostenson CG, Humphreys K, Wahlestedt C, et al. (2004) Single nucleotide polymorphisms in the proximal promoter region of the adiponectin (APM1) gene are associated with type 2 diabetes in Swedish caucasians. Diabetes 53 Suppl 1: S31–35.
15. Schwarz PE, Towers GW, Fischer S, Govindarajalu S, Schulze J, et al. (2006) Hypoadiponectinemia is associated with progression toward type 2 diabetes and genetic variation in the ADIPOQ gene promoter. Diabetes Care 29: 1645–1650.
16. Subbaramaiah K, Howe LR, Zhou XK, Yang P, Hudis CA, et al. (2012) Pioglitazone, a PPARγ agonist, suppresses CYP19 transcription: evidence for involvement of 15-hydroxyprostaglandin dehydrogenase and BRCA1. Cancer Prev Res 5: 1183–1194.
17. Menzaghi C, Ercolino T, Di Paola R, Berg AH, Warram JH, et al. (2002) A haplotype at the adiponectin locus is associated with obesity and other features of the insulin resistance syndrome. Diabetes 51: 2306–2312.
18. Hasani-Ranjbar S, Amoli MM, Tabatabaei-Malazy O, Rumi Y, Tavakkoly-Bazzaz J, et al. (2012) Effect of adiponectin gene polymorphisms on waist circumference in patients with diabetes. J Diabetes Metab Disord 11: 14.
19. Daien CI, Morel J (2014) Predictive Factors of Response to Biological Disease Modifying Antirheumatic Drugs: Towards Personalized Medicine. Mediators Inflamm 2014: 386148.
20. Hayes DF, Markus HS, Leslie RD, Topol EJ (2014) Personalized medicine: risk prediction, targeted therapies and mobile health technology. BMC Med 12: 37.

4

An Interaction between a *FNDC5* Variant and Obesity Modulates Glucose Metabolism in a Chinese Han Population

Shanshan Tang, Rong Zhang, Feng Jiang, Jie Wang, Miao Chen, Danfeng Peng, Jing Yan, Yuqian Bao, Cheng Hu, Weiping Jia*

Shanghai Diabetes Institute, Department of Endocrinology and Metabolism, Shanghai Key Laboratory of Diabetes Mellitus, Shanghai Clinical Center for Diabetes, Shanghai Jiao Tong University Affiliated Sixth People's Hospital, Shanghai, PR China

Abstract

Background: To investigate the impact of common variants of *FNDC5* on type 2 diabetes and clinical traits related to glucose metabolism in a large Chinese population sample.

Methods: Three tagging single nucleotide polymorphisms within the region of the *FNDC5* gene were selected and genotyped in 6822 participants. Detailed clinical investigations and biochemistry measurements were carried out in all of the participants. Subjects without diabetes were classified into normal weight and overweight/obese subgroups according to body mass index (BMI).

Results: None of the SNPs were associated with either the risk of type 2 diabetes in all of the participants or with any of the clinical quantitative traits in the controls with normal glucose regulation. Subgroup analysis showed that in controls with normal weight (BMI <25 kg/m^2), the rs16835198 major allele G was significantly associated with fasting insulin levels, and that each additional copy of the allele resulted in a 0.0178 mU/L increment of the values ($p = 0.046$). Moreover, after adjusting for confounding variables, there were trends towards correlation of rs16835198 with HOMA-insulin resistance (HOMA-IR) ($p = 0.057$) and low-density lipoprotein cholesterol (LDL-C) levels ($p = 0.083$). In overweight/obese subjects (BMI ≥ 25 Kg/m^2), we noted rs16835198 showed trends towards association with fasting insulin ($p = 0.057$) and HOMA-IR levels ($p = 0.091$), both of which declined with additional copies of the major allele G. Moreover, rs16835198 was significantly associated with high-density lipoprotein cholesterol (HDL-C) levels ($p = 0.013$), and HOMA-β cell function ($p = 0.028$) in the overweight/obese subjects. Finally, we observed a significant interaction between BMI-rs16835198 and fasting insulin levels in the control group ($p = 0.003$).

Conclusions: Our data indicate that the effect of the common *FNDC5* SNP rs16835198 on fasting insulin was significantly modified by BMI in the Chinese Han population.

Editor: Yanqiao Zhang, Northeast Ohio Medical University, United States of America

Funding: This work was funded by grants from the Key Program of the Shanghai Municipality for Basic Research (11JC1409600), National 863 program (2012AA02A509), National Science Foundation of China (81322010, 81170735, 81200582 and 81300691), National Major Scientific and Technological Special Project for "Significant New Drugs Development" (2011ZX09307-001-02) and Key Discipline of Public Health of Shanghai (12GWZX0104), the Innovation Fund for PhD Students (BXJ201340) from the Shanghai Jiao Tong University School of Medicine, Excellent Young Medical Expert of Shanghai (XYQ2011041), Shanghai Talent Development Grant (2012041), and National Young Top Talent Supporting Program. The authors appreciate all the participants of this research study. The authors gratefully acknowledge the skillful technical support of all nursing and medical staff at the Shanghai Clinical Center for Diabetes. The funders had no role in study design, data collection and analysis, decision to publish, or preparation of the manuscript.

Competing Interests: The authors have declared that no competing interests exist.

* Email: wpjia@sjtu.edu.cn

Introduction

Diabetes is a major public health concern, and changes in diet and lifestyle have accelerated the rise in the incidence of this disease to pandemic proportions in many countries worldwide, including China. According to the national epidemiological survey conducted in 2008, China has the largest number of diabetics in any single country [1], of which 90% have type 2 diabetes. It is acknowledged that insulin resistance plays an important role in the pathogenesis of diabetes as well as obesity. In recent decades, with the global prevalence of obesity rising, the burden of chronic metabolic disorders has been boosted even further [2].

Physical exercise is recognized not only as an indispensable component of lifestyle intervention but also, increasingly, as a cornerstone for non-pharmacological therapy in ameliorating obesity and insulin resistance [3,4]. As the largest organ in the body, skeletal muscle is increasingly considered an important endocrine organ that interacts with adipose tissue, pancreas, and

Table 1. Clinical characteristics of the study sample population.

	Cases of type2 diabetes	Controls	Controls	
			Normal weight	Overweight/obesity
Samples(n)	3410	3412	2387	1022
Male/female (n)	1812/1597	1364/2048	920/1467	442/580
Age (years)	60.33±12.49	51.41±14.39	50.53±14.86	53.45±12.96
BMI (kg/m^2)	24.20 (22.00,26.60)	23.23 (21.27,27.68)	22.07 (20.55,23.45)	26.78 (25.81,28.23)
Fasting plasma glucose(mmol/L)	12.78 (9.00,16.00)	5.02 (4.70,5.40)	5.00 (4.64,5.38)	5.10 (4.73,5.46)
2-h plasma glucose (mmol/L)	17.00 (13.00,22.00)	5.42 (4.60,6.30)	5.30 (4.53,6.20)	5.70 (4.80,6.60)
Total cholesterol (mmol/L)	4.70 (4.00,5.50)	4.70 (4.04,5.35)	4.60 (3.97,5.30)	4.86 (4.20,5.50)
Triglyceride(mmol/L)	1.49 (0.99,2.18)	1.25 (0.87,1.82)	1.13 (0.80,1.64)	1.61 (1.11,2.26)
HDL-C (mmol/L)	1.11 (0.94,1.33)	1.33 (1.13,1.51)	1.36 (1.18,1.55)	1.25 (1.05,1.43)
LDL -C (mmol/L)	2.97 (2.42,3.57)	3.04 (2.49,3.61)	2.98 (2.42,3.53)	3.20 (2.64,3.80)

Data are shown as n or median (interquartile range).
BMI, body mass index; HDL-C, high-density lipoprotein cholesterol; LDL-C, low-density lipoprotein cholesterol.

liver to modulate metabolism through the beneficial effects of exercise [5–7]. In addition, skeletal muscle secretes metabolically active myokines such as irisin [8], which is encoded by the *FNDC5* (*FRCP2, PeP*) gene in both mice and humans [9,10]. Irisin undergoes proteolytic cleavage to yield a mature 112 aa polypeptide, which is secreted in response to physical exercise [8]. Irisin is expressed in fat, kidney, lung, and liver [11], with peak expression levels in skeletal muscle, where it is regulated by peroxisome proliferator-activated receptor γ (PPARγ) coactivator 1α (PGC1-α), an exercise-responsive mediator that is involved in energy metabolism [8]. Irisin has been shown in mice to induce the transformation of white adipose tissue to brown adipose tissue by induction of the *Ucp1* and *Cidea* genes, implying its potential as therapeutic for combat obesity, diabetes and other disease could be ameliorate by exercise [8,12,13]. Up to now, two previous genetic studies have investigated the association of common SNPs in *FNDC5* with insulin sensitivity and glucose metabolism [14,15]. In addition, although irisin is a myokine known to be closely related with obesity, its impact on the relationship between glycolipid metabolism and BMI is not clearly defined. Given the lack of data implicating *FNDC5* variants in human metabolic disease, we set out to examine the association between *FNDC5* variants and a range of metabolic parameters in a large Chinese Han population.

Materials and Methods

Ethics statement

The study was approved by the Ethics Committee of Shanghai Jiao Tong University Affiliated Sixth People's Hospital and in accordance with the Declaration of Helsinki. Written informed consent was obtained from each participant.

Subjects recruitments

The overall study group totally comprised 6822 participants of Han Chinese ancestry residing in Shanghai. Detailed information regarding this study population was described in detail previously [16–18]. Among them, 3410 participants were unrelated individ-

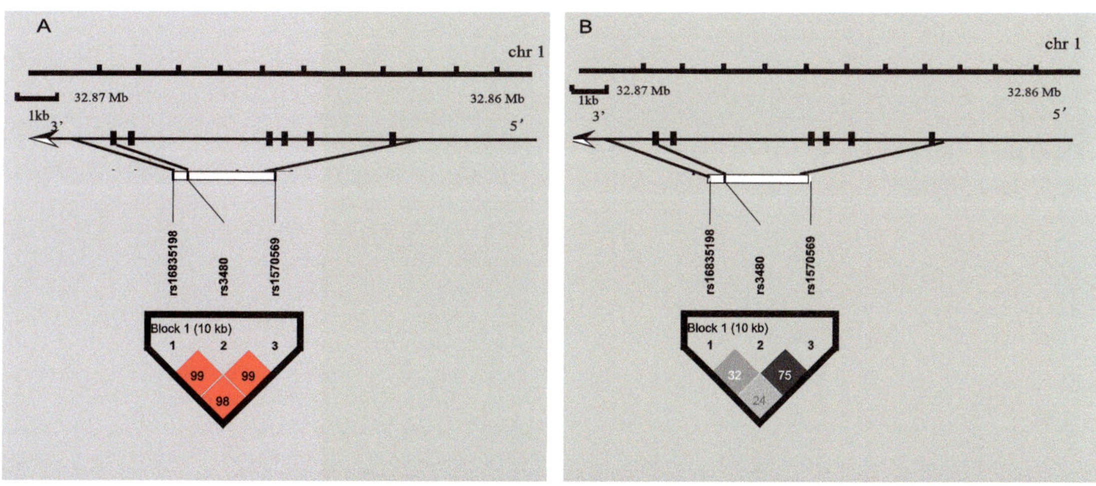

Figure 1. Linkage disequilibrium maps for SNPs genotyped in the region of the *FNDC5* gene. A. Shades of red demonstrate the strength of the pairwise linkage disequilibrium based on D' and numbers represent the value of D' expressed as a percentage. B. Shades of grey show the strength of the pairwise linkage disequilibrium based on r^2 and numbers indicate the value of r^2 expressed as a percentage.

Table 2. Associations of *FNDC5* SNPs with type 2 diabetes.

SNP	Chr. Position (Build 104)	Major/minor allele	Cases of type2 diabetes (n = 3410)		Controls (n = 3412)		OR for major allele (95%CI)	*p* value for major allele	OR for genotype (95%CI)	*p* value for genotype (*p**)
			Major allele frequencies	Genotype count 11/12/22#	Major allele frequencies	Genotype count 11/12/22#				
rs16835198	33326681	G/T	0.518	929/1661/807	0.519	899/1735/768	0.995(0.930,1.064)	0.880	0.995(0.930,1.064)	0.880(0.929)
rs3480	33328165	A/G	0.734	1855/1275/267	0.742	1874/1306/225	0.957(0.887,1.034)	0.265	0.958(0.888,1.034)	0.269(0.205)
rs1570569	33336956	G/T	0.782	2088/1126/175	0.790	2121/1122/153	0.956(0.930,1.064)	0.286	0.957(0.882,1.038)	0.290(0.240)

The additive model was used in the association analyses between genotype and type 2 diabetes.
#11, major allele homozygotes; 12, heterozygotes; 22, minor allele homozygotes.
*Adjusted for age, gender and BMI.

uals with type 2 diabetes, defined according to 1999 WHO criteria (fasting plasma glucose ≥7.0 mmol/l and/or 2-h postchallenge plasma glucose ≥11.1 mmol/l), and who were recruited from the clinical inpatient database of Shanghai Diabetes Institute [19]. The remaining 3412 participants were unrelated controls with normal glucose tolerance as assessed by 75 g oral glucose tolerant tests (OGTTs), and a negative family history of diabetes, and who were selected from community-based epidemiological studies of diabetes and related metabolic diseases. Using 1999 WHO criteria [20], BMI was used to divide individuals with normal blood glucose into two groups, namely: normal weight (BMI<25 Kg/m^2), and overweight/obese (BMI≥25 Kg/m^2). The clinical characteristics of all participants are shown in Table 1.

Clinical measurements

All participants underwent a detailed clinical investigation as described previously [21,22]. In summary, anthropometric parameters such as height, weight, waist and hip circumference were measured. Body mass index (BMI) was calculated as weight in kilograms divided by height in meters squared. Controls were subjected to standard OGTTs involving administration of 75 g glucose in the morning after an overnight fast. Blood samples were obtained at baseline and 2 h time points during the OGTT. Plasma glucose, serum insulin and serum lipid profiles were also measured. Insulin resistance index and β cell function were estimated using the homeostasis model assessment (HOMA), which was calculated using fasting plasma glucose and insulin levels [23]. In addition, Insulin sensitivity from the OGTT was also estimated according to the insulin sensitivity index (ISI) proposed by Gutt *et al.* [24]: ISI = [75000+ (fasting plasma glucose −2 h plasma glucose) × 0.19×weight]/120/mean plasma glucose/$\log_{10}$ mean insulin.

Single nucleotide polymorphism (SNP) selection and genotyping

Using the HapMap Phase III (release 27) Han Chinese database and a threshold of $r^2 \geq 0.8$, we selected three tagging SNPs in a region encompassing the *FNDC5* gene and its 10 kb up- and downstream sequences. These three tagging SNPs tagged 100% of SNPs (5/5 SNPs in the HapMap Chinese Han sample) with a minor allele frequency (MAF) of >0.05. All SNPs were genotyped by primer extension of multiplex products with detection by matrix-assisted laser desorption ionization–time of flight mass spectroscopy, using a MassARRAY Compact Analyzer (Sequenom, San Diego, CA, USA) with an overall call rate of 99.6%.

Statistical analysis

For each variant, the Hardy-Weinberg equilibrium test was performed separately in the cases and controls prior to association analysis. SNPs failing this test ($p<0.05$ in the controls) were excluded. Pairwise linkage disequilibrium including |D'| and r^2 was estimated using Haploview (version 4.2). Allele and genotype distributions between the cases and control subjects were compared with χ^2 test or logistic regression [25], and odds ratios (ORs) with 95% confidence intervals (CIs) were calculated. All skewly distributed quantitative traits [including fasting plasma glucose, 2 h plasma glucose, fasting insulin, 2 h insulin, triglycerides, total cholesterol, low-density lipoprotein cholesterol (LDL-C), high-density lipoprotein cholesterol (HDL-C), estimated ISI, HOMA for β-cell function and insulin resistance] were logarithmically transformed to approximate univariate normality. Quantitative traits were analyzed in the control group by linear regression under an additive genetic model adjusted for age,

Table 3. Association analyses of rs16835198 with clinical characteristics in normal weight controls.

rs16835198	**TT (n = 537)**	**GT (n = 1192)**	**GG(n = 650)**	**β**	**SE**	***p***	***p****
Age (years)	50.36±15.25	50.51±14.42	50.66±15.39	0.1513	0.4327	0.727	/
BMI (kg/m^2)	22.06 (20.52,23.34)	22.10 (20.58,23.45)	22.07(20.50,23.52)	0.0014	0.0012	0.261	/
Fasting plasma glucose(mmol/L)	5.03 (4.70,5.40)	5.00 (4.62,5.35)	5.00 (4.65,5.35)	-0.0004	0.0013	0.739	0.572
2-h plasma glucose (mmol/L)	5.49(4.54,6.21)	5.30 (4.52,6.20)	5.20 (4.55,6.12)	−0.0027	0.0028	0.328	0.211
Fasting insulin (mU/L)	5.46(3.94,7.65)	5.63 (4.07,7.73)	5.77 (3.98,7.94)	0.0178	0.0089	**0.046**	*0.059*
2-h insulin (mU/L)	24.21(15.45,43.63)	25.79 (13.50,41.75)	23.05 (14.08,41.29)	−0.0049	0.0124	0.691	0.498
Total cholesterol (mmol/L)	4.60(3.97,5.30)	4.65 (4.00,5.30)	4.55 (3.91,5.26)	−0.0027	0.0029	0.339	0.190
Triglyceride (mmol/L)	1.12 (0.83,1.64)	1.13 (0.81,1.62)	1.13(0.77,1.66)	−0.0027	0.0066	0.684	0.514
HDL-C (mmol/L)	1.37 (1.21,1.55)	1.36 (1.19,1.55)	1.35(1.15,1.56)	−0.0033	0.0028	0.238	0.198
LDL-C (mmol/L)	2.98(2.45,3.48)	3.01 (2.46,3.58)	2.91 (2.36,3.53)	−0.0060	0.0039	0.119	*0.057*
HOMA-IR	1.17 (0.85,1.71)	1.23 (0.86,1.66)	1.23 (0.83,1.72)	0.0172	0.0093	*0.064*	*0.083*
HOMA-B	80.00 (54.90,121.33)	84.81 (60.67,128.29)	87.07 (61.36,126.40)	0.0158	0.0102	0.124	0.128
Gutt-ISI	691.58(563.64,889.09)	697.61(573.72,903.39)	707.89(583.82,886.08)	0.0013	0.0054	0.813	0.589

Data are shown as mean±SD or median (interquartile range).
BMI, body mass index; HDL-C, high-density lipoprotein cholesterol; LDL-C, low-density lipoprotein cholesterol; HOMA-IR, homeostasis assessment model of insulin resistance; HOMA-B, homeostasis assessment model of β-cell function; Gutt-ISI, insulin sensitivity index proposed by Gutt.
p values <0.05 are shown in bold, *p* values <0.1 are shown in italics.
*Adjusted for age, gender and BMI.

Table 4. Association analyses of rs16835198 with clinical characteristics in overweight and obese controls.

rs16835198	**TT (n = 229)**	**GT (n = 543)**	**GG(n = 248)**	**β**	**SE**	***p***	***p****
Age (years)	53.69±13.01	53.66±12.78	52.68±13.34	−0.5141	0.5938	0.387	/
BMI (kg/m^2)	26.77 (25.73,28.38)	26.76 (25.78,28.13)	26.81(25.90,28.26)	−0.0563	0.0954	0.555	/
Fasting plasma glucose(mmol/L)	5.06 (4.70,5.40)	5.10 (4.77,5.44)	5.10 (4.73,5.48)	0.0007	0.0020	0.706	0.613
2-h plasma glucose (mmol/L)	5.70(4.90,6.57)	5.80 (4.80,6.60)	5.66 (4.75,6.70)	0.0025	0.0042	0.549	0.334
Fasting insulin (mU/L)	8.43(5.83,11.38)	7.47 (5.22,10.50)	7.03 (5.04,10.18)	−0.0267	0.0140	*0.057*	*0.054*
2-h insulin (mU/L)	31.34(18.99,60.36)	37.22 (19.77,56.06)	35.34 (19.52,60.18)	0.0125	0.0197	0.528	0.437
Total cholesterol (mmol/L)	4.90(4.20,5.52)	4.85 (4.18,5.54)	4.81 (4.30,5.40)	0.0018	0.0042	0.669	0.469
Triglyceride (mmol/L)	1.64 (1.09,2.26)	1.58 (1.10,2.25)	1.64(1.16,2.30)	−0.0029	0.0108	0.793	0.580
HDL-C (mmol/L)	1.22 (1.00,1.44)	1.24 (1.06,1.41)	1.29(1.10,1.46)	0.0113	0.0045	**0.013**	**0.001**
LDL-C (mmol/L)	3.24(2.62,3.81)	3.18 (2.63,3.80)	3.20 (2.71,3.79)	0.0022	0.0059	0.707	0.550
HOMA-IR	1.89 (1.26,2.46)	1.67 (1.12,2.40)	1.59 (1.12,2.24)	−0.0245	0.0145	*0.091*	*0.089*
HOMA-B	123.31 (75.64,181.55)	104.67 (72.25,156.83)	95.79 (74.31,147.13)	−0.0344	0.0157	**0.028**	**0.025**
Gutt-ISI	635.63(490.54,793.14)	584.37(487.26,741.31)	602.96(473.75,750.12)	−0.0079	0.0079	0.317	0.238

Data are shown as mean±SD or median (interquartile range).
BMI, body mass index; HDL-C, high-density lipoprotein cholesterol; LDL-C, low-density lipoprotein cholesterol; HOMA-IR, homeostasis assessment model of insulin resistance; HOMA-B, homeostasis assessment model of β-cell function; Gutt-ISI, insulin sensitivity index proposed by Gutt.
p values <0.05 are shown in bold, *p* values <0.1 are shown in italics.
*Adjusted for age, gender and BMI.

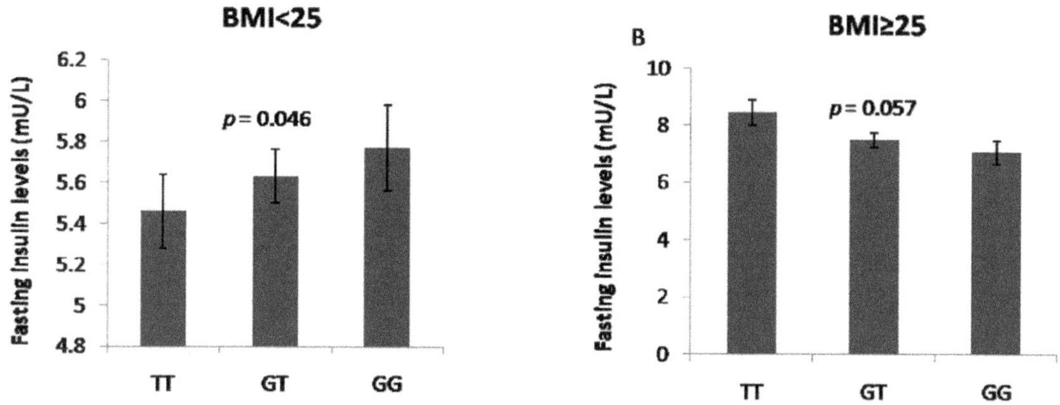

Figure 2. Association between the SNP rs16835198 and fasting insulin levels in BMI-specific controls, under the additive genetic model. The p value for interaction between rs16835198-BMI on fasting insulin was 0.003. A. Normal weight controls (BMI <25). B. Overweight/obesity controls (BMI ≥25).

gender and BMI as potential confounders. Both BMI-pooled analysis and BMI-specific analysis were conducted. All statistical analyses were performed using SAS for Windows (version 8.0; SAS Institute, Cary, NC, USA). The interaction analysis was accounted using PLINK (version 1.05). A two tailed p-value of 0.05 was considered statistically significant.

Quanto was used to calculate the statistical power [26]. Based on the assumption that the population risk was 9.6%, and a two-side α of 0.05, for SNPs in our sample with a minor allele frequency over 0.2, we had over 80% power to detect the minimum OR of 1.13 under the additive model.

Results

All the three SNPs were in Hardy-Weinberg equilibrium in the control population ($p>0.05$). Linkage disequilibrium analysis for these SNPs was shown in Figure 1. One haplotype block was constructed in this region. Single SNP association analysis failed to detect a significant association between any of the three SNP and type 2 diabetes, with a minimum p value of 0.265 for rs3480. Similarly, logistic regression analysis found no association between any SNP and type 2 diabetes (Table 2). To determine the effect of these SNPs on clinical characteristics in the control participants, we next performed genotype-phenotype analyses using an additive genetic model. As shown in the Supporting Information (Table S1 in File S1), none of the SNPs were significantly associated with quantitative traits related to glucose and lipid metabolism in the control population.

To examine the effects of *FNDC5* SNPs on glycolipid metabolism parameters in subjects with different BMI, we then analyzed the distribution of these SNPs in two BMI-based subgroups of individuals with normal glucose regulation, namely, overweight/obese or normal weight. In the normal weight subgroup (BMI <25 Kg/m^2), rs16835198 major allele G was significantly associated with a 0.0178 mU/L increment in fasting insulin levels for each additional allele copy ($p = 0.046$). Moreover, after adjustment for confounding variables, this SNP exhibited trends towards association with HOMA-IR ($p = 0.057$) and serum LDL-C levels ($p = 0.083$) in the same subgroup (Table 3). However, opposite association was observed in overweight/obese subgroup (BMI ≥25 Kg/m^2) subgroup, with each additional copy of major allele (G) exhibiting lower values than TT homozygotes ($p = 0.057$ for fasting insulin, $p = 0.091$ for HOMA-IR, respectively). Moreover, rs16835198 was also significantly associated with HDL-C and HOMA-β cell function levels in the overweight/obese subgroup both before ($p = 0.013$, 0.028, respectively) and after ($p = 0.001$, 0.025, respectively) adjusting for these covariates (Table 4). Finally, we noted a conflict between the SNP rs16835198 and fasting insulin levels in the different subgroups (Figure 2). When we tested the SNP-BMI interaction in participants with normal glucose regulation, a significant interaction between rs16835198-BMI and fasting insulin levels was observed ($p = 0.003$). Results regarding the association between the other two SNPs and clinical traits in BMI-specific subgroups are shown in Supporting Information (Table S2 and S3 in File S1).

Discussion

In the present study, three tagging SNPs in the region of the *FNDC5* gene, which encodes the myokine irisin, were tested for their association with type 2 diabetes and related quantitative traits in a Chinese Han population. We found that the effect of the common SNP rs16835198 on fasting insulin was significantly modified by BMI.

Irisin was originally characterized as a regulator of brown-fat-like development in specific depots of white adipose tissue, whose overexpression in mice resulted in increased energy expenditure, improved glucose tolerance, and modest but significant weight loss [8]. Irisin has since been linked to a variety of disorders, including obesity, anorexia nervosa, insulin sensitivity, nonalcoholic fatty liver disease and chronic kidney disease [27–30]. Despite these reports, to the best of our knowledge, the relationship between variants of *FNDC5* and the risk of type 2 diabetes and related clinical parameters in the Chinese population has not been previously evaluated. Here, we found that rs16835198 was significantly associated with the levels of fasting insulin in normal weight subjects without diabetes, and that the presence of the major allele G had an insulin-desensitizing effect on these individuals. Nevertheless, an opposite trend towards association of rs16835198 with fasting insulin and HOMA-IR levels was observed in overweight/obese controls. That is to say, the association of fasting insulin levels with this SNP in specific BMI-defined subgroups indicates that BMI contributes to the effect of this SNP on glycolipid metabolism. Moreover, we also detected that with each additional copy of the major allele G of rs16835198, HOMA-β cell function levels decreased significantly in overweight/obese controls, which means this SNP also influence β cell function in this part of subjects. However, so far, there is no unambiguous functional study focus on whether BMI modified the association between variants within *FNDC5* and glycolipid metabolism. The exact mechanisms underlying the results should be worthy for further investigation.

In contrast, a previous study in Southern German Caucasians indicated that the effect of SNPs rs16835198 and rs726344 on insulin sensitivity and resistance was not BMI-dependent [14]. However, rs726344 was excluded from our study, due to its extremely low minor allele frequency (MAF = 0), as estimated from the HapMap Chinese database. Additionally, we also observed that rs3480 had a trend towards association with HDL and LDL levels in the overweight/obesity participants (Table S3 in File S1), rather than fasting insulin values, which is not consistent with the latest study performed in Japan [15]. These results reiterate the relationship of genetic architecture with ethnicity, and further highlight the importance of perform genetic analyses in multiple populations with distinct genetic backgrounds.

The present study has some limitations. Firstly, we didn't detect the circulating irisin levels in our samples, which may enhance the conclusion and make the article more interesting. Secondly, as our patients with diabetes were not newly diagnosed and were treated with anti-diabetic drugs and/or insulin, we cannot perform the association between the SNPs in *FNDC5* and clinical parameters in patients. Thirdly, due to lacking of functional study, the inner mechanism is still unclear. Therefore, it is imperative to extend studies of the influence of *FNDC5* variants on type 2 diabetes and metabolic traits in other Chinese populations.

Conclusion

Our data suggest that the contribution of the common *FNDC5* SNP rs16835198 to fasting insulin is significantly modified by BMI. Further investigations with larger East Asian origin populations are necessary to confirm and further characterize our observations.

Supporting Information

File S1 Table S1, association between SNPs in *FNDC5* and clinical characteristics in the normal glucose tolerant group. **Table S2,** Association analyses of the rs3480 and rs1570569 genotypes with clinical characteristics in normal weight controls. **Table S3,** Association analyses of the rs3480 and rs1570569 genotypes with clinical characteristics in overweight and obese individuals.

Author Contributions

Conceived and designed the experiments: CH WJ. Performed the experiments: ST. Analyzed the data: ST. Contributed reagents/materials/analysis tools: RZ FJ JW YB. Contributed to the writing of the manuscript: ST. Participated in samples collection: MC DP JY.

References

1. Yang W, Lu J, Weng J, Jia W, Ji L, et al. (2010) Prevalence of diabetes among men and women in China. N Engl J Med 362: 1090–101.
2. Tuomilehto J, Lindstrom J, Eriksson JG, Valle TT, Hamalainen H, et al. (2001) Prevention of type 2 diabetes mellitus by changes in lifestyle among subjects with impaired glucose tolerance. N Engl J Med 344: 1343–50.
3. Thompson D, Karpe F, Lafontan M, Frayn K (2012) Physical activity and exercise in the regulation of human adipose tissue physiology. Physiol Rev 92: 157–91.
4. Roque FR, Hernanz R, Salaices M, Briones AM (2013) Exercise training and cardiometabolic diseases: focus on the vascular system. Curr Hypertens Rep 15: 204–14.
5. Pedersen BK, Febbraio MA (2012) Muscles, exercise and obesity: skeletal muscle as a secretory organ. Nat Rev Endocrinol 8: 457–65.
6. Pedersen BK (2009) The diseasome of physical inactivity-and the role of myokines in muscle-fat cross talk. J Physiol 587: 5559–68.
7. Handschin C, Choi CS, Chin S, Kim S, Kawamori D, et al. (2007) Abnormal glucose homeostasis in skeletal muscle-specific PGC-1alpha knockout mice reveals skeletal muscle-pancreatic beta cell crosstalk. J Clin Invest 117: 3463–74.
8. Bostrom P, Wu J, Jedrychowski MP, Korde A, Ye L, et al. (2012) A PGC1-alpha-dependent myokine that drives brown-fat-like development of white fat and thermogenesis. Nature 481: 463–8.
9. Teufel A, Malik N, Mukhopadhyay M, Westphal H (2002) Frcp1 and Frcp2, two novel fibronectin type III repeat containing genes. Gene 297: 79–83.
10. Ferrer-Martinez A, Ruiz-Lozano P, Chien KR (2002) Mouse PeP: a novel peroxisomal protein linked to myoblast differentiation and development. Dev Dyn 224: 154–67.
11. Huh JY, Panagiotou G, Mougios V, Brinkoetter M, Vamvini MT, et al. (2012) FNDC5 and irisin in humans: I. Predictors of circulating concentrations in serum and plasma and II. mRNA expression and circulating concentrations in response to weight loss and exercise. Metabolism 61: 1725–38.
12. Polyzos SA, Kountouras J, Shields K, Mantzoros CS (2013) Irisin: a renaissance in metabolism? Metabolism 62: 1037–44.
13. Lee P, Linderman JD, Smith S, Brychta RJ, Wang J, et al. (2014) Irisin and FGF21 Are Cold-Induced Endocrine Activators of Brown Fat Function in Humans. Cell Metab 19: 302–9.
14. Staiger H, Bohm A, Scheler M, Berti L, Machann J, et al. (2013) Common genetic variation in the human FNDC5 locus, encoding the novel muscle-derived browning' factor irisin, determines insulin sensitivity. PLoS One 8: e61903.
15. Tanisawa K, Taniguchi H, Sun X, Ito T, Cao ZB, et al. (2014) Common single nucleotide polymorphisms in the FNDC5 gene are associated with glucose metabolism but do not affect serum irisin levels in Japanese men with low fitness levels. Metabolism 63: 574–83.
16. Hu C, Zhang R, Wang C, Yu W, Lu J, et al. (2010) Effects of GCK, GCKR, G6PC2 and MTNR1B variants on glucose metabolism and insulin secretion. PLoS One 5: e11761.
17. Hu C, Wang C, Zhang R, Ng MC, Bao Y, et al. (2010) Association of genetic variants of NOS1AP with type 2 diabetes in a Chinese population. Diabetologia 53: 290–8.
18. Hu C, Zhang R, Wang C, Wang J, Ma X, et al. (2010) Variants from GIPR, TCF7L2, DGKB, MADD, CRY2, GLIS3, PROX1, SLC30A8 and IGF1 are associated with glucose metabolism in the Chinese. PLoS One 5: e15542.
19. Alberti KG, Zimmet PZ (1998) Definition, diagnosis and classification of diabetes mellitus and its complications. Part 1: diagnosis and classification of diabetes mellitus provisional report of a WHO consultation. Diabet Med 15: 539–53.
20. (2000) Obesity: preventing and managing the global epidemic. Report of a WHO consultation. World Health Organ Tech Rep Ser 894: i–xii, 1–253.
21. Jia WP, Pang C, Chen L, Bao YQ, Lu JX, et al. (2007) Epidemiological characteristics of diabetes mellitus and impaired glucose regulation in a Chinese adult population: the Shanghai Diabetes Studies, a cross-sectional 3-year follow-up study in Shanghai urban communities. Diabetologia 50: 286–92.
22. Jiang S, Fang Q, Yu W, Zhang R, Hu C, et al. (2012) Genetic variations in APPL2 are associated with overweight and obesity in a Chinese population with normal glucose tolerance. BMC Med Genet 13: 22.
23. Matthews DR, Hosker JP, Rudenski AS, Naylor BA, Treacher DF, et al. (1985) Homeostasis model assessment: insulin resistance and beta-cell function from fasting plasma glucose and insulin concentrations in man. Diabetologia 28: 412–9.
24. Gutt M, Davis CL, Spitzer SB, Llabre MM, Kumar M, et al. (2000) Validation of the insulin sensitivity index (ISI(0,120)): comparison with other measures. Diabetes Res Clin Pract 47: 177–84.
25. Purcell S, Neale B, Todd-Brown K, Thomas L, Ferreira MA, et al. (2007) PLINK: a tool set for whole-genome association and population-based linkage analyses. Am J Hum Genet 81: 559–75.
26. Gauderman WJ (2002) Sample size requirements for matched case-control studies of gene-environment interaction. Stat Med 21: 35–50.
27. Stengel A, Hofmann T, Goebel-Stengel M, Elbelt U, Kobelt P, et al. (2013) Circulating levels of irisin in patients with anorexia nervosa and different stages of obesity-correlation with body mass index. Peptides 39: 125–30.
28. Liu JJ, Wong MD, Toy WC, Tan CS, Liu S, et al. (2013) Lower circulating irisin is associated with type 2 diabetes mellitus. J Diabetes Complications 27: 365–9.
29. Polyzos SA, Kountouras J, Anastasilakis AD, Geladari EV, Mantzoros CS (2014) Irisin in patients with nonalcoholic fatty liver disease. Metabolism 63: 207–17.
30. Wen MS, Wang CY, Lin SL, Hung KC (2013) Decrease in irisin in patients with chronic kidney disease. PLoS One 8: e64025.

Fluid Overload, Pulse Wave Velocity, and Ratio of Brachial Pre-Ejection Period to Ejection Time in Diabetic and Non-Diabetic Chronic Kidney Disease

Yi-Chun Tsai[1,2,4], Yi-Wen Chiu[2,4], Hung-Tien Kuo[2,4], Szu-Chia Chen[4,5], Shang-Jyh Hwang[1,2,4,6], Tzu-Hui Chen[3], Mei-Chuan Kuo[1,2,4]*, Hung-Chun Chen[2,4]

1 Graduate Institute of Clinical Medicine, Kaohsiung Medical University, Kaohsiung, Taiwan, **2** Division of Nephrology, Kaohsiung Medical University Hospital, Kaohsiung, Taiwan, **3** Department of Nursing, Kaohsiung Medical University Hospital, Kaohsiung, Taiwan, **4** Faculty of Renal Care, Kaohsiung Medical University, Kaohsiung, Taiwan, **5** Department of Internal Medicine, Kaohsiung Municipal Hsiao-Kang Hospital, Kaohsiung, Taiwan, **6** Institute of Population Sciences, National Health Research Institutes, Miaoli, Taiwan

Abstract

Fluid overload is one of the characteristics in chronic kidney disease (CKD). Changes in extracellular fluid volume are associated with progression of diabetic nephropathy. Not only diabetes but also fluid overload is associated with cardiovascular risk factors The aim of the study was to assess the interaction between fluid overload, diabetes, and cardiovascular risk factors, including arterial stiffness and left ventricular function in 480 patients with stages 4–5 CKD. Fluid status was determined by bioimpedance spectroscopy method, Body Composition Monitor. Brachial-ankle pulse wave velocity (baPWV), as a good parameter of arterial stiffness, and brachial pre-ejection period (bPEP)/brachial ejection time (bET), correlated with impaired left ventricular function were measured by ankle-brachial index (ABI)-form device. Of all patients, 207 (43.9%) were diabetic and 240 (50%) had fluid overload. For non-diabetic CKD, fluid overload was associated with being female ($\beta = -2.87$, $P = 0.003$), heart disease ($\beta = 2.69$, $P = 0.04$), high baPWV ($\beta = 0.27$, $P = 0.04$), low hemoglobin ($\beta = -1.10$, $P < 0.001$), and low serum albumin ($\beta = -5.21$, $P < 0.001$) in multivariate analysis. For diabetic CKD, fluid overload was associated with diuretics use ($\beta = 3.69$, $P = 0.003$), high mean arterial pressure ($\beta = 0.14$, $P = 0.01$), low bPEP/ET ($\beta = -0.19$, $P = 0.03$), low hemoglobin ($\beta = -1.55$, $P = 0.001$), and low serum albumin ($\beta = -9.46$, $P < 0.001$). In conclusion, baPWV is associated with fluid overload in non-diabetic CKD and bPEP/bET is associated with fluid overload in diabetic CKD. Early and accurate assessment of these associated cardiovascular risk factors may improve the effects of entire care in late CKD.

Editor: Giuseppe Remuzzi, Mario Negri Institute for Pharmacological Research and Azienda Ospedaliera Ospedali Riuniti di Bergamo, Italy

Funding: Dr. Tsai's research was supported by the Kaohsiung Medical University Faculty of Renal Care and a grant from the Kaohsiung Medical University Research Foundation (KMU-Q103011). The author(s) received no specific funding for this work. The funders had no role in study design, data collection and analysis, decision to publish, or preparation of the manuscript.

Competing Interests: The authors have declared that no competing interests exist.

* Email: mechku@cc.kmu.edu.tw

Introduction

Cardiovascular disease (CVD) is the major cause of morbidity and mortality in patients with chronic kidney disease (CKD). The presentation of fluid overload is often noticed in patients with CKD, and excess fluid status induces elevated arterial pressure, left ventricular hypertrophy, and associated cardiovascular sequelae [1,2]. Hung et al. indicated a significant association of fluid overload with cardiovascular risk factors, such as diabetes, systolic blood pressure, and arterial stiffness in CKD patients not on dialysis [3]. Previous studies reported that fluid overload was a predictor of cardiovascular mortality in patients on dialysis [4–7]. Fluid overload is not only a characteristic but also a clinical indicator of cardiovascular burden.

On the other hand, diabetic CKD patients have a greater risk of commencing dialysis, and higher all-cause and cardiovascular mortality than non-diabetic CKD patients [8]. This is probably the result that more advanced atherosclerotic change of vascular or cardiac level in diabetic CKD or vascular disease in non-diabetic CKD is not necessarily atherosclerotic. Additionally, diabetics are more likely to have fluid overload than non-diabetics [9], and progression of diabetic nephropathy would contribute to the increase in extracellular fluid volume [10]. An interaction between fluid overload, diabetes, and vascular injury or cardiac dysfunction might exist in CKD. Accumulating evidence shows that pulse wave velocity (PWV), which can be easily measured by a clinical device, the ankle-brachial index (ABI)-form, has been regarded as a clinical indicator of arterial stiffness [11,12]. Cardiac dysfunction is frequently evaluated by echocardiography; however, its application in predicting cardiovascular events is limited because echocardiography is time-consuming and operator-dependent [13]. The ratio of brachial pre-ejection period (bPEP) and brachial ejection time (bET), measured easily by ABI device, was reported to have a significant correlation with impaired left ventricular systolic function [14]. Chen et al. found that bPEP/bET was an independent predictor for all-cause and cardiovascular mortality in CKD patients on or not on dialysis [13,15]. Hence, the aim of this study is to evaluate the relationship between fluid overload, diabetes, and baPWV or bPEP/bET and whether baPWV or bPEP/bET could be used as simple clinically available measures for risk stratification in late CKD.

Materials and Methods

Study Participants

All 612 of CKD stages 4–5 patients were invited to participate in the study from January 2011 to December 2011 at one hospital in Southern Taiwan. The study protocol was approved by the Institutional Review Board of the Kaohsiung Medical University Hospital. All patients had been enrolled in our integrated CKD program for more than 3 months (30.9±27.0 months). CKD was staged according to K/DOQI definitions and the estimated glomerular filtration rate (eGFR) was calculated using the equation of the 4-variable Modification of Diet in Renal Disease (MDRD) Study (CKD stage 3, eGFR: 30~59 ml/min/1.73 m^2; CKD stage 4, eGFR: 15~29 ml/min/1.73 m^2; CKD stage 5, eGFR<15 ml/min/1.73 m^2) [16]. Of all patients, we excluded 115 with disabilities, 12 with impaired skin integrity, and 5 with pacemaker implantation. Four hundred and eighty patients were enrolled and scheduled for a study interview after informed consent.

Ethics Statement

The study protocol was approved by the Institutional Review Board of the Kaohsiung Medical University Hospital (KMUH-IRB-990125). Informed consents were obtained in written form from patients and all clinical investigations were conducted according to the principles expressed in the Declaration of Helsinki. The patients gave consent for the publication of the clinical details.

Measurement of fluid status

Fluid status was measured once by a bioimpedance spectroscopy method, Body Composition Monitor (BCM, Fresenius Medical Care) at enrollment. BCM has been validated extensively against all available gold-standard methods in the general and dialysis populations [17–20]. The information of normohydrated lean tissue, normohydrated adipose tissue, and extracellular fluid overload in whole body based on the difference of impedance in each tissue is provided by BCM. Fluid overload can be calculated from the difference between the normal expected and measured extracellular water (ECW) [21]. Fluid overload value, ECW, intracellular water (ICW) and total body water (TBW) were determined from the measured impedance data based on the model of Moissl et al [22,23]. The relative hydration status (ΔHS = fluid overload/ECW) has been used as an indicator of fluid status in a previous study [5]. In the present study, "Fluid overload" was defined as ΔHS of 7% or more corresponding to the value of 90th percentile for the normal reference population when the fluid status was measured with the same technology [3,22,23].

Assessment of baPWV, bPEP, and bET

Brachial-ankle pulse wave velocity (baPWV), as a good parameter of arterial stiffness, was measured by the ABI-form device, which automatically and simultaneously measured blood pressures in both arms and ankles using an oscillometric method [11,12], at the same time of fluid measurement for each patient. For measuring PWV, pulse waves obtained from the brachial and tibial arteries were recorded simultaneously, and the transmission time (ΔTba), which was defined as the time interval between the initial increase in brachial and ankle waveforms, was determined. The transmission distance from the brachium to ankle was calculated according to body height. The path length from the suprasternal notch to the brachium(Lb) was obtained using the following equation: Lb = 0.2195×height of the patient (in cm)–2.0734. The path length from the suprasternal notch to the ankle(La) was obtained using the following equation: La = (0.8129×height of the patient [in cm]+12.328). Finally, the following equation was used to automatically obtain baPWV: baPWV = (La–Lb)/ΔTba [24]. After obtaining bilateral PWV values, the higher one was used as representative for each subject. Additionally, bPEP, and bET was also measured by the ABI-form device.

The bET was automatically measured from the foot to the dicrotic notch (equivalent to the incisura on the downstroke of the aortic pressure wave contour produced by the closure of aortic valve) of the pulse volume waveform. The total electromechanical systolic interval (QS2) was measured from the onset of the QRS complex on the electrocardiogram to the first high-frequency vibration of the aortic component of the second heart sound on the phonocardiogram. The bPEP was also automatically calculated by subtracting the bET from the QS2 [13,15,25].

Data Collection

Demographic and clinical data of patients were obtained from interviews and medical records at enrollment. Blood and urine samples were obtained at the same time of fluid status measurement. Patients were asked to fast for at least 12 hours before blood sample collection for the biochemistry study. Protein in urine was measured using an immediate semiquantitative urine protein dipstick test and graded as negative, trace, 1+, 2+, 3+, or 4+. The body mass index was calculated as the ratio of weight in kilograms divided by square of height in meters. Blood pressure was recorded as the mean of two consecutive measurements with 5-minute intervals, using one single calibrated device. Mean arterial pressure was calculated as 2/3 diastolic blood pressure plus 1/3 systolic blood pressure. Diabetes was defined as those with a medical history through chart review. Cardiovascular disease was defined as a history of heart failure, acute or chronic ischemic heart disease, and myocardial infarction. Information regarding patient's medications including diuretics, HMG-CoA reductase inhibitors (statins), anti-hypertensive drugs, including calcium channel blocker, β-blocker, and angiotensin converting enzyme inhibitor, and angiotensin II receptor blocker within 3 months before enrollment was obtained from medical records.

Statistical Analysis

The study population was further classified into two groups according to the presence or absence of diabetes. Continuous variables were expressed as mean ± SD or median (25th, 75th percentile), as appropriate, and categorical variables were expressed as percentages. Skewed distribution continuous variables were log-transformed to attain normal distribution. The significance of differences in continuous variables between groups was tested using independent t-test or the Mann-Whitney U analysis, as appropriate. The difference in the distribution of categorical variables was tested using the Chi-square test. Linear regression models were utilized to evaluate the determinants of fluid overload in diabetes and non-diabetes. All the variables in Table 1 tested by univariate analysis and those variables with P-value less than 0.05 were selected in multivariate analysis. Statistical analyses were conducted using SPSS 18.0 for Windows (SPSS Inc., Chicago, Illinois) and some graphs were made by GraphPad Prism 5.0 (GraphPad Software Inc., San Diego CA,

Table 1. The clinical characteristics of study subjects stratified by Diabetes Mellitus.

	Entire Cohort (n = 480)	Non-diabetes (n = 269)	Diabetes (n = 211)	P-value
Demographic variables				
Age, year	65.4±12.7	65.6±13.9	65.0±10.9	0.57
Sex (male), %	54.6	50.9	59.2	0.07
Smoke, %	20.4	16.0	26.1	0.002
Alcohol, %	9.8	9.8	8.5	0.49
Cardiovascular disease, %	18.5	14.1	24.2	0.01
Hypertension, %	84.8	75.8	96.2	<0.001
Hyperlipidemia, %	52.7	42.0	66.4	<0.001
CKD stage 4, %	49.2	49.1	49.3	0.96
5	50.8	50.9	50.7	
Body Mass Index, kg/m^2	24.4±3.8	23.4±3.2	25.6±4.1	<0.001
Mean arterial pressure, mmHg	96.9±11.9	95.4±11.6	98.8±12.0	0.002
baPWV (cm/s)	1863.7±393.1	1782.6±365.1	1963.7±403.2	<0.001
bPEP/bET	0.4±0.1	0.4±0.1	0.3±0.1	0.01
Body Composition				
Lean tissue Index (kg/m^2)	13.7±2.6	13.7±2.6	13.8±2.7	0.56
Fat tissue Index (kg/m^2)	9.9±4.2	9.2±3.8	10.7±4.5	<0.001
Total body water (L)	32.6±6.6	31.7±6.0	34.1±7.2	<0.001
Intracellular water (L)	17.1±3.6	16.9±3.6	17.4±3.7	0.12
Extracellular water (L)	15.6±3.5	14.8±2.9	16.7±4.1	<0.001
ECW/ICW	0.9±0.1	0.9±0.1	1.0±0.2	<0.001
ECW/TBW (%)	47.7±3.5	46.9±3.2	48.9±3.5	<0.001
OH (L)	1.0(2)	0.9(1)	1.7(3)	<0.001
Relative hydration status[a] (%)	50	41.2	61.1	<0.001
Medications				
Diuretics, %	29.4	16.0	46.4	<0.001
Statin, %	31.0	23.4	40.8	<0.001
Hypertension medication, %	79.6	69.5	92.4	<0.001
Laboratory parameters				
eGFR, ml/min/1.73 m^2	15.3±7.5	15.3±7.6	15.4±7.5	0.89
Hemoglobin, g/dl	10.4±1.7	10.4±1.8	10.5±1.7	0.53
Albumin, g/dl	4.0±0.5	4.1±0.4	3.9±0.5	<0.001
Calcium-Phosphate product, mg^2/dl^2	38.5(34.2,44.0)	38.3(33.6,43.3)	39.2(34.8,45.4)	0.09
Uric acid, mg/dl	7.7±1.7	7.4±1.7	8.0±1.7	<0.001
Cholesterol, mg/dl	180(153,210)	179(153,210)	181(153,209)	0.91
Triglyceride, mg/dl	116(80,166)	104(75,151)	136(90,191)	<0.001
C-reactive protein, mg/L	1.3(0.6,3.6)	1.2(0.6,3.2)	1.8(0.7,4.4)	0.05
Urine protein[b] >1+, %	49.8	36.8	67.0	<0.001

Notes: Data are expressed as number (percentage) for categorical variables and mean ± SD or median (25th, 75th percentile) for continuous variables, as appropriate. Abbreviations: CKD, chronic kidney disease; baPWV, brachial-ankle pulse wave velocity; bPEP/bET, brachial prolonged pre-ejection period/brachial shorted ejection time; ECW, extracellular water; ICW, intracellular water; TBW, total body water; ACEI, angiotensin converting enzyme inhibitors; ARB, angiotensin II receptor blockers; eGFR, estimated glomerular filtration rate.

[a]Relative hydration status (△HS) was defined as OH/extracellular water.

[b]Urine protein was measured using dipstick test.

USA). Statistical significance was set at a two-sided p-value of less than 0.05.

Results

Characteristics of Entire Cohort

The comparison of clinical characteristics between groups based on the presence or absence of diabetes is shown in Table 1. A total of 211 (44.0%) had diabetes. The mean age was 65.4±12.7 years.

The median of OH (overhydration) value was 1.0 L. Diabetic patients had higher prevalence of cardiovascular disease (24.2%), hypertension (96.2%), and hyperlipidemia (66.4%) than non-diabetes. Diabetic patients had higher body mass index (25.6±4.1 kg/m^2), mean arterial pressure (98.8±12.0 mmHg), fat tissue index (10.7±4.5 kg/m^2), TBW (34.1±7.2 L), ECW (16.7±4.1 L), ECW/TBW (48.9±3.5%), and OH (1.7 L) than non-diabetic patients. Diabetic patients with fluid overload received more diuretics, statin, and anti-hypertension treatment. Higher baPWV, and lower bPEP/bET were found in diabetic patients than non-diabetic patients. Uric acid levels and the degree of proteinuria were higher and serum albumin was lower in diabetic patients than in non-diabetic patients.

Different zones can be identified in the plot of mean arterial pressure (Y-axis) versus relative hydration status (ΔHS) (X-axis), of normovolemic and normotensive patients (40.9%, zone A), fluid-overloaded and hypertensive patients (14.0%, zone B), fluid-overloaded but normo- or hypotensive patients (36.0%, zone C), hypertensive and normovolemic patients (9.1%, zone D), in Figure 1. Figure 1A shows a substantial scatter of baPWV quartiles, and the proportion of baPWV quartile 4 was the highest in zone B (36.4%) than other zones (P<0.001). Figure 1B shows that the proportion of diabetes was higher in zone B (59.7%) and C (51.7%) than other zones (P<0.001). There was no significant difference of gender distribution among zones (Figure 1C).

Determinants of fluid overload (relative hydration status, ΔHS) in non-diabetic CKD

Figure 2 shows a positive association of baPWV and fluid overload in non-diabetic CKD (r = 0.488, P<0.001). The determinants of fluid overload in non-diabetic patients are reported in Table 2. ΔHS correlated positively with age, heart disease, diuretics use, anti-hypertension drug use, baPWV, and urine protein, but negatively with the male gender, body mass index, eGFR, serum albumin, cholesterol, and hemoglobin levels in univariate linear regression analysis. Further multivariate analysis showed that increased ΔHS was associated with being female (β = –2.87, P = 0.003), heart disease (β = 2.69, P = 0.04), high baPWV (β = 0.27, P = 0.04), low hemoglobin (β = –1.10, P< 0.001), and low serum albumin (β = –5.21, P<0.001).

Determinants of fluid overload (relative hydration status, ΔHS) in diabetic CKD

Figure 3 shows a negative association of bPEP/bET and fluid overload in diabetic CKD (r = –0.251, P = 0.01). The determinants of fluid overload in diabetic patients are reported in Table 3. ΔHS correlated positively with diuretics use, anti-hypertensive drug use, mean arterial pressure, and urine protein, but negatively with age, male, body mass index, bPEP/bET, eGFR, serum albumin, and hemoglobin levels in univariate linear regression analysis. Further multivariate analysis showed that increased ΔHS was associated with diuretics use (β = 3.69, P = 0.003), high mean arterial pressure (β = 0.14, P = 0.01), low bPEP/bET (β = –0.19, P = 0.03), low hemoglobin (β = –1.55, P = 0.001), and low serum albumin (β = –9.46, P<0.001).

Discussion

The aim of this study was to evaluate the relationship between fluid overload, diabetes and baPWV or bPEP/bET in patients with stages 4–5 CKD. Fluid overload was associated with baPWV, a clinical indicator of arterial stiffness, in non-diabetic CKD. Conversely, instead of baPWV, fluid overload was associated with

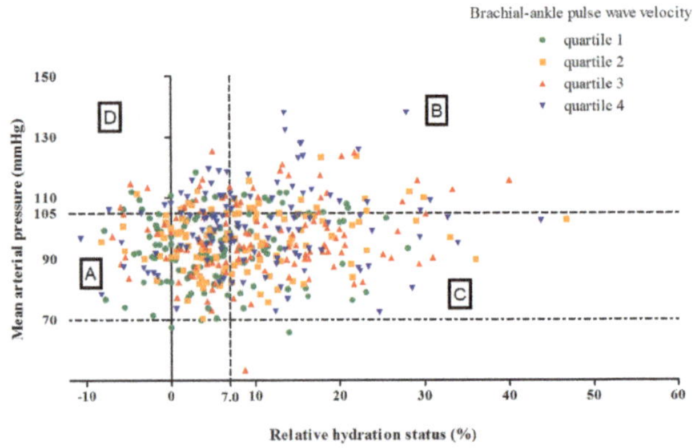

Figure 1B

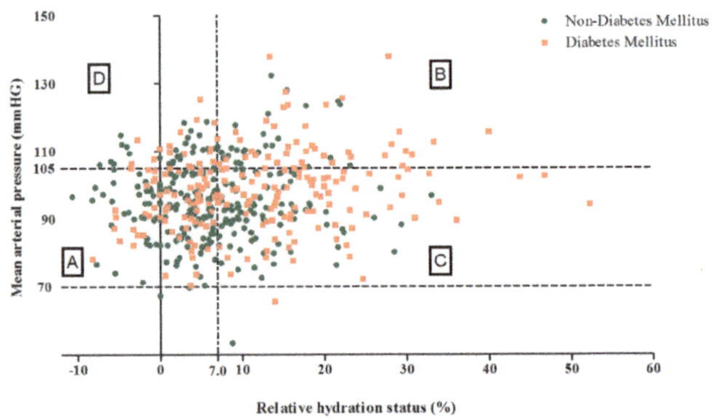

Figure 1C

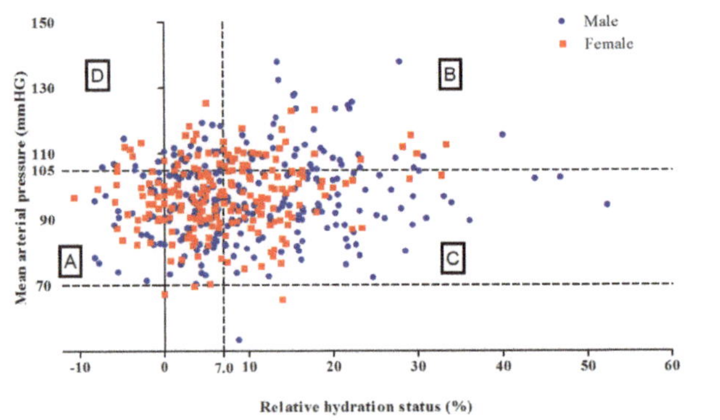

Figure 1. Scatter plot of brachial-ankle pulse wave velocity (1A), diabetes (1B), and gender (1C) between relative hydration status (%) in the X-axis and mean arterial pressure (mmHg) in the Y-axis in all study subjects.

bPEP/bET, a marker of left ventricular systolic function, in diabetic CKD.

Fluid overload may have an influence on vasculature and lead to vascular remodeling, characterized by dilatation of muscular and elastic type arteries and increased wall thickness, thereby inducing arterial stiffness and consequent cardiovascular sequelae [26]. Previous reports demonstrated that baPWV was associated with fluid overload in CKD [3,27]. On the other hand, diabetes has profound effects on vasculature, and baPWV appears to be associated with clinical variants of diabetes and microvascular and macrovascular complications [28–30]. There might be an interaction between fluid overload, baPWV, and diabetes. In the

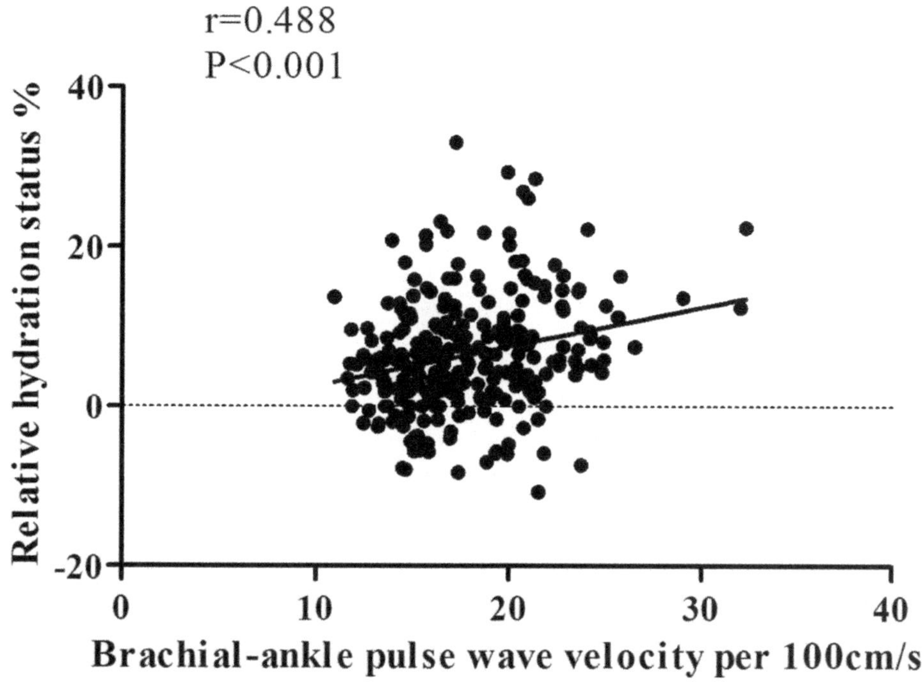

Figure 2. Relative hydration status was positively correlated with ratio of pulse wave velocity in non-diabetic chronic kidney disease.

Table 2. The determinants of relative hydration status in non-diabetic chronic kidney disease patients.

	Univariate		Multivariate	
	β (95%CI)	P-value	β (95%CI)	P-value
Clinical characteristics				
Age, year	0.12(0.06,0.18)	<0.001	0.01(−0.07,0.09)	0.7
Sex (male), %	−2.24(−3.97,−0.52)	0.01	−2.87(−4.76,−0.98)	0.003
Heart disease, %	4.43(1.99,6.86)	<0.001	2.69(0.13,5.25)	0.04
Diuretics, %	4.26(1.94,6.58)	<0.001	1.63(−0.69,3.96)	0.1
Anti-Hypertension drug, %	1.96(0.07,3.85)	0.04	0.64(−1.20,2.49)	0.5
Bady mass index, kg/m^2	−0.29(−0.56,−0.02)	0.03	−0.19(−0.46,0.08)	0.2
Mean arterial pressure, mmHg	0.02(−0.05,0.10)	0.5	–	–
baPWV, per100 cm/s	0.49(0.25,0.72)	<0.001	0.27(0.01,0.54)	0.04
bPEP/bET, ×100	0.05(−0.09,0.19)	0.48	–	–
Laboratory parameters				
eGFR, ml/min/1.73 m^2	−0.15(−0.26,−0.03)	0.01	−0.07(−0.21,0.07)	0.3
Hemoglobin, g/dl	−1.17(−1.65,−0.69)	<0.001	−1.10(−1.66,−0.53)	<0.001
Albumin, g/dl	−8.49(−10.63,−6.35)	<0.001	−5.21(−7.74,−2.68)	<0.001
Log Calcium-phosphate product, mg^2/dl^2	0.96(−9.27,11.20)	0.8	–	–
Uric acid, mg/dl	0.53(−0.01,1.06)	0.05	–	–
Log Cholesterol, mg/dl	−13.24(−22.34,4.14)	0.005	−3.32(−12.38,5.75)	0.4
C-reactive protein, mg/L	0.06(−0.02,0.14)	0.1	–	–
Urine protein >1+, %	1.004(1.001,1.007)	0.023	1.28(−0.64,3.20)	0.2

Abbreviations: baPWV, brachial-ankle pulse wave velocity; bPEP/bET, brachial prolonged pre-ejection period/brachial shorted ejection time; eGFR, estimated glomerular filtration rate.

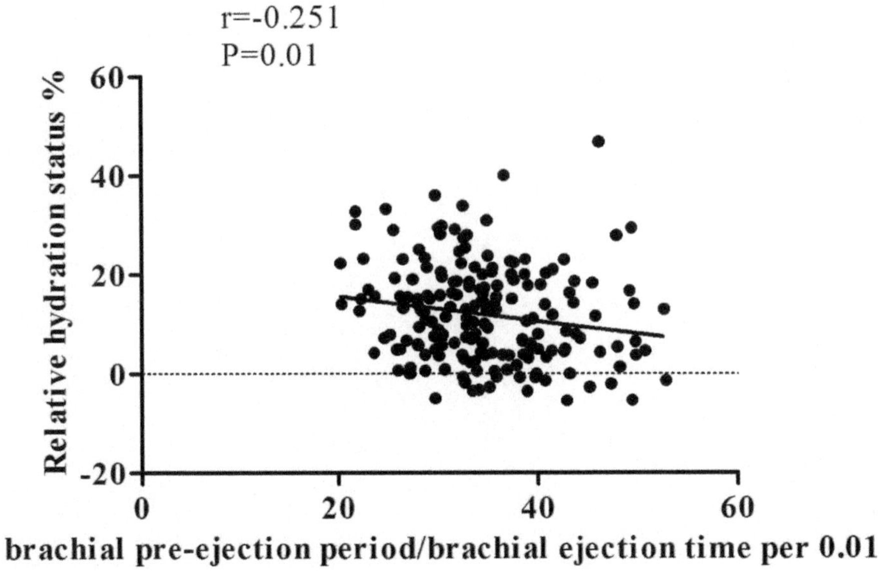

Figure 3. Relative hydration status was negatively correlated with ratio of brachial pre-ejection period to ejection time in diabetic chronic kidney disease.

present study, a positive correlation between fluid overload and baPWV was found in multivariate analysis of all subjects ($\beta = 0.30$, $P = 0.02$). However, there was no interaction between diabetes and baPWV in the analysis of the determinants of fluid overload. Hence, we divided all subjects into non-diabetes and diabetes groups to analyze the relationship between fluid overload and baPWV respectively and found a significant association between

Table 3. The determinants of relative hydration status in diabetic chronic kidney disease patients.

	Univariate		Multivariate	
	β (95%CI)	P-value	β (95%CI)	P-value
Clinical characteristics				
Age, year	−0.21(−0.34,−0.08)	0.001	−0.08(−0.20,0.04)	0.2
Sex (male), %	−3.26(−6.13,−0.40)	0.02	−2.06(−4.62,0.48)	0.1
Heart disease, %	0.42(−2.91,3.75)	0.8	–	–
Diuretics, %	4.45(1.66,7.24)	0.002	3.69(1.23,6.14)	0.003
Hypertension medication, %	5.98(0.66,11.30)	0.03	1.94(−2.43,6.32)	0.3
Body mass index, kg/m^2	−0.46(−0.81,−0.12)	0.009	−0.01(−0.32,0.31)	0.9
Mean arterial pressure, mmHg	0.16(0.05,0.28)	0.006	0.14(0.03,0.24)	0.01
baPWV, per100 cm/s	0.23(−0.12,0.57)	0.2	–	–
bPEP/bET, ×100	−0.25(−0.45,−0.05)	0.01	−0.19(−0.37,−0.02)	0.03
Laboratory parameters				
eGFR, ml/min/1.73 m^2	−0.24(−0.42,−0.05)	0.01	0.09(−0.10,0.27)	0.4
Hemoglobin, g/dl	−1.88(−2.68,−1.07)	<0.001	−1.55(−2.41,−0.68)	0.001
Albumin, g/dl	−12.88(−15.38,−10.37)	<0.001	−9.46(−12.21,−6.71)	<0.001
Log Calcium-phosphate product, mg^2/dl^2	0.08(−17.99,18.16)	0.9	–	–
Uric acid, mg/dl	0.28(−0.61,1.17)	0.5	–	–
Log Cholesterol, mg/dl	−9.73(−22.86,3.40)	0.1	–	–
C-reactive protein, mg/L	0.02(−0.23,0.27)	0.8	–	–
Urine protein >1+, %	1.004(1.001,1.007)	0.023	1.59(−1.35,4.53)	0.2

Abbreviations: baPWV, brachial-ankle pulse wave velocity; bPEP/bET, brachial prolonged pre-ejection period/brachial shorted ejection time; eGFR, estimated glomerular filtration rate.

fluid overload and baPWV in non-diabetic CKD, not in diabetic CKD.

Interestingly, instead of baPWV, low bPEP/bET, which has a significant correlation with impaired left ventricular ejection fraction [14], is correlated with fluid overload in diabetic CKD patients. This study also used the echocardiographic examination to evaluate cardiac function in 184 subjects and found that left ventricular ejection fraction was significantly correlated with fluid overload in diabetic CKD ($\beta = -0.21$, $P = 0.002$), not in non-diabetic CKD ($\beta = -0.02$, $P = 0.4$). These findings suggest that fluid overload may have different levels of influences on CKD patients depending on the presence or absence of diabetes. Fluid overload is correlated with vascular level alterations in non-diabetic CKD, and with cardiac level modifications in diabetic CKD.

Cardiovascular dysfunction progresses with arterial-cardiac interactions [31]. The arterial-cardiac compensatory adaptations maintain cardiac performance with enhanced contractility [32]. Fluid overload alters and blunts the arterial-cardiac response, leading to hemodynamic instability [32]. The difference of rates of progression of dysfunction between the heart and the vasculature may explain our results. Probably, the phenomenon of fluid overload directly affecting cardiac function beyond vasculature in diabetic CKD exists. Arterial stiffness may occur in early diabetic CKD and then fluid overload may subsequently have effect on left ventricular systolic dysfunction in late diabetic CKD. Further study is needed to evaluate the mechanisms between fluid overload, arterial stiffness and cardiac dysfunction in diabetic CKD.

Due to the strong association of fluid overload and adverse outcomes [27], precise measurement of fluid status is important in clinical practice of CKD patients. Traditional physical examination is not enough to detect slight variations of fluid status. Accumulating evidence suggests that multifrequency spectroscopic bioimpedance can provides information of increases in fluid status and associated body composition. Besides, using a non-invasive ABI-form device, clinicians can easily obtain the value of baPWV, a reliable marker of arterial stiffness, and bPEP/bET, a surrogate of left ventricular systolic function. These inexpensive and convenient tools might assist clinicians in assessing the risk of renal progression and cardiovascular morbidity and mortality earlier.

The present study has some limitations that must be considered. This study was conducted at a single center. Fluid status, baPWV, bPEP/bET, clinical parameters, and the use of drugs were measured only once at enrollment. The association of time-varying baPWV, bPEP/bET, clinical parameters, and the use of drugs with time-varying fluid status could not be estimated. Additionally, our findings show the relative weak correlation between bPEP/bET and fluid overload in diabetic CKD. The weak correlation between fluid overload and bPEP/bET is probably related to the relatively small sample size of diabetic patients. Based on the association of bPEP/bET with cardiac function, we performed subgroup analysis to analyze the relationship between bPEP/bET and fluid overload in the heart disease group and the result was consistent ($\beta = -0.46$, $P = 0.03$). However, there was no significant correlation between bPEP/bET and fluid overload in the non-heart disease group. We need a large population study to evaluate the interaction between bPEP/bET, cardiac function and diabetes in a CKD cohort.

In conclusion, our study evaluates a relationship between fluid overload, diabetes, and arterial stiffness or cardiac function in late CKD patients. Fluid overload is correlated with arterial stiffness in non-diabetic CKD, and with left ventricular dysfunction in diabetic CKD. Fluid overload probably has distinct arterial-cardiac influences on CKD patients in the presence or absence of diabetes. Early and accurate assessment of these associated cardiovascular risk factors may improve the effects of entire care in late CKD patients.

Acknowledgments

The authors thank the from the staff of the Statistical Analysis Laboratory, Department of Medical Research, Kaohsiung Medical University Hospital, Kaohsiung Medical University for their assistance.

Author Contributions

Conceived and designed the experiments: YCT MCK. Performed the experiments: YCT THC. Analyzed the data: YCT YWC. Contributed reagents/materials/analysis tools: YWC HTK SCC SJH HCC. Contributed to the writing of the manuscript: YCT MCK.

References

1. Wizemann V, Schilling M (1995) Dilemma of assessing volume state–the use and the limitations of a clinical score. Nephrol Dial Transplant 10: 2114–2117.
2. Wizemann V, Leibinger A, Mueller K, Nilson A (1995) Influence of hydration state on plasma volume changes during ultrafiltration. Artif Organs 19: 416–419.
3. Hung SC, Kuo KL, Peng CH, Wu CH, Lien YC, et al. (2014) Volume overload correlates with cardiovascular risk factors in patients with chronic kidney disease. Kidney Int 85: 703–9.
4. Saran R, Bragg-Gresham JL, Levin NW, Twardowski ZJ, Wizemann V, et al. (2006) Longer treatment time and slower ultrafiltration in hemodialysis: associations with reduced mortality in the DOPPS. Kidney Int 69: 1222–1228.
5. Wizemann V, Wabel P, Chamney P, Zaluska W, Moissl U, et al. (2009) The mortality risk of overhydration in haemodialysis patients. Nephrol Dial Transplant 24: 1574–1579.
6. Paniagua R, Ventura MD, Avila-Diaz M, Hinojosa-Heredia H, Mendez-Duran A, et al. (2010) NT-proBNP, fluid volume overload and dialysis modality are independent predictors of mortality in ESRD patients. Nephrol Dial Transplant 25: 551–557.
7. Movilli E, Gaggia P, Zubani R, Camerini C, Vizzardi V, et al. (2007) Association between high ultrafiltration rates and mortality in uraemic patients on regular haemodialysis. A 5-year prospective observational multicentre study. Nephrol Dial Transplant 22: 3547–3552.
8. Fox CS, Matsushita K, Woodward M, Bilo HJ, Chalmers J, et al. (2012) Chronic Kidney Disease Prognosis Consortium: Associations of kidney disease measures with mortality and end-stage renal disease in individuals with and without diabetes: a meta-analysis. Lancet 380: 1662–1673.
9. Tsai YC, Tsai JC, Chiu YW, Kuo HT, Chen SC, et al. (2013) Is fluid overload more important than diabetes in renal progression in late chronic kidney disease? PLoS One 8: e82566.
10. Tucker BJ, Collins RC, Ziegler MG, Blantz RC(1991) Disassociation between glomerular hyperfiltration and extracellular volume in diabetic rats. Kidney Int 39: 1176–1183.
11. Yokoyama H, Shoji T, Kimoto E, Shinohara K, Tanaka S, et al. (2003) Pulse wave velocity in lower-limb arteries among diabetic patients with peripheral arterial disease. J Atheroscler Thromb 10: 253–258.
12. Yamashina A, Tomiyama H, Takeda K, Tsuda H, Arai T, et al. (2002) Validity, reproducibility, and clinical significance of noninvasive brachial-ankle pulse wave velocity measurement. Hypertens Res 25: 359–364.
13. Chen SC, Chang JM, Tsai JC, Lin TH, Hsu PC, et al. (2010) A systolic parameter defined as the ratio of brachial pre-ejection period to brachial ejection time predicts cardiovascular events in patients with chronic kidney disease. Circ J 74: 2206–2210.
14. Su HM, Lin TH, Lee CS, Lee HC, Chu CY, et al. (2009) Myocardial performance index derived from brachial-ankle pulse wave velocity: A novel and feasible parameter in evaluation of cardiac performance. Am J Hypertens 22: 871–876.
15. Chen SC, Chang JM, Tsai JC, Hsu PC, Lin TH, et al. (2010) A new systolic parameter defined as the ratio of brachial pre-ejection period to brachial ejection time predicts overall and cardiovascular mortality in hemodialysis patients. Hypertens Res 33: 492–498.
16. Levey AS, Bosch JP, Lewis JB, Greene T, Rogers N, et al. (1999) A more accurate.

17. Wabel P, Chamney P, Moissl U, Jirka T (2009) Importance of whole-body bioimpedance spectroscopy for the management of fluid balance. Blood Purif 27: 75–80.
18. Crepaldi C, Soni S, Chionh CY, Wabel P, Cruz DN, et al. (2009) Application of body composition monitoring to peritoneal dialysis patients. Contrib Nephrol 163: 1–6.
19. Wizemann V, Rode C, Wabel P (2008) Whole-body spectroscopy (BCM) in the.
20. Moissl UM, Wabel P, Chamney PW, Bosaeus I, Levin NW, et al. (2006) Body fluid volume determination via body composition spectroscopy in health and disease. Physiol Meas 27: 921–933.
21. Hur E, Usta M, Toz H, Asci G, Wabel P, et al. (2013) Effect of fluid management guided by bioimpedance spectroscopy on cardiovascular parameters in hemodialysis patients: a randomized controlled trial. Am J Kidney Dis 61: 957–965.
22. Wieskotten S, Heinke S, Wabel P, Moissl U, Becker J, et al. (2008) Bioimpedance-based identification of malnutrition using fuzzy logic. Physiol Meas 29: 639–654.
23. Van Biesen W, Williams JD, Covic AC, Fan S, Claes K, et al. (2011) Fluid status in peritoneal dialysis patients: the European Body Composition Monitoring (EuroBCM) study cohort. PLoS One. 6: e17148.
24. Chen SC, Chang JM, Liu WC, Huang JC, Chen YY, et al. (2012) Decrease in ankle-brachial index over time and cardiovascular outcomes in patients with hemodialysis. Am J Med Sci 344: 457–461.
25. Chen SC, Chang JM, Liu WC, Tsai JC, Chen LI, et al. (2011) Significant correlation between ratio of brachial pre-ejection period to ejection time and left ventricular ejection fraction and mass index in patients with chronic kidney disease. Nephrol Dial Transplant 26: 1895–1902.
26. Zheng D, Cheng LT, Zhuang Z, Gu Y, Tang LJ, et al. (2009) Correlation between.
27. Tsai YC, Tsai JC, Chen SC, Chiu YW, Hwang SJ, et al. (2014) Association of Fluid Overload With Kidney Disease Progression in Advanced CKD: A Prospective Cohort Study. Am J Kidney Dis 63: 68–75.
28. Kimoto E, Shoji T, Shinohara K, Inaba M, Okuno Y, et al. (2003) Preferential stiffening of central over peripheral arteries in type 2 diabetes. Diabetes 52: 448–52.
29. Tsuchikura S, Shoji T, Kimoto E, Shinohara K, Hatsuda S, et al. (2010) Central versus peripheral arterial stiffness in association with coronary, cerebral and peripheral arterial disease. Atherosclerosis 211: 480–5.
30. Kim WJ, Park CY, Park SE, Rhee EJ, Lee WY, et al. (2012) The association between regional arterial stiffness and diabetic retinopathy in type 2 diabetes. Atherosclerosis 225: 237–241.
31. Moody WE, Edwards NC, Chue CD, Ferro CJ, Townend JN (2013) Arterial disease in chronic kidney disease. Heart 99: 365–372.
32. Chen CH, Nakayama M, Nevo E, Fetics BJ, Maughan WL, et al. (1998) Coupled systolic-ventricular and vascular stiffening with age: implications for pressure regulation and cardiac reserve in the elderly. J Am Coll Cardiol 32: 1221–7.

6

Inhibition of Kidney Proximal Tubular Glucose Reabsorption Does Not Prevent against Diabetic Nephropathy in Type 1 Diabetic eNOS Knockout Mice

Muralikrishna Gangadharan Komala, Simon Gross, Harshini Mudaliar, Chunling Huang, Katherine Pegg, Amanda Mather, Sylvie Shen, Carol A. Pollock, Usha Panchapakesan*

Renal Research Lab, Kolling Institute of Medical Research, Sydney University, Royal North Shore Hospital, St Leonards, Australia

Abstract

Background and Objective: Sodium glucose cotransporter 2 (SGLT2) is the main luminal glucose transporter in the kidney. SGLT2 inhibition results in glycosuria and improved glycaemic control. Drugs inhibiting this transporter have recently been approved for clinical use and have been suggested to have potential renoprotective benefits by limiting glycotoxicity in the proximal tubule. We aimed to determine the renoprotective benefits of empagliflozin, an SGLT2 inhibitor, independent of its glucose lowering effect.

Research Design and Methods: We induced diabetes using a low dose streptozotocin protocol in 7–8 week old endothelial nitric oxide (eNOS) synthase knockout mice. We measured fasting blood glucose on a monthly basis, terminal urinary albumin/creatinine ratio. Renal histology was assessed for inflammatory and fibrotic changes. Renal cortical mRNA transcription of inflammatory and profibrotic cytokines, glucose transporters and protein expression of SGLT2 and GLUT1 were determined. Outcomes were compared to diabetic animals receiving the angiotensin receptor blocker telmisartan (current best practice).

Results: Diabetic mice had high matched blood glucose levels. Empagliflozin did not attenuate diabetes-induced albuminuria, unlike telmisartan. Empagliflozin did not improve glomerulosclerosis, tubular atrophy, tubulointerstitial inflammation or fibrosis, while telmisartan attenuated these. Empagliflozin did not modify tubular toll-like receptor-2 expression in diabetic mice. Empagliflozin did not reduce the upregulation of macrophage chemoattractant protein-1 (MCP-1), transforming growth factor β1 and fibronectin mRNA observed in the diabetic animals, while telmisartan decreased transcription of MCP-1 and fibronectin. Empagliflozin increased GLUT1 mRNA expression and telmisartan increased SGLT2 mRNA expression in comparison to untreated diabetic mice. However no significant difference was found in protein expression of GLUT1 or SGLT2 among the different groups.

Conclusion: Hence SGLT2 inhibition does not have renoprotective benefits independent of glucose lowering.

Editor: Nick Ashton, The University of Manchester, United Kingdom

Funding: The study was funded by a Research Grant from the National Health and Medical Research Council, Australia (APP1004926, https://www.nhmrc.gov.au). MGK received Research Entry Scholarship from the Jacquot Foundation through the Royal Australasian College of Physicians. The study drug empagliflozin and telmisartan was supplied by Boehringer Ingelheim, Germany, and they partially funded the project. The funders had no role in study design, data collection and analysis, decision to publish, or preparation of the manuscript.

Competing Interests: The study drug empagliflozin and telmisartan was supplied by Boehringer Ingelheim, Germany, and they partially funded the project. However, they were not involved in study design or interpretation of results.

* Email: usha.panchapakesan@sydney.edu.au

Introduction

Diabetic nephropathy is the commonest cause of chronic kidney disease worldwide [1]. Current best practice in the management of diabetic nephropathy involves tight glycaemic and blood pressure control, which includes specific blockade of the renin, angiotensin aldosterone systems [2,3]. Although treatment options for patients have expanded in recent years, this has not translated to a reduction in the incidence of diabetic nephropathy [4]. Hence there is a need for novel agents that confer renoprotection.

Sodium glucose cotransporter 2 inhibitors (SGLT2i) are novel diabetic agents that block glucose entry into the kidney proximal tubular cell (PTC), resulting in glycosuria and lowering of blood

Table 1. Physical and clinical parameters.

	Control (n = 12)	Control +empagliflozin (n = 8)	Diabetic (n = 12)	Diabetic +empagliflozin (n = 10)	Diabetic +telmisartan (n = 7)
Gain in weight (gram)	5.4±0.5	3.9±1.0	2.4±0.7**	0.8±0.6**	3.1±0.6*
Left kidney/body weight ratio (%)	0.77±0.04	0.80±0.03	0.91±0.06	0.82±0.08	0.89±0.08
Average blood sugar (mmol/L)	11.0±0.3	11.5±0.4	21.1±0.4**	22.1±0.6**	22.9±0.7**
Systolic BP (mm Hg)	120±2	128±4	117±2	122±6	118±10
24 hour urine glucose excretion (μmol/day)	2.6±0.3	456.5±74.4	3038.0±864.8*	3551.0±35.9**	3462.0±320.4**
Mid experimental albumin/creatinine ratio (μg/mg)	133±25	197±48	987±336*	463±136	180±121
Terminal albumin/creatinine ratio (μg/mg)	224±36	290±56	1474±388*	1697±596*	80±30#

Data are mean ± standard error of mean.
* = P<0.05 vs control group,
** = P<0.001 vs control group,
# = P<0.05 vs diabetic group.

glucose levels and have the added advantage of not inducing weight gain or hypoglycaemia [5,6].

SGLTs are located on the luminal aspect of the proximal tubule (PT) and able to transport sodium and glucose from the ultrafiltrate into the cell due to a sodium concentration gradient, generated by the basolateral Na, K-ATPase pump [7]. Sodium glucose cotransporter 2 (SGLT2) is the major luminal glucose transporter located in the S1 and S2 segments of the PT, whilst sodium glucose cotransporter 1 (SGLT1) in the S3 segment contributes to less than 10% of total luminal glucose transport [8]. On the basolateral side of the cell, glucose is then passively transported via facilitative glucose transporters (GLUTs) into the vasculature. In the early segments of the kidney PT, SGLT2 on the apical membrane is coupled with GLUT2 on the basolateral side and together they reabsorb upto 90% of filtered glucose under normoglycaemic conditions [8].

Hyperglycaemia induces activation of various pathways, which stimulates the production of proinflammatory and profibrotic cytokines relevant in diabetic nephropathy including TGFβ. The effects of high glucose are predominantly mediated through the hypertrophic and profibrotic cytokine, TGFβ which is overexpressed in diabetic nephropathy [9]. There is clear evidence of the damaging effects of TGFβ on PTC growth and function [10–12]. We and others have also shown evidence for TGFβ induced activation of the innate immunity pathway in diabetic nephropathy, in particular Toll like receptor 2 (TLR2) and its endogenous ligand High Mobility Group Box 1 (HMGB1) [13,14]. We have previously defined the effects of high glucose in mediating inflammatory and profibrotic effects in the PTC [15,16] and the specific effects of increased PTC sodium transport in early diabetes [17,18]. Hence it is well established that high intracellular glucose alters intracellular metabolism and promotes inflammatory and profibrotic cytokines resulting in the development of diabetic nephropathy [12,15,19].

We have previously shown using human kidney PTC *in vitro* that empagliflozin, an SGLT2i (provided by Boehringer Ingelheim, Germany), was able to reduce high glucose induced tubular expression of inflammatory and fibrotic markers. In the short term, this occurred without a compensatory increase in SGLT1 or GLUT2 expression [20].

This provided proof of concept to extend these studies to a validated small animal model of diabetic nephropathy. An important aspect of our experimental design was to match glucose levels in all diabetic groups, so that any observed renal outcomes could be interpreted independent of the glucose lowering effect of empagliflozin, which has confounded the interpretation of previous studies to date. This was achieved by using a 5 day low dose protocol of intraperitoneal streptozotocin to induce diabetes [21] and long acting insulin in the diabetic mice to match glucose levels among all the experimental limbs.

Materials and Methods

Animal Model

Male *enos* knockout mice on a C57BL/6 background were purchased from Jackson laboratory, USA. Mice were housed singly in filter top cages in a pathogen free facility and had free access to standard chow and drinking water. Diabetes was induced by a low-dose streptozotocin (STZ) protocol. Mice received intraperitoneal injections of STZ (55 mg/kg daily for 5 days) at 7–8 weeks of age. Control mice received citrate buffer injections (pH 4.5). Blood glucose was tested using a glucometer (Accuchek Nano, Roche) two weeks after STZ through tail vein blood collection. Diabetes was defined by blood glucose greater than 16 mmol/L after a six-hour daytime fast. Mice with levels below 16 mmol/L were excluded from the study. Fasting blood glucose levels were measured monthly. Long acting insulin (Insulin Glargine, Sanofi Aventis, Australia) was initiated as required from 10 weeks of age and was administered thrice weekly if the blood sugar exceeded 28 mmol/L or if they had lost weight greater than 25% from baseline. The study was approved by the Royal North Shore Hospital Ethics Committee (protocol number 1101-003A). The Australian Code of Practice for the Care and Use of Animals for Scientific Purposes was followed in this study. Animals were anaesthetised using short inhalational anaesthesia with 2% isoflurane for minor procedures. Animals were euthanised under 2% isoflurane anaesthesia using cardiac puncture terminally.

Experimental Design

The SGLT2i empagliflozin (provided by Boehringer-Ingelheim Germany) was administered by daily oral gavage (Instech Lab,

Table 2. PCR primer sequences.

Target	Forward	Reverse	Source
MCP-1	GCCTGCTGTTCACAGTTGC	CAGGTGAGTGGGGCGTTA	Sigma
Collagen IV	TTAAAGGACTCCAGGGACCAC	CCCACTGAGCCTGTCACAC	Sigma
Fibronectin	CACGGAGGCCACCATTACT	CTTCAGGGCAATGACGTAGAT	Sigma
TGFβ	TCAGACATTCGGGAAGCAGT	ACGCCAGGAATTGTTGCTAT	Sigma
Actin	AAGGCCAAGCGTGAAAAGAT	GTGGTAGGACCAGAGGCATAC	Sigma
GLUT1	AACATGGAACCACCGCTACG	GTGGTGAGTGTGGTGGATGG	Sigma
GLUT2	ATCGCCCTCTGCTTCCAGTAC	GAACACGTAAGGCCCAAGGA	Sigma
SGLT1	Mm00451203_m1 (Applied Biosystems)		
SGLT2	Mm00453831_m1 (Applied Biosystems)		

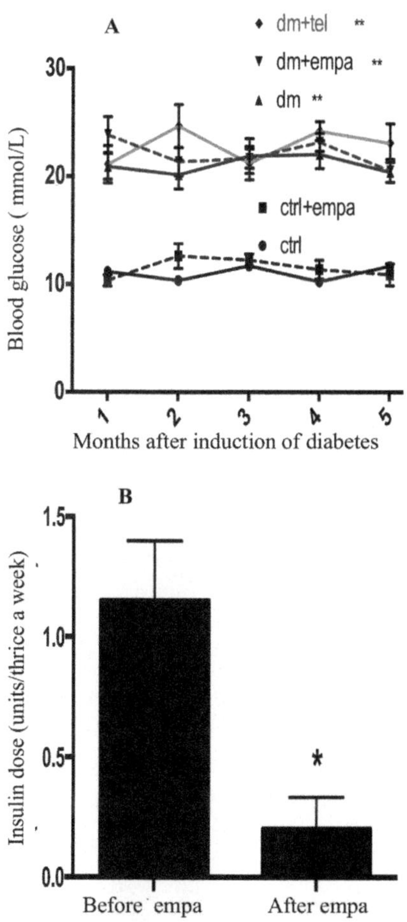

Figure 1. Blood glucose levels among diabetic mice were matched throughout the study and showed similar glucose levels among the diabetic mice at 1, 2, 3, 4 and 5 months post diabetes induction and were significantly higher than control mice (A). Empagliflozin reduced insulin requirement in diabetic mice (B). The comparison was made between average insulin requirement per dose administered thrice weekly, before and after initiation of empagliflozin. Data are expressed as mean ± SEM with * = P<0.05 and ** = P<0.001 vs ctrl.

USA) using 1% hydroxyethylcellulose (Sigma Aldrich) as a vehicle. Current best practice is renin-angiotensin-aldosterone blockade. Hence telmisartan (Boehringer-Ingelheim, Germany) at a dose of 3 mg/kg/day was administered in drinking water as a comparative limb. Empagliflozin and telmisartan were initiated at 13 weeks of age. Mice were killed at 32 weeks of age. The groups were as below.

1. Control (ctrl, n = 12)
2. Control receiving empagliflozin 10 mg/kg daily (ctrl+empa, n = 8)
3. Diabetic (dm, n = 12)
4. Diabetic receiving empagliflozin 10 mg/kg daily (dm+empa, n = 10)
5. Diabetic receiving telmisartan, 3 mg/kg in drinking water (dm+tel = 7)

Measurement of Physiological Parameters

Body weight was assessed monthly. Blood pressure was measured using a noninvasive tail vein cuff method (CODA BP apparatus, Kent Scientific, USA) preterminally (Table 1).

Urine Biochemistry

Urine was collected at three different time points (48 hour post initiation of treatment, 4–6 weeks after initiation of treatment using metabolic cages and terminally using bladder puncture). Urine creatinine was measured using a picric acid method (Creatinine Companion, Exocell Inc., USA). Urinary glucose was measured using Abbot Architect C16000 analyser. Urine albumin was measured using Elisa (Albuwel, Exocell Inc., USA).

Kidney Tissue Harvest

The unperfused left kidney was harvested and snap frozen after embedding in OCT compound. The right kidney was perfused with phosphate buffered saline (PBS) followed by 4% paraformaldehyde (PFA) and subsequently fixed in 10% neutral buffered formalin for 24–48 hours.

Histology

Formalin fixed paraffin embedded (FFPE) kidney sections were stained with Masson's Trichrome, Sirius Red and Periodic Acid Schiff. Assessment of histological change was done in a blinded manner. The Glomerulosclerotic index (GSI) was calculated based on previously described methodology [22]. Atrophic tubules were

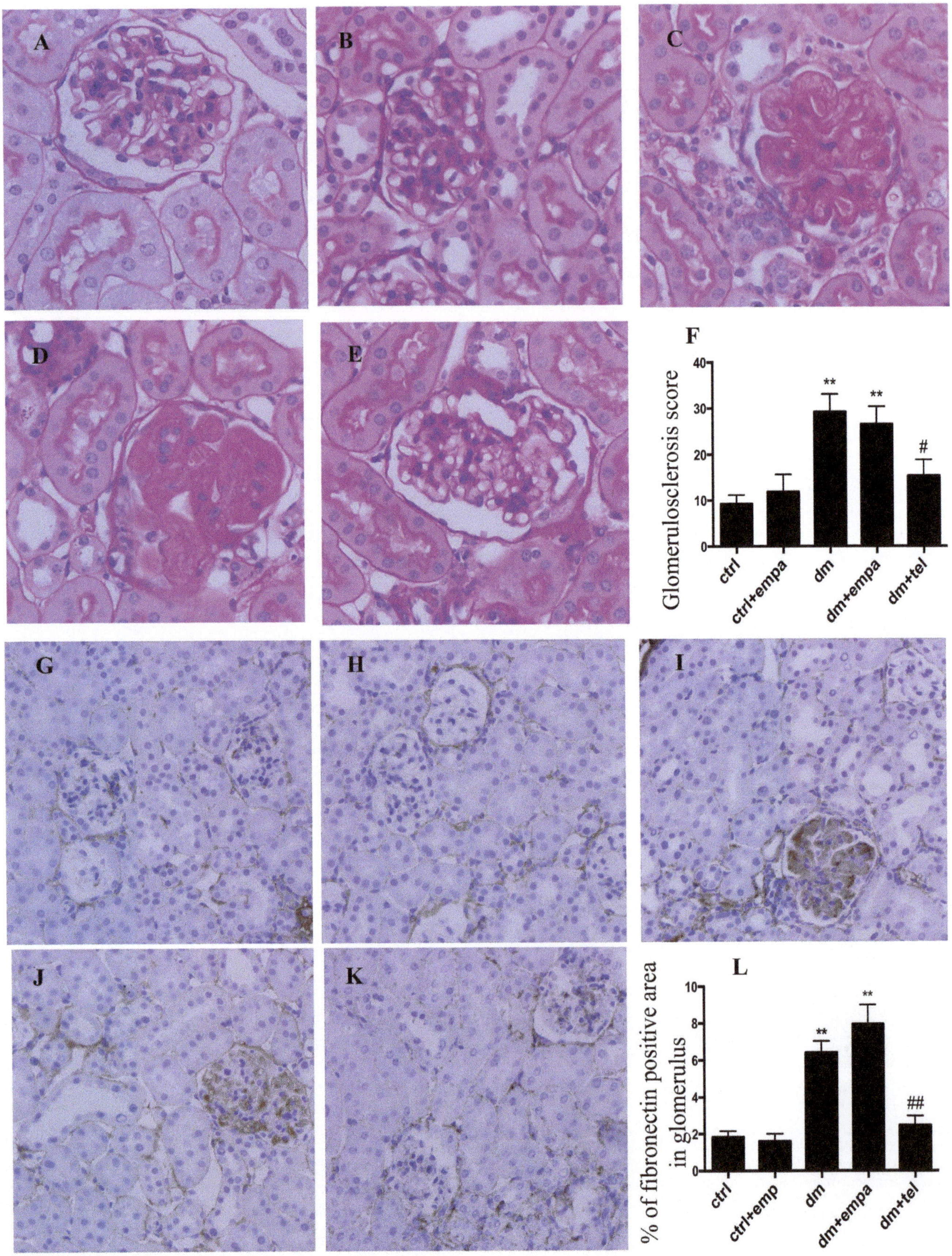
A
B
C
D
E
F
Glomerulosclerosis score
40
30
20
10
0
**
**
#
ctrl
ctrl+empa
dm
dm+empa
dm+tel
G
H
I
J
K
L
% of fibronectin positive area in glomerulus
10
8
6
4
2
0
**
**
##
ctrl
ctrl+emp
dm
dm+empa
dm+tel

Figure 2. Diabetic mice demonstrated increased glomerulosclerosis and glomerular fibronectin deposition, which was improved by telmisartan but not by empagliflozin. Representative photographs of PAS stained sections for A) ctrl, B) ctrl + empa, C) dm, D) dm + empa and E) dm + tel groups and quantification of glomerulosclerosis by glomerulosclerotic index (F). Representative photographs of immunohistochemistry for glomerular fibronectin in G) ctrl, H) ctrl + empa, I) dm, J) dm + empa and K) dm + tel groups and quantification of glomerular fibronectin by Image J (L) (Magnification = original X400). Data are expressed as mean ± SEM with ** = P<0.001 vs ctrl, # = P<0.05 vs dm and ## = P<0.001 vs dm.

defined by dilatation, epithelial shedding and thinning of epithelium. Tubular damage was scored by counting the number of atrophic tubules per 400 tubules at X 200 magnification.

Immunohistochemistry for fibronectin and TLR2 were done on 4 micron paraffin embedded sections using rabbit anti mouse fibronectin (F3468, Sigma Aldrich, USA) at a concentration of 1:2000 and rabbit anti mouse TLR2 (Imgenex, San Diego, California) at a concentration of 1:250. The chromogenic reaction was carried out with 3, 3′-diaminobenzidine chromogen (Dako, Australia) solution for 10 minutes. Immunohistochemistry for F4/80 staining was done on 10 micron frozen section slides. They were incubated with rat anti mouse F4/80 (MCA497R, ABD Serotec, USA) at a concentration of 1:100 for one hour followed by HRP tagged goat anti Rat antibody at a concentration of 1:200 (ABD Serotec, USA).

F4/80 positive cells per high power field was counted and averaged for each slide. The degree of interstitial collagen content in Masson's and Sirius red stains were assessed in a blinded manner using Image J by identifying the percentage of interstitial collagen positive region at X 200 magnification in 5 randomly selected regions. Glomerular fibronectin was quantified using Image J at X 400 magnification after selecting 10–15 glomeruli at random and quantifying the percentage of fibronectin positive area in each glomerulus.

Real Time PCR Experiments

Total RNA was extracted from kidney tissue using Trizol. cDNA was synthesised using Superscript III (Life Technologies) first strand synthesis. The cDNA was subjected to standard curve measurement to ensure efficiency prior to real time PCR, which was done using SYBR green (Life Technologies, Australia) for MCP-1, fibronectin, TGFβ, collagen IV, GLUT1 and GLUT2 using actin as the endogenous control. PCR for SGLT2 and SGLT1 were done using Taqman PCR Universal Mastermix (Applied Biosystems). The RTPCR was performed on the AB7900 machine (Applied Biosystems, Australia). Gene expression was quantified relative to actin. The primers are listed in Table 2.

Western Blot

Frozen tissue was homogenized with Quiagen Tissue Ruptur in 1.5 ml of cold 20 mM HEPES buffer, pH 7.2, containing 1 mM EGTA, 210 mM mannitol, 70 mM sucrose and centrifuged at 1.500×g for 5 min at 4°C. Samples were then analysed by SDS gel electrophoresis (Novex, Life technologies, Australia) and electroblotted to Hybond Nitrocellulose membranes (Amersham Pharmacia Biotech, Bucks, UK). Membranes were then probed with primary antibodies to GLUT1 (ab652, Abcam, Cambridge, UK), SGLT2 (sc98975, Santa Cruz, USA) and actin (Santa Cruz, USA). Proteins were visualized using Luminata Western HRP Substrate (Millipore) in a LAS 4000 image reader (GE Healthcare Life Sciences). Analysis was performed using Image J software (NIH, USA).

Statistical Analysis

Statistical analysis was done using Graph Prism 6. Data are expressed as mean ± standard error of mean. A P value <0.05 was considered statistically significant. Significance was assessed using paired t- test for analysing the difference in insulin requirement of diabetic mice before and after initiation of empagliflozin. Blood glucose profile during the study was measured using repeated measures Anova. Anova with Bonferroni's correction for multiple comparisons was used for all other statistical analysis.

Results

Diabetic Mice had Similar Fasting Glucose Levels

The blood glucose levels were measured monthly, starting two weeks after induction of diabetes and average values were calculated over the duration of the experiment for all groups. The diabetic mice displayed significantly elevated blood glucose levels at 21.4 mmol/L after induction with streptozotocin (Table 1) maintained with long acting insulin and empagliflozin treatments, while the glucose level was matched in all the diabetic limbs throughout the experiment (Figure 1A) as planned.

Empagliflozin Induced Glycosuria in Non Diabetic Mice

The control + empagliflozin group displayed nearly 200 fold increase in urinary glucose levels compared to the control mice (Table 1). The urinary glucose excretion among all diabetic mice was significantly higher than control mice (Table 1).

Empagliflozin Reduced Insulin Requirement and Accentuated Poor Weight Gain in Diabetic Mice

Comparisons were made between the thrice weekly insulin dose of diabetic mice in the diabetic + empagliflozin group, before and after initiation of empagliflozin. The insulin requirements of the diabetic mice were significantly reduced after initiation of empagliflozin (Figure 1B). All diabetic mice had poor weight gain which was pronounced in the diabetic + empagliflozin group (Table 1).

Telmisartan but Not Empagliflozin Reduced Terminal Urinary Albumin Excretion in Diabetic Mice

The terminal urinary albumin to creatinine ratio was elevated in the diabetic mice. Treatment with empagliflozin did not improve albuminuria in diabetic mice. This was significantly reduced by treatment with telmisartan in diabetic mice. In the early stages of the illness, SGLT2 inhibition shows a non significant trend towards improving albuminuria in diabetic mice, which is not maintained as the disease progresses (Table 1).

Telmisartan but not empagliflozin reduced the degree of glomerulosclerosis and glomerular fibronectin deposition in diabetic mice

The untreated diabetic mice (Figure 2C) developed significant glomerulosclerosis in comparison with control mice (Figure 2A) Treatment with empagliflozin showed no improvement in the glomerulosclerotic index in diabetic mice (Figure 2D), whereas diabetics treated with telmisartan (Figure 2E) had significantly

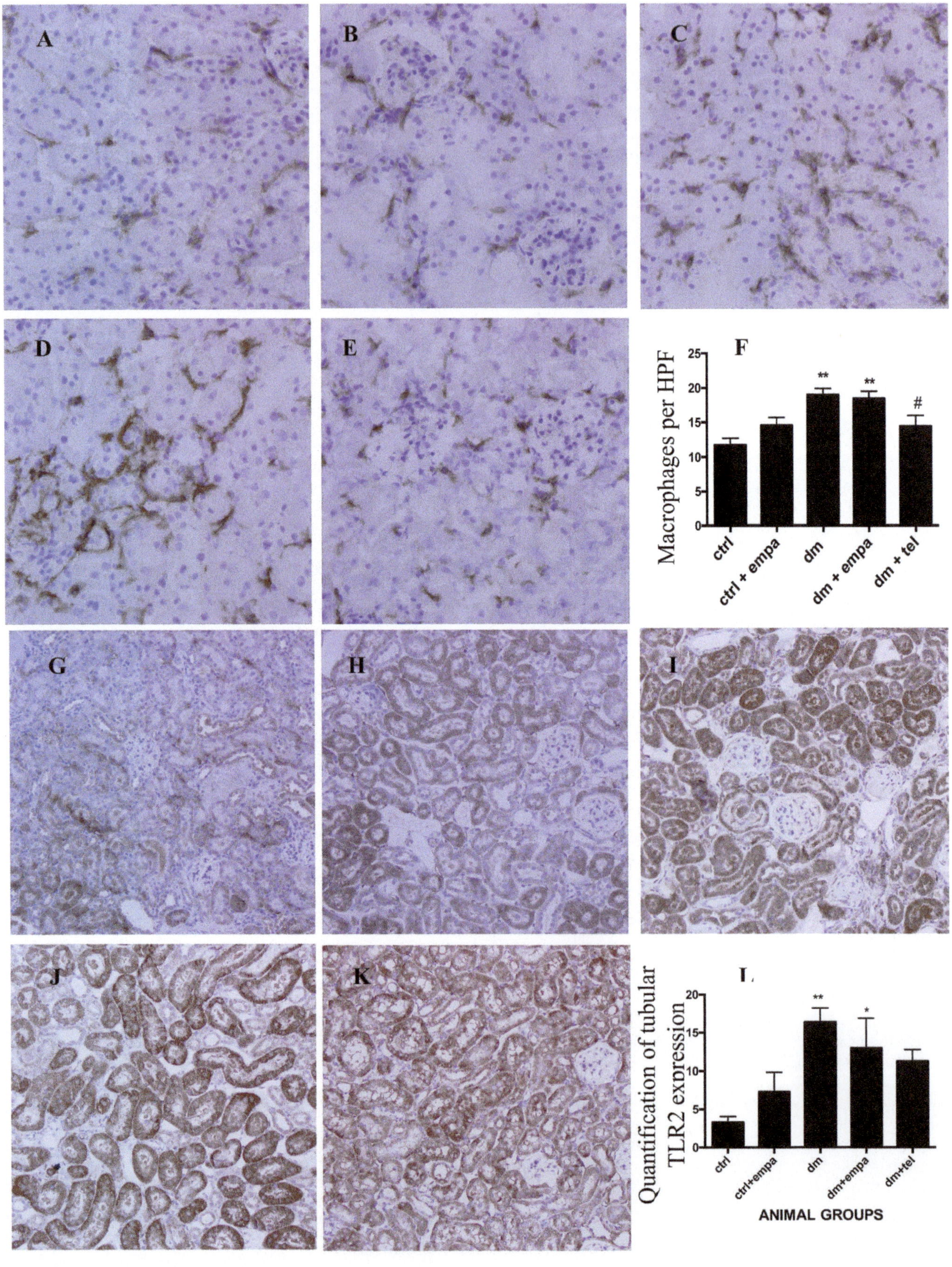
A
B
C
D
E
F
Macrophages per HPF
0
5
10
15
20
25
**
**
#
ctrl
ctrl + empa
dm
dm + empa
dm + tel
G
H
I
J
K
Quantification of tubular TLR2 expression
0
5
10
15
20
**
*
ctrl
ctrl+empa
dm
dm+empa
dm+tel
ANIMAL GROUPS

Figure 3. Diabetic animals demonstrated increased tubulointerstitial inflammation, which was not ameliorated by empagliflozin. Representative photographs of immunohistochemistry for tubulointerstitial F4/80 stain for activated macrophages in A) ctrl, B) ctrl + empa, C) dm, D) dm + empa, E) dm + tel groups (Magnification = original X 400) and quantification of F4/80 positive cells in tubulointerstitium (F) which was done by calculating the average number of F4/80 positive cells per high power field (HPF) in each group. Representative photographs of immunohistochemistry for tubular TLR2 in G) ctrl, H) ctrl + empa, I) dm, J) dm + empa, K) dm + tel groups (Magnification = original X 200) and quantification of tubular TLR2 expression by Image J (L). (Data are expressed as mean ± SEM with * = $P<0.05$ vs ctrl, ** = $P<0.001$ vs ctrl and # = $P<0.05$ vs dm).

lower glomerulosclerotic scores. The diabetic mice (Figure 2I) developed significant glomerular fibronectin deposition in comparison with control mice (Figure 2G). There was no improvement with concurrent empagliflozin therapy (Figure 2J), while telmisartan was associated with a significant reduction in glomerular fibronectin deposition in diabetic mice (Figure 2K).

Empagliflozin did not reduce tubulointerstitial inflammation in diabetic mice

The diabetic mice (Figure 3C) developed significantly increased tubulointerstitial infiltration of activated macrophages, demonstrated by F4/80 staining, compared to controls (Figure 3A). Concurrent treatment with empagliflozin did not improve this in diabetic mice (Figure 3D). However, telmisartan therapy significantly reduced macrophage infiltration in diabetic (Figure 3E). The diabetic mice also displayed increased tubular expression of TLR2 (Figure 3I). Empagliflozin did not modify the upregulation of TLR2 while telmisartan treated diabetic mice showed TLR2 expression not significantly different to that in control mice (Figure 3J and K).

Telmisartan but not empagliflozin reduced the degree of tubular atrophy and tubulointerstitial fibrosis in diabetic mice

The diabetic mice (Figure 4C) developed significant tubular atrophy in comparison with control mice (Figure 4A). Empagliflozin did not reduce tubular atrophy (Figure 4D), while temisartan treated diabetic mice showed tubular atrophy not significantly different to control mice (Figure 4E). The degree of interstitial fibrosis was assessed by Sirius Red sensitive collagen staining (Figures 4G-K) and Masson's staining (Figures 4M-Q). The diabetic mice showed a non significant trend towards increased collagen deposition with the sirius red stain. However with the masson's stain, the diabetic mice had significantly increased collagen deposition (Figure 4O), which was not improved by empagliflozin (Figure 4P). Telmisartan treated diabetic mice showed tubulointerstitial fibrosis not significantly different to that of control mice (Figure 4Q).

Empagliflozin did not improve the renal cortical transcription of inflammatory or profibrotic cytokines in diabetic mice

To determine whether empagliflozin or telmisartan modulated the cortical transcription of MCP-1, collagen IV, fibronectin and TGFβ in diabetes, we performed real time PCR from RNA derived from renal cortical tissue. The transcription of MCP-1, fibronectin and TGFβ was increased in diabetic mice and was unchanged by empagliflozin (Figure 5). Diabetic mice treated with telmisartan displayed MCP-1 (Figure 5A) and fibronectin (Figure 5D) transcription, which was not significantly different to control mice although TGFβ transcription was noted to be increased in this group (Figure 5C). No change was noted in the transcription of collagen IV between control and diabetic mice (Figure 5B).

Empagliflozin significantly increased GLUT1 transcription in diabetic mice although no difference was noted in GLUT1 protein expression

There was no difference in mRNA transcription of any glucose transporters between diabetic and non diabetic mice (Figure 6). Empagliflozin treated diabetic mice showed a significant increase in GLUT1 transcription compared to other diabetic mice (Figure 6A) and telmisartan treated diabetic mice showed increased SGLT2 transcription compared to diabetic mice (Figure 6D). However there was no difference in either SGLT2 or GLUT1 protein expression among the different groups (Figure 6E-H).

Discussion

To our knowledge this is the first study to evaluate the renoprotective effects of SGLT2 inhibition independent of glucose lowering. We used a type 1 diabetic enos knockout mouse model, validated by the Animal Models of Diabetic Complications Consortium (AMDCC) [21], with matched glycaemia across experimental groups. Although we have previously demonstrated that empagliflozin reduced high glucose induced expression of inflammatory and fibrotic markers in *in vitro* studies of human kidney PTC, our results show that it did not confer renoprotection in this *in vivo* model. This was in contrast to the renoprotection afforded by the angiotensin receptor blocker (ARB) telmisartan.

The strength of our study is based on the determination of renal parameters in a setting of matched high blood glucose levels among diabetic groups. In our study, empagliflozin caused a 200 fold increase in glycosuria in control mice compared to control mice not receiving the drug, which confirms that empagliflozin was absorbed and achieved sufficient concentration in the lumen to actively inhibit PTC SGLT2. Furthermore the diabetic mice receiving empagliflozin had less insulin requirements and less weight gain reflecting the efficacy of empagliflozin in inducing glycosuria in our model. As the effectiveness of SGLT2 inhibition is dependent on the creatinine clearance with decreased efficiency as creatinine clearance decreases we would expect the efficacy to decrease as the severity of diabetic nephropathy increases [23].

In contrast to our findings, there are recent animal studies wherein SGLT2 inhibitors have shown significant renal benefit [24,25]. There are however important differences in these studies from our current study. In the study by Nagata et al, a type 2 diabetic model was used and diabetic mice treated with the SGLT2i tofogliflozin had lower plasma glucose levels, making interpretation of renal benefit independent of glucose lowering difficult. The second study by Kojima et al utilized older (> I year old) type 2 diabetic rats with established diabetic nephropathy and showed that although matched for glucose levels the diabetic mice receiving the SGLT2i luseogliflozin had better renal outcomes than the mice receiving insulin. The mice receiving insulin had 10 fold higher plasma insulin levels. Studies have shown that insulin itself can increase TGFβ-1 gene expression by mesangial cells [26] and can promote glomerular and interstitial fibrosis [27]. Furthermore, in a recent publication, Wright et al has described

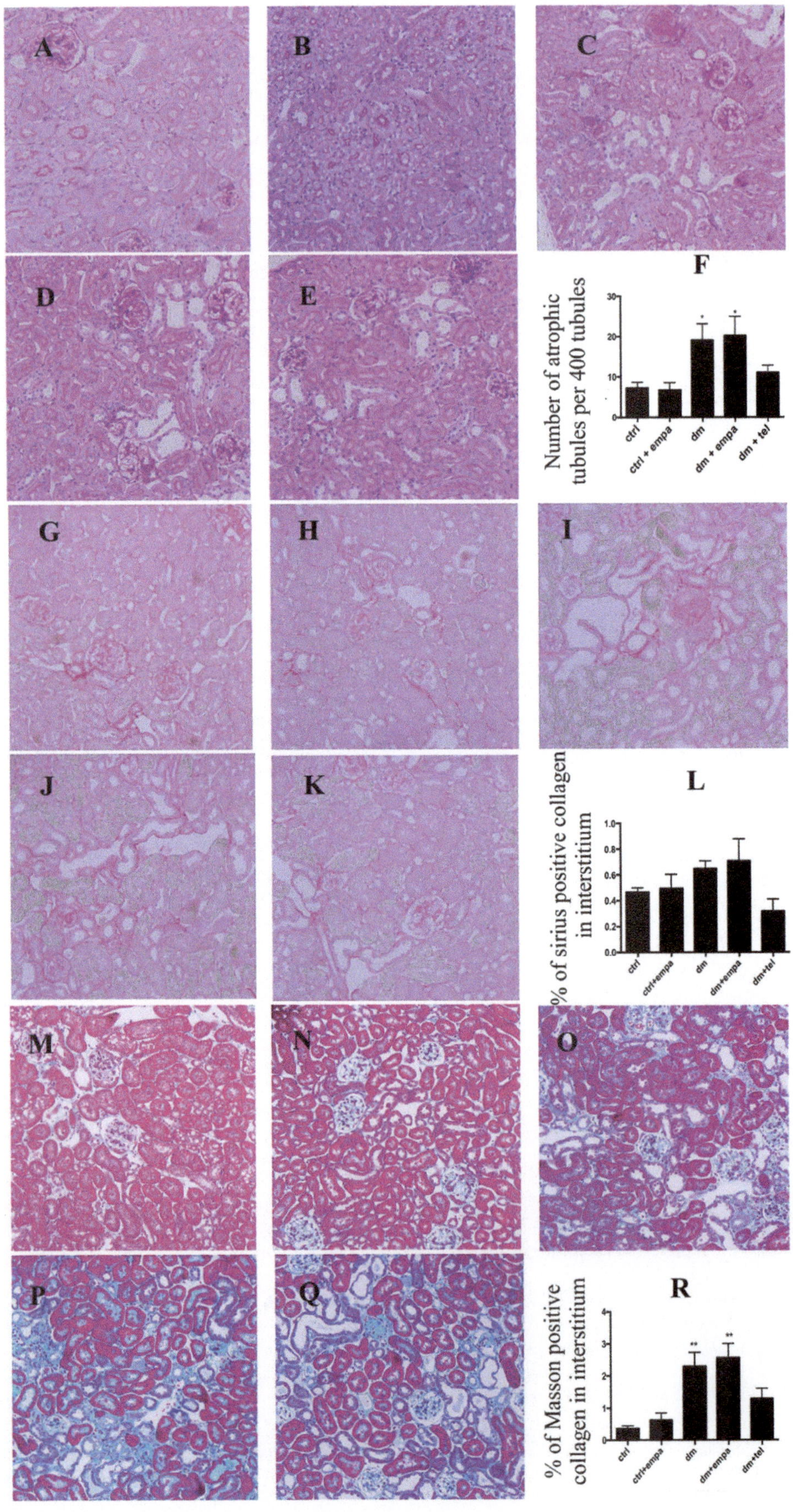
A
B
C
D
E
F
Number of atrophic tubules per 400 tubules
30
20
10
0
ctrl
ctrl + empa
dm
dm + empa
dm + tel
G
H
I
J
K
L
% of sirius positive collagen in interstitium
1.0
0.8
0.6
0.4
0.2
0.0
ctrl
ctrl+empa
dm
dm+empa
dm+tel
M
N
O
P
Q
R
% of Masson positive collagen in interstitium
4
3
2
1
0
ctrl
ctrl+empa
dm
dm+empa
dm+tel

Figure 4. Diabetic mice demonstrated tubular atrophy and tubulointerstitial fibrosis, which was not improved by empagliflozin and partially reduced by telmisartan. Representative photographs of PAS stained sections of tubulointerstitium in A) ctrl, B) ctrl + empa, C) dm, D) dm + empa, E) dm + tel groups and F) Quantification of tubular atrophy in all groups was done by counting the number of atrophic tubules per 400 tubule count (Data are expressed as mean ± SEM with * = P<0.05 vs ctrl). Representative photographs of tubulointerstitial picrosirius red stain in G) ctrl, H) ctrl + empa, I) dm, J) dm + empa, K) dm + tel groups and L) Quantification of tubulointerstitial Sirius red positive collagen content by Image J. Representative photographs of Masson's stain in M) ctrl, N) ctrl + empa, O) dm, P) dm + empa, Q) dm + tel groups and R) Quantification of Masson's positive collagen content by Image J (Magnification = original X 200). (Data are expressed as mean ± SEM with * = P<0.05 vs ctrl, ** = P<0.001 vs ctrl).

the probable role of insulin as an agonist in stimulating SGLT2 activity through activation of protein kinase A and C [28]. This would explain an increase in glucose reabsorption in type 2 diabetic mice with high insulin levels and provide an explanation for better outcomes with SGLT2 inhibition in this model. Current data available from the registration trials of SGLT2 inhibitors is limited, but suggests a stable reduction in estimated GFR than reverts to baseline after cessation of the drug. This occurs in association with a reduction in albuminuria. However, renoprotective benefits cannot be concluded from available clinical data.

Our studies are consistent with two recent studies by Vallon et al. The first study used SGLT2 knockout mice showing that although there was an improvement in glucose control and glomerular hyperfiltration, there was no improvement in kidney growth or injury [29]. An important difference between our own study and this study is that there was an improvement in blood glucose among mice treated with empagliflozin. Moreover it was noted that after 18 weeks of diabetes, no increase in TGFβ expression was observed in the renal cortex by their group. Conversely, we did demonstrate increased transcription of TGFβ

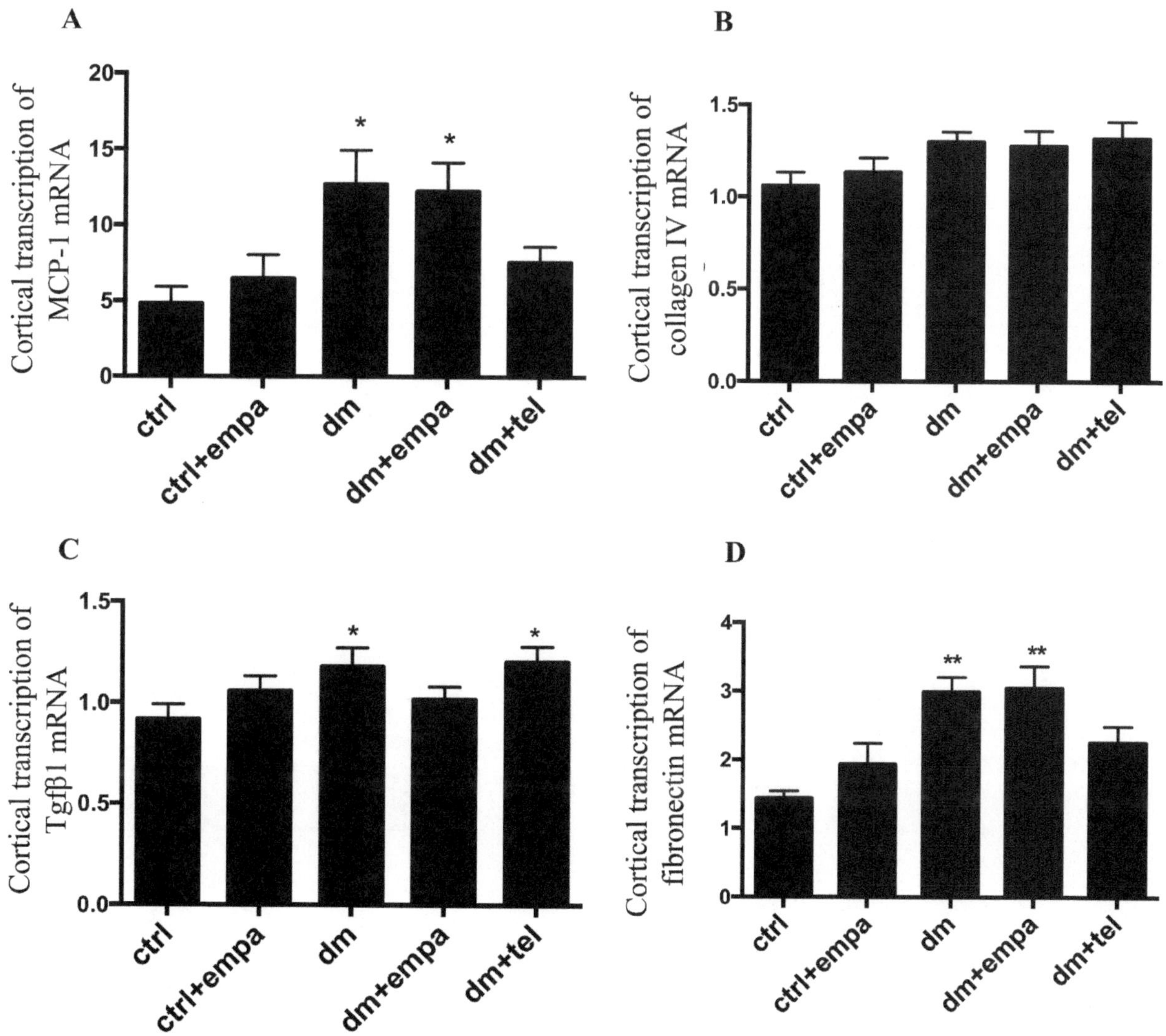

Figure 5. Diabetic mice showed increased renal cortical transcription of inflammatory and fibrotic cytokines, which was not improved by empagliflozin. Real time PCR results for Renal cortical transcription of A) MCP-1, B) Collagen 4, C) TGFβ and D) Fibronectin relative to actin (Data are expressed as mean ± SEM with * = P<0.05 vs ctrl and ** = P<0.001 vs ctrl).

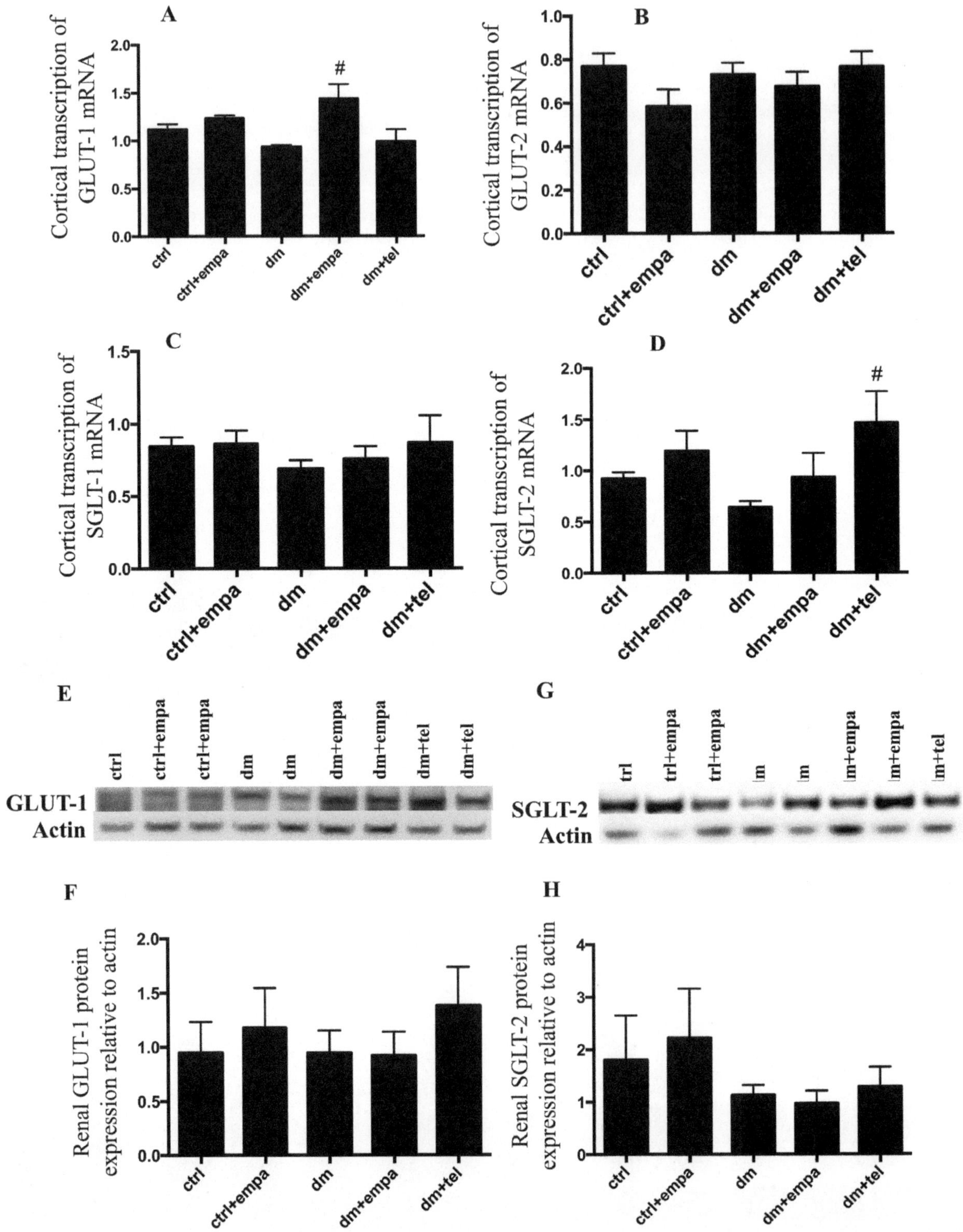

Figure 6. Empagliflozin increased renal GLUT1 transcription in comparison with untreated diabetic mice although renal protein expression of GLUT1 and SGLT2 were unchanged. Real time PCR results for A) GLUT1, B) GLUT2, C) SGLT1 and D) SGLT2 expressed relative to actin. Expression levels of renal GLUT1 protein (E and F) and SGLT2 (G and H) relative to actin (Data are expressed as mean ± SEM with # = $P<0.05$ vs dm).

in the renal cortex of diabetic animals although there was no statistically significant improvement with empagliflozin. Similar to Vallon's study, we found a statistically non significant trend towards decreased SGLT2 protein expression in diabetic mice, which may have contributed to reduced renoprotection by empagliflozin. However this cannot explain the significant diabetic changes in empagliflozin treated mice in contrast to improvement in the telmisartan group. The second study by Vallon et al in Akita mice, a type 1 model of diabetes, demonstrated that empagliflozin was effective in reducing GFR independent of blood glucose but the reduction in albuminuria, kidney growth and inflammation was thought to be the result of concomitant glucose lowering [30]. Our study in contrast was designed to evaluate renal outcome independent of glucose levels, which has been a confounding variable in all studies to date.

There are several possible reasons for our findings. Firstly, as the blood glucose levels were similarly elevated among all diabetic mice, this has resulted in glomerular injury, as SGLT2 inhibition does not prevent glucose entry into the glomerular compartment. It is known that progressive glomerular injury can cause tubulointerstitial damage through a number of different mechanisms including misdirected filtration (filtrate leakage external to the tubular lumen), obstructed filtration and proteinuria as a result of damage to the glomerular filtration barrier [31]. This then initiates a cycle of progressive tubulointerstitial injury, which is not prevented by blocking glucose entry into the PTC. Secondly, the lack of renoprotection seen in our study could be the result of incomplete inhibition of glucose reabsorption by empagliflozin. We know that SGLT2 inhibition only prevents reabsorption of 40% of glucose and this could be due to multiple reasons [32]. GLUT1 is a major glucose transporter in mesangial cells and is a facilitative transporter of glucose in the S3 segment of the basolateral aspect of the tubular cell with bidirectional transport properties [33]. It is possible that hyperglycaemia could influence the movement of glucose into the tubular cell from the basolateral aspect and is not modified by empagliflozin. This is not dependent on an increase in GLUT1 protein expression.

The diabetic mice in our model had matched high glucose levels, which is not reflective of the well controlled diabetic patient. However this was necessary in the design of the experiment to test the hypothesis whether SGLT2 inhibition can offer renoprotection independent of glucose lowering. There is evidence to suggest that SGLT2i can reduce diabetic nephropathy when glycaemic control is optimal in a Type 2 diabetic animal model and is even more pronounced when used in combination with an angiotensin receptor blocker [25]. However this could have been due to glucose lowering rather than specific SGLT2 inhibition. In summary, we have shown that although empagliflozin reduces high glucose induced inflammatory and fibrotic markers in vitro; it does not have renoprotective benefits independent of glucose lowering in vivo.

Supporting Information

Data S1 Analysis results for physical parameters, histology and PCR.

Acknowledgments

We are grateful for the support provided by Sue Smith from Histology Core Laboratory and Sergey Kurdyukov from Genomics Core Laboratory, Kolling Institute, for their technical advice, to Pacific Laboratory Medicine Services (PALMS) of the Royal North Shore Hospital, St Leonards, NSW, Australia for support with performing urine biochemistry and to the Department of Anatomical Pathology for PAS and Masson staining of kidney tissue sections

Part of the results of the study were presented in abstract form at the World Congress of Nephrology, June 2013 at Hong Kong and at the Annual Scientific Meeting of the Australian and New Zealand Society of Nephrology, September 2013 at Brisbane, Australia.

Author Contributions

Conceived and designed the experiments: MGK CP AM SS UP. Performed the experiments: MGK HM CH SG KP. Analyzed the data: MGK UP. Contributed reagents/materials/analysis tools: MGK UP CAP. Wrote the paper: MGK UP CAP.

References

1. Reutens AT, Atkins RC (2011) Epidemiology of diabetic nephropathy. Contrib Nephrol 170: 1–7.
2. Holman RR, Paul SK, Bethel MA, Matthews DR, Neil HA (2008) 10-year follow-up of intensive glucose control in type 2 diabetes. N Engl J Med 359: 1577–1589.
3. Evans M, Bain SC, Hogan S, Bilous RW, Collaborative Study Group p (2012) Irbesartan delays progression of nephropathy as measured by estimated glomerular filtration rate: post hoc analysis of the Irbesartan Diabetic Nephropathy Trial. Nephrol Dial Transplant 27: 2255–2263.
4. de Boer IH, Rue TC, Hall YN, Heagerty PJ, Weiss NS, et al. (2011) Temporal trends in the prevalence of diabetic kidney disease in the United States. JAMA 305: 2532–2539.
5. Ghosh RK, Ghosh SM, Chawla S, Jasdanwala SA (2011) SGLT2 Inhibitors: A New Emerging Therapeutic Class in the Treatment of Type 2 Diabetes Mellitus. J Clin Pharmacol 0091270011400604 [pii] 10.1177/0091270011400604 [doi].
6. Vallon V, Sharma K (2010) Sodium-glucose transport: role in diabetes mellitus and potential clinical implications. Current opinion in nephrology and hypertension 19: 425–431.
7. Mather A, Pollock C (2011) Glucose handling by the kidney. Kidney international Supplement 10.1038/ki.2010.509: S1–6.
8. Mather A, Pollock C (2010) Renal glucose transporters: novel targets for hyperglycemia management. Nature reviews Nephrology 6: 307–311.
9. Ziyadeh FN (2004) Mediators of diabetic renal disease: the case for tgf-Beta as the major mediator. J Am Soc Nephrol 15 Suppl 1: S55–57.
10. Holian J, Qi W, Kelly DJ, Zhang Y, Mreich E, et al. (2008) Role of Kruppel-like factor 6 in transforming growth factor-beta1-induced epithelial-mesenchymal transition of proximal tubule cells. American journal of physiology Renal physiology 295: F1388–1396.
11. Qi W, Twigg S, Chen X, Polhill TS, Poronnik P, et al. (2005) Integrated actions of transforming growth factor-beta1 and connective tissue growth factor in renal fibrosis. American journal of physiology Renal physiology 288: F800–809.
12. Johnson DW, Saunders HJ, Brew BK, Poronnik P, Cook DI, et al. (1998) TGF-beta 1 dissociates human proximal tubule cell growth and Na(+)-H+ exchange activity. Kidney Int 53: 1601–1607.
13. Lin M, Yiu WH, Wu HJ, Chan LY, Leung JC, et al. (2012) Toll-like receptor 4 promotes tubular inflammation in diabetic nephropathy. J Am Soc Nephrol 23: 86–102.
14. Mudaliar H, Pollock C, Komala MG, Chadban S, Wu H, et al. (2013) The role of Toll-like receptor proteins (TLR) 2 and 4 in mediating inflammation in proximal tubules. Am J Physiol Renal Physiol 305: F143–154.
15. Panchapakesan U, Pollock CA, Chen XM (2004) The effect of high glucose and PPAR-gamma agonists on PPAR-gamma expression and function in HK-2 cells. American journal of physiology Renal physiology 287: F528–534.
16. Panchapakesan U, Sumual S, Pollock CA, Chen X (2005) PPARgamma agonists exert antifibrotic effects in renal tubular cells exposed to high glucose. American journal of physiology Renal physiology 289: F1153–1158.
17. Pollock CA, Field MJ, Bostrom TE, Dyne M, Gyory AZ, et al. (1991) Proximal tubular cell sodium concentration in early diabetic nephropathy assessed by electron microprobe analysis. Pflugers Arch 418: 14–17.
18. Pollock CA, Lawrence JR, Field MJ (1991) Tubular sodium handling and tubuloglomerular feedback in experimental diabetes mellitus. Am J Physiol 260: F946–952.
19. Qi W, Chen X, Holian J, Mreich E, Twigg S, et al. (2006) Transforming growth factor-beta1 differentially mediates fibronectin and inflammatory cytokine expression in kidney tubular cells. American journal of physiology Renal physiology 291: F1070–1077.

20. Panchapakesan U, Pegg K, Gross S, Komala MG, Mudaliar H, et al. (2013) Effects of SGLT2 inhibition in human kidney proximal tubular cells–renoprotection in diabetic nephropathy? PLoS One 8: e54442.
21. Brosius FC, 3rd, Alpers CE, Bottinger EP, Breyer MD, Coffman TM, et al. (2009) Mouse models of diabetic nephropathy. Journal of the American Society of Nephrology: JASN 20: 2503–2512.
22. Maric C, Sandberg K, Hinojosa-Laborde C (2004) Glomerulosclerosis and tubulointerstitial fibrosis are attenuated with 17beta-estradiol in the aging Dahl salt sensitive rat. J Am Soc Nephrol 15: 1546–1556.
23. Yale JF, Bakris G, Cariou B, Yue D, David-Neto E, et al. (2013) Efficacy and safety of canagliflozin in subjects with type 2 diabetes and chronic kidney disease. Diabetes Obes Metab 15: 463–473.
24. Nagata T, Fukuzawa T, Takeda M, Fukazawa M, Mori T, et al. (2013) Tofogliflozin, a novel sodium-glucose co-transporter 2 inhibitor, improves renal and pancreatic function in db/db mice. Br J Pharmacol 10.1111/bph.12269.
25. Kojima N, Williams JM, Takahashi T, Miyata N, Roman RJ (2013) Effects of a new SGLT2 inhibitor, luseogliflozin, on diabetic nephropathy in T2DN rats. J Pharmacol Exp Ther 345: 464–472.
26. Anderson PW, Zhang XY, Tian J, Correale JD, Xi XP, et al. (1996) Insulin and angiotensin II are additive in stimulating TGF-beta 1 and matrix mRNAs in mesangial cells. Kidney Int 50: 745–753.
27. Sarafidis PA, Ruilope LM (2006) Insulin resistance, hyperinsulinemia, and renal injury: mechanisms and implications. Am J Nephrol 26: 232–244.
28. Ghezzi C, Wright EM (2012) Regulation of the human Na+-dependent glucose cotransporter hSGLT2. Am J Physiol Cell Physiol 303: C348–354.
29. Vallon V, Rose M, Gerasimova M, Satriano J, Platt KA, et al. (2013) Knockout of Na-glucose transporter SGLT2 attenuates hyperglycemia and glomerular hyperfiltration but not kidney growth or injury in diabetes mellitus. Am J Physiol Renal Physiol 304: F156–167.
30. Vallon V, Gerasimova M, Rose M, Masuda T, Satriano J, et al. (2013) SGLT2 Inhibitor Empagliflozin Reduces Renal Growth and Albuminuria in Proportion to Hyperglycemia and Prevents Glomerular Hyperfiltration in Diabetic Akita Mice. Am J Physiol Renal Physiol 10.1152/ajprenal.00520.2013.
31. Hodgkins KS, Schnaper HW (2012) Tubulointerstitial injury and the progression of chronic kidney disease. Pediatr Nephrol 27: 901–909.
32. Powell DR, DaCosta CM, Gay J, Ding ZM, Smith M, et al. (2013) Improved glycemic control in mice lacking Sglt1 and Sglt2. American journal of physiology Endocrinology and metabolism 304: E117–130.
33. Zhao FQ, Keating AF (2007) Functional properties and genomics of glucose transporters. Curr Genomics 8: 113–128.

Investigation of Variants in UCP2 in Chinese Type 2 Diabetes and Diabetic Retinopathy

Yinchen Shen[1]☯, Zujia Wen[2]☯, Ning Wang[1]*, Zhi Zheng[1], Kun Liu[1], Xin Xia[1], Qing Gu[1], Yongyong Shi[2], Xun Xu[1]

1 Department of Ophthalmology, Shanghai First People's Hospital, Shanghai Jiao Tong University, Shanghai, People's Republic of China, Shanghai Key Laboratory of Fundus Disease, Shanghai, People's Republic of China, **2** Bio-X Institutes, Key Laboratory for the Genetics of Developmental and Neuropsychiatric Disorders (Ministry of Education), Shanghai Jiao Tong University, Shanghai, People's Republic of China

Abstract

Purpose: The aim of this study was to investigate variants in *UCP2* genes in type 2 diabetes mellitus (DM) and diabetic retinopathy (DR) in Chinese population.

Materials and Methods: We conducted a single nucleotide polymorphism-based and haplotype-based case-control study between the variants of *UCP2* and DM and between the variants of *UCP2* and DR in 479 Chinese patients with type 2 DM and 479 control subjects without DM. Two SNPs (rs660339 and rs659366) were selected as genetic markers.

Results: The risk allele C at *UCP2* rs660339 was closely associated with DM in Chinese population. There was significant difference in rs660339 between DM and controls (P = 0.0016; OR [95%CI] = 1.37 (1.14–1.65)). Subjects who were homozygous of the C allele were more likely to develop DM. The frequency of C allele was higher in DM (58%) than in control (51%). But this locus didn't have a definite effect on the onset of non-proliferative diabetic retinopathy (NPDR) (P = 0.44; OR [95%CI] = 0.80 (0.56–1.14)) and proliferative diabetic retinopathy (PDR) (P = 1.00; OR [95%CI] = 0.99 (0.74–1.34)) comparing to subjects with DM without retinopathy (DWR), respectively. Moreover, the *UCP2* rs659366 polymorphism showed no significant difference between DM and control (P = 0.66; OR [95%CI] = 1.10 (0.91–1.32)). However, there was a significant difference between PDR and DWR (P = 0.016; OR [95%CI] = 0.66 (0.49–0.90)), but there was no difference between NPDR and DWR (P = 1.00; OR [95%CI] = 0.96 (0.67–1.37)). Participants who carried the G allele at rs659366 were more likely to develop PDR. For the haplotype, C-A was present more frequently in DM than in control (16% vs 7%), indicating that it was risky, and T-A was present less in DM than in control (29% vs 35%). Haplotype frequencies in DR and DWR showed no significant difference (P = 0.068).

Conclusion: It was indicated that *UCP2* may be implicated in the pathogenesis of type 2 DM and DR in Chinese population.

Editor: Junwen Wang, The University of Hong Kong, Hong Kong

Funding: This work was sponsored by grants from the National Natural Science Foundation of China (No. 81100679; No. 81273424), Major Basic Research Development Program of China (973 Program) (No. 2011CB707500) and Shanghai Guide Fund for Medical Projects (No. 124119a9600). The funders had no role in study design, data collection and analysis, decision to publish, or preparation of the manuscript.

Competing Interests: The authors have declared that no competing interests exist.

* Email: drwangning@126.com

☯ These authors contributed equally to this work.

Introduction

Diabetic retinopathy (DR) is a common sight-threatening microvascular complication affecting patients with diabetes mellitus (DM) and it is a major cause of new cases of blindness [1]. In the United States, an estimated 25.8 million children and adults or approximately 8.3% of the population, have diabetes [2]. Meanwhile, according to a recent epidemiological survey in China, the overall prevalence of diabetes was estimated to be 11.6% in Chinese adult population [3]. With such incidence, and prevalence of DM increasing worldwide, DR is expected to reach epidemic proportions.

Many diabetes-induced metabolic abnormalities are implicated in the development of DR, and appear to be mostly influenced by elevated oxidative stress [4]. Consequently, different candidate genes of oxidative stress were paid special attention to [5]. Several genetic and functional studies have implicated the important role of oxidative stress genes in the pathogenesis of retinopathy in diabetes [6–8]. However, the exact mechanism underlying its development remains unclear. There is considerable evidence that in patients with diabetes, mitochondrial reactive oxygen species (ROS) generation, especially at high blood glucose levels, is one of the main sources of oxidative stress [9,10]. Some antioxidant defense mechanisms exist to neutralize ROS and prevent harm. One of these is represented by human uncoupling proteins (UCPs).

Table 1. Demographic characteristics of the patients with DM and control subjects.

	Control	DWR	DR
No. of subjects	479	155	324
Male: female	203: 276	78: 77	139: 185
Age (years)	58.74±12.22	60.15±10.90	58.15±12.52
Duration of diabetes (years)	—	10.61±6.77	11.42±6.93
Fasting blood glucose (mmol/L)	—	8.40±2.52	8.76±3.11
Systolic blood pressure (mmHg)	128.55±16.66	129.72±16.19	130.63±16.52
Diastolic blood pressure (mmHg)	76.90±9.24	78.50±8.30	77.89±9.29
BMI (kg/m^2)	24.33±3.56	24.69±3.19	24.90±3.03

The results are expressed as mean ± SD.

UCPs are mitochondrial transporters present in the inner membrane of mitochondria which are considered pivotal regulators of energy and glucose homeostasis [11]. They belong to the mitochondrial anion carrier gene family and as suggested by their name, UCPs can uncouple ATP production from mitochondrial respiration by causing proton leak [12]. Recent studies demonstrated that UCPs can prevent mitochondrial hyperpolarization and formation of ROS [13]. A group of five different UCPs have been identified. These proteins have distinct tissue distributions and functions. Among them, *UCP2* is widely expressed in almost all mammalian tissues including white adipose tissue, liver, kidney, pancreatic islets, macrophages and retinal endothelial cells and pericytes [14]. Recently, the relationships between *UCP2* polymorphisms and susceptibility for type 2 DM [15–17], obesity [18] and cardiovascular disease [19] have been investigated. Several variants including Ala55Val polymorphism (rs660339) in the exon 4 and −866G/A polymorphism (rs659366) in the promoter region were paid specific attention to, however, the results were contradicting [15–17]. Limited studies about the association between *UCP2* polymorphisms and DM in Chinese population have found no significant differences [20]. In addition, no study has investigated the relationship between these two polymorphisms and the risk of DR in Chinese population.

Considering the role of *UCP2* in the protection against oxidative stress, we conducted an association analysis between variants of *UCP2* and DM and between variants of *UCP2* and DR in subjects with type 2 DM in Chinese population.

Materials and Methods

Subjects

The study population comprised of 479 unrelated patients with type 2 diabetes mellitus (mean age ± SD, 58.80±12.02; ratio of male to female, 45.3:54.7) and 479 unrelated controls subjects without DM (mean age ± SD, 58.74±12.22; ratio of male to female, 42.4:57.6), all of Han Chinese ethnicity. The subjects with DM were randomly recruited from the data bank in the department of ophthalmology of Shanghai First People's Hospital, Shanghai Jiao Tong University. The diagnosis of diabetes was based on criteria outlined by the American Diabetes Association in 1997. Control subjects without DM were chosen from a population of the outpatient of Shanghai First People's Hospital, Shanghai Jiao Tong University. The inclusion criteria of the control group was healthy blood donors of Chinese ancestry who did not have DM or family history for this disease. This study was approved by the Ethics committee of Shanghai First People's Hospital, Shanghai Jiao Tong University, Shanghai, China (permit number: 2013KY095). An informed consent process was established following the guidelines of the Helsinki Declaration, and consent forms were signed by all subjects.

We obtained blood samples from all the 958 subjects for DNA extraction. All subjects with DM underwent a standard ophthalmic examination, including measurement of visual acuity, slit-lamp biomicroscopy and dilated fundus examination. The evaluation of DR was according to the diagnostic criteria of the American Academy of Ophthalmology (AAO) 2001 Annual Meeting.

Among the 479 subjects with DM, there were 324 patients with DR (n = 215 of proliferative diabetic retinopathy (PDR) and n = 109 of non-proliferative diabetic retinopathy (NPDR)), 155 subjects with DM without retinopathy (DWR). The data of patients' age, gender, duration of diabetes, fasting blood glucose levels, systolic blood pressure, diastolic blood pressure, height and weight were all recorded.

Age, gender, systolic blood pressure, diastolic blood pressure and BMI were comparable in the control, DWR and DR groups. Besides, there was no significant difference in the duration of diabetes and the fasting blood glucose between DWR and DR groups ($P>0.05$). Demographic characteristics of all patients included in the study were shown in Table 1.

Genotyping

We selected rs660339 in the exon 4, and rs659366 in the promoter region of *UCP2* gene for our study. Genomic DNA was extracted from venous blood using standard phenol-chloroform extraction for the genotyping of these two polymorphisms. PCR amplifications producing two genomic segments, rs659366 and for rs660339, were performed on the GeneAmp PCR 9700 System (Applied Biosystems, ABI, USA) in a 15.0 µl reaction containing 10 ng genomic DNA,1.2 U Taq polymerase, 0.2 µl of each primer (10 PM), 1.5 µl PCR buffer (10×, Qiagen), and 1.5 µl dNTPs (each 2 mM). Amplification conditions consisted of an initial 3 min at 95°C, 35 cycles of 30 sec at 94°C, and 30 sec at 57°C for the two segments. We then genotyped the two variants using DNA sequencing on an ABI 3100 genetic analyzer using the BigDye Terminator Cycle Sequencing Kit (Applied Biosystems, ABI, USA). The primers and the sequence number definition of *UCP2* were constructed on the basis of NC_000006. Primer sequences were listed in the Table S1.

Table 2. Distributions of genotypes and alleles for the two variants in the DM and controls.

SNP site	Samples	N	Allele		$\chi2$	p	OR (95%CI)	Genotype			$\chi2$	P
			C	**T**				**CC**	**CT**	**TT**		
rs660339	DM	472	551(58%)	393(42%)	11.20	**0.0016**	1.37(1.14–1.65)	166(35%)	219(46%)	87(19%)	10.69	**0.01**
	Control	441	446(51%)	436(49%)				121(28%)	204(46%)	116(26%)		
			A	**G**				**AA**	**AG**	**GG**		
rs659366	DM	454	411(45%)	497(55%)	0.96	0.66	1.10(0.91–1.32)	97(21%)	217(48%)	140(31%)	1.14	1.00
	Control	448	385(43%)	511(57%)				90(20%)	205(46%)	153(34%)		

P value were calculated between DM and control.

Table 3. Distributions of genotypes and alleles for the two variants in the DR and DWR.

SNP site	Samples	N	Allele		$\chi2$	p	OR (95%CI)	Genotype			$\chi2$	P
			C	**T**				**CC**	**CT**	**TT**		
rs660339	DR	317	366(58%)	268(42%)	0.33	0.57	0.92(0.70–1.22)	106(33%)	154(49%)	57(18%)	1.92	0.38
	DWR	155	185(60%)	125(40%)				60(39%)	65(42%)	30(19%)		
			A	**G**				**AA**	**AG**	**GG**		
rs659366	DR	305	262(43%)	348(57%)	4.02	**0.045**	0.75(0.57–0.99)	59(19%)	144(47%)	102(34%)	3.89	0.14
	DWR	149	149(50%)	149(50%)				38(26%)	73(49%)	38(25%)		

P value were calculated between DR and DWR.

Table 4. Distributions of genotypes and alleles for the two variants in NPDR, PDR and DWR.

SNP site	Samples	N	Allele		$\chi 2$	P	OR (95%CI)	Genotype			$\chi 2$	P
			C	T				CC	CT	TT		
rs660339	NPDR	106	115(54%)	97(46%)	1.52	0.44	0.80(0.56–1.14)	33(31%)	49(46%)	24(23%)	1.61	0.90
	PDR	211	251(60%)	171(40%)	0.003	1.00	0.99(0.74–1.34)	73(34%)	105(50%)	33(16%)	2.31	0.62
	DWR	155	185(60%)	125(40%)				60(39%)	65(42%)	30(19%)		
			A	G				AA	AG	GG		
rs659366	NPDR	102	100(49%)	104(51%)	0.05	1.00	0.96(0.67–1.37)	23(23%)	54(53%)	25(24%)	0.43	1.00
	PDR	203	162(40%)	244(60%)	7.11	**0.016**	0.66(0.49–0.90)	36(18%)	90(44%)	77(38%)	6.93	0.06
	DWR	149	149(50%)	149(50%)				38(26%)	73(49%)	38(25%)		

P value were calculated between NPDR or PDR and DWR, respectively.

Statistical analysis

The parameters, allele and genotype frequencies, Hardy-Weinberg equilibrium (HWE), pair-wised linkage disequilibrium, and haplotype analysis were conducted online using a software platform called SHEsis (http://analysis.bio-x.cn) [21]. A case-control format was adopted for data analysis. The P values of allele and genotype frequencies were obtained based on chi-square distribution. We adjusted the P values using the Bonferroni correction. The threshold value of HWE was set at 0.05. Haplotype analysis was conducted using the PLEM algorithm, and those haplotypes that exhibited a frequency less than 0.03 were abandoned.

Results

Totally, 479 subjects with DM and 479 controls were enrolled in our study. All of the polymorphisms investigated were proved to be in HWE. The results of HWE testing were showed in the Table S2. The total number of samples genotyped differed between the variants because not all were capable of being amplified with PCR.

Two polymorphisms of *UCP2* (rs660339 and rs659366) were genotyped by sequencing in the 958 subjects. The frequency distribution of the alleles and genotypes were present in Table 2, Table 3 and Table 4.

When Bonferroni corrections were strictly adopted, there was significant difference in rs660339 between DM and controls (P = 0.0016; OR [95%CI] = 1.37 (1.14–1.65)). The frequency of C allele was higher in DM (58%) than in control (51%). The percentage of genotype CC at rs660339 were higher in DM (35%) and than in control subjects (28%) ($P < 0.05$). Multiple comparison for the 3 genotypes (CC, CT, TT) showed that there were significant differences between CC and TT ($\chi 2 = 10.688$, $P = 0.001$) and between CT and TT ($\chi 2 = 4.364$, $P = 0.037$), but no difference was found between CC and CT ($\chi 2 = 2.535$, $P = 0.111$). The results of multiple comparison were showed in the Table S3. It suggested that the risk allele C was closely associated with type 2 DM in Chinese population. Moreover, rs659366 showed no significant difference between DM and control (P = 0.66; OR [95%CI] = 1.10 (0.91–1.32)). We observed no significant difference in genotype distribution at rs659366 between DM and control group ($P > 0.05$) (Table 2).

To investigate the association between *UCP2* variants and DR, we found no significant difference between DR and DWR (P = 0.57; OR [95%CI] = 0.92 (0.70–1.22)) for rs660339. Nevertheless, for rs659366, there was a significant difference between DR and DWR (P = 0.045; OR [95%CI] = 0.75 (0.57–0.99)). For the genotype distribution analysis, we found no significant difference between DR and DWR at rs660339 and rs659366 (Table 3).

Then, we further compared the distribution of alleles between DR subtypes (NPDR, PDR) and DWR. For rs660339, we found no significant difference neither between NPDR and DWR (P = 0.44; OR [95%CI] = 0.80 (0.56–1.14)) nor between PDR and DWR (P = 1.00; OR [95%CI] = 0.99 (0.74–1.34)). Interestingly, for rs659366, there was a significant difference between PDR and DWR (P = 0.016; OR [95%CI] = 0.66 (0.49–0.90)). But, there was no difference between NPDR and DWR (P = 1.00; OR [95%CI] = 0.96 (0.67–1.37)). For the genotype distribution analysis, we found no significant difference among NPDR, PDR and DWR groups at rs660339 and rs659366. However, participants who were homozygous for the G allele at rs659366 were more likely to develop PDR but there was no statistical significance (P = 0.06) (Table 4).

Table 5. The estimated haplotype frequencies in DM and control.

Haplotype	DM	Control	Chi-square	OR(95%CI)	Global P value
C-A	140.5(16%)	58.0(7%)	31.97	2.48(1.79–3.42)	**P<0.001** ($df=3$, $\chi2=34.76$)
C-G	385.5(43%)	361.0(44%)	0.04	0.98(0.81–1.19)	
T-A	263.5(29%)	294.0(35%)	7.11	0.76(0.62–0.93)	
T-G	106.5(12%)	117.0(14%)	1.88	0.82(0.62–1.09)	

Within *UCP2*, pair-wised linkage disequilibrium analysis in DM case showed rs660339 was in moderate linkage disequilibrium ($D' = 0.52$) with rs659366 (Table S4).

For the haplotype analysis, one significant association was noted for C-A haplotype that was present two times frequently in DM than in control (16% vs 7%), indicating that it was risky. Another significant association was T-A haplotype which was present less frequently in DM than in control (29% vs 35%) (Table 5). Moreover, haplotype frequencies in DR and DWR showed no significant difference ($P = 0.068$) (Table 6).

Discussion

DM and its chronic complications are complex diseases associated with both genetic and environmental risk factors [22]. Considering the important role of *UCP2* in ROS formation by mitochondria, the relationship between *UCP2* locus and susceptibility for DM and its chronic complications [15–17,23–26] has been investigated. Over the past few years, several studies have suggested that there was an association between the *UCP2*-866G/A (rs659366) and Ala55Val (rs660339) polymorphisms and the risk of type 2 DM [15–17]. However, the results showed significant between-study variation. Prior studies examining these two variants in the *UCP2* gene have produced controversial results [15–17]: population of different races, ethnic backgrounds, and environmental exposures might influence the final result. Moreover, the evidence in Chinese population was quite limited. Recent study conducted in Hubei Han Chinese have reported no significant association between *UCP2* polymorphisms and type 2 DM [20]. Therefore, we found it still necessary to enlarge the sample size and conduct further investigation about the effects of *UCP2* genetic polymorphisms on type 2 DM.

In this study, we genotyped rs659366 and rs660339 of *UCP2* in 958 participants. The SNP analysis demonstrated that the C allele of rs660339 had significantly higher frequency in DM ($P = 0.0016$; OR [95%CI] = 1.37 (1.14–1.65)) than in control subjects, indicating that the risk C allele was related with the onset of DM in Chinese population. Meanwhile, participants who were homozygous for the C allele at rs660339 were more likely to develop DM. Haplotype analysis demonstrated that C-A haplotype was present two times more in DM than in control, while T-A haplotype was present less frequently in DM than in control, indicating that C was risky. The result of haplotype analysis was in accordance with those of allele and genotype analysis between DM and control. Our result complied with prior studies conducted by Lee et al. [11] and Vimaleswaran et al. [27] in Asian ethnicity. Nevertheless, the *UCP2* rs659366 polymorphism showed no significant difference between DM and control ($P = 0.66$; OR [95%CI] = 1.10 (0.91–1.32)). Other studies conducted in Asian ethnicity have reported different results [11,27–30]. Some indicated that patients with G alleles at rs659366 were more likely to suffer from DM [11], and the others showed no significant difference [27–30]. According to a recent meta-analysis of seventeen published articles, rs659366 was not a candidate for susceptibility to type 2 DM in any ethnic population, however, rs660339 was type 2 DM susceptibility loci in population of Asian, but not European descent [31]. Our study has consolidated these findings in Chinese population.

As a severe sight-threatening microvascular complication of DM, DR represents a major cause of new cases of blindness in adults [32]. There already had evidence showed that longer duration of diabetes, poorer control of blood glucose and elevated blood pressure were the major factors responsible for the onset and progression of DR. However, DR still occurs in subjects with normal glucose and blood pressure [33]. In addition, the prevalence of DR also showed racial differences and familial clustering indicating that genetic factors may have a significant effect in promoting the severity and the speed of onset of retinopathy in patients with DM [34]. Thus, identifying the genes contributing to the susceptibility of DR is quite important. Experimental research demonstrated that an overproduction of ROS was a triggering cause in the pathogenesis of diabetic complications. *UCP2* can protect retinal vascular endothelial cells from damage by inhibiting the overproduction of mitochondrial ROS [35], a phenomenon that revealed the important role of *UCP2* in DR. Although the genetic association between *UCP2* and DM has already been investigated, how *UCP2* polymorphsms influence the onset of DR still requires more evidences based on case-control genetic study. Crispim D et al. [23] has reported an association between the polymorphisms of *UCP2* and PDR in

Table 6. The estimated haplotype frequencies in DR and DWR.

Haplotype	DR	DWR	Chi-square	OR(95%CI)	Global P value
C-A	86.1 (14%)	53.9 (18%)	2.07	0.76(0.52–1.11)	P = 0.068 ($df=3$, $\chi2=10.21$)
C-G	258.9(43%)	127.1 (43%)	0.04	1.03(0.78–1.36)	
T-A	168.9(29%)	95.1(32%)	1.28	0.84(0.62–1.14)	
T-G	84.1(14%)	21.9(7%)	8.55	2.06(1.26–3.37)	

subjects with both type 2 and type 1 DM in European ancestry. However, there was no evidence about the relationship between *UCP2* and DR in Asian population. Therefore, we examined the two common *UCP2* gene polymorphisms, rs660339 and rs659366 variants, in Chinese participants to try to confirm this association.

For rs660339, we found no significant difference for the SNP analysis between DR and DWR. Although Crispim D et al. [23] indicated that type 2 DM patients with PDR presented higher frequencies of the T allele than type 2 DM patients without this complication, we observed no significant difference between NPDR or PDR and DWR, respectively. We guess that their result might only be limited to European ethnicity. Besides, for *UCP2* rs659366 polymorphism, there was a significant difference between DR and DWR. It was interesting that when we compared the SNP distributions in DR subtypes and DWR, we observed a significant difference between PDR and DWR, but there was no difference between NPDR and DWR. Participants who were homozygous for the G allele at rs659366 were more likely to develop PDR, indicating that the risk G allele was associated with the onset of PDR. When Bonferroni corrections were strictly adopted, we found that haplotype frequencies in DR and DWR showed no significant difference. In previous studies, Rudofsky et al. [24] reported no association of the rs659366 polymorphism with DR in a sample of Caucasian type 2 DM patients. However, Crispim D et al. [23] found that type 2 DM patients with PDR presented higher frequency of A allele. Our finding contradicted with prior studies in European ethnicity probably due to a racial difference, and our preliminary results need further consolidation by larger sample studies. It is worth pointing out that most studies focused on the genetic epidemiology of *UCP2* gene, and its function or protein expression changes by the influence of gene mutations were rarely investigated. Recently, one study indicated that the presence of the −866A/55Val/Ins haplotype was associated with decreased *UCP2* gene expression in human retina [36], which shed light on further research.

In conclusion, we examined the frequencies of two common polymorphisms in *UCP2*, rs660339 and rs659366, in the type 2 DM patients consist of NPDR, PDR, DWR and also control subjects without DM. The result indicated that homozygous of the C allele at *UCP2* rs660339 were more likely to develop DM, but this locus doesn't have a definite effect on the onset of NPDR and PDR. Moreover, the *UCP2* rs659366 polymorphism demonstrated a modest relationship with DM, but the DR patients who were homozygous for the G allele at rs659366 were more likely to develop PDR. Although the genetic susceptibilities to DR and to DM were sometimes similar, the difference still existed.

SNPs in the *UCP2* may be implicated in the pathogenesis of type 2 DM and DR in Chinese population. As far as our knowledge concerns, this is the first genetic study showing that *UCP2* polymorphisms are associated with DR in Asian population. However, this is a preliminary study and further functional studies are required to confirm its effect in human retinal cells.

Supporting Information

Table S1 Primers used in PCR for each of the two polymorphisms.

Table S2 Hardy-Weinberg equilibrium testing.

Table S3 Multiple comparison of genotypes distribution in rs660339 between DM and control.

Table S4 Linkage disequilibrium between SNPs in our samples, showing D'(above the diagonal) and r2(below the diagonal).

Author Contributions

Conceived and designed the experiments: YS ZW NW X. Xu. Performed the experiments: YS ZW NW ZZ KL X. Xia QG. Analyzed the data: YS NW. Contributed reagents/materials/analysis tools: ZW QG YS. Wrote the paper: YS NW.

References

1. Yau JW, Rogers SL, Kawasaki R, Lamoureux EL, Kowalski JW, et al. (2012) Global prevalence and major risk factors of diabetic retinopathy. Diabetes care 35: 556–564.
2. Threatt J, Williamson JF, Huynh K, Davis RM (2013) Ocular disease, knowledge and technology applications in patients with diabetes. Am J Med Sci 345: 266–270.
3. Xu Y, Wang L, He J, Bi Y, Li M, et al. (2013) Prevalence and control of diabetes in Chinese adults. JAMA 310: 948–959.
4. Kowluru RA, Chan PS (2007) Oxidative stress and diabetic retinopathy. Exp Diabetes Res 2007: 43603.
5. Petrovič D (2013) Candidate genes for proliferative diabetic retinopathy. Biomed Res Int 2013: 540416.
6. Santos JM, Tewari S, Kowluru RA (2012) A compensatory mechanism protects retinal mitochondria from initial insult in diabetic retinopathy. Free Radic Biol Med 53: 1729–1737.
7. Cilenšek I, Mankoč S, Petrovič MG, Petrovič D (2012) GSTT1 null genotype is a risk factor for diabetic retinopathy in Caucasians with type 2 diabetes, whereas GSTM1 null genotype might confer protection against retinopathy. Dis Markers 32: 93–99.
8. Kanwar M, Chan PS, Kern TS, Kowluru RA (2007) Oxidative damage in the retinal mitochondria of diabetic mice: possible protection by superoxide dismutase. Invest Ophthalmol Vis Sci 48: 3805–3811.
9. Nishikawa T, Edelstein D, Du XL, Yamagishi S, Matsumura T, et al. (2000) Normalizing mitochondrial superoxide production blocks three pathways of hyperglycaemic damage. Nature 404: 787–790.
10. Piconi L, Quagliaro L, Ceriello A (2003) Oxidative stress in diabetes. Clin Chem Lab Med 41: 1144–1149.
11. Lee HJ, Ryu HJ, Shin HD, Park BL, Kim JY, et al. (2008) Associations between polymorphisms in the mitochondrial uncoupling proteins (UCPs) with T2DM. Clin Chim Acta 398: 27–33.
12. Adams SH (2000) Uncoupling protein homologs: emerging views of physiological function. J Nutr 130: 711–714.
13. Skulachev VP (1998) Uncoupling: new approaches to an old problem of bioenergetics. Biochim Biophys Acta 1363: 100–124.
14. Duval C, Nègre-Salvayre A, Dogilo A, Salvayre R, Pénicaud L, et al. (2002) Increased reactive oxygen species production with antisense oligonucleotides directed against uncoupling protein 2 in murine endothelial cells. Biochem Cell Biol 80: 757–764.
15. Yu X, Jacobs DR Jr, Schreiner PJ, Gross MD, Steffes MW, et al. (2005) The uncoupling protein 2 Ala55Val polymorphism is associated with diabetes mellitus: the CARDIA study. Clin Chem 51: 1451–1456.
16. D'Adamo M, Perego L, Cardellini M, Marini MA, Frontoni S, et al. (2004) The −866A/A genotype in the promoter of the human uncoupling protein 2 gene is associated with insulin resistance and increased risk of type 2 diabetes. Diabetes 53: 1905–1910.
17. Bulotta A, Ludovico O, Coco A, Di Paola R, Quattrone A, et al. (2005) The common -866G/A polymorphism in the promoter region of the UCP-2 gene is associated with reduced risk of type 2 diabetes in Caucasians from Italy. J Clin Endocrinola Metab 90: 1176–1180.
18. Oktavianthi S, Trimarsanto H, Febinia CA, Suastika K, Saraswati MR, et al. (2012) Uncoupling protein 2 gene polymorphisms are associated with obesity. Cardiovasc Diabetol 11: 41.
19. Gioli-Pereira L, Santos PC, Sugaya LS, Ferreira NE, Krieger JE, et al. (2013) Association between UCP2 A55V polymorphism and risk of cardiovascular events in patients with multi-vessel coronary arterial disease. BMC Med Genet 14: 40.
20. Qin LJ, Wen J, Qu YL, Huang QY (2013) Lack of association of functional UCP2 −866G/A and Ala55Val polymorphisms and type 2 diabetes in the Chinese population based on a case-control study and a meta-analysis. Genet Mol Res 12: 3324–3334.

21. Shi YY, He L (2005) SHEsis, a powerful software platform for analyses of linkage disequilibrium, haplotype construction, and genetic association at polymorphism loci. Cell Res 15: 97–98.
22. Souza BM, Assmann TS, Kliemann LM, Gross JL, Canani LH, et al. (2011) The role of uncoupling protein 2 (UCP2) on the development of type 2 diabetes mellitus and its chronic complications. Arq Bras Endocrinol Metabol 55: 239–248.
23. Crispim D, Fagundes NJ, dos Santos KG, Rheinheimer J, Bouças AP, et al. (2010) Polymorphisms of the UCP2 gene are associated with proliferative diabetic retinopathy in patients with diabetes mellitus. Clin Endocrinol (Oxf) 72: 612–619.
24. Rudofsky G Jr, Schrödter A, Voron'ko OE, Schlotterer A, Humpert PM, et al. (2007) Promoter polymorphisms of UCP1, UCP2, and UCP3 are not associated with diabetic microvascular complications in type 2 diabetes. Horm Metab Res 39: 306–309.
25. Rudofsky G, Schroedter A, Schlotterer A, Voron'ko OE, Schlimme M, et al. (2006) Functional polymorphisms of UCP2 and UCP3 are associated with a reduced prevalence of diabetic neuropathy in patients with type 1 diabetes. Diabetes Care 29: 89–94.
26. Lindholm E, Klannemark M, Agardh E, Groop L, Agardh CD (2004) Putative role of polymorphisms in UCP1-3 genes for diabetic nephropathy. J Diabetes Complications 18: 103–107.
27. Vimaleswaran KS, Radha V, Ghosh S, Majumder PP, Sathyanarayana Rao MR, et al. (2011) Uncoupling protein 2 and 3 gene polymorphisms and their association with type 2 diabetes in Asian Indians. Diabetes Technol Ther 13: 19–25.
28. Sasahara M, Nishi M, Kawashima H, Ueda K, Sakagashira S, et al. (2004) Uncoupling protein 2 promoter polymorphism− 866G/A affects its expression in beta-cells and modulates clinical profiles of Japanese type 2 diabetic patients. Diabetes 53: 482–485.
29. Hsu YH, Niu T, Song Y, Tinker L, Kuller LH, et al. (2008) Genetic variants in the UCP2-UCP3 gene cluster and risk of diabetes in the Women's Health Initiative Observational Study. Diabetes 57: 1101–1107.
30. Heidari J, Akrami SM, Heshmat R, Amiri P, Fakhrzadeh H, et al. (2010) Association study of the-866G/A UCP2 gene promoter polymorphism with type 2 diabetes and obesity in a Tehran population: a case control study. Arch Iran Med 13: 384–390.
31. Xu K, Zhang M, Cui D, Fu Y, Qian L, et al. (2011) UCP2 −866G/A and Ala55Val, and UCP3 −55C/T polymorphisms in association with type 2 diabetes susceptibility: a meta-analysis study. Diabetologia 54: 2315–2324.
32. Fong DS, Aiello L, Gardner TW, King GL, Blankenship G, et al. (2004) Retinopathy in diabetes. Diabetes Care 27: 84–87.
33. Klein R, Klein BE, Moss SE, Davis MD, DeMets DL (1984) The Wisconsin epidemiologic study of diabetic retinopathy. II. Prevalence and risk of diabetic retinopathy when age at diagnosis is less than 30 years. Arch Ophthalmol 102: 520–526.
34. Liew G, Klein R, Wong TY (2008)The role of genetics in susceptibility to diabetic retinopathy. Int Ophthalmol Clin 49: 35–52.
35. He Y, Wang N, Shen Y, Zheng Z, Xu X (2014) Inhibition of high glucose-induced apoptosis by uncoupling protein 2 in human umbilical vein endothelial cells. Int J Mol Med 33: 1275–1281.
36. de Souza BM, Assmann TS, Kliemann LM, Marcon AS, Gross JL, et al. (2012) The presence of the −866A/55Val/Ins haplotype in the uncoupling protein 2 (UCP2) gene is associated with decreased UCP2 gene expression in human retina. Exp Eye Res 94: 49–55.

Defects in the Acquisition of Tumor-Killing Capability of CD8$^+$ Cytotoxic T Cells in Streptozotocin-Induced Diabetic Mice

Shu-Ching Chen[1], Yu-Chia Su[2], Ya-Ting Lu[3], Patrick Chow-In Ko[4], Pei-Yu Chang[1], Hung-Ju Lin[3], Hong-Nerng Ho[5], Yo-Ping Lai[3]*

1 Department of Medical Research, National Taiwan University Hospital, Taipei, Taiwan, **2** National Laboratory Animal Center, National Applied Research Laboratories, Taipei, Taiwan, **3** Department of Internal Medicine, National Taiwan University Hospital, Taipei, Taiwan, **4** Department of Emergency Medicine, National Taiwan University Hospital, Taipei, Taiwan, **5** Department of Obstetrics and Gynecology, National Taiwan University, College of Medicine, Taipei, Taiwan

Abstract

Emerging evidences have shown that diabetes mellitus not only raises risk but also heightens mortality rate of cancer. It is not clear, however, whether antitumor CD8$^+$ cytotoxic T lymphocyte (CTL) response is down-modulated in diabetic hosts. We investigated the impact of hyperglycemia on CTLs' acquisition of tumor-killing capability by utilizing streptozotocin-induced diabetic (STZ-diabetic) mice. Murine diabetes was induced by intraperitoneal injection of STZ (200 mg/kg) in C57BL/6 mice, 2C-T cell receptor (TCR) transgenic and P14-TCR transgenic mice. The study found that, despite harboring intact proliferative capacity measured with CFSE labeling and MTT assay, STZ-diabetic CD8$^+$ CTLs displayed impaired effector functions. After stimulation, STZ-diabetic CD8$^+$ CTLs produced less perforin and TNFα assessed by intracellular staining, as well as expressed less CD103 protein. Furthermore, adoptive transfer of STZ-diabetic P14 CD8$^+$ effector cells showed an insufficient recruitment to the B16.gp33 melanoma and inadequate production of perforin, granzyme B and TNFα determined by immunohistochemistry in the tumor milieu. As a result, STZ-diabetic CD8$^+$ effector cells were neither able to eliminate tumor nor to improve survival of tumor-bearing mice. Taken together, our data suggest that CD8$^+$ CTLs are crippled to infiltrate into tumors and thus fail to acquire tumor-killing capability in STZ-diabetic hosts.

Editor: George Kassiotis, MRC National Institute for Medical Research, United Kingdom

Funding: The study was supported by grants from National Science Council (NSC 99-2314-B-002-081-MY3), National Taiwan University Hospital (NTUH. 98P22) and Liver Disease Prevention and Treatment Research Foundation. The funders had no role in study design, data collection and analysis, decision to publish, or preparation of the manuscript.

Competing Interests: The authors have declared that no competing interests exist.

* Email: yopinglai@ntu.edu.tw

Introduction

Diabetes and cancer are severe health concerns of worldwide significance. According to the estimation of World Health Organization, 347 million people worldwide have diabetes. In addition to severe complications caused by chronic hyperglycemia, epidemiological studies show that diabetic patients have higher risk of cancer [1–6], suggesting that diabetic patients carry impaired anti-tumor immunity.

CTL plays a cardinal role in anti-tumor defense. Upon activation, naïve CD8$^+$ T cells are driven to clonal expansion and differentiation into the CTLs that exert cytokine production and tumor-lysis activity [7–10]. Glucose is essential fuel for T cell activation, proliferation, and acquisition of effector functions [11–15]. Chronic exposure to hyperglycemia may result in delayed response to antigen stimulation and failure to eliminate implanted ultraviolet-induced tumors [16–21]. The hypothesis is proposed that diabetes may cause defective CD8$^+$ T cell responses that render diabetic hosts bearing poor tumor control. Nevertheless, two important questions remain unanswered. First, whether the diabetic condition hinders CD8$^+$ T cell activation and differentiation into functional effector cells remains undefined. Second, it remains elusive in what extent of CD8$^+$ T cells that are hampered by acute hyperglycemia.

STZ is used to induce diabetes by damaging pancreatic β-cells, resulting in insulin deficiency and consequently hyperglycemia [22,23]. To investigate whether diabetes causes CD8$^+$ T cell impairment, we used STZ-diabetic murine model to examine CD8$^+$ T cell activation and differentiation both *in vitro* and *in vivo*. Furthermore, to evaluate anti-tumor immunity of STZ-diabetic CD8$^+$ T cells, the effector functions at early and late differentiation stages were checked *in vitro*. Finally, we used murine melanoma model to assess tumor-killing capability of STZ-diabetic CD8$^+$ T cells by monitoring tumor size and mice survival.

Materials and Methods

Ethical statements

All animal procedures in this study were followed guideline of the Use of Laboratory Animals published by National Taiwan University (NTU) and approved by Institutional Animal Care and

Use Committee (IACUC) of College of Medicine and College of Public Health of NTU (Permit Number: 20100131). Mice were housed on a 12 h light–dark cycle, with the dark cycle occurring from 8:00 P.M. to 8:00 A.M in a specific pathogen-free environment of the animal center at NTU hospital. The mice enrolled in the study were monitored at least three times per week. All surgery was performed under sodium pentobarbital (30–90 mg/kg, intraperitoneal injection) anesthesia, and all efforts were made to minimize suffering. The humane endpoint criteria were set following IACUC guidelines, including the body weight loss of no more than 20% of pre-procedural weight, tumor size reaching 20 mm in diameter. At the end of experiment, mice were sacrificed by euthanasia with carbon dioxide gas inhalation. The spleens and tumors were collected after sacrifice of the mice.

Mice

Male C57BL/6, B10.A, CD45.1, 2C and P14 TCR-transgenic mice at age of 6–8 weeks were obtained from animal center at NTU Hospital. The mice used in this study included more than

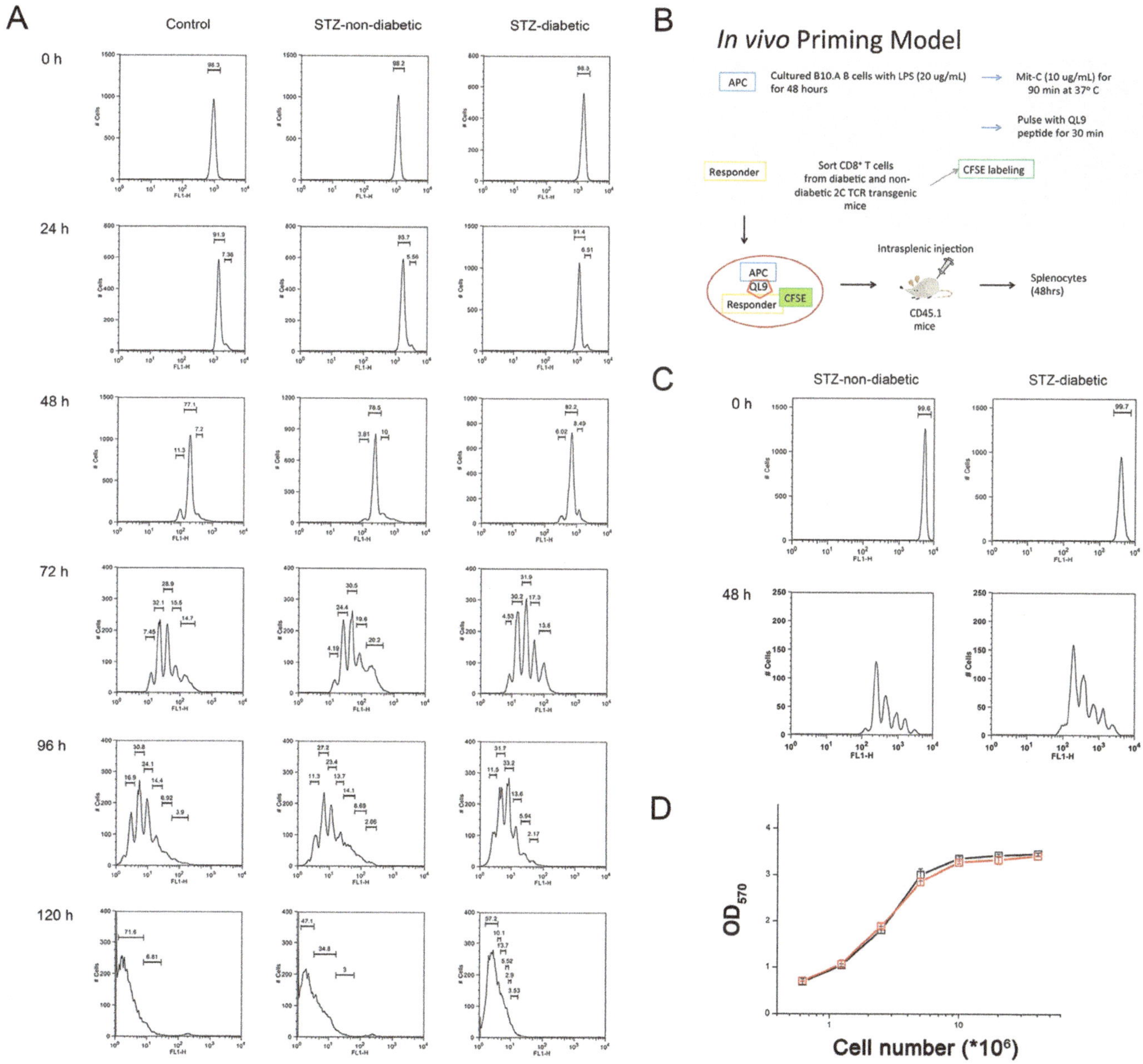

Figure 1. CD8⁺ T cell proliferation following stimulation. (A) CFSE-labeled STZ-diabetic, STZ-non-diabetic and control naïve CD8⁺ T cells from C57BL/6 mice were stimulated by anti-CD3/CD28 antibodies *in vitro* at the indicated time (24, 48, 72, 96 and 120 hours) and cell divisions were analyzed by flow cytometry. (B) *In vivo* CD8⁺ T cell priming model. (C) CFSE-labeled STZ-diabetic or STZ-non-diabetic 2C CD8⁺ T cells were co-administered with QL9-pulsed B10.A B blast cells into the spleen of healthy CD45.1 mice. Forty eight hours after priming, the splenocytes of CD45.1 mice were stained with PE anti-mouse CD45.2 antibody and cell divisions were analyzed by flow cytometry. (D) Five-day antigen-stimulated 2C CD8⁺ T cells from STZ-diabetic (red line) and STZ-non-diabetic (black line) mice were cultured in IL-2-containing medium for 24 hours, followed by MTT assay. Mit C, mitomycin C. APC, antigen-presenting cells. The data represent three independent experiments.

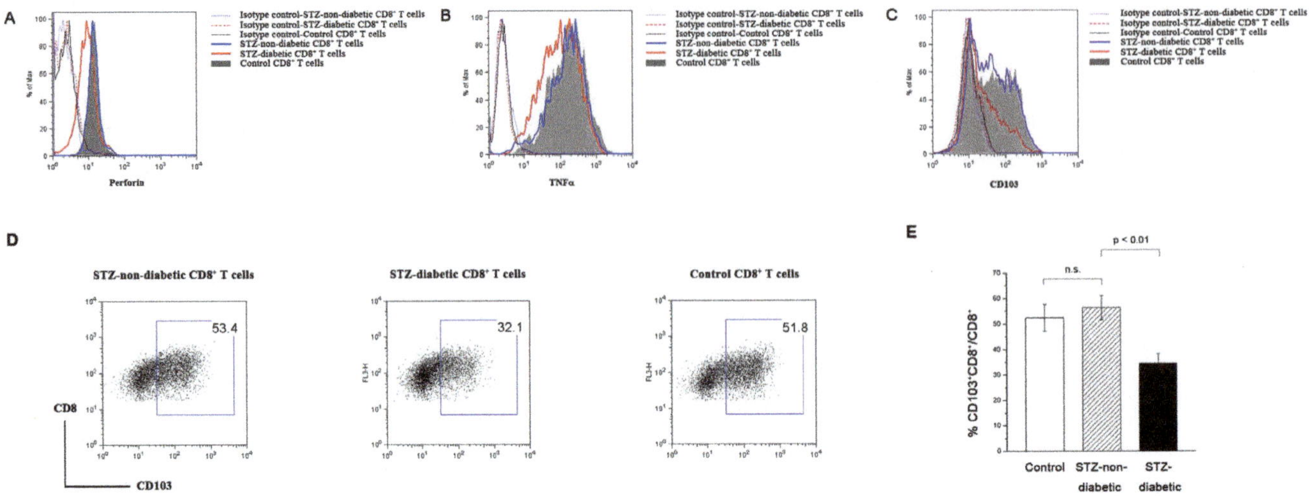

Figure 2. Effector functions of STZ-diabetic CD8$^+$ T cells. (A, B) Naïve CD8$^+$ T cells from STZ-diabetic (red line), STZ-non-diabetic (blue line) and control (gray-filled) C57BL/6 mice were stimulated by anti-CD3/CD28 antibodies *in vitro*. At 24 and 72 hours after stimulation, the production of perforin and TNFα was checked by intracellular staining and analyzed by flow cytometry. (C) At 120 hours of antigenic stimulation, 2C CD8$^+$ T cells from STZ-diabetic (red line) and STZ-non-diabetic (gray-filled) mice were harvested and surface CD103 expression was checked and analyzed by flow cytometry. Staining of isotype control for the three experimental groups was shown: STZ-non-diabetic (blue dot), STZ-diabetic (red dash) and control (black line) mice. (D) CD103-positive population was gated in 5 day-stimulated 2C CD8$^+$ T cells from STZ-non-diabetic, STZ-diabetic and control mice. (E) CD103-positive percentage in 5 day-stimulated 2C CD8$^+$ T cells was analyzed from the three experimental groups. Data are representative of three independent experiments with three to five mice per time point.

eight mice in each group and all experiments were repeated for at least three independent times.

Antibodies and reagents

Anti-mouse CD3 (clone 145-2C11) and anti-CD28 (clone 37.51) antibodies were prepared in our laboratory. DMEM, penicillin and streptomycin from GIBCO Inc. (Grand Island, NY, USA); fetal bovine serum (FBS) from HyClone Inc. (Logan, UT, USA); anti-mouse antibodies including FITC anti-CD3, -IFNγ and -granzyme B, PE anti-CD4, -CD19 and -perforin, PE-Cy5 anti-CD8 and APC anti-CD45.2 antibodies from eBioscience (San Diego, CA, USA); PE anti-TNFα and -CD103 antibodies from BioLegend (San Diego, CA, USA); STZ, Mitomycin C, LPS, MTT, phorbol myristic acid (PMA), Ionomycin and Brefeldin A from Sigma (St. Louis, MO, USA); CFSE from Molecular Probes (Eugene, OR, USA); QL9 (QLSPFPFDL) and KM9 (KAVTNFATM) peptides from AnaSpec, Inc. (San Jose, CA, USA) were purchased.

Diabetes development

Diabetes was induced by intraperitoneal injection of STZ (200 mg/kg) into male mice as described previously [22,23]. Blood glucose and weight were measured before and after STZ administration. Blood glucose level above 400 mg/dL was defined as diabetes.

Cell preparation and culture conditions

Naïve (CD62L^{hi}CD44^{lo}) CD8$^+$ T cells were obtained from spleens of mice by positive isolation of CD8$^+$ T cells [24], and further by sorting on FACSAria (BD Bioscience, San Jose, CA, USA) through service provided by Flow Cytometric Analyzing and Sorting Core Facility (First Core Laboratory, NTU, College of Medicine). Cells culture was set up in DMEM containing 10% FBS and 5×10^{-5} M 2-Mercaptoethanol. To activate CD8$^+$ T cells, the naïve cells were stimulated by anti-CD3/CD28 antibodies for the indicated time. For activating 2C TCR-transgenic (2C) CD8$^+$ T cells, the cells were stimulated by mitomycin C-treated [25] LPS-stimulated B10.A B blasts [26] and QL9 peptide. Cells were grown in 5% CO_2 humidified air at 37°C. For *in vivo* priming, naïve 2C CD8$^+$ T cells mixed with QL9-pulsed B10.A B blast cells were injected into the spleens of CD45.1 mice.

Cell proliferation assays

CFSE (carboxyfluorescein succinimidyl ester) labeling. CFSE (5 mM) was added to the cells (10×10^6 cells/mL) according to the manufacturer's instructions.

MTT (3-[4,5-dimethylthiazol-2-yl]-2,5-diphenyltetrazolium bromide) assay. Cells were incubated with MTT (1 mg/mL) for 4 hours. The formazan was solubilized by dimethyl sulfoxide and colorimetric absorbance was quantified by measuring optical density (OD) at 570 nm by a spectrophotometer (Tecan Group Ltd., Mannedorf, Switzerland).

Intracellular cytokine staining

After 6-hour culture with PMA (10 ng/mL)/Ionomycine (1 μg/mL) and 4-hour culture with Brefeldin A (10 μg/mL), the cells were fixed and permeabilized with cytofix-cytoperm kit (BD Biosciences) and stained with specific antibodies according to the manufacturer's instructions.

B16.gp33 melanoma model with adoptive transfer of P14 CD8$^+$ effector cells

B16.gp33 cells derived from B16 melanoma cells and genetically modified to express gene encoding amino acid 33–41 of glycoprotein from lymphocytic choriomeningitis virus (LCMV) were kindly provided by Dr. Hanspeter Pircher [27] and cultured in DMEM supplemented with 10% FBS and 200 μg/mL G418. Following subcutaneous inoculation of B16.gp33 cells (1×10^6 cells/mouse), the tumor diameter and survival of mice

A

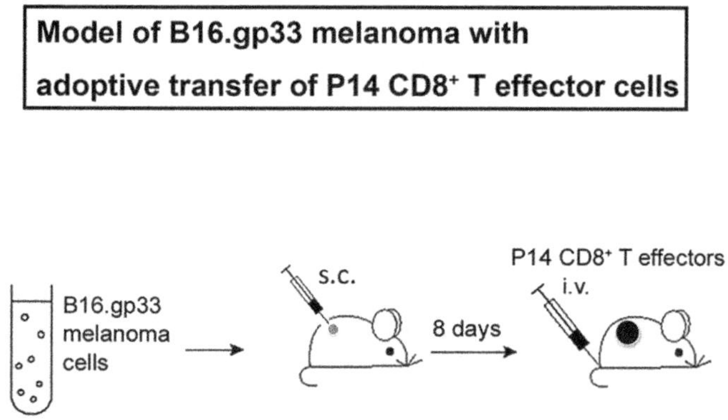
Model of B16.gp33 melanoma with
adoptive transfer of P14 CD8⁺ T effector cells
B16.gp33
melanoma
cells
s.c.
8 days
P14 CD8⁺ T effectors
i.v.

B

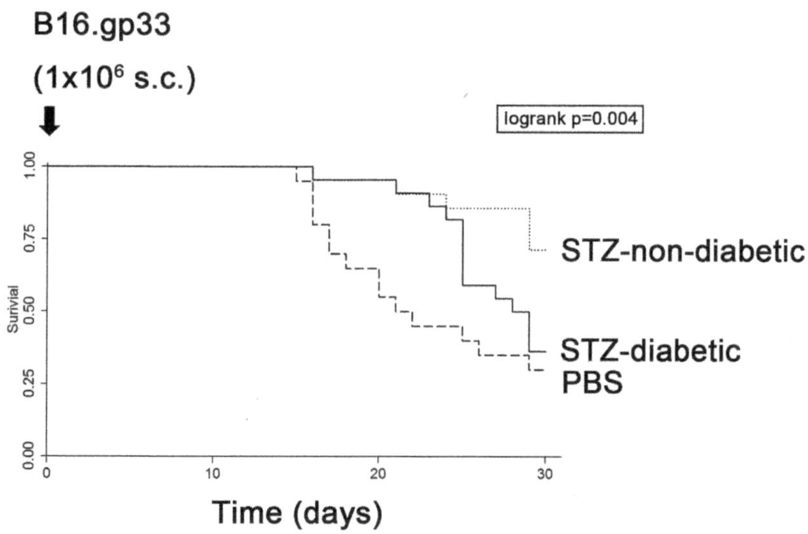
B16.gp33
(1x10⁶ s.c.)
logrank p=0.004
Surivial
STZ-non-diabetic
STZ-diabetic
PBS
Time (days)

C

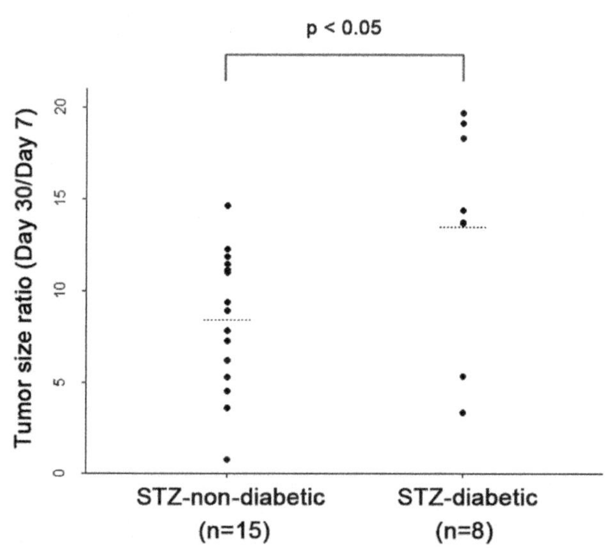
p < 0.05
Tumor size ratio (Day 30/Day 7)
STZ-non-diabetic
(n=15)
STZ-diabetic
(n=8)

Figure 3. Impaired anti-tumor immunity of STZ-diabetic CTLs. (A) Murine model of B16.gp33 melanoma with adoptive transfer of P14 $CD8^+$ T effector cells. (B) After adoptive transfer of STZ-diabetic (n = 22) or STZ-non-diabetic (n = 21) P14 $CD8^+$ T effector cells into B16.gp33 melanoma-bearing C57BL/6 mice, the survival time of the mice was recorded. Tumor-bearing mice with PBS but not T cells injection were considered as the controls (n = 20). (C) Tumor size of the mice that survived on day 30 after tumor inoculation. The increased fold of tumor size was calculated as tumor size at day 30 divided by that at day 7.

were recorded. P14 CTLs specific for LCMV gp33 in the context of $H\text{-}2D^b$ were generated by activating the P14 naïve $CD8^+$ T cells with mitomycin C-treated LPS-activated syngeneic B cell blasts and KM9 peptide, followed by harvest and cultured in recombinant human IL-2 (100 IU/mL)-containing medium as previously described [28]. The P14 CTLs in 1 X PBS (1×10^7 cells/0.15 mL/mouse) were injected intravenously into the mice that had B16.gp33 tumor inoculation for 8 days.

Detection of TNFα granzyme B and perforin in tumor-infiltrating lymphocytes

At 16 hours after transfer of P14 CTLs, the tumors were processed for cryosections and subjected to immunohistochemical staining by 2 μg/mL of FITC anti-granzyme B, PE anti-TNFα, PE anti-perforin and APC anti-CD45.2 antibodies.

Statistical analysis

Experiments were performed independently for at least three times. The percentage of $CD103^+$ cells in $CD8^+$ T cells between three groups was analyzed by unpaired Student's *t*-test. The difference of relative distribution of immune cells and increased fold of tumor size between two groups was analyzed by Student's *t*-test. The survival difference between two groups was analyzed by logrank test. The general linear model was fitted for the unbalanced data to assess the difference of CD 45.2^+ cell infiltration between two groups. Statistical significance was set at a p value of less than 0.05.

Results

STZ-diabetic mice and relative distribution of $CD8^+$ T cells in peripheral lymphoid tissues

C57BL/6 male mice at the age of 6–8 weeks were administered with STZ intraperitoneally. Twenty days after STZ injection, blood glucose level was significantly increased (>400 mg/dL vs. non-diabetic control: 142.9±16.5 mg/dL, $p<0.05$) and weight was significantly decreased (18.5±1.7 g vs. 25.4±1.7 g, $p<0.05$) in STZ-diabetic mice (n = 22) compared to non-diabetic control mice (n = 15). The splenocytes of STZ-diabetic and C57BL/6 control mice were immune-phenotyped and analyzed by flow cytometry to study the relative distribution of $CD8^+$ T cells in peripheral lymphoid tissues in diabetic condition, showing no significant difference between STZ-diabetic and control mice. To investigate whether the numbers of naïve $CD62L^{hi}CD44^{lo}CD8^+$ T cells were changed in STZ-diabetic mice, the expression of CD62L and CD44 proteins in $CD3^+CD8^+$ T cells were further inspected. It showed that naïve $CD8^+$ T cells still remained a significant population in the spleen of STZ-diabetic mice (data not shown).

Proliferation of STZ-diabetic $CD8^+$ T cells after activation

To investigate STZ-diabetic $CD8^+$ T cell activation, CFSE-labeled naïve $CD8^+$ T cells from STZ-diabetic and control C57BL/6 mice were stimulated by anti-CD3/CD28 antibodies *in vitro*, respectively, and harvested at indicated time for analyzing cell proliferation. It showed that, as control cells, STZ-diabetic $CD8^+$ T cells had high proliferative capability (Figure 1A). To further study diabetic $CD8^+$ T cell activation by specific antigenic peptide, the cell proliferation following *in vivo* priming was assessed (Figure 1B). It revealed that after priming for 48 hours, more than 50% of both STZ-diabetic and STZ-non-diabetic 2C $CD8^+$ T cells had 3–4 cell divisions (Figure 1C), indicating that STZ-diabetic $CD8^+$ T cells still attain proliferative capability upon stimulation *in vivo*. To further study the proliferative capability in late activated stage, 5-day stimulated 2C $CD8^+$ T cells were cultured in IL-2-containing medium for 24 hours and cell proliferation was analyzed, revealing no significant difference between STZ-diabetic and STZ-non-diabetic groups (Figure 1D). Taken together, the results indicated that as non-diabetic cells, the STZ-diabetic $CD8^+$ T cells possess proliferative potential.

Effector function of STZ-diabetic $CD8^+$ T cells

The anti-CD3/CD28-stimulated $CD8^+$ T cells from STZ-diabetic and non-diabetic control C57BL/6 mice were harvested at indicated time for checking the effector function. Significant production of IL-2, IFNγ and Granzyme B was observed in all groups (data not shown). However, STZ-diabetic $CD8^+$ T cells produced less perforin and TNFα at 24–72 hours after stimulation (Figures 2A and 2B), indicating an impaired effector function at early differentiation stage. Besides, expression of CD103protein was significantly lower in STZ-diabetic 2C $CD8^+$ T cells on day 5 following stimulation (Figure 2C). Of note, fewer $CD103^+$ cells were present in STZ-diabetic $CD8^+$ T cell population (Figures 2D and 2E), implying accumulation deficit of diabetic CTLs in tumor and thereby compromising anti-tumor immunity.

Anti-tumor immunity of STZ-induced diabetic $CD8^+$ T cells

To investigate tumor-killing capability of STZ-diabetic $CD8^+$ T cells *in vivo*, B16-gp33 melanoma cells were subcutaneously inoculated, followed by adoptive transfer of the tumor-specific P14 $CD8^+$ effector cells intravenously (Figure 3A). All the mice developed tumor and 70% of the PBS control group (14/20) died of tumor burden whereas, only 29% of the mice with adoptive transfer of STZ-non-diabetic P14 $CD8^+$ effector cells died (6/21) during the experimental observation period. It showed that adoptive transfer of STZ-non-diabetic P14 $CD8^+$ effector cells caused a prolonged survival from 36% (8/22 mice of STZ-diabetic group) to 71% (15/21 mice of STZ-non-diabetic group) of tumor-bearing mice on 30 days after tumor inoculation (Figure 3B, $p<0.01$). By contrast, transfer of the STZ-diabetic P14 $CD8^+$ effector cells did not show beneficial effect on survival (8/22 mice of STZ-diabetic group vs. 6/20 mice of PBS injection group). Furthermore, smaller tumor size was revealed in STZ-non-diabetic P14 $CD8^+$ effector cells-treated group (Figure 3C, $p<0.05$). Taken together, STZ-diabetic $CD8^+$ T cells are defective in tumor eradication *in vivo*. To elucidate the tumor-infiltrating efficacy of tumor-specific T cells, the tumor was removed and intra-tumor $CD45.2^+$ cells was analyzed by immunohistochemical staining at 16 hours after adoptive transfer of P14 $CD8^+$ effector cells ($CD45.2^+$) into tumor-bearing CD45.1 mice, (Figure 4A). Significantly fewer $CD45.2^+$ cells were found in the tumor of mice receiving STZ-diabetic P14 $CD8^+$ effector cells than STZ-non-diabetic group (Figure 4B), STZ-diabetic: 24.8, 95% confidence

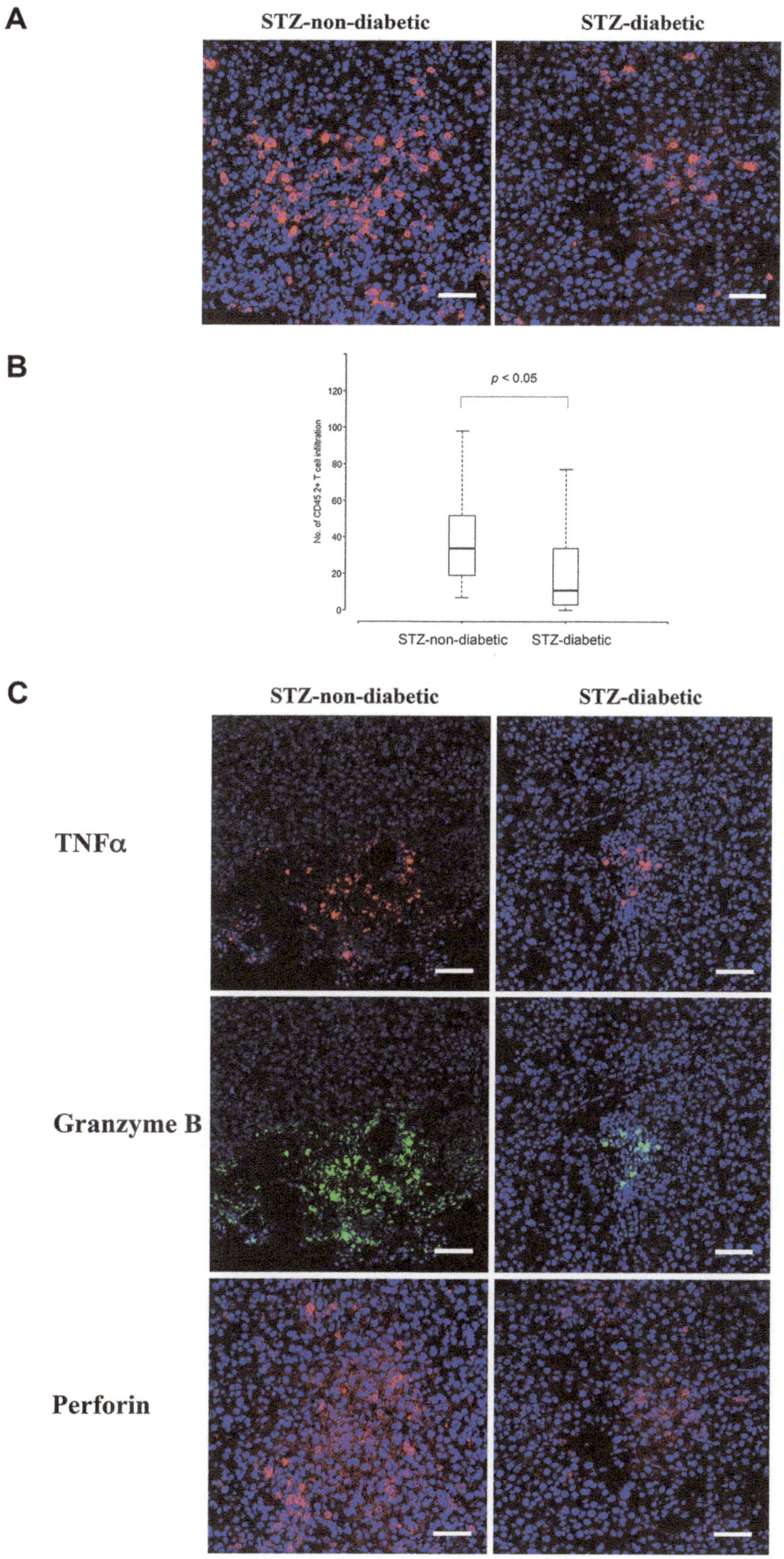
A
STZ-non-diabetic
STZ-diabetic
B
p < 0.05
No. of CD45.2+ T cell infiltration
0
20
40
60
80
100
120
STZ-non-diabetic
STZ-diabetic
C
STZ-non-diabetic
STZ-diabetic
TNFα
Granzyme B
Perforin

Figure 4. Infiltration and cytotoxicity of STZ-diabetic CTLs in tumor. (A, B) Assessment of the tumor-specific CTL infiltration in the tumor. Sixteen hours after adoptive transfer of STZ-diabetic or STZ-non-diabetic P14 $CD8^+$ T effector cells into tumor-bearing CD45.1 mice, the tumors were processed for cryosections and stained by APC anti-mouse CD45.2 antibody and Hoechst 33342. (C) The production of TNFα, granzyme B and perforin by STZ-diabetic or STZ-non-diabetic P14 CTLs was monitored by immunostaining the tumors with specific antibodies and Hoechst 33342, and were visualized by a Zeiss LSM 510 confocal microscope. Scale bar: 50 μm.

interval (CI), 14.8–34.8; STZ-non-diabetic: 43.7, 95% CI, 34.4–52.9; $p<0.01$. the difference: 18.9, 95% CI, 5.3–32.5; $p<0.01$). Moreover, there were significantly fewer perforin-, granzyme B- and TNFα-producing cells in the tumor of mice receiving STZ-diabetic P14 $CD8^+$ effector cells than STZ-non-diabetic group (Figure 4C). Therefore, STZ-diabetic P14 T cells had impaired effector function and were ineffective against tumor burden *in vivo*.

Discussion

Diabetic patients have an increased incidence of cancers [1–6], suggesting that diabetes hampers anti-tumor CTL function. Considerable evidence has accumulated supporting the importance of abundant tumor-infiltrating CTLs for better outcomes in various types of cancers [29–31]. Therefore, appropriate intra-tumor migration of CTLs is a prerequisite for antitumor surveillance. Our data showed that adoptive transfer of STZ-diabetic $CD8^+$ effector cells resulted in fewer tumor-infiltrating T cells as well as less production of perforin, Granzyme B and TNFα *in situ*. It is plausible that, in addition to defective cytotoxicity, the intra-tumor migration of STZ-diabetic CTLs is impeded.

Recent reports have shown that TNFα can promote influx of tumor-reactive T cells by remodeling intra-tumor vessels [32–34], and thereby exerts a local immunomodulatory function in tumor microenvironment. Our study showed that the less production of intra-tumor TNFα in STZ-diabetic $CD8^+$ T cells-treated mice may lead to insufficient infiltration of tumor-reactive CTLs. Furthermore, anti-tumor defense requires recognition of tumor antigens by CTLs' TCRs and strengthening CTL/tumor cell contacts by LFA-1-ICAM-1 and/or CD103-E-cadherin interaction [35–39]. This firm adhesion constructed by CD103-E-cadherin interaction is crucial for CTLs to kill tumor cells especially when tumors do not express ICAM-1 [37,39]. It ensures tumor killing by promoting the maturation of immunological synapse and polarized release of cytokine and lytic granules. Thus, significantly less expression of CD103 protein on STZ-diabetic CTLs revealed in our study may cripple CTLs' intratumor migration and firm retention in tumors, leading to insufficient cytokine production and cytotoxicity toward tumor cells.

The findings from the current study strongly suggest that the effect of diabetes on $CD8^+$ T cell function should be reconsidered more precisely. Overall, these results provide values for identifying STZ-induced diabetes may hamper the CTL function as a result of impaired cell differentiation. The enfeebled CTLs with inadequate CD103 expression show ineffective tumor infiltration and insufficient production of the cytotoxic mediators. The elucidation of how effector functions of STZ-diabetic $CD8^+$ T cells are impeded will optimize strategies for advancing tumor-killing capability and inducing protective antitumor immunity in diabetic hosts.

Supporting Information

Checklist S1 The Arrive Guidelines Checklist for Animal Research reports *in vivo* experiments of this study.

Acknowledgments

We thank Dr. Chung-Jiuan Jeng for critical review of the manuscript. We are grateful for Yu-Ching Lin for excellent technical assistance. We appreciate the service provided by the Flow Cytometric Analyzing and Sorting Core Facility of the First Core Laboratory, College of Medicine, National Taiwan University.

Author Contributions

Conceived and designed the experiments: SCC YPL. Performed the experiments: SCC YCS YTL PYC. Analyzed the data: SCC YCS YTL PYC HJL. Contributed reagents/materials/analysis tools: PCIK HNH. Wrote the paper: SCC YPL.

References

1. Giovannucci E, Harlan DM, Archer MC, Bergenstal RM, Gapstur SM, et al. (2010) Diabetes and cancer: a consensus report. Diabetes Care 33: 1674–1685.
2. Stattin P, Bjor O, Ferrari P, Lukanova A, Lenner P, et al. (2007) Prospective study of hyperglycemia and cancer risk. Diabetes Care 30: 561–567.
3. Connolly GC, Safadjou S, Chen R, Nduaguba A, Dunne R, et al. (2012) Diabetes mellitus is associated with the presence of metastatic spread at disease presentation in hepatocellular carcinoma. Cancer Invest 30: 698–702.
4. Chen HF, Liu MD, Chen P, Chen LH, Chang YH, et al. (2013) Risks of Breast and Endometrial Cancer in Women with Diabetes: A Population-Based Cohort Study. PLoS One 8: e67420.
5. Williams JC, Walsh DA, Jackson JF (1984) Colon carcinoma and diabetes mellitus. Cancer 54: 3070–3071.
6. La Vecchia C, D'Avanzo B, Negri E, Franceschi S (1991) History of selected diseases and the risk of colorectal cancer. Eur J Cancer 27: 582–586.
7. Kaech SM, Hemby S, Kersh E, Ahmed R (2002) Molecular and functional profiling of memory CD8 T cell differentiation. Cell 111: 837–851.
8. Lyman MA, Aung S, Biggs JA, Sherman LA (2004) A spontaneously arising pancreatic tumor does not promote the differentiation of naive CD8+ T lymphocytes into effector CTL. J Immunol 172: 6558–6567.
9. Klebanoff CA, Gattinoni L, Torabi-Parizi P, Kerstann K, Cardones AR, et al. (2005) Central memory self/tumor-reactive CD8+ T cells confer superior antitumor immunity compared with effector memory T cells. Proc Natl Acad Sci U S A 102: 9571–9576.
10. Milstein O, Hagin D, Lask A, Reich-Zeliger S, Shezen E, et al. (2011) CTLs respond with activation and granule secretion when serving as targets for T-cell recognition. Blood 117: 1042–1052.
11. Maciver NJ, Jacobs SR, Wieman HL, Wofford JA, Coloff JL, et al. (2008) Glucose metabolism in lymphocytes is a regulated process with significant effects on immune cell function and survival. J Leukoc Biol 84: 949–957.
12. Bental M, Deutsch C (1993) Metabolic changes in activated T cells: an NMR study of human peripheral blood lymphocytes. Magn Reson Med 29: 317–326.
13. Jacobs SR, Herman CE, Maciver NJ, Wofford JA, Wieman HL, et al. (2008) Glucose uptake is limiting in T cell activation and requires CD28-mediated Akt-dependent and independent pathways. J Immunol 180: 4476–4486.
14. MacIver NJ, Michalek RD, Rathmell JC (2013) Metabolic regulation of T lymphocytes. Annu Rev Immunol 31: 259–283.
15. Fox CJ, Hammerman PS, Thompson CB (2005) Fuel feeds function: energy metabolism and the T-cell response. Nat Rev Immunol 5: 844–852.
16. Stentz FB, Kitabchi AE (2003) Activated T lymphocytes in Type 2 diabetes: implications from in vitro studies. Curr Drug Targets 4: 493–503.
17. De Maria R, Todaro M, Stassi G, Di Blasi F, Giordano M, et al. (1994) Defective T cell receptor/CD3 complex signaling in human type I diabetes. Eur J Immunol 24: 999–1002.
18. Delespesse G, Duchateau J, Bastenie PA, Lauvaux JP, Collet H, et al. (1974) Cell-mediated immunity in diabetes mellitus. Clin Exp Immunol 18: 461–467.
19. Eibl N, Spatz M, Fischer GF, Mayr WR, Samstag A, et al. (2002) Impaired primary immune response in type-1 diabetes: results from a controlled vaccination study. Clin Immunol 103: 249–259.

20. Mahmoud AA, Rodman HM, Mandel MA, Warren KS (1976) Induced and spontaneous diabetes mellitus and suppression of cell-mediated immunologic responses. Granuloma formation, delayed dermal reactivity and allograft rejection. J Clin Invest 57: 362–367.
21. Diepersloot RJ, Bouter KP, Beyer WE, Hoekstra JB, Masurel N (1987) Humoral immune response and delayed type hypersensitivity to influenza vaccine in patients with diabetes mellitus. Diabetologia 30: 397–401.
22. Rakieten N, Rakieten ML, Nadkarni MV (1963) Studies on the diabetogenic action of streptozotocin (NSC-37917). Cancer Chemother Rep 29: 91–98.
23. Junod A, Lambert AE, Stauffacher W, Renold AE (1969) Diabetogenic action of streptozotocin: relationship of dose to metabolic response. J Clin Invest 48: 2129–2139.
24. Lai YP, Lin CC, Liao WJ, Tang CY, Chen SC (2009) CD4+ T cell-derived IL-2 signals during early priming advances primary CD8+ T cell responses. PLoS One 4: e7766.
25. Janeway CA Jr, Ron J, Katz ME (1987) The B cell is the initiating antigen-presenting cell in peripheral lymph nodes. J Immunol 138: 1051–1055.
26. Kakiuchi T, Chesnut RW, Grey HM (1983) B cells as antigen-presenting cells: the requirement for B cell activation. J Immunol 131: 109–114.
27. Prevost-Blondel A, Zimmermann C, Stemmer C, Kulmburg P, Rosenthal FM, et al. (1998) Tumor-infiltrating lymphocytes exhibiting high ex vivo cytolytic activity fail to prevent murine melanoma tumor growth in vivo. J Immunol 161: 2187–2194.
28. Castellino F, Huang AY, Altan-Bonnet G, Stoll S, Scheinecker C, et al. (2006) Chemokines enhance immunity by guiding naive CD8+ T cells to sites of CD4+ T cell-dendritic cell interaction. Nature 440: 890–895.
29. Fridman WH, Pages F, Sautes-Fridman C, Galon J (2012) The immune contexture in human tumours: impact on clinical outcome. Nat Rev Cancer 12: 298–306.
30. Naito Y, Saito K, Shiiba K, Ohuchi A, Saigenji K, et al. (1998) CD8+ T cells infiltrated within cancer cell nests as a prognostic factor in human colorectal cancer. Cancer Res 58: 3491–3494.
31. Mahmoud SM, Paish EC, Powe DG, Macmillan RD, Grainge MJ, et al. (2011) Tumor-infiltrating CD8+ lymphocytes predict clinical outcome in breast cancer. J Clin Oncol 29: 1949–1955.
32. Johansson A, Hamzah J, Payne CJ, Ganss R (2012) Tumor-targeted TNFalpha stabilizes tumor vessels and enhances active immunotherapy. Proc Natl Acad Sci U S A 109: 7841–7846.
33. Ganss R, Ryschich E, Klar E, Arnold B, Hammerling GJ (2002) Combination of T-cell therapy and trigger of inflammation induces remodeling of the vasculature and tumor eradication. Cancer Res 62: 1462–1470.
34. Johansson A, Hamzah J, Ganss R (2012) Intratumoral TNFalpha improves immunotherapy. Oncoimmunology 1: 1395–1397.
35. Anikeeva N, Somersalo K, Sims TN, Thomas VK, Dustin ML, et al. (2005) Distinct role of lymphocyte function-associated antigen-1 in mediating effective cytolytic activity by cytotoxic T lymphocytes. Proc Natl Acad Sci U S A 102: 6437–6442.
36. Springer TA, Dustin ML (2012) Integrin inside-out signaling and the immunological synapse. Curr Opin Cell Biol 24: 107–115.
37. Le Floc'h A, Jalil A, Vergnon I, Le Maux Chansac B, Lazar V, et al. (2007) Alpha E beta 7 integrin interaction with E-cadherin promotes antitumor CTL activity by triggering lytic granule polarization and exocytosis. J Exp Med 204: 559–570.
38. Franciszkiewicz K, Le Floc'h A, Jalil A, Vigant F, Robert T, et al. (2009) Intratumoral induction of CD103 triggers tumor-specific CTL function and CCR5-dependent T-cell retention. Cancer Res 69: 6249–6255.
39. Franciszkiewicz K, Le Floc'h A, Boutet M, Vergnon I, Schmitt A, et al. (2013) CD103 or LFA-1 engagement at the immune synapse between cytotoxic T cells and tumor cells promotes maturation and regulates T-cell effector functions. Cancer Res 73: 617–628.

Multicenter Epidemiological Study to Assess the Population of CKD Patients in Greece: Results from the PRESTAR Study

Konstantinos Sombolos[1], Demitrios Tsakiris[2], John Boletis[3], Demetrios Vlahakos[4], Kostas C. Siamopoulos[5], Vassilios Vargemezis[6], Pavlos Nikolaidis[7], Christos Iatrou[8], Eugene Dafnis[9], Konstantinos Xynos[10], Christos Argyropoulos[11]*

1 Nephrology Clinic, Papanikolaou Hospital, Thessaloniki, Greece, **2** Nephrology Clinic, Papageorgiou Hospital, Thessaloniki, Greece, **3** Nephrology Clinic, Laiko Hospital, Athens, Greece, **4** Nephrology Clinic, ATTIKON University Hospital, Athens, Greece, **5** Nephrology Clinic, Ioannina University Hospital, Ioannina, Greece, **6** Nephrology Clinic, Alexandroupoli University Hospital, Alexandroupoli, Greece, **7** Nephrology Clinic, AHEPA Hospital, Thessaloniki, Greece, **8** Center for Nephrology, G Papadakis, Nikea Hospital, Athens, Greece, **9** Nephrology Clinic, PE.PA.G.N.I, Crete University Hospital, Iraklio, Greece, **10** AbbVie Pharmaceuticals, Chicago, Illinois, United States of America, **11** AbbVie Pharmaceuticals SA, Athens, Greece

Abstract

Background: Chronic Kidney Disease (CKD) is a relatively common condition not only associated with increased morbidity and mortality but also fuelling End Stage Renal Disease (ESRD). Among developed nations, Greece has one of the highest ESRD incidence rates, yet there is limited understanding of the epidemiology of earlier stages of CKD.

Methods: Cross-sectional survey of pre-dialysis CKD outpatients in nephrology clinics in the National Health Care system between October 2009 and October 2010. Demographics, cause of CKD, blood pressure, level of renal function, duration of CKD and nephrology care, and specialty of referral physician were collected and analyzed. Different methods for estimating renal function (Cockroft-Gault [CG], CKD-Epi and MDRD) and staging CKD were assessed for agreement.

Results: A total of 1,501 patients in 9 centers were enrolled. Diabetic nephropathy was the most common nephrologist assigned cause of CKD (29.7%). In total, 36.5% of patients had self-referred to the nephrologist; patients with diabetes or serum creatinine above 220 μmol/l (eGFR<40 ml/min/1.73 m^2) were more likely to have been referred by a physician. Agreement between MDRD and CKD-Epi, but not between CG, the other estimating equations, was excellent. There was substantial heterogeneity with respect to renal diagnoses, referral patterns and blood pressure among participating centers.

Conclusions: In this first epidemiologic assessment of CKD in Greece, we documented delayed referral and high rates of self-referral among patients with CKD. eGFR reporting, currently offered by a limited number of laboratories, may facilitate detection of CKD at an earlier, more treatable stage.

Editor: Emmanuel A. Burdmann, University of Sao Paulo Medical School, Brazil

Funding: The PRESTAR (PRospective Epidemiology STudy Aiming to Register CKD Patients Stage 3, 4, and 5 not on Hemodialysis Followed by Nephrologists) study was designed and funded by the Greek Affiliate of Abbott Laboratories. AbbVie reviewed the manuscript for potential issues pertaining to Intellectual Property rights protection and for scientific content. Abbott and AbbVie Laboratories Sales and Marketing personnel did not influence the content development of this manuscript in any way, including through discussions with the external authors (SK, DT, JB, DV, KS, VV, PV, CI, ED). The funder provided support in the form of salaries for authors CA & KX, designed the study and provided funding for data collection and analysis and participated in the decision to publish and the preparation of the manuscript. The specific roles of these authors are articulated in the "author contributions" section.

Competing Interests: Drs. SK, DT, JB, DV, KS, VV, PV, CI, and ED are clinician investigators responsible for enrolling patients and collecting the data; they all received investigator fees for their participation in PRESTAR. Dr. KX is a former Abbott (now AbbVie) employee and may own Abbott/AbbVie stock, while Dr. CA was an Abbott Laboratories Hellas (now AbbVie Pharmaceuticals SA) Medical Affairs contractor. Abbott Laboratories funded this study. There are no patents, products in development or marketed products to declare.

* Email: argchris@hotmail.com

Introduction

Chronic Kidney Disease (CKD) is a relatively common condition associated with increased morbidity and mortality, mainly due to cardiovascular causes [1,2]. The increasing prevalence of risk factors for CKD such as obesity, diabetes and hypertension appears to fuel an emergent CKD epidemic on a global scale [3]. Contrary to patients with End Stage Renal Disease (ESRD), the care of patients with pre-dialysis CKD is primarily being overseen by general medicine, primary care physicians (PCPs), with specialist (nephrologist) input provided for patients with advanced stages of CKD [4–6]. These practice patterns translate to substantial missed opportunities to optimize care of patients with CKD in terms of disease education, selection of dialysis modality, pre-emptive transplantation, and implementing plans for the timely creation and maturation of dialysis access [7–9]. Furthermore, referral and [10–12] treatment in nephrology clinics has been shown to decrease the rate of progression of CKD and optimize the treatment of CKD complications [13].

In spite of these advantages, our understanding of how patients are referred for pre-dialysis nephrology consultation is limited, especially in settings in which formal partnerships between PCPs and nephrologists and referral recommendations for patients with CKD are not in place [14]. Furthermore, such information is rarely available on a country-wide basis, limiting the possibility of linking pre-dialysis practices to dialysis treatment pattern and outcomes in national registries. This is particularly important in settings characterized by high incidence of ESRD, given the toll the disease exacts on patients, caregivers and healthcare systems. Greece has one of the highest ESRD incidence rates [15] among industrialized nations, yet there is limited understanding of the epidemiology of earlier stages of CKD at the national level. In this cross-sectional, multicenter assessment, we describe the patient characteristics, causes of CKD and distribution of renal function in outpatients of nephrology clinics in the Greek National Healthcare System. Additionally, we characterize the referral patterns in relation to diagnosis of renal disease and the level of renal function, and describe center specific variations in these parameters. Finally, we examine the relative performance of different equations for estimated Glomerular Filtration Rate (eGFR) in the Greek CKD population.

Subjects and Methods

Design and Participants

This is a multicentre, observational, cross-sectional epidemiological study conducted in 9 outpatient Nephrology Clinics of the National Health System from across the different regions of Greece from October 2009 to October 2010. Centers were selected for participation based on previous workload and catchment area that included both urban and rural segments of the population. The sample size for the study was selected to ensure that the percentage of CKD 3–5 patients will be estimated with a degree of error of 2.3% when the expected percentage is 70%. Patients were eligible to participate in the study if they were older than 18 years, able to give informed consent, established patients of the clinic, not currently receiving renal replacement therapy. Patients with acute kidney injury/acute renal failure and patients with neoplasms or any other serious disease with projected life expectancy of less than 12 months were excluded from the study to ensure that only medically stable outpatients could be observed. During the course of the study the following data were collected from consecutive patients: demographics, cause of CKD assigned by the treating consultant nephrologist, day of first diagnosis of CKD and first nephrology visit, intervening period between first diagnosis and the study visit and between first nephrology visit and the study visit, specialty of referring physician, blood pressure, weight and height and laboratory values of blood urea nitrogen, creatinine and PTH available for physician review during the study visit. Field collected data were used to derive body mass index (BMI) and different estimates of renal function (estimated creatinine clearance by Cockroft-Gault (CG), CG normalized to Body Surface Area (CG-BSA) and estimated glomerular filtration rate (eGFR) according to the CKD-Epi and the MDRD equations (the latter modified to use standardized creatinine values which was almost invariably used by Greek clinical laboratories during the study). For this study, renal function was classified by CKD stage according to the numerical cutoffs in the NKF classification system for estimates normalized to BSA (MDRD, CKD-Epi, CG-BSA) as well as the CG equation. This study was conducted in accordance with a pre-specified protocol and applicable local regulations and guidelines. The protocol was prospectively registered with the National Medicines Organization (registration code EE 25/01-09/09) and approved by the Institutional Review Board of each participating center (Hospital Scientific Committee of Papanikolaou General Hospital Decision of the 3rd Meeting/31-3-2009, Hospital Scientific Committee of Papageorgiou General Hospital Decision of the 131th Meeting/25-05-2009, Hospital Scientific Committee of Laiko Hospital Decision: 114/3-6-09, Hospital Scientific Committee of Attikon University Hospital Decision of the 2nd Meeting/16-03-2009, Hospital Scientific Committee of University Hospital of Ioannina Decision: 196/30-6-2009, Hospital Scientific Committee of University Hospital of Alexandroupoli Decision: 378/9-06-2009, Hospital Scientific Committee of AHEPA Hospital Decision: 257/6-5-2009, Hospital Scientific Committee of Crete University Hospital Decision: 3564/5-5-2009), and each participant provided written informed consent before patient enrollment.

Statistical Methods

Descriptive statistical methods were used to summarize the distribution of all variables: for continuous variables the mean and the standard deviation, and for categorical variables the frequencies of responses at each level were reported. Unadjusted assessments were carried out with the Kruskal Wallis test (continuous responses) and the chi-square test (discrete responses). The pair-wise agreement between estimating equations for renal function was examined by means of Bland Altman plots [16]. We assessed agreement between CKD stages based on all other estimating equations compared to the CKD-Epi with the Spearman correlation coefficient. Regression methods were used to examine the relationship between renal function at the time of the study visit and other covariates, using when appropriate, penalized splines for semi-parametric modeling [17]. Center wise comparisons were carried out by random effect models and portrayed as forest plots, while model heterogeneity was assessed by means of the I^2 statistic. All analyses were performed with SAS v9.1 (table generation) and R v2.12.1 (meta-analyses and figures).

Results

Patient Characteristics and Comparison of Renal Function Estimating Equations

The study included 1501 patients from 9 outpatient nephrology clinics, with a range of 80–300 patients per clinic. Patients on average were older (mean age 66.2±14.6 years, median: 69.6 years), predominantly male (54. 9%), slightly overweight (median BMI: 27.8 kg/m^2). The three most commonly assigned causes of CKD were: diabetic nephropathy (29.7%), hypertensive vascular disease (25.3%) and glomerular diseases (16.3%). The average time interval since the initial diagnosis of CKD was 4.4±5.5 years, while the average time interval since the initial nephrology consultation was 3.0±3.7 years. Other patient characteristics are shown in Table 1.

Average eGFR (by CKD-Epi) was 40.9±23.9 ml/min/1.73 m^2, similar to the MDRD estimate (39.9±22.1 ml/min/1.73 m^2). Estimating renal function by CG, or GC normalized to BSA (CGBSA) resulted in higher numerical values (Figure 1A) than either MDRD or CKD-Epi. Agreement was best between CKD-Epi and MDRD (Figure 1B, average bias 1 ml/min/1.73 m^2, although MDRD yielded lower estimates for values> 60 ml/min/1.73 m^2) and worse between CG and CKD-Epi (Figure 1C); normalization of CG to BSA (CGBSA) improved agreement (Figure 1D, average bias −3.7 ml/min/1.73 m^2).

Table 1. Patient characteristics.

Age (yrs)	66.2 (14.6)
Gender (Male)	824 (55%)
Time since initial diagnosis of renal disease (yrs)	4.4±5.5
Time since initial nephrology consultation (yrs)	3.0±3.7
Systolic Blood Pressure (mmHg)	137.1±17.8
Diastolic Blood Pressure (mmHg)	80.5±10.4
Cause of CKD	
Diabetic Nephropathy	445 (29.7)
Hypertensive Vascular Disease	380 (25.3)
Glomerular Disease	244 (16.3)
Interstitial Nephropathy	75 (5.0)
Solitary kidney post nephrectomy	61 (4.1)
Arterial Hypertension – Congestive Heart Failure	56 (3.7)
Obstructive Nephropathy	38 (2.5)
Polycystic Kidney Disease	35 (2.3)
Autoimmune Disease	29 (1.9)
Nephrolithiasis	28 (1.9)
Dysplastic/Hypoplastic Disease	21 (1.4)
Malignancy	12 (0.8)
Post infectious	7 (0.5)
Drug Related	4 (0.3)
Others	115 (7.7)
Weight (kg)	77.9±15.5
Height (cm)	164.7±9.4
Body Mass Index (BMI, kg/m^2)	28.8±5.5
Body Surface Area (BSA, m^2)	1.84±0.20
Blood Urea Nitrogen (mmol/l)	80.9±45.8
Serum creatinine (μmol/l)	176.8±97.2
eGFR (by CKD-Epi, ml/min/1.73 m^2)	40.9±23.9

Data are given as Mean ±SD or n (%) unless stated otherwise.

Approximately 44% of all patients would be classified as having CKD Stage 3 irrespective of the estimating equation used, while CG and CGBSA classification led to higher prevalence estimates of stages 1–2 in the study population (Figure 2). The correlation between CKD stages based on different estimating equations was highest between MDRD and CKD-Epi (Spearman's ρ 0.96) and lowest between MDRD and CG (Spearman's ρ 0.82).

Renal Function, Cause of CKD and Referral Patterns

The level of renal function (eGFR) in nephrology outpatients appeared to differ according to the renal diagnosis, with diabetic patients having lower eGFR, while patients with glomerular disease having higher eGFR (Table 2). Overall, 63.2% (948/1501) of all CKD patients had been referred to a nephrologist by a physician, most commonly an internist (48.0% of referred patients), a diabetologist or a cardiologist in the overall population and across the different CKD stages (Table 3).

The likelihood of a patient being referred to a nephrologist were assessed as a function of serum creatinine concentration (Figure 3A) and eGFR (Figure 3B) adjusted for the time the patient had spent under nephrology care. The odds ratio of a referral increased as serum creatinine increased above 88.4 μmol/l (1 mg/dl) and peaked around 150 μmol/l and remained relatively stable until 220 μmol/l, to increase thereafter. Stated in other terms, the patients were much more likely to be referred for a creatinine concentration exceeding 220 μmol/l (~2.5 mg/dl) than at lower creatinine values. Viewed as a function of eGFR, the odds of a nephrology referral were a monotonic (decreasing) function of the estimated GFR, so that patients with eGFR< 40 ml/min/1.73 m^2 were more likely to have been referred to a specialist than to have self-referred.

In unadjusted analyses examining renal diagnosis and likelihood of referral, patients with diabetes were more likely to had been referred to a nephrologist by another physician (Odds Ratio 1.82, 95% CI 1.61–2.06, p<0.001), while patients with glomerular and interstitial disease were less likely to have been referred (Table 4). In analyses adjusting for age, gender, SBP, DBP, eGFR (CKD-Epi), center, and time spent under nephrology care, patients with diabetes were more likely to have been referred to a nephrologist (OR: 1.73, 95% CI: 1.25–2.38, p = 0.036), while patients with polycystic kidney disease were less likely to have been referred (OR: 0.69, 95% CI: 0.48–0.97, p = 0.032). Age was not independently associated with lower odds of nephrology referral (p>0.10).

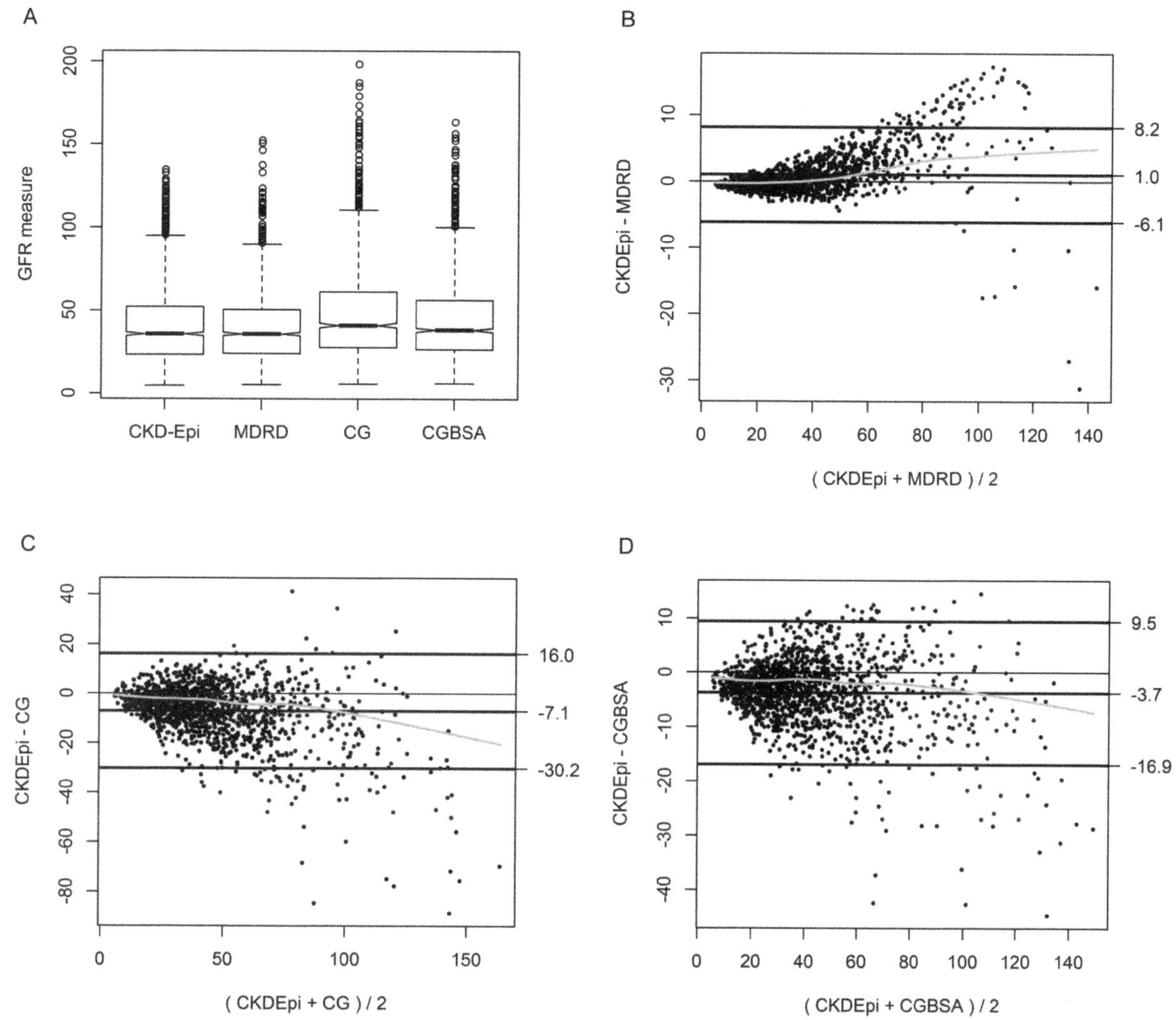

Figure 1. Estimating equations for renal function in the PreSTAR study (A) Box whisker plots of individual estimates based on the CKD Epi (CKD-Epi), MDRD, Cockroft Gault (CG) and Cockroft Gault normalized to Body Surface Area (CGBSA). The thick horizontal line is the median estimate, the bottom and top of each box are the 25th and 75th percentiles, the thin horizontal lines are the most extreme data points within 1.5 times the interquartile range, while the outliers are shown as circles. (B–D) Bland Altman (BA) plot of the MDRD (B), CG(C) and CGBSA against CKD-Epi (D). Each BA plot shows the difference between the two levels of renal function (y-axis) against their average (x-axis) for each patient. The three thick black lines demarcate the bias and the upper and lower limits of agreement, while the thin horizontal line is the zero bias line. In each plot, the gray line is a non-parametric estimate of the constancy of the bias across the range of possible values.

Center level variations

Large center-wise variations and heterogeneity were observed in a number of characteristics of the outpatients attending nephrology clinics (Figure 4): percentage of patients with diabetes (I^2: 89.19%, $p<0.001$), CKD-Epi eGFR (I^2: 95.74%, $p<0.001$) SBP (I^2: 88.58%, $p<0.001$), DBP (I^2: 93.56%, $p<0.001$), BMI (I^2: 90.4%, $p<0.001$), percentage of patients referred by a physician (I^2: 97.62%, $p<0.001$), and time under care in the nephrology clinic(I^2: 96.16%, $p<0.001$).

Discussion

The purpose of this research was to report for the first time the characteristics of the outpatients attending the nephrology clinics of the Greek National Health System (GHNS). We found that a large proportion of patients had referred themselves to nephrologists, with the likelihood of self-referral increasing with higher eGFR levels. Diabetic patients were more likely to have been referred by a physician, even after adjusting for eGFR and other factors. There appears to be some heterogeneity at the center level with respect to the proportion of diabetic patients and self-referrals and the level of blood pressure.

The findings of this report need to be interpreted in light of several factors operating in the Greek healthcare system: a) patients have direct access to laboratory results, irrespective of the public or private ownership of the laboratory, b) lack of automatic eGFR reporting by the laboratories, c) lack of consensus guidelines for referrals to specialists, and finally d) extremely low barriers limiting patient access to specialty care in the outpatient clinics of the GNHS.

Direct patient access to laboratory results, along with their reference range, probably explains the large percentage of self-referrals in this study. Under this scenario, it is very likely that small changes in serum creatinine levels or dipstick positive

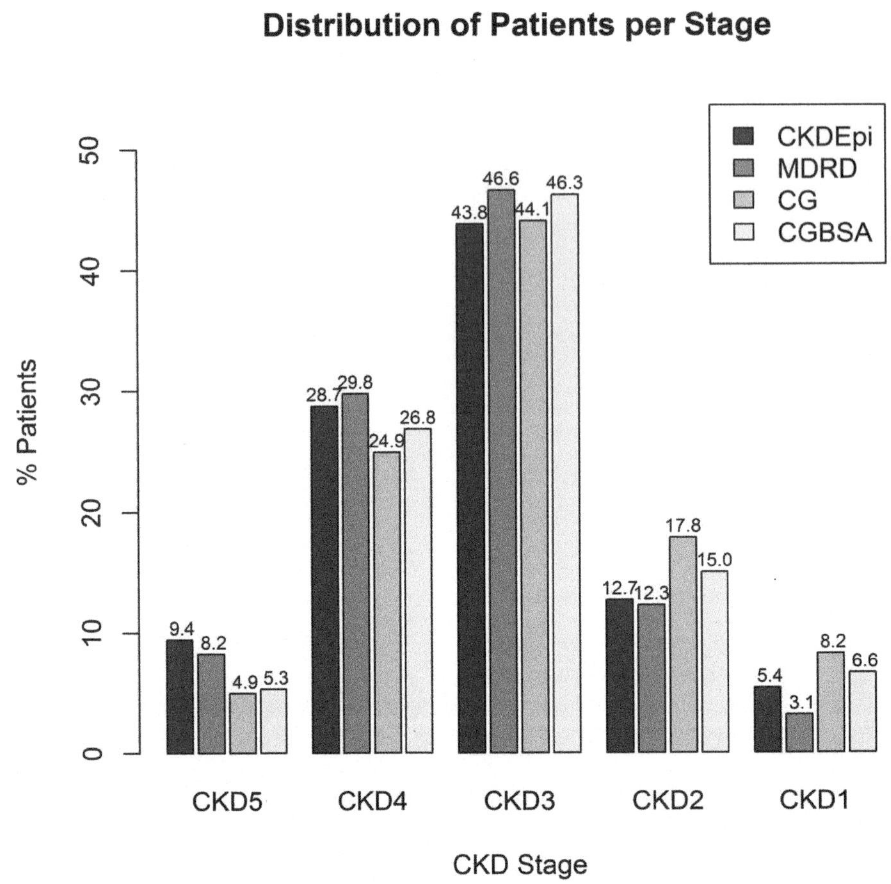

Figure 2. Distribution of stages of CKD in PRESTAR according to different estimating equations, CKD-Epi, MDRD, Cockroft Gault (CG), CG normalized to Body Surface Area (CGBSA).

albuminuria are interpreted by patients as indicating a potential problem with their kidneys. This in turn will prompt them to seek specialty evaluation in the GHNS, which by design does not have a gatekeeper mechanism to restrict access and only commissions a small fee for specialty evaluation. Hence many patients with relatively preserved renal function, but some form of renal pathology, will end up being evaluated by a nephrologist. From this perspective, direct patient access to creatinine test results may provide a less costly alternative to screening programs [9,18] for the identification of patients who may benefit from specialty care [19].

On the other hand, patients referred to a nephrologist by another physician had lower levels of eGFR, implying that either renal disease is under-recognized or some form of filtering of patients by referring physicians is taking place. Such a filtering has been observed in other settings, in which only a small minority (27%) of patients with CKD would be identified as such by their primary providers [20], while large increases in serum creatinine (36%) are used as triggers for patient referral. As very few laboratories currently report eGFR in Greece, we postulate that recognition of renal impairment by non-nephrologists is largely based on serum creatinine concentration, which is an insensitive marker of renal dysfunction [21]. This hypothesis is supported by our finding that the odds of referral as a function of serum creatinine level exceeds parity only when serum creatinine increases above the upper limit of normal (~110 μmol/l) but substantially increases only when creatinine is higher than 220 μmol/l (~2.5 mg/dl), or approximately two times the upper

Table 2. Renal function (eGFR by CKD-Epi in ml/min/1.73 m^2) according to presence or absence of renal diagnosis.

Renal Diagnosis	Present	Absent	P-value
Diabetic Nephropathy	34±18	45±28	<0.001
Hypertensive Vascular Disease	38±19	43±27	0.089
Glomerular Disease	52±29	40±24	<0.001
Interstitial Nephropathy	42±26	42±26	0.830
Polycystic Kidney Disease	48±24	42±26	0.047

Table 3. Specialty of physicians referring patients to Greek National Health System Outpatient Nephrology Clinics.

	Stage 1	Stage 2	Stage 3	Stage 4	Stage 5	All
Referring Specialty	**51 (100%)**	**106 (100%)**	**425 (100%)**	**265 (100%)**	**101 (100%)**	**948 (100%)**
Internal Medicine	26 (51.0)	47 (44.3)	194 (45.6)	138 (52.1)	50 (49.5)	455 (48.0)
Diabetology	1 (2.0)	12 (11.3)	43 (10.1)	30 (11.3)	10 (9.9)	96 (10.1)
Cardiology	0 (0.0)	2 (1.9%)	50 (11.8)	23 (8.7)	9 (8.9)	84 (8.9)
Urology	4 (7.8)	9 (8.5)	31 (7.3)	17 (6.4)	4 (4.0)	65 (6.9)
Endocrinology	1 (2.0)	9 (8.5)	26 (6.1)	15 (5.7)	7 (6.9)	58 (6.1)
General Surgery	2 (3.9)	4 (3.8)	18 (4.2)	8 (3.0)	1 (1.0)	33 (3.5)
Rheumatology	2 (3.9)	5 (4.7)	10 (2.4)	6 (2.3)	3 (3.0)	26 (2.7)
Hematology	3 (5.9)	3 (2.8)	12 (2.8)	2 (0.8)	2 (2.0)	22 (2.3)
GP/Family Medicine	0 (0.0)	2 (1.9)	5 (1.2)	7 (2.6)	2 (2.0)	16 (1.7)
Nephrology	1 (2.0)	3 (2.8)	9 (2.1)	2 (0.8)	1 (1.0)	16 (1.7)
Pulmonary Medicine	0 (0.0)	3 (2.8)	5 (1.2)	4 (1.5)	1 (1.0)	13 (1.4)
Neurology	0 (0.0)	1 (0.9)	3 (0.7)	2 (0.8)	2 (2.0)	8 (0.8)
Vascular Surgery	0 (0.0)	1 (0.9)	3 (0.7)	3 (1.1)	1 (1.0)	8 (0.8)
All others	11 (21.5)	5 (4.7)	16 (3.8)	8 (3.0)	8 (7.9)	48 (4.8)

The number of patients (N = 948) in this table differs from the total number of patients in the study (N = 1501), because N = 1501−948 = 553 patients were self-referrals. Data are given as n(%).

limit of normal. This level, clearly understood to warrant specialty evaluation in the pre-eGFR days [22], coincides with the putative "point of no return" of many renal diseases [23,24] suggesting that some patients may in fact receive sub-optimal care due to such filtering. In contrast, self-referring patients do not seem to apply such filtering, seeking specialty evaluation even when creatinine has increased just above the range of normal values reported by the laboratory. This finding is no different from previous reports showing that non nephrologists will refer late, i.e. after creatinine is higher than 177 μmol/l(~2.0 mg/dl) [25], a pattern which may be due to limited awareness of the need for early specialty evaluation and care [25–31]. Alternatively such late referrals can be due to perceptions of the nephrologist role as one of transitioning the patient with advanced CKD towards a plan for ESRD management when eGFR declines below 30 ml/min/ 1.73 m^2 [32]. In that regards, automatic eGFR reporting, which has been shown to aid the identification of subtle renal impairment [33–35], increase the prescription rate of nephro-protective ACEis/ARBs [33,36,37] and the probability of specialty referral [38], may be viewed as an important tool for the management of CKD patients by primary care practitioners. On the other hand, eGFR reporting may increase the number of inappropriate evaluations and the nephrologist workload [39], as patients are seen at higher levels of eGFR. Nevertheless, recent evaluations have shown that although consults increase [36,40], the proportion of inappropriate consults does not invariably go up [40,41],

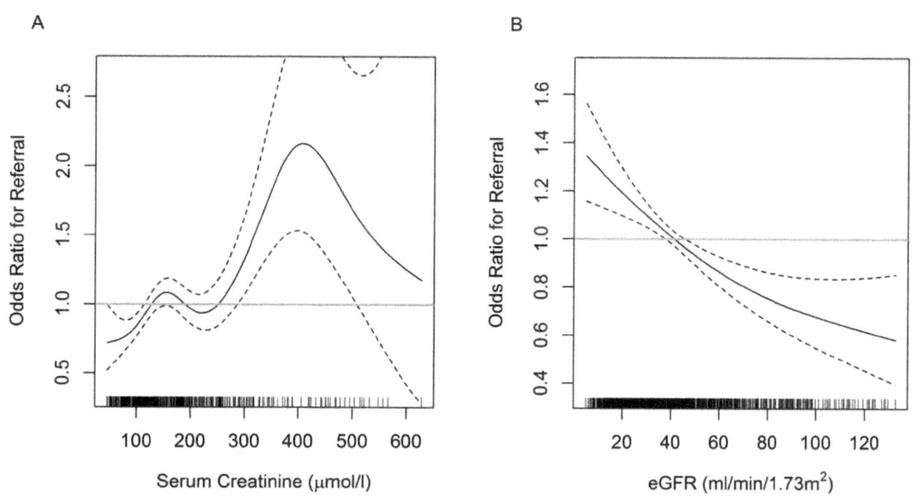

Figure 3. Adjusted odds of a patient having been referred to a nephrologist by a specialist in relation to serum creatinine (A) and eGFR (CKD-Epi), (B) during the study visit. Models were adjusted for age, gender, race, presence of diabetic renal disease, center, systolic and diastolic blood pressure and time the patient had been under nephrology care. Solid black line: estimated adjusted odds ratio, dashed black lines: associated pointwise 95% confidence internal, gray horizontal line: corresponds to an odds ratio of one.

Table 4. Likelihood of a physician referral to a nephrologist by renal diagnosis.

	Unadjusted Analyses			Adjusted Analyses		
Renal Diagnosis	**OR**	**95% CI**	**P**	**OR**	**95% CI**	**P**
Diabetic Nephropathy	1.82	1.43–2.32	<0.001	1.73	1.25–2.39	<0.001
Hypertensive Vascular Disease	0.82	0.65–1.05	0.12	0.40	0.16–1.00	0.051
Glomerular Disease	0.46	0.35–0.61	<0.001	0.73	0.50–1.07	0.10
Interstitial Nephropathy	0.57	0.36–0.91	0.02	0.97	0.52–1.81	0.92
Polycystic Kidney Disease	0.60	0.31–1.18	0.14	0.69	0.49–0.97	0.032

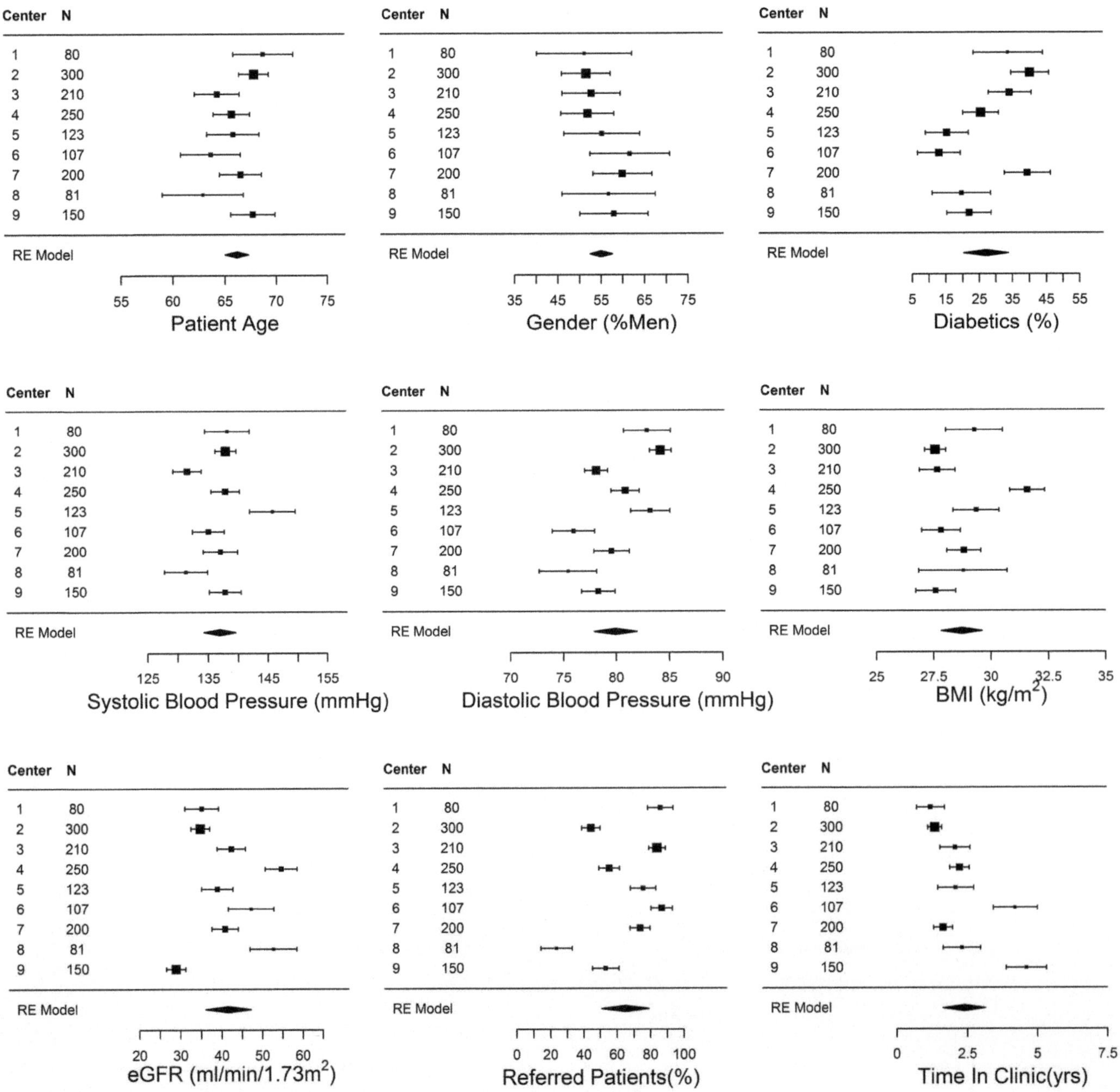

Figure 4. Center wise variations in patient demographics, blood pressure, renal function, diabetes and percentage of referred patients (Could number of patients in each center be added as a footnote?).

the reported eGFR does not influence the rate of consults among patients without CKD, and the additional workload is modest (23 additional consults per nephrologist per year) [42].

Early nephrology referral has been associated with slower disease progression and a 45% reduction in the risk of death [43], and is thus an important aspect of a comprehensive CKD population health care program. Furthermore, patients referred late have inferior control of risk factors for CKD progression, CKD complications, uremic cardiomyopathy and worse patient survival [44,45] when they reach dialysis [7,46]. On the other hand, specialty referral has been shown to lead to higher rates of prescriptions for ACEis/ARBs [47], NSAID avoidance [48], stabilization or improvement in renal function decline CKD [12,43,49] and improved survival among patients with consistent nephrology follow-up [50,51].

Since eGFR reporting may be a valuable component for the optimization of pre-dialysis CKD care and it is currently not implemented on a large scale in the Greek health care system, we explored the utility of different estimating equations for either GFR or creatinine clearance. Assuming the CKD-Epi equation as the emerging gold standard [52,53], our analyses highlight potential pitfalls of the other methods including the imprecision of the MDRD at higher levels of eGFR, the large bias of the CG (moderated somewhat by scaling the result to BSA) and the potential for misclassification at earlier CKD stages. This is particularly important from the perspective of public health expenditure in Greece, as therapies targeting complications of CKD stages 3–5 are currently fully reimbursed without any patient copayment (currently standing at 25% of the price of non CKD related therapies) Hence accurate staging of CKD is important for both early identification and public health budget optimization, goals that can be attained by widespread adoption of the CKD-Epi equation in the GNHS.

In this report, we also observed center variations in a number of characteristics relating to diagnosis, pathway to specialty evaluation, and blood pressure levels of CKD patients under nephrology care. Since the participating centers in this study cover both rural and urban segments of the Greek population, it is possible that some of these differences directly reflect some heterogeneity in the distribution of risk factors for CKD, local practice patterns of referring physicians and nephrologists and models of cooperation between them. Nevertheless, the fact that such differences do exist, suggest a missed opportunity for standardizing care at a national level by e.g. CKD diagnosis and treatment educational programs aiming at non-specialists and promotion and adoption of guidelines specifying thresholds for appropriate referral and blood pressure targets.

The findings and interpretations in this report should be interpreted in light of certain limitations. First, the cross-sectional design of the study precludes drawing conclusions about the rate of renal function decline over time among study participants. Second, we did not have access to referring physicians' records so we cannot explain the apparent channeling bias in referring patients with diabetes to a nephrologist. This pattern may reflect the limited understanding of the subtle manifestations of a wide spectrum of renal pathology by non-specialists, the sensitization of non-nephrologists to the renal complications of diabetes [54], or possibly a skewed view by non-specialists about the benefits of nephrologist co-management [13,49,55–57]. A study of referring physicians could help us understand these referral patterns, suggesting one possible way for filling this knowledge gap. Third, even though the MDRD and CKD-Epi equations have been evaluated in a number of different populations and cohorts, no direct validation exists for the Greek population, so that the comparison between these equations should not be viewed as one of a method against a gold standard. Finally our study was conducted before the 2012 KDIGO classification of CKD stages along the two dimensions of eGFR and albuminuria categories, and thus we did not collect data about abnormal urinary biomarkers (proteinuria, albuminuria or even hematuria) in our patients. Hence, we cannot exclude the likelihood that such abnormalities drive nephrology referrals at higher levels of eGFR especially for patients with glomerular disease who are more likely to manifest proteinuria and/or hematuria.

In summary, we have undertaken the first national cross-sectional evaluation of non-dialysis dependent CKD patients in outpatient nephrology clinics of the Greek National Health System. We found that many patients appear to be referred late by physicians, while self-referred patients consult a nephrologist at a higher level of renal function possibly due to direct access to test results. To reduce the burden of ESRD in Greece, with the 8th highest incidence rate in the world [15], which during the current financial crisis bears the cost of providing unfunded dialysis services to a large number of uninsured individuals including illegal immigrants future initiatives should focus on the adoption of eGFR reporting in order to facilitate early detection, appropriate confirmatory testing, and prescription of reno-protective medications in order to reduce the progression to dialysis dependency.

Acknowledgments

We would like to thank the patients and the staff in the hospital centers for their participation as well as Abbott Laboratories Hellas clinical research staff for their valuable contribution during the execution of this study.

Author Contributions

Conceived and designed the experiments: KX. Performed the experiments: KS DT JB DV KCS VV PN CI ED. Analyzed the data: CA. Wrote the paper: KS DT JB DV KCS VV PN CI ED KX CA.

References

1. Yang M, Fox CH, Vassalotti J, Choi M (2011) Complications of progression of CKD. Adv Chronic Kidney Dis 18: 400–405. doi: 10.1053/j.ackd.2011.10.001.
2. Locatelli F, Vecchio LD, Pozzoni P (2002) The importance of early detection of chronic kidney disease. Nephrol Dial Transplant 17 Suppl 11: 2–7.
3. Stenvinkel P (2010) Chronic kidney disease: a public health priority and harbinger of premature cardiovascular disease. J Intern Med 268: 456–467. doi: 10.1111/j.1365-2796.2010.02269.x.
4. Campbell KH, Smith SG, Hemmerich J, Stankus N, Fox C, et al. (2011) Patient and provider determinants of nephrology referral in older adults with severe chronic kidney disease: a survey of provider decision making. BMC Nephrol 12: 47. doi: 10.1186/1471-2369-12-47.
5. Kinchen KS, Sadler J, Fink N, Brookmeyer R, Klag MJ, et al. (2002) The timing of specialist evaluation in chronic kidney disease and mortality. Ann Intern Med 137: 479–486.
6. Richards N, Harris K, Whitfield M, O'Donoghue D, Lewis R, et al. (2008) The impact of population-based identification of chronic kidney disease using estimated glomerular filtration rate (eGFR) reporting. Nephrol Dial Transplant 23: 556–561. doi: 10.1093/ndt/gfm839.
7. De Jager DJ, Voormolen N, Krediet RT, Dekker FW, Boeschoten EW, et al. (2011) Association between time of referral and survival in the first year of dialysis in diabetics and the elderly. Nephrol Dial Transplant 26: 652–658. doi: 10.1093/ndt/gfq438.
8. Lenz O, Mekala DP, Patel DV, Fornoni A, Metz D, et al. (2005) Barriers to successful care for chronic kidney disease. BMC Nephrol 6: 11. doi: 10.1186/1471-2369-6-11.
9. Stolk M, McCoy C (2011) Chronic kidney disease: screening, follow-up and referral. Med Health R I 94: 63–65.
10. Gøransson LG, Bergrem H (2001) Consequences of late referral of patients with end-stage renal disease. J Intern Med 250: 154–159.

11. Levin A (2000) Consequences of late referral on patient outcomes. Nephrol Dial Transplant 15 Suppl 3: 8–13.
12. Black C, Sharma P, Scotland G, McCullough K, McGurn D, et al. (2010) Early referral strategies for management of people with markers of renal disease: a systematic review of the evidence of clinical effectiveness, cost-effectiveness and economic analysis. Health Technol Assess 14: 1–184. doi: 10.3310/hta14210.
13. Orlando LA, Owen WF, Matchar DB (2007) Relationship between nephrologist care and progression of chronic kidney disease. N C Med J 68: 9–16.
14. Abdel-Kader K, Fischer GS, Li J, Moore CG, Hess R, et al. (2011) Automated clinical reminders for primary care providers in the care of CKD: a small cluster-randomized controlled trial. Am J Kidney Dis 58: 894–902. doi: 10.1053/j.ajkd.2011.08.028.
15. U S Renal Data System (2011) International Comparisons. USRDS 2011 Annual Data Report: Atlas of Chronic Kidney Disease and End-Stage Renal Disease in the United States. Bethesda, MD: National Institutes of Health, National Institute of Diabetes and Digestive and Kidney Diseases.
16. Bland JM, Altman DG (1986) Statistical methods for assessing agreement between two methods of clinical measurement. Lancet 1: 307–310.
17. Ruppert D, Wand MP, Carroll RJ (2009) Semiparametric regression during 2003-2007. Electron J Stat 3: 1193–1256. doi: 10.1214/09-EJS525.
18. Jurkovitz CT, Elliott D, Li S, Saab G, Bomback AS, et al. (2012) Physician utilization, risk-factor control, and CKD progression among participants in the Kidney Early Evaluation Program (KEEP). Am J Kidney Dis 59: S24–S33. doi: 10.1053/j.ajkd.2011.11.019.
19. Cheung CK, Bhandari S (2009) Perspectives on eGFR reporting from the interface between primary and secondary care. Clin J Am Soc Nephrol 4: 258–260. doi: 10.2215/CJN.05151008.
20. Aakre KM, Thue G, Svarstad E, Skadberg Ø, Sandberg S (2011) Laboratory investigation and follow-up of chronic kidney disease stage 3 in primary care. Clin Chim Acta 412: 1138–1142. doi: 10.1016/j.cca.2011.03.004.
21. Swedko PJ, Clark HD, Paramsothy K, Akbari A (2003) Serum creatinine is an inadequate screening test for renal failure in elderly patients. Arch Intern Med 163: 356–360.
22. Mendelssohn DC, Barrett BJ, Brownscombe LM, Ethier J, Greenberg DE, et al. (1999) Elevated levels of serum creatinine: recommendations for management and referral. CMAJ 161: 413–417.
23. Maschio G, Oldrizzi L, Rugiu C (1991) Is there a "point of no return" in progressive renal disease? J Am Soc Nephrol 2: 832–840.
24. Komatsu H, Fujimoto S, Sato Y, Hara S, Yamada K, et al. (2005) "Point of no return (PNR)" in progressive IgA nephropathy: significance of blood pressure and proteinuria management up to PNR. J Nephrol 18: 690–695.
25. Tamba K, Kusano E, Tabei K, Kajii E, Asano Y (2009) Physicians make different decisions from nephrologists at serum creatinine 2.0 mg/dl. Clin Exp Nephrol 13: 447–451. doi: 10.1007/s10157-009-0176-4.
26. Agrawal V, Ghosh AK, Barnes MA, McCullough PA (2009) Perception of indications for nephrology referral among internal medicine residents: a national online survey. Clin J Am Soc Nephrol 4: 323–328. doi: 10.2215/CJN.03510708.
27. Boulware LE, Troll MU, Jaar BG, Myers DI, Powe NR (2006) Identification and referral of patients with progressive CKD: a national study. Am J Kidney Dis 48: 192–204. doi: 10.1053/j.ajkd.2006.04.073.
28. Diamantidis CJ, Powe NR, Jaar BG, Greer RC, Troll MU, et al. (2011) Primary care-specialist collaboration in the care of patients with chronic kidney disease. Clin J Am Soc Nephrol 6: 334–343. doi: 10.2215/CJN.06240710.
29. Lenz O, Fornoni A (2006) Chronic kidney disease care delivered by US family medicine and internal medicine trainees: results from an online survey. BMC Med 4: 30. doi: 10.1186/1741-7015-4-30.
30. Navaneethan SD, Kandula P, Jeevanantham V, Nally JV Jr, Liebman SE (2010) Referral patterns of primary care physicians for chronic kidney disease in general population and geriatric patients. Clin Nephrol 73: 260–267.
31. Finkelstein FO, Story K, Firanek C, Barre P, Takano T, et al. (2008) Perceived knowledge among patients cared for by nephrologists about chronic kidney disease and end-stage renal disease therapies. Kidney Int 74: 1178–1184. doi: 10.1038/ki.2008.376.
32. Coritsidis GN, Linden E, Stern AS (2011) The role of the primary care physician in managing early stages of chronic kidney disease. Postgrad Med 123: 177–185. doi: 10.3810/pgm.2011.09.2473.
33. Wyatt C, Konduri V, Eng J, Rohatgi R (2007) Reporting of estimated GFR in the primary care clinic. Am J Kidney Dis 49: 634–641. doi: 10.1053/j.ajkd.2007.02.258.
34. Phillips LA, Donovan KL, Phillips AO (2009) Renal quality outcomes framework and eGFR: impact on secondary care. QJM 102: 415–423. doi: 10.1093/qjmed/hcp030.
35. Akbari A, Swedko PJ, Clark HD, Hogg W, Lemelin J, et al. (2004) Detection of chronic kidney disease with laboratory reporting of estimated glomerular filtration rate and an educational program. Arch Intern Med 164: 1788–1792. doi: 10.1001/archinte.164.16.1788.
36. Kagoma YK, Weir MA, Iansavichus AV, Hemmelgarn BR, Akbari A, et al. (2011) Impact of estimated GFR reporting on patients, clinicians, and health-care systems: a systematic review. Am J Kidney Dis 57: 592–601. doi: 10.1053/j.ajkd.2010.08.029.
37. Jain AK, Cuerden MS, McLeod I, Hemmelgarn B, Akbari A, et al. (2012) Reporting of the estimated glomerular filtration rate was associated with increased use of angiotensin-converting enzyme inhibitors and angiotensin-II receptor blockers in CKD. Kidney Int 81: 1248–1253. doi: 10.1038/ki.2012.18.
38. Jain AK, McLeod I, Huo C, Cuerden MS, Akbari A, et al. (2009) When laboratories report estimated glomerular filtration rates in addition to serum creatinines, nephrology consults increase. Kidney Int 76: 318–323. doi: 10.1038/ki.2009.158.
39. Jain A, Hemmelgarn BR (2011) Impact of estimated glomerular filtration rate reporting on nephrology referrals: a review of the literature. Curr Opin Nephrol Hypertens 20: 218–223. doi: 10.1097/MNH.0b013e3283446193.
40. Noble E, Johnson DW, Gray N, Hollett P, Hawley CM, et al. (2008) The impact of automated eGFR reporting and education on nephrology service referrals. Nephrol Dial Transplant 23: 3845–3850. doi: 10.1093/ndt/gfn385.
41. Akbari A, Grimshaw J, Stacey D, Hogg W, Ramsay T, et al. (2012) Change in appropriate referrals to nephrologists after the introduction of automatic reporting of the estimated glomerular filtration rate. CMAJ 184: E269–E276. doi: 10.1503/cmaj.110678.
42. Hemmelgarn BR, Zhang J, Manns BJ, James MT, Quinn RR, et al. (2010) Nephrology visits and health care resource use before and after reporting estimated glomerular filtration rate. JAMA 303: 1151–1158. doi: 10.1001/jama.2010.303.
43. Jones C, Roderick P, Harris S, Rogerson M (2006) Decline in kidney function before and after nephrology referral and the effect on survival in moderate to advanced chronic kidney disease. Nephrol Dial Transplant 21: 2133–2143. doi: 10.1093/ndt/gfl198.
44. Herget-Rosenthal S, Quellmann T, Linden C, Hollenbeck M, Jankowski V, et al. (2010) How does late nephrological co-management impact chronic kidney disease? - an observational study. Int J Clin Pract 64: 1784–1792. doi: 10.1111/j.1742-1241.2010.02535.x.
45. Shin SJ, Kim HW, Chung S, Chung HW, Lee SJ, et al. (2007) Late referral to a nephrologist increases the risk of uremia-related cardiac hypertrophy in patients on hemodialysis. Nephron Clin Pract 107: c139–c146. doi: 10.1159/000110034.
46. Hasegawa T, Bragg-Gresham JL, Yamazaki S, Fukuhara S, Akizawa T, et al. (2009) Greater first-year survival on hemodialysis in facilities in which patients are provided earlier and more frequent pre-nephrology visits. Clin J Am Soc Nephrol 4: 595–602. doi: 10.2215/CJN.03540708.
47. Chen S-C, Chang J-M, Chou M-C, Lin M-Y, Chen J-H, et al. (2008) Slowing renal function decline in chronic kidney disease patients after nephrology referral. Nephrology (Carlton) 13: 730–736. doi: 10.1111/j.1440-1797.2008.01023.x.
48. Abdel-Kader K, Fischer GS, Johnston JR, Gu C, Moore CG, et al. (2011) Characterizing pre-dialysis care in the era of eGFR reporting: a cohort study. BMC Nephrol 12: 12. doi: 10.1186/1471-2369-12-12.
49. Meran S, Don K, Shah N, Donovan K, Riley S, et al. (2011) Impact of chronic kidney disease management in primary care. QJM 104: 27–34. doi: 10.1093/qjmed/hcq151.
50. Tseng C-L, Kern EFO, Miller DR, Tiwari A, Maney M, et al. (2008) Survival benefit of nephrologic care in patients with diabetes mellitus and chronic kidney disease. Arch Intern Med 168: 55–62. doi: 10.1001/archinternmed.2007.9.
51. Chen S-C, Hwang S-J, Tsai J-C, Liu W-C, Hwang S-C, et al. (2010) Early nephrology referral is associated with prolonged survival in hemodialysis patients even after exclusion of lead-time bias. Am J Med Sci 339: 123–126. doi: 10.1097/MAJ.0b013e3181c0678a.
52. O'Callaghan CA, Shine B, Lasserson DS (2011) Chronic kidney disease: a large-scale population-based study of the effects of introducing the CKD-EPI formula for eGFR reporting. BMJ Open 1: e000308. doi: 10.1136/bmjopen-2011-000308.
53. Stevens LA, Padala S, Levey AS (2010) Advances in glomerular filtration rate-estimating equations. Curr Opin Nephrol Hypertens 19: 298–307. doi: 10.1097/MNH.0b013e32833893e2.
54. Davis Giardina T, Singh H (2011) Should patients get direct access to their laboratory test results? An answer with many questions. JAMA 306: 2502–2503. doi: 10.1001/jama.2011.1797.
55. Campbell GA, Bolton WK (2011) Referral and comanagement of the patient with CKD. Adv Chronic Kidney Dis 18: 420–427. doi: 10.1053/j.ackd.2011.10.006.
56. Bayliss EA, Bhardwaja B, Ross C, Beck A, Lanese DM (2011) Multidisciplinary team care may slow the rate of decline in renal function. Clin J Am Soc Nephrol 6: 704–710. doi: 10.2215/CJN.06610810.
57. Mondry A, Zhu A-L, Loh M, Vo TD, Hahn K (2004) Active collaboration with primary care providers increases specialist referral in chronic renal disease. BMC Nephrol 5: 16. doi: 10.1186/1471-2369-5-16.

Leucocyte Telomere Length and Risk of Type 2 Diabetes Mellitus: New Prospective Cohort Study and Literature-Based Meta-Analysis

Peter Willeit[1,2*⁹], Julia Raschenberger[3⁹], Emma E. Heydon[2], Sotirios Tsimikas[4], Margot Haun[3], Agnes Mayr[5], Siegfried Weger[6], Joseph L. Witztum[4], Adam S. Butterworth[2], Johann Willeit[1], Florian Kronenberg[3], Stefan Kiechl[1*]

1 Department of Neurology, Innsbruck Medical University, Innsbruck, Austria, **2** Department of Public Health and Primary Care, University of Cambridge, Cambridge, United Kingdom, **3** Division of Genetic Epidemiology, Innsbruck Medical University, Innsbruck, Austria, **4** Department of Medicine, University of California San Diego, La Jolla, United States of America, **5** Department of Laboratory Medicine, Bruneck Hospital, Bruneck, Italy, **6** Department of Internal Medicine, Bruneck Hospital, Bruneck, Italy

Abstract

Background: Short telomeres have been linked to various age-related diseases. We aimed to assess the association of telomere length with incident type 2 diabetes mellitus (T2DM) in prospective cohort studies.

Methods: Leucocyte relative telomere length (RTL) was measured using quantitative polymerase chain reaction in 684 participants of the prospective population-based Bruneck Study (1995 baseline), with repeat RTL measurements performed in 2005 (n = 558) and 2010 (n = 479). Hazard ratios for T2DM were calculated across quartiles of baseline RTL using Cox regression models adjusted for age, sex, body-mass index, smoking, socio-economic status, physical activity, alcohol consumption, high-density lipoprotein cholesterol, log high-sensitivity C-reactive protein, and waist-hip ratio. Separate analyses corrected hazard ratios for within-person variability using multivariate regression calibration of repeated measurements. To contextualise findings, we systematically sought PubMed, Web of Science and EMBASE for relevant articles and pooled results using random-effects meta-analysis.

Results: Over 15 years of follow-up, 44 out of 606 participants free of diabetes at baseline developed incident T2DM. The adjusted hazard ratio for T2DM comparing the bottom vs. the top quartile of baseline RTL (i.e. shortest vs. longest) was 2.00 (95% confidence interval: 0.90 to 4.49; P = 0.091), and 2.31 comparing the bottom quartile vs. the remainder (1.21 to 4.41; P = 0.011). The corresponding hazard ratios corrected for within-person RTL variability were 3.22 (1.27 to 8.14; P = 0.014) and 2.86 (1.45 to 5.65; P = 0.003). In a random-effects meta-analysis of three prospective cohort studies involving 6,991 participants and 2,011 incident T2DM events, the pooled relative risk was 1.31 (1.07 to 1.60; P = 0.010; $I^2 = 69\%$).

Conclusions/Interpretation: Low RTL is independently associated with the risk of incident T2DM. To avoid regression dilution biases in observed associations of RTL with disease risk, future studies should implement methods correcting for within-person variability in RTL. The causal role of short telomeres in T2DM development remains to be determined.

Editor: Arthur J. Lustig, Tulane University Health Sciences Center, United States of America

Funding: This project was funded by a grant of the 'Tiroler Wissenschaftsfonds', Austria. The Bruneck Study was supported by the 'Pustertaler Verein zur Prävention von Herz- und Hirngefaesserkrankungen, Gesundheitsbezirk Bruneck' and the 'Assessorat für Gesundheit', Province of Bolzano, Italy. The funders had no role in study design, data collection and analysis, decision to publish, or preparation of the manuscript.

Competing Interests: The authors have declared that no competing interests exist.

* Email: pwilleit@outlook.com (PW); stefan.kiechl@i-med.ac.at (SK)

⁹ These authors contributed equally to this work.

Introduction

Telomeres are the extreme ends of eukaryotic chromosomes, stabilising and protecting the chromosome from degradation [1,2]. Telomeres shorten with each cellular division, accelerated by inflammation and oxidative stress, and, below a critical length, the apoptotic programme of the cell is induced [1,3].

Short telomeres are associated with increased risk of several age-related diseases [2] such as cardiovascular diseases [4–8] and cancer [9–11]. It has been suggested that biological ageing reflected by telomere length is also related to the development of type 2 diabetes (T2DM) [12]. Proposed pathophysiological mechanisms include a reduction in beta-cell mass [13], impaired insulin secretion [14] and adipocyte insulin resistance elicited by cellular senescence [15]. On the other hand, diabetic patients suffer from elevated levels of oxidative stress [16], which in turn leads to telomere attrition [17]. To disentangle these two effects and establish a temporal relationship, it is crucial to investigate the association of telomere length with risk of new-onset T2DM in studies with a prospective design. In such studies, telomere length is assessed before the diabetes diagnosis (although subclinical pre-diabetic changes may already be present). Furthermore, because telomere length fluctuates considerably over time [18–27], studies are needed that take into account the within-person variability of telomere length. Such analyses use repeated measurements instead of single baseline measurements to predict "long-term average" telomere length and therefore help estimate the "true" aetiological association with T2DM risk.

Our aims were three-fold. First, to assess the association of baseline leucocyte relative telomere length (RTL) with new-onset T2DM in the prospective population-based Bruneck Study. Second, to correct association estimates for long-term within-person variability of RTL. Third, to contextualise findings in a literature-based meta-analysis of all prospective evidence available to date.

Material and Methods

The Bruneck Study

The Bruneck Study is a prospective, population-based survey conducted in 1,000 individuals aged 40 to 79 years (125 per sex and decade of life). In 1990, participants were randomly selected from the inhabitants of the town of Bruneck (South Tyrol, Italy) and were examined every five years between 1990 and 2010 [5,10,19,28,29]. Participation rates exceeded 90% at all surveys. In the present study, we used leucocyte RTL measurements available from the surveys in 1995, 2005 and 2010 (n = 684, 558, and 479, respectively). Full medical records were available for review for all individuals, including those who did not participate in or died during follow up (100% follow up for clinical endpoints). The study protocol was approved by the local ethic committee of Bolzano ('Comitato etico del comprensorio sanitario di Bolzano'; approval number 28–2010). All participants gave informed written informed consent before taking part and the study complies with the Declaration of Helsinki.

Clinical history and examination at baseline

We assessed risk factors by validated standard procedures as previously described [5,28]. Waist and hip circumferences were assessed with a plastic tape measure at the levels of the umbilicus and the greater trochanters respectively. We defined socioeconomic status on a three-category scale (low, medium or high) on the basis of information about occupational status and educational level of the person with the highest income in the household. High socioeconomic status was assumed if the participant had ≥12 years of education or an occupation with an average monthly income ≥$2,000 (baseline salary before tax). Low socioeconomic status was defined by ≤8 years of education or an average monthly income ≤$1,000. Physical activity was assessed using the validated Baeke Score [30]. Oxidation-specific biomarkers and other laboratory parameters were measured as previously described [31]. HbA1c was quantified using high performance liquid chromatography (DCCT-aligned assay). We estimated the degree of insulin resistance by homeostasis model assessment (HOMA-IR) using the formula fasting plasma glucose in mmol/l × fasting serum insulin in mU/l divided by 22.5 [32], with higher HOMA-IR values indicating higher insulin resistance. LDL cholesterol was estimated using the Friedewald equation [33].

Measurement of leucocyte telomere length

Genomic DNA from the Bruneck Study blood samples was extracted from frozen EDTA-blood samples with the Invisorb Blood Universal Kit. DNA concentrations were measured with the Tecan NanoQuant infinite M200. Samples were normalised in 96-well microtiter plates. Leucocyte RTL was measured in a single laboratory by a single person within a short time period using a quantitative polymerase chain reaction (qPCR) approach developed by Cawthon [34] to measure T/S-ratios. The protocol was modified with regard to control samples and data processing as recently described [35]. T/S-ratios are proportional to individual telomere length. The composition of singleplex PCRs for telomere (T) and housekeeping gene (S) PCRs was identical. DNA samples were run in 15 μl reactions containing 1× Quantifast TM SYBR Green PCR mastermix (Qiagen), 10 ng of DNA, 1 μM of telomere primer or 250 nm of housekeeping gene 36B4 primer. The primer sequences (5′→3′) were: tel1b CGGTTTGTTTGG-GTTTGGGTTTGGGTTTGGGTTTGGGTT; tel2b GGCTT-GCCTTACCCTTACCCTTACCCTTACCCTTACCCT; 36B4u CAGCAAGTGGGAAGGTGTAATCC; 36B4d CCCATTCTA-TCATCAACGGGTACAA [5]. Each qPCR was carried out in 384-well format which was vertically segmented in two parts: one for the telomeres (T) and one for the housekeeping gene 36B4 (S). Each qPCR plate contained the standard DNA, a quality control (commercially available DNA-Human Genomic DNA, Roche), and a non-template control. All samples, standards, and controls were analysed in quadruplicate. All sample transfers and dilution steps were performed with a Tecan robotic workstation. Relative qPCR was carried out on an Applied Biosystems Taqman Fast Real-Time PCR 7900HT System. The thermal cycling began with the initial polymerase activation step (10 min at 95°C) and was followed by 40 cycles of 95°C for 15 s, 60°C for 1 min. The relative quantities were determined by the efficiency correction method [36], which does not require calibration curves and includes the individual real-time PCR efficiencies. Efficiencies were computed for all replicates of each sample. To check PCR data for outliers, the coefficients of variation (intra-assay CVs) were assessed for the Ct-values and the efficiency-values of quadruplicates in each gene. All single outlying values (CV>5%) were removed from further analyses. Further details were already published before [35]. Although RTL of samples from 1995 and 2005 was already measured before [5,10], we reanalysed all samples of all time points together with the newly extracted samples from 2010 to avoid a measurement error over the time period. In addition, RTL measurement of samples of the same participant of all available time points were positioned on the same 384-well qPCR plate. After each qPCR run a melting curve analysis was performed to verify the specificity and identity of the products. The inter-assay coefficient of variation of T/S-ratios of the quality control, which was positioned on each 384-well plate (a total of 37 plates), was 11.8%. The laboratory personnel who performed the RTL measurements were blinded to the participants' status and outcome.

Definition of type 2 diabetes mellitus

We established the diagnosis of T2DM according to the 1997 American Diabetes Association criteria (fasting glucose ≥126 mg/dl, i.e. ≥7 mmol/l) or when the subjects had a clinical diagnosis of T2DM and received anti-diabetic treatment [37]. Impaired fasting glucose was defined as a fasting glucose level of 100 to <126 mg/dl (i.e. 5.6 to <7.0 mmol/l). Self-reported T2DM status was confirmed by reviewing the medical records of the subject's general practitioners and Bruneck Hospital. A major strength of the Bruneck Study is that virtually all participants living in the

Characteristic	Mean (SD) or n (%)	Standardised mean difference (95% CI) in RTL per SD increase or compared to reference group
Questionnaire-based and anthropometric measures		
Age, years	63 (11)	-0.22 (-0.30, -0.15)***
Sex		
Male	335 (49%)	[Reference]
Female	349 (51%)	0.11 (-0.04, 0.25)
Body mass index, kg/m^2	26 (4)	0.01 (-0.06, 0.08)
Current smoker		
Never/Ex	551 (81%)	[Reference]
Current	133 (19%)	-0.16 (-0.35, 0.03)
Socioeconomic status		
Low	412 (60%)	[Reference]
Middle	156 (23%)	-0.02 (-0.21, 0.17)
High	116 (17%)	0.12 (-0.08, 0.33)
Physical activity, Baeke score	2.4 (0.9)	-0.03 (-0.11, 0.05)
Alcohol consumption, g/d	23 (31)	-0.08 (-0.17, 0.01)
Lipid markers		
HDL cholesterol, mg/dl	59 (17)	-0.04 (-0.11, 0.04)
LDL cholesterol, mg/dl	144 (38)	0.05 (-0.03, 0.12)
Log Lp(a), mg/dl	2.5 (1.4)	-0.02 (-0.09, 0.05)
Markers of inflammation		
Log hsCRP, mg/l	-1.7 (1.0)	0.07 (-0.01, 0.14)
Fibrinogen, mg/dl	290 (78)	0.05 (-0.02, 0.13)
Leukocyte count per µl	6457 (1713)	-0.06 (-0.13, 0.01)
Log IL-6, ng/l	1.4 (1.0)	0.02 (-0.05, 0.10)
alpha1-Antitrypsin, mg/dl	200 (37)	-0.00 (-0.08, 0.07)
Markers of oxidative stress		
Log OxPL/apoB, RLU	8.8 (0.9)	0.04 (-0.03, 0.12)
Log OxPL/apoB, ratio	-2.6 (0.9)	0.04 (-0.03, 0.12)
MDA-LDL IgG, RLU	9.6 (0.5)	0.02 (-0.05, 0.10)
MDA-LDL IgM, RLU	9.6 (0.5)	0.03 (-0.04, 0.11)
Cu-OxLDL IgG, RLU	9.0 (0.5)	0.04 (-0.04, 0.11)
Cu-OxLDL IgM, RLU	8.3 (0.6)	0.04 (-0.04, 0.12)
ApoB-IC IgG, RLU	7006 (3843)	-0.00 (-0.08, 0.07)
ApoB-IC IgM, RLU	5112 (2796)	0.04 (-0.04, 0.11)
Ferritin, ng/ml	136 (172)	-0.02 (-0.10, 0.05)
Ceruloplasmin, mg/dl	27 (5)	0.07 (-0.01, 0.15)
Uric acid, mg/dl	4.7 (1.3)	0.02 (-0.06, 0.10)
Markers of dysglycaemia		
Fasting plasma glucose, mg/dl	102 (25)	-0.01 (-0.08, 0.07)
Urine glucose, mg/dl	116 (60)	-0.05 (-0.12, 0.03)
Log HOMA-IR	1.1 (0.6)	-0.03 (-0.10, 0.05)
HbA1c, %	5.8 (3.7)	-0.00 (-0.07, 0.07)

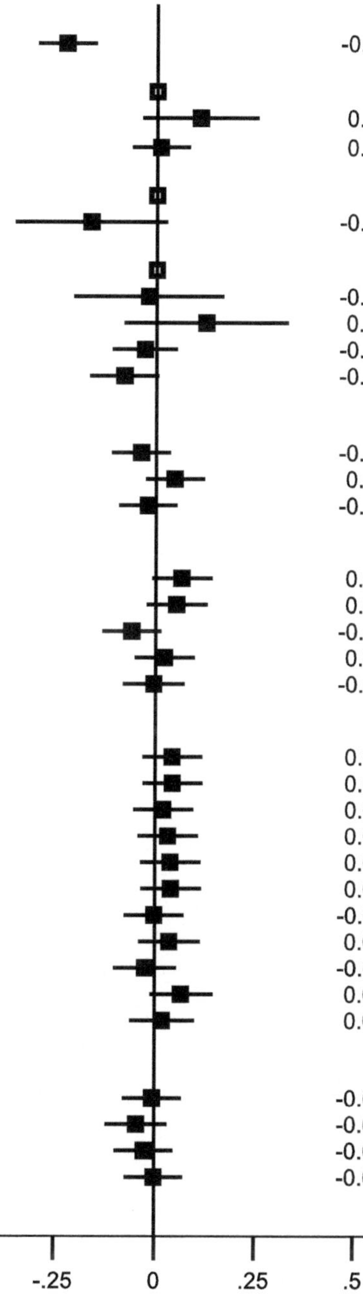

Figure 1. Baseline characteristics of the Bruneck Study population and their cross-sectional association with leucocyte relative telomere length (1995, n = 684). Standardised mean differences in leucocyte relative telomere length were adjusted for age and sex. Asterisks indicate level of statistical significance: *P≤0.05; **P≤0.01; ***P≤0.001. The mean (SD) of HbA1c was 5.8% (3.7%) in DCCT-derived units and 40 mmol/mol (17 mmol/mol) in SI units. Abbreviations: ApoB, apolipoprotein B; ApoB-IC, apoB-immune complexes; CI, confidence interval; Cu-OxLDL, copper-oxidised low-density lipoprotein; HbA1c, glycated haemoglobin; HDL, high-density lipoprotein; HOMA-IR, homeostatic model assessment of insulin resistance; hsCRP, high-sensitivity C-reactive protein; IgG, immunoglobulin G; IgM, immunoglobulin M; LDL, low-density lipoprotein; RTL, relative telomere length; MDA, malondialdehyde; OxPL/apoB, oxidised phospholipids on apolipoprotein B-100; SD, standard deviation; RLU, relative light unit; SMD, standardised mean difference; WHR, waist-hip ratio.

survey area are referred to the same hospital and the network existing between hospital and practitioners allows retrieval of full medical information. There were no cases of type 1 diabetes mellitus in this cohort.

Literature-based meta-analysis

Prospective studies of the association of telomere length with the risk of incident T2DM were sought using the databases PubMed, Web of Science and EMBASE. The search strategy combined

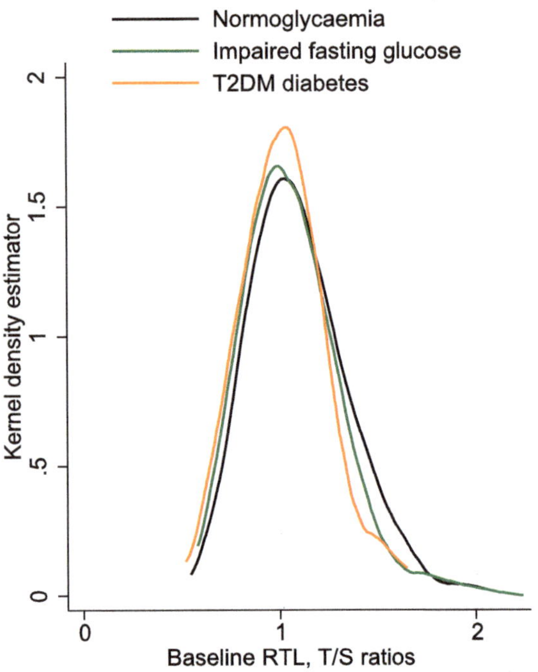

Figure 2. Distribution of baseline leucocyte relative telomere length in the Bruneck Study according to different disease states (1995, n = 684). Abbreviations: RTL, relative telomere length; T2DM, type 2 diabetes mellitus. There were 390 participants with normoglycaemia, 216 participants with impaired fasting glucose, and 78 participants with a clinical diagnosis of T2DM.

keywords related to the exposure of interest ("telomere" or "telomeres"), the outcome ("diabetes") and the study design ("cohort" or "prospective" or "longitudinal" or "hazard" or "risk" or "odds"). We included articles published before March 26th 2014 and applied no language restrictions. We scanned the reference lists of identified studies and reviews for any additional relevant articles. Because of their vulnerability to reverse causation biases, retrospective case-control studies were excluded from the meta-analysis (whereas nested case-control studies conducted within prospective cohort studies were included). Study level characteristics and participant characteristics were extracted using a standardised data extraction form, including information on: geographic location, population source, year of baseline survey, number of participants, mean age and age range, percentage of males, telomere length assay method, number of incident T2DM cases, duration of follow-up, and reported measures of association (i.e. hazard ratios, odds ratios, or other measures of relative risk) with corresponding confidence intervals and degree of adjustment for confounders. If studies had reported measures of association for different degree of adjustment, the most adjusted estimate was used in the meta-analysis. We assessed the quality of the included studies with the Newcastle-Ottawa scale, a quality score ranging from zero to nine points [38].

Statistical analysis

The statistical analysis was conducted according to a pre-specified analysis plan. Continuous variables were summarised as means (standard deviations) or medians (interquartile ranges), and dichotomous variables as numbers (percentages). Cross-sectional associations between RTL and other participant characteristics were determined using unadjusted and age- and sex-adjusted linear regression. To quantify within-person variability of RTL, regression dilution ratios were calculated using information from all available RTL measurements in 1995, 2005 and 2010 [39].

Table 1. Association of leucocyte relative telomere length with incident type 2 diabetes mellitus in the Bruneck Study (n = 606, 44 events).

Exposure/adjustment	Quartile 1 (Longest RTL)	Quartile 2	Quartile 3	Quartile 4 (Shortest RTL)	Quartile 4 vs. remainder
Baseline RTL					
Median (range) of RTL, T/S ratios	1.35 (1.21–3.87)	1.13 (1.05–1.21)	0.98 (0.92–1.05)	0.82 (0.52–0.91)	
Incidence rate of T2DM per 1,000 person-years	5.2 (2.9, 9.4)	3.1 (1.4, 6.9)	5.4 (3.0, 9.8)	10.6 (6.5, 17.2)	
Hazard ratio for T2DM (95% CI)					
Adjusted for age and sex	1.00 [Reference]	0.58 (0.22, 1.58)	0.95 (0.41, 2.22)	1.89 (0.85, 4.18)	2.21 (1.17, 4.16)*
Plus BMI, smoking, SES, and physical activity	1.00 [Reference]	0.57 (0.21, 1.56)	0.96 (0.41, 2.24)	1.89 (0.85, 4.21)	2.22 (1.17, 4.21)*
Plus alcohol consumption, HDL-C, log hsCRP, and WHR	1.00 [Reference]	0.58 (0.21, 1.58)	0.99 (0.42, 2.32)	2.00 (0.90, 4.49)	2.31 (1.21, 4.41)*
Long-term average RTL					
Median (range) of RTL, T/S ratios	1.29 (1.18–2.94)	1.12 (1.06–1.18)	1.02 (0.97–1.06)	0.89 (0.63–0.96)	
Incidence rate of T2DM per 1,000 person-years	3.6 (1.8, 7.3)	5.0 (2.7, 9.4)	4.5 (2.3, 8.6)	12.2 (7.6, 19.6)	
Hazard ratio for T2DM (95% CI)					
Adjusted for age and sex	1.00 [Reference]	1.36 (0.53, 3.45)	1.16 (0.44, 3.05)	3.24 (1.29, 8.15)*	2.76 (1.41, 5.41)**
Plus BMI, smoking, SES, and physical activity	1.00 [Reference]	1.24 (0.48, 3.20)	1.10 (0.41, 2.92)	3.05 (1.21, 7.70)*	2.73 (1.39, 5.36)**
Plus alcohol consumption, HDL-C, log hsCRP, and WHR	1.00 [Reference]	1.25 (0.49, 3.23)	1.11 (0.42, 2.94)	3.22 (1.27, 8.14)*	2.86 (1.45, 5.65)**

Asterisks indicate level of statistical significance: *P≤0.05; **P≤0.01; ***P≤0.001. Abbreviations: BMI, body mass index; HDL-C, high density lipoprotein cholesterol; hsCRP; high-sensitivity C-reactive protein; RTL, relative telomere length; SES, socio-economic status; T2DM, type 2 diabetes mellitus; WHR, waist-hip ratio. Participants with a baseline history of type 2 diabetes mellitus were excluded from the analysis (n = 78).

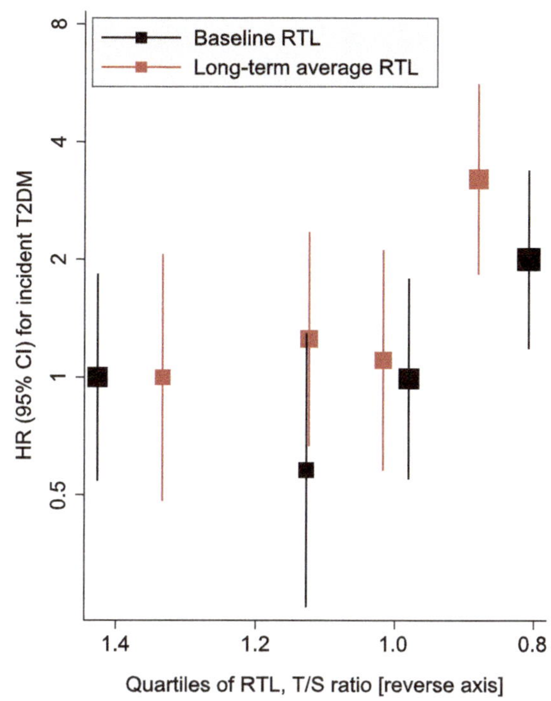

Figure 3. Association of leucocyte relative telomere length an risk of type 2 diabetes mellitus in the Bruneck Study (n = 606, 44 events over follow-up 1995–2010). Cox models were adjusted for age, sex, body mass index, smoking, socio-economic status, physical activity, alcohol consumption, high density lipoprotein cholesterol, log high-sensitivity C-reactive protein, and waist-hip ratio. Abbreviations: CI, confidence interval; HR, hazard ratio; RTL, relative telomere length; T2DM, type 2 diabetes mellitus.

Regression dilution ratios can range from 0 to 1, with 1 indicating absence of within-person variability. Long-term average RTL was estimated by multivariate linear-mixed regression calibration model that allowed for a random intercept at the participant level [40].

The time-to-event analysis excluded participants with baseline T2DM. Person-years of follow-up were accrued from the baseline in 1995 until diagnosis of T2DM, death or October 1, 2010, whichever came first. Cox proportional hazard models were used to assess the association between RTL and T2DM incidence. Following a previous report of a possible threshold effect in associations of RTL with T2DM risk [41], we categorised study participants into groups of RTL quartiles and compared T2DM risk across these groups. The analyses were progressively adjusted for age, sex, body mass index, smoking, socio-economic status, physical activity, alcohol consumption, high-density lipoprotein cholesterol, log high-sensitivity C-reactive protein, and waist-hip ratio. The proportional hazards assumption was tested and confirmed using Schoenfeld residuals. To assess effect modification by sex, subsidiary analyses used interaction term between sex and RTL quartiles and tested for interaction with a likelihood ratio test. For the literature-based meta-analysis, we did not need to rescale published relative risks (RRs), because all eligible studies reported RRs on the same scale, i.e. for a comparison of extreme RTL quartiles. Hazard ratios (HRs) and odds ratios were assumed to approximate the same measure of RR. Reported RRs were pooled using random-effects meta-analysis. Heterogeneity between studies was quantified using the I^2 statistic and tested by a standard χ^2 test [42]. Potential publication and small-study bias was formally assessed using Egger's test [43]. All analyses were conducted with Stata 12.0. A two-sided P value ≤0.05 was considered statistically significant. The presentation of results follows the recommendations by the STROBE and PRISMA guidelines (see **Checklists S1** and **S2**).

Results

Baseline characteristics

The median RTL at baseline was 1.05 T/S ratios (interquartile range: 0.92–1.21). **Figure 1** summarises baseline characteristics of the study population (n = 684). The mean age of study participants was 63 years (SD, 11) and 49% were men. The multivariable adjusted regression dilution ratio of RTL was 0.68 (95% confidence interval: 0.61 to 0.76). We investigated the age- and sex-adjusted cross-sectional association at baseline between several characteristics and standardised RTL (**Figure 1**). The strongest association was observed with age. On average, every one standard deviation older age (11 years) was associated with 0.22 shorter standardised RTL (−0.30 to −0.15; $P = 2\times10^{-9}$). There was no significant correlation of RTL with other parameters, including markers of inflammation, oxidative stress and hyperglycaemia (all P>0.05).

We further investigated whether baseline RTL differed according to baseline T2DM status (**Figure 2**). We observed no significant difference in RTL across the groups of normoglycaemic participants (n = 390), participants with impaired fasting glucose levels (n = 216), and participants with a clinical diagnosis of T2DM (n = 78) ($P_{trend} = 0.346$).

Association of leucocyte telomere length with risk of incident type 2 diabetes mellitus

The Cox regression analyses excluded 78 participants with a baseline diagnosis of T2DM. Between 1995 and 2010, 44 of the 606 individuals in the study population developed T2DM (incidence rate, 5.8 per 1,000 person years [4.3 to 7.8]). **Table 1** compares T2DM risk across quartiles of decreasing RTL. In a comparison of the bottom vs. top quartile of baseline RTL, the age- and sex-adjusted HR was 1.89 (0.85 to 4.18; P = 0.116). The most adjusted model yielded a HR of 2.00 (0.90 to 4.49; P = 0.091). In a comparison of the bottom quartile of baseline RTL vs. the remainder, the respective HRs were 2.21 (1.17 to 4.16; P = 0.015) and 2.31 (1.21 to 4.41; P = 0.011). **Table 1** also shows analyses using long-term average RTL. In the most adjusted model, participants in the bottom quartile of long-term average RTL had a HR of 3.22 (1.27, to 8.14; P = 0.014) compared with the top RTL quartile and 2.86 (1.45 to 5.65; P = 0.002) compared with all other quartiles. We observed that increases in T2DM risk were confined to the bottom RTL quartile (particularly when using long-term average RTL), in line with a possible threshold effect (**Figure 3**). Results were similar in analyses that excluded the first five years of follow-up (data not shown). There was no evidence for differential associations in women and men (likelihood-ratio tests for interaction: P = 0.776 for baseline RTL; P = 0.571 for long-term average RTL).

Subsidiary analysis evaluated the association of a baseline diagnosis of T2DM with RTL change over 15 years. There was no significant difference in RTL dynamics according to baseline T2DM status (mean standardised RTL change in participants with vs. without T2DM at baseline [95% confidence interval]: −0.068 [−0.450 to 0.314]; P = 0.727). This analysis had limited power because it included only 400 study participants with RTL measurements available both in 1995 and 2010, of which only 20 had T2DM at baseline.

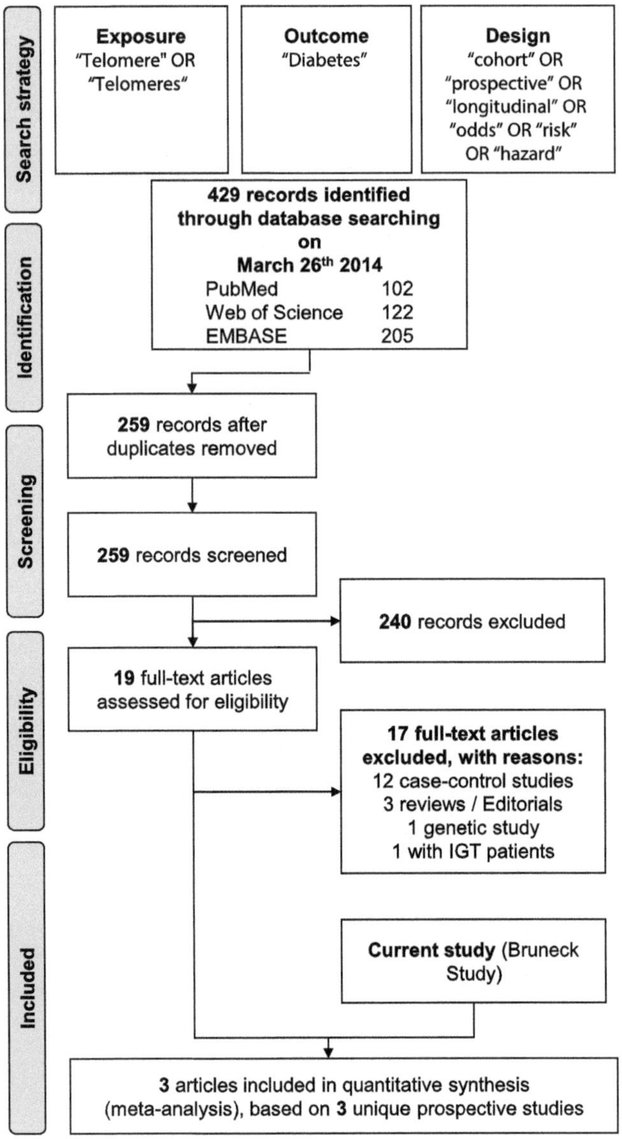

Figure 4. Study flow diagram of the literature-based meta-analysis. The figure is based on the 2009 PRISMA flow diagram template (available from http://www.prisma-statement.org/statement.htm).

Literature-based meta-analysis

Our literature search retrieved 429 records (**Figure 4**). We excluded 170 duplicate records and 240 records on the basis of their title and abstract. We carefully checked the full-text of the remaining 19 records and excluded a further 17 articles, including 12 case-control studies and 1 study that selectively recruited participants with impaired glucose tolerance [44]. Finally, together with the Bruneck Study, we identified three relevant prospective studies eligible for inclusion in the literature-based meta-analysis [41,45].

The characteristics of the three studies are summarised in **Figure 5**. The Strong Heart Family Study is a multigenerational study of American Indian families in four states of the USA, which recorded 292 incident T2DM events over a mean of 5.5 years (defined according to the 1997 American Diabetes Association criteria) [41]. The observational arm of the Women's Health Initiative used a nested case-control analysis that included 1,675 incident cases of T2DM (defined based on self-report or T2DM hospitalisation) [45]. Overall, information from the three studies was available on 6,991 participants and 2,011 incident T2DM events recorded over a weighted mean of 6.6 years. Baseline age of participants ranged from 14 to 93 years; 18% were male. The reported multivariable adjusted RRs for T2DM were quantitatively similar in the Bruneck Study and the Strong Heart Family Study (**Figure 5**). The pooled RR for all three studies was 1.31 (1.07 to 1.60; $P = 0.010$) for a comparison of the bottom vs. the top quartile of baseline RTL. Between-study heterogeneity was moderate with an I^2 of 69% (0% to 91%) (**Figure 5**). There was no evidence of publication bias ($P = 0.460$). We could not calculate a pooled RR corrected for long-term variability, because such an estimate was only available for the Bruneck Study.

Discussion

In the present report, we demonstrate a significant positive association between shorter leucocyte telomeres and T2DM risk. In the Bruneck Study, the increase in risk appeared to be confined to the bottom quartile of RTL (i.e. participants with the shortest RTL) and was particularly evident in analyses correcting for long-term variability in RTL. In a pooled analysis of published reports from three prospective cohort studies, we estimated that people in the bottom RTL quartile had a 31% (7 to 60%) higher risk of developing T2DM than those in the longest RTL quartile.

RTL is a dynamic measure that may decrease but also increase over time [18–27]. Possible sources of variability in measured RTL include the (i) cumulative effect of environmental and behavioural exposures, (ii) varying telomerase activity, (iii) stress-induced repopulation of peripheral blood by recently dividing hematopoietic bone marrow cells, (iv) shifts in the cellular composition of peripheral blood leucocytes (differential blood count) and release of leucocyte subpopulations during acute infections [46,47] (i.e. "true variation"), and (v) measurement error. Previous epidemiological studies on RTL and T2DM risk have not been able to correct for RTL variability, potentially yielding biased estimates. The Bruneck study, which made such a correction on the basis of up to three repeated measurements taken over a follow-up time of 15 years, indicates an independent association of shorter telomeres with T2DM, of greater magnitude than previously reported. The within-person variability of RTL was comparable to that of commonly measured cardio-metabolic risk markers, such as blood pressure or high-sensitivity C-reactive protein. It was lower than previously reported [19] because we further optimised our technique for RTL quantification, including consistent DNA extraction method and re-measurement in quadruplicate.

Previous studies have suggested a possible threshold effect of associations of RTL with age-related diseases, including T2DM [41]. Our study independently confirms this hypothesis, demonstrating an elevation in T2DM risk only in the quartile of participants with the shortest telomeres. As suggested by Zhao *et al.* [41], one intriguing biological explanation for this finding could be the crossing of the "Hayflick limit" [3], beyond which cells cease to divide and undergo apoptosis. Furthermore, several pieces of evidence support that short telomeres play an important role in T2DM pathogenesis, rather than being an epiphenomenon of a pre-diabetic metabolic state. In mice, deletion of the telomerase RNA component (TERC) lowers the replication capacity of beta-cells and thereby leads to a reduced islet mass and failure to produce adequate amounts of insulin in response to glucose stimulation and high fat diet [13]. It has also been proposed that short telomeres impede insulin secretion through inhibition of

Study name	Location	Population source	n	Age range, years	% of males	NOS scale	No. of T2DM events	Length of follow-up, years	Level of adjustment* (Age, Sex, Body mass index, Smoking, SES, Physical activity, Alcohol consumption, Further adjustment)	Relative risk (95% CI) for T2DM comparing the bottom vs. the top quartile of leukocyte RTL
Bruneck Study	Italy	Population register	606	45-84	49	9	44	15.0†	■ ■ ■ ■ ■ ■ ■ +2	2.00 (0.90, 4.49)
Strong Heart Family Study	USA	American Indian families	2328	14-93	40	8	292	5.5‡	■ ■ ■ □ □ □ □ +3	1.83 (1.26, 2.66)
WHI Observational Study	USA	Population register$	4057	50-79	0	6	1675	6.0†	■ x ■ ■ □ ■ ■ +3	1.08 (0.84, 1.38)
Overall			**6991**	**14-93**	**18**		**2011**	**6.6**		**1.31 (1.07, 1.60) [P=0.010] I^2=69%**

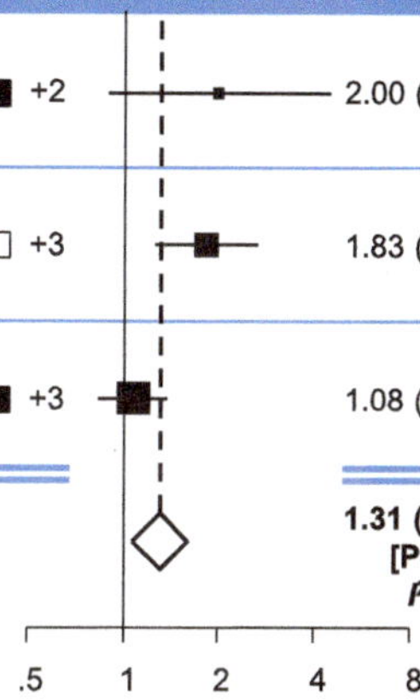

Figure 5. Description and meta-analysis of published data from three prospective cohort studies on the association of short telomeres and risk of type 2 diabetes mellitus. Published relative risks were pooled by random-effects meta-analysis. In the Bruneck Study and the Strong Heart Family Study, type 2 diabetes was defined according to the 1997 American Diabetes Association criteria. In the WHI Observational Study, diabetes was defined based on self-report and hospitalisation for type 2 diabetes. All three studies measured telomere length with a quantitative polymerase chain reaction technique. *Reported relative risks were additionally adjusted for two variables in the Bruneck Study (HDL cholesterol and log hsCRP), three variables in the Strong Heart Family Study (age^2, fasting glucose, total triglycerides), and three variables in the Women's Health Initiative Observational Study (date of blood collection, clinical centre, hormone therapy). †Max. ‡Mean. $The Women's Health Initiative Observational Study involved postmenopausal women who proved to be ineligible or unwilling to be randomised as part of the Women's Health Initiative Clinical Trial. Abbreviations: CI, confidence interval; NOS, Newcastle-Ottawa Scale for assessing the quality of nonrandomised studies in meta-analyses; T2DM, type 2 diabetes mellitus; WHI, Women's Health Initiative.

calcium-mediated exocytosis [14]. In adipocytes, cellular senescence leads to insulin resistance, which is reversible by inhibition of p53 activity [15]. In a study of 22,715 women and 1,445 incident T2DM events, Zee *et al.* have shown that genetic variants related to telomere pathways are associated with T2DM risk [48]. On the other hand, evidence suggests that diabetes has a marked impact on telomere length dynamics. High levels of oxidative stress observed in diabetes patients [16] accelerate telomere attrition because the high guanine content of telomeres makes them particularly vulnerable to reactive oxygen species [17]. Xu *et al.* demonstrated that new-borns have significantly shorter telomeres if their mother suffered from gestational diabetes [49]. However, the Nurses' Health Study has quantified genetic predisposition to T2DM with a risk score combining 36 genetic variants and ruled out a strong causal impact of T2DM on telomere dynamics (although the study was powered to only detect effects of ≥9% explained variability) [50].

To place our findings in context of the currently available epidemiological literature, we performed a systematic literature review and meta-analysis of the available published evidence from prospective cohort studies on the topic. The pooled RR for a comparison of bottom vs. top quartiles of telomere length (i.e. shortest vs. longest) involving data from 6,991 participants and 2,011 incident T2DM cases was 1.31 (1.07 to 1.60). In contrast to an earlier meta-analysis [12], we excluded articles reporting on case-control studies, thereby limiting the effect of reverse causation biases in our analysis. However, because the present evaluation was based on observational studies, we cannot fully exclude the possibility that our estimates are confounded by other factors or the consequence of the often extended lag time between manifestation and diagnosis of T2DM.

Our study has several strengths. First, the Bruneck Study is representative of the general population (with a recruitment process using municipal registers and with a response rate>90%). It therefore crucially expands our knowledge from select populations (i.e. populations from specific ethnic backgrounds or other non-representative samples) to the healthy general community. Second, the Bruneck cohort is extremely well-characterised with 100% follow-up over 15 years and high-quality ascertainment of both clinical endpoints and potential confounders. The detailed characterisation of the study participants helped us estimate independent associations adjusted for a large panel of proposed risk markers for T2DM, including adiposity measures, smoking, social class, and physical activity. Third, the present study had a prospective design and used rigorous baseline examinations to exclude all individuals with T2DM at baseline, thereby minimising any reverse causation biases. Supplementary analyses that excluded the first five years of follow-up yielded qualitatively similar results. Fourth, to enhance validity of the measurement, we extracted all available DNA samples with the same DNA extraction kit. Although samples taken in 1995 and 2005 had been previously analysed [5,10], samples from all three time points were reanalysed simultaneously to avoid a measurement error over the time period. In addition, a bias according to the ascertainment of RTL on different qPCR plates was avoided by positioning the available DNA samples from a single individual from different time points side by side on the same plate. To maximise accuracy, RTL measurements were performed in quadruplicate, in an intensively standardised and automated manner, and within a short period of time by personnel blinded to the characteristics and outcome of the study participants. We have demonstrated previously that RTL measurement using qPCR, as performed in the Bruneck Study, is highly correlated with measurement of absolute telomere length using a Southern Blot technique ($r = 0.765$) [5]. Fifth, we were able to model long-term average RTL and provide effect estimates for T2DM corrected for fluctuations in RTL over time. Finally, we performed a comprehensive literature review and combined data from previously published prospective studies.

Our study also has potential limitations. First, the Bruneck Study population was entirely Caucasian and therefore findings are only generalizable to this ethnicity. Previous investigations by the Nurses' Health Study on differences by ethnicity (Caucasian, African Americans, Hispanic, and Asian) have shown generally comparable associations of RTL with T2DM incidence [45]. Second, telomere length was measured in circulating blood leucocytes only. More precise assessments and comparisons of telomere length in different tissues (e.g. liver, muscle, adipose tissue, and pancreas) would be helpful to better understand the role of telomeres in disease development but, clearly, this is not feasible in large population studies. Third, the number of incident T2DM events was low in the Bruneck Study limiting our ability to conduct more detailed investigations (e.g. extensive subgroup analyses), although major findings were independently confirmed in the literature-based meta-analysis. Fourth, the meta-analyses of published data used single baseline measurements of RTL to study the association with subsequent T2DM. Our analysis of RTL reproducibility over up to 15 years suggests that previous studies could have substantially underestimated potential associations with T2DM. Finally, because the present evidence is limited to observational studies in primarily adult populations, no judgement on the causal involvement of telomere length in T2DM can be made on the basis of the present report.

Conclusion

Low RTL is independently associated with the risk of incident T2DM. To avoid regression dilution bias in observed associations of RTL with disease risk, future studies should implement methods correcting for within-person variability in RTL. Whether there is a causal involvement of telomeres in T2DM development remains to be determined.

Supporting Information

Checklist S1 STROBE Statement—Checklist of items that should be included in reports of cohort studies.

Checklist S2 PRISMA 2009 Checklist.

File S1 Underlying data for Figure 1, 3 and 5.

Author Contributions

Conceived and designed the experiments: PW AM SW JW FK SK. Performed the experiments: JR ST MH JLW FK. Analyzed the data: PW. Wrote the paper: PW JR EEH ST MH AM SW JLW ASB JW FK SK. Collected data on baseline characteristics and disease incidence of the Bruneck Study participants: PW AM SW JW SK.

References

1. Blackburn EH (1991) Structure and function of telomeres. Nature 350: 569–573.
2. Calado RT, Young NS (2009) Telomere diseases. N Engl J Med 361: 2353–2365.
3. Hayflick L (1965) The limited in vitro lifetime of human diploid cell strains. Exp Cell Res 37: 614–636.
4. Weischer M, Bojesen SE, Cawthon RM, Freiberg JJ, Tybjærg-Hansen A, et al. (2012) Short telomere length, myocardial infarction, ischemic heart disease, and early death. Arterioscler Thromb Vasc Biol 32: 822–829.
5. Willeit P, Willeit J, Brandstätter A, Ehrlenbach S, Mayr A, et al. (2010) Cellular aging reflected by leukocyte telomere length predicts advanced atherosclerosis and cardiovascular disease risk. Arterioscler Thromb Vasc Biol 30: 1649–1656.
6. Zee RY, Michaud SE, Germer S, Ridker PM (2009) Association of shorter mean telomere length with risk of incident myocardial infarction: a prospective, nested case-control approach. Clin Chim Acta 403: 139–141.
7. Brouilette SW, Moore JS, McMahon AD, Thompson JR, Ford I, et al. (2007) Telomere length, risk of coronary heart disease, and statin treatment in the West of Scotland Primary Prevention Study: a nested case-control study. Lancet 369: 107–114.
8. Haycock PC, Heydon EE, Kaptoge S, Butterworth AS, Thompson A, et al. (2014) Leucocyte telomere length and risk of cardiovascular disease: systematic review and meta-analysis. BMJ 349: g4227.
9. Wentzensen IM, Mirabello L, Pfeiffer RM, Savage SA (2011) The association of telomere length and cancer: a meta-analysis. Cancer Epidemiol Biomarkers Prev 20: 1238–1250.
10. Willeit P, Willeit J, Mayr A, Weger S, Oberhollenzer F, et al. (2010) Telomere length and risk of incident cancer and cancer mortality. JAMA 304: 69–75.
11. Ma H, Zhou Z, Wei S, Liu Z, Pooley KA, et al. (2011) Shortened telomere length is associated with increased risk of cancer: a meta-analysis. PLoS One 6: e20466.
12. Zhao J, Miao K, Wang H, Ding H, Wang DW (2013) Association between telomere length and type 2 diabetes mellitus: a meta-analysis. PLoS One 8: e79993.
13. Kuhlow D, Florian S, von Figura G, Weimer S, Schulz N, et al. (2010) Telomerase deficiency impairs glucose metabolism and insulin secretion. Aging (Albany NY) 2: 650–658.
14. Guo N, Parry EM, Li LS, Kembou F, Lauder N, et al. (2011) Short telomeres compromise β-cell signaling and survival. PLoS One 6: e17858.
15. Minamino T, Orimo M, Shimizu I, Kunieda T, Yokoyama M, et al. (2009) A crucial role for adipose tissue p53 in the regulation of insulin resistance. Nat Med 15: 1082–1087.
16. Roberts CK, Sindhu KK (2009) Oxidative stress and metabolic syndrome. Life Sci 84: 705–712.
17. Houben JM, Moonen HJ, van Schooten FJ, Hageman GJ (2008) Telomere length assessment: biomarker of chronic oxidative stress? Free Radic Biol Med 44: 235–246.
18. Weischer M, Bojesen SE, Nordestgaard BG (2014) Telomere shortening unrelated to smoking, body weight, physical activity, and alcohol intake: 4,576 general population individuals with repeat measurements 10 years apart. PLoS Genet 10: e1004191.
19. Willeit P, Willeit J, Kloss-Brandstätter A, Kronenberg F, Kiechl S (2011) Fifteen-year follow-up of association between telomere length and incident cancer and cancer mortality. JAMA 306: 42–44.
20. Svenson U, Nordfjäll K, Baird D, Roger L, Osterman P, et al. (2011) Blood cell telomere length is a dynamic feature. PLoS One 6: e21485.
21. Huzen J, Wong LS, van Veldhuisen DJ, Samani NJ, Zwinderman AH, et al. (2014) Telomere length loss due to smoking and metabolic traits. J Intern Med 275: 155–163.
22. Rehkopf DH, Dow WH, Rosero-Bixby L, Lin J, Epel ES, et al. (2014) Seasonal variation of peripheral blood leukocyte telomere length in Costa Rica: A population-based observational study. Am J Hum Biol 26: 367–375.
23. Epel ES, Merkin SS, Cawthon R, Blackburn EH, Adler NE, et al. (2009) The rate of leukocyte telomere shortening predicts mortality from cardiovascular disease in elderly men. Aging (Albany NY) 1: 81–88.
24. Nordfjäll K, Svenson U, Norrback KF, Adolfsson R, Lenner P, et al. (2009) The individual blood cell telomere attrition rate is telomere length dependent. PLoS Genet 5: e1000375.
25. Aviv A, Chen W, Gardner JP, Kimura M, Brimacombe M, et al. (2009) Leukocyte telomere dynamics: longitudinal findings among young adults in the Bogalusa Heart Study. Am J Epidemiol 169: 323–329.
26. Chen W, Kimura M, Kim S, Cao X, Srinivasan SR, et al. (2011) Longitudinal versus cross-sectional evaluations of leukocyte telomere length dynamics: age-dependent telomere shortening is the rule. J Gerontol A Biol Sci Med Sci 66: 312–319.

27. Farzaneh-Far R, Lin J, Epel E, Lapham K, Blackburn E, et al. (2010) Telomere length trajectory and its determinants in persons with coronary artery disease: longitudinal findings from the heart and soul study. PLoS One 5: e8612.
28. Kiechl S, Lorenz E, Reindl M, Wiedermann CJ, Oberhollenzer F, et al. (2002) Toll-like receptor 4 polymorphisms and atherogenesis. N Engl J Med 347: 185–192.
29. Kloss-Brandstätter A, Willeit P, Lamina C, Kiechl S, Kronenberg F (2010) Correlation between baseline telomere length and shortening over time–spurious or true? Int J Epidemiol 40: 840–841.
30. Baecke JA, Burema J, Frijters JE (1982) A short questionnaire for the measurement of habitual physical activity in epidemiological studies. Am J Clin Nutr 36: 936–942.
31. Tsimikas S, Willeit P, Willeit J, Santer P, Mayr M, et al. (2012) Oxidation-specific biomarkers, prospective 15-year cardiovascular and stroke outcomes, and net reclassification of cardiovascular events. J Am Coll Cardiol 60: 2218–2229.
32. Bonora E, Targher G, Alberiche M, Bonadonna RC, Saggiani F, et al. (2000) Homeostasis model assessment closely mirrors the glucose clamp technique in the assessment of insulin sensitivity: studies in subjects with various degrees of glucose tolerance and insulin sensitivity. Diabetes Care 23: 57–63.
33. Friedewald WT, Levy RI, Fredrickson DS (1972) Estimation of the concentration of low-density lipoprotein cholesterol in plasma, without use of the preparative ultracentrifuge. Clin Chem 18: 499–502.
34. Cawthon RM (2002) Telomere measurement by quantitative PCR. Nucleic Acids Res 30: e47.
35. Raschenberger J, Kollerits B, Hammerer-Lercher A, Rantner B, Stadler M, et al. (2013) The association of relative telomere length with symptomatic peripheral arterial disease: results from the CAVASIC study. Atherosclerosis 229: 469–474.
36. Pfaffl MW (2001) A new mathematical model for relative quantification in real-time RT-PCR. Nucleic Acids Res 29: e45.
37. Genuth S, Alberti KG, Bennett P, Buse J, Defronzo R, et al. (2003) Follow-up report on the diagnosis of diabetes mellitus. Diabetes Care 26: 3160–3167.
38. Wells G, Shea B, Peterson J, Welch V, Losos M, et al. (2000) The Newcastle-Ottawa Scale (NOS) for assessing the quality of nonrandomised studies in meta-analyses. Available: http://www.ohri.ca/programs/clinical_epidemiology/oxford.htm. Accessed 12 May 2014.
39. Wood AM, White I, Thompson SG, Lewington S, Danesh J (2006) Regression dilution methods for meta-analysis: assessing long-term variability in plasma fibrinogen among 27,247 adults in 15 prospective studies. Int J Epidemiol 35: 1570–1578.
40. Fibrinogen Studies Collaboration (2009) Correcting for multivariate measurement error by regression calibration in meta-analyses of epidemiological studies. Stat Med 28: 1067–1092.
41. Zhao J, Zhu Y, Lin J, Matsuguchi T, Blackburn E, et al. (2014) Short leukocyte telomere length predicts risk of diabetes in american indians: the strong heart family study. Diabetes 63: 354–362.
42. Higgins JP, Thompson SG, Deeks JJ, Altman DG (2003) Measuring inconsistency in meta-analyses. BMJ 327: 557–560.
43. Egger M, Smith GD, Schneider M, Minder C (1997) Bias in meta-analysis detected by a simple, graphical test. BMJ 315: 629–634.
44. Hovatta I, de Mello VD, Kananen L, Lindström J, Eriksson JG, et al. (2012) Leukocyte telomere length in the Finnish Diabetes Prevention Study. PLoS One 7: e34948.
45. You NC, Chen BH, Song Y, Lu X, Chen Y, et al. (2012) A prospective study of leukocyte telomere length and risk of type 2 diabetes in postmenopausal women. Diabetes 61: 2998–3004.
46. Cohen S, Janicki-Deverts D, Turner RB, Casselbrant ML, Li-Korotky HS, et al. (2013) Association between telomere length and experimentally induced upper respiratory viral infection in healthy adults. JAMA 309: 699–705.
47. Lin J, Epel E, Cheon J, Kroenke C, Sinclair E, et al. (2010) Analyses and comparisons of telomerase activity and telomere length in human T and B cells: insights for epidemiology of telomere maintenance. J Immunol Methods 352: 71–80.
48. Zee RY, Ridker PM, Chasman DI (2011) Genetic variants of 11 telomere-pathway gene loci and the risk of incident type 2 diabetes mellitus: the Women's Genome Health Study. Atherosclerosis 218: 144–146.
49. Xu J, Ye J, Wu Y, Zhang H, Luo Q, et al. (2014) Reduced fetal telomere length in gestational diabetes. PLoS One 9: e86161.
50. Du M, Prescott J, Cornelis MC, Hankinson SE, Giovannucci E, et al. (2013) Genetic predisposition to higher body mass index or type 2 diabetes and leukocyte telomere length in the Nurses' Health Study. PLoS One 8: e52240.

GTP Cyclohydrolase I Gene Polymorphisms Are Associated with Endothelial Dysfunction and Oxidative Stress in Patients with Type 2 Diabetes Mellitus

Pawel P. Wolkow[1,2], Wladyslaw Kosiniak-Kamysz[3], Grzegorz Osmenda[3], Grzegorz Wilk[3], Beata Bujak-Gizycka[1,2], Adam Ignacak[3], Mihir Kanitkar[4], Malgorzata Walus-Miarka[5], David G. Harrison[4], Ryszard Korbut[2], Maciej T. Malecki[5,6], Tomasz J. Guzik[3,7]*

1 Centre for Medical Genomics OMICRON, Jagiellonian University Medical College, Krakow, Poland, **2** Department of Pharmacology, Jagiellonian University Medical College, Krakow, Poland, **3** Department of Internal and Agricultural Medicine, Jagiellonian University Medical College, Krakow, Poland, **4** Department of Clinical Pharmacology, Vanderbilt University, Nashville, TN, United States of America, **5** Department of Metabolic Diseases, Jagiellonian University Medical College, Krakow, Poland, **6** University Hospital, Krakow, Poland, **7** Institute of Cardiovascular and Medical Sciences, University of Glasgow, Glasgow, United Kingdom

Abstract

Background: The genetic background of atherosclerosis in type 2 diabetes mellitus (T2DM) is complex and poorly understood. Studying genetic components of intermediate phenotypes, such as endothelial dysfunction and oxidative stress, may aid in identifying novel genetic components for atherosclerosis in diabetic patients.

Methods: Five polymorphisms forming two haplotype blocks within the GTP cyclohydrolase 1 gene, encoding a rate limiting enzyme in tetrahydrobiopterin synthesis, were studied in the context of flow and nitroglycerin mediated dilation (FMD and NMD), intima-media thickness (IMT), and plasma concentrations of von Willebrand factor (vWF) and malondialdehyde (MDA).

Results: Rs841 was associated with FMD ($p = 0.01$), while polymorphisms Rs10483639, Rs841, Rs3783641 (which form a single haplotype) were associated with both MDA ($p = 0.012$, $p = 0.0015$ and $p = 0.003$, respectively) and vWF concentrations ($p = 0.016$, $p = 0.03$ and $p = 0.045$, respectively). In addition, polymorphism Rs8007267 was also associated with MDA ($p = 0.006$). Haplotype analysis confirmed the association of both haplotypes with studied variables.

Conclusions: Genetic variation of the GCH1 gene is associated with endothelial dysfunction and oxidative stress in T2DM patients.

Editor: Paolo Fiorina, Children's Hospital Boston/Harvard Medical School, United States of America

Funding: This study was supported by the Foundation for Polish Science Welcome/02/09 Grant and by the Wellcome Trust Senior International Research Fellowship. PW and TJG were supported by grants from the Polish National Center of Science (NCN) including No N402 096 32/3258 and No N402 468937. The funders had no role in study design, data collection and analysis, decision to publish, or preparation of the manuscript.

Competing Interests: The authors have declared that no competing interests exist.

* Email: t.guzik@uj.edu.pl

Introduction

Atherosclerosis and its clinical manifestations, such as myocardial infarction and stroke, are the major causes of mortality in type 2 diabetes mellitus (T2DM) patients [1]. While major clinical and biochemical risk factors are well known, several large randomized clinical trials show ineffectiveness of intensive therapies in the prevention of cardiovascular mortality in T2DM [2–4], suggesting that not all therapeutic options have already been exploited. This may be related to the complexity of the pathogenesis of atherosclerosis, which is initiated and modified by numerous genetic and environmental risk factors, many of which remain unknown. Use of quantitative phenotypes, rather than dichotomized presence of atherosclerosis or its clinical complications as outcome variables, may increase the power to detect significant genetic associations. In addition, intermediate quantitative phenotypes are usually associated with a single predominant pathomechanism of atherosclerosis [5]. Thus, studies involving such phenotypes are less prone to confounding by concomitant factors [6]. The most important mechanisms of atherosclerosis include lipid accumulation in the arterial wall [7], endothelial dysfunction [8], imbalance in redox homeostasis [9] and chronic inflammation [10]. While all of these mechanisms are important, endothelial dysfunction seems to precede the development of atherosclerotic plaque both locally [11] and systemically [12]. More importantly, endothelial dysfunction in human vessels from diabetic subjects is primarily caused by increased oxidative stress, which results primarily from the uncoupling of endothelial nitric oxide synthase (eNOS) [13]. In T2DM patients, uncoupled eNOS contributes to net superoxide excess, rather than producing protective nitric oxide (NO). This phenomenon is caused by the loss of bioavailability of the eNOS co-factor - tetrahydrobiopterin (BH_4) and can be reversed by BH_4 supplementation [13]. The mechanism for decreased bioavailability of BH_4 in T2DM is not known. Several recent studies have shown that BH_4 levels may be modified by genetic variability of the GTP-cyclohydrolase 1 (GCH1) gene located on chromosome 14 in humans and encoding a rate limiting enzyme in the complex process of tetrahydrobiopterin synthesis [14–16]. In the present study, we searched for the association between the polymorphisms within the GCH1 gene and selected intermediate, quantitative phenotypes related to atherosclerosis in T2DM patients. These included endothelial dysfunction (flow mediated dilation – FMD) and its biochemical parameter (von Willebrand factor – vWF), measures of oxidative stress (malondialdehyde levels – MDA), and subclinical atherosclerosis (intima-media thickness – IMT).

Materials and Methods

Study population

The study population consisted of 182 consecutive patients diagnosed with T2DM and followed up in an outpatient setting at the Department of Metabolic Diseases, University Hospital, Krakow, Poland. During patient recruitment, the WHO definitions and criteria of diabetes diagnosis were used [17]. All patients were white Caucasians and inhabitants of southeastern Poland. Upon examination, demographic data and information about the course of their disease, family history, past and current treatments and lifestyle habits were obtained. Only patients with clinical diagnosis of T2DM and no insulin therapy, within the first year of initial diagnosis, were included in this study. Blood for DNA isolation and biochemical measurements, including MDA and vWF plasma concentrations, was obtained by antecubital venipuncture. Vasodilation and IMT were measured ultrasonographically with an 8 MHz probe by a single researcher, blinded to other data. Diagnosis of diabetic complications and biochemical measurements were performed as previously described [17]. The study was approved by the Bioethics Committee of the Jagiellonian University. All patients provided informed consent.

Assessment of endothelial function

Endothelial function was assessed by flow mediated dilation (FMD) measurement as described and validated by our laboratory before [17,18]. Measurements were performed with the Toshiba Xario Diagnostic Ultrasound System and an 8MHz linear transducer. Briefly, measurements were recorded before 5 minute-long brachial artery occlusion and then subsequently 1, 2 and 5 minutes after cuff deflation. Measurements during diastole were recorded and maximal dilation (usually detected within ca. 60–120 sec) was analyzed and reported. Maximal nitroglycerine mediated dilation (NMD) was measured to study non-endothelium dependent vasodilations. vWF concentration in plasma was analyzed using a commercial ELISA kit from DAKO (Glostrup, Denmark).

Measurement of IMT

Measurement of IMT was performed as previously described [17,18] at 12 different points along the right and left common carotid artery. Mean (IMTmean) and maximal IMT (IMTmax) were calculated.

MDA determination

MDA in plasma was determined using liquid chromatography with mass detection (HPLC/MS, LCQ Finnigan Matt). These tests were performed at the Department of Pharmacology JUMC by a modified method described by Sim et al. [19]. Plasma samples were incubated with NaOH to liberate bound MDA and perchloric acid to precipitate proteins. The supernatant was then subjected to extraction twice with n-hexane. The separated organic phase was analyzed by HPLC/MS.

Genotyping

Polymorphisms in the GCH1 gene were selected for genotyping based on the existing literature [20,21]. The GCH1 gene spans slightly over 60 kb on human chromosome 14 (physical location 54,378,474–54,439,292 on March 2006 build of human genome according to UCSC genome browser). Linkage disequilibrium (LD) in a European (Tuscany, Italy) and European descent (Utah, USA) populations (CEU + TSI) from HapMap data [22] is shown in Figure 1A. These populations combined are probably the best available approximation of LD extent for White Caucasians, such as a Polish population from Central Europe. Data show the existence of two haplotype blocks of very tight LD, extending beyond the gene boundaries. The boundary between these two blocks is localized in the second intron, dividing the gene into two thirds in the 5′-end block and one third in the 3′-end block. Therefore, the polymorphisms for this association study were selected from both haplotype blocks (Figure 1B). DNA was isolated from peripheral blood leukocytes using a guanidinium thiocyanate method (DNAzol, Life Technologies).

Polymorphisms rs10483639, rs841, rs3783641, rs10137071, and rs8007267 were determined using commercially available kits ABI TaqMan SNP Genotyping pre-designed assays (Applied Biosystems, USA). End-point fluorescence was determined using Applied Biosystems 7900HT Fast Real-Time PCR System (Applied Biosystems, USA).

Statistical analysis

Data for statistical analysis were analyzed with SAS ver. 9.3 (Cary, USA). Deviations of genotype frequencies of studied polymorphisms from Hardy-Weinberg equilibrium were tested using a modified Chi-square test, implemented in the SAS Genetics module. An extent of LD between the studied polymorphisms was calculated and presented graphically with Haploview ver. 4.1. Patients with different genotypes were compared for differences in continuous variables using the Wilcoxon test and in categorical variables using Chi-square or Fisher's exact test. To compare the effect of polymorphisms and haplotype blocks on quantitative outcome variables, we used PLINK ver. 1.06 with association tests based on Wald statistic. Univariate tests of association were used for individual polymorphisms and haplotype blocks, multivariate tests for combinations of polymorphisms and clinical variables. The following clinical variables, potential confounders of association between genetic factors and outcome variables, were tested: age and sex of patients, characteristics of T2DM, risk factors of atherosclerosis and medication used. P values of less than 0.05 were considered statistically significant.

Results

Study population

Clinical characteristics of patients are summarized in Table 1. These data include demographic characteristics (sex and age), major risk factors for atherosclerosis, current therapies, history of

A.

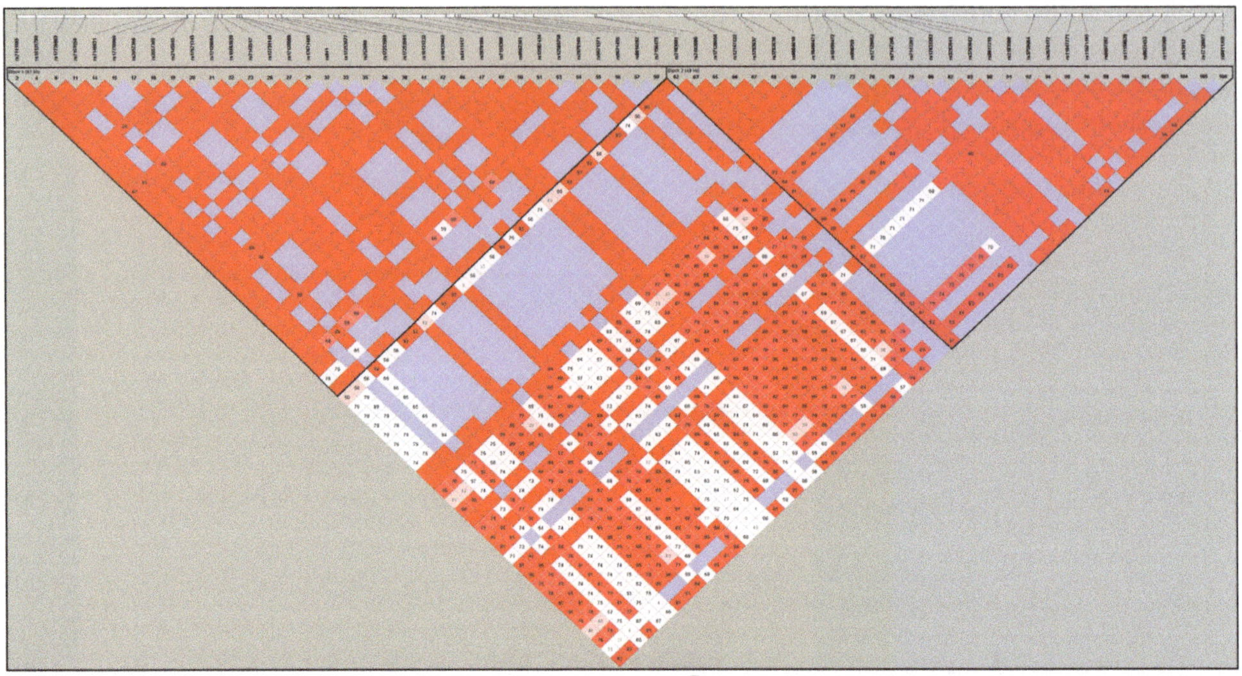

B.

Polymorphism	Location (GCH1 locus) 55 308 724 (3'end) – 55 369 542 (5'end)*	Minor allele freq. (%)
1. rs10483639	55 306 457	18.2
2. rs841	55 310 492	16.8
3. rs3783641	55 360 139	17.9
4. rs10137071	55 370 340	7,6
5. rs8007267	55 378 991	16.4

* UCSC Genome Browser (Feb 2009 assembly).

C.

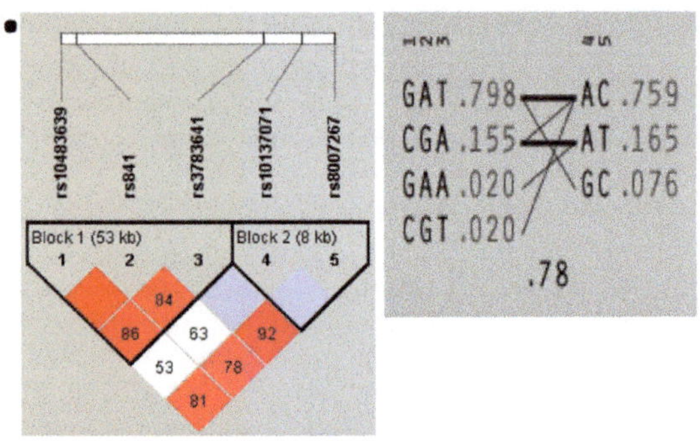

Figure 1. LD within GCH1 gene locus. (A) Extent of LD between polymorphisms at the GCH1 gene locus, based on HapMap Phase II data. Two black triangles designate two haplotype blocks of tight LD. (B) Physical location and minor allele frequency of 5 genotyped polymorphisms from GCH1 locus according to UCSC Genome Browser (Feb 2009 assembly). (C) LD analysis between 5 polymorphisms, genotyped in T2DM subjects from the Polish population, forms two separate haplotype blocks. Data were analyzed and visualized with Haploview ver. 4.2. Haplotype blocks were defined based on the solid spine of LD rule. Numeric values represent Lewontin's D' between pairs of polymorphisms.

diabetes and its complications, cardiovascular diseases, lipid profile, and outcome phenotypes (FMD, NMD, vWF, and MDA).

LD in GCH1 gene in T2DM patients in Poland

The physical location of 5 genotyped polymorphisms on chromosome 14 is described in Figure 1B. Linkage analysis of genotyping data obtained in our study population revealed the existence of 2 haplotype blocks, similar to the results obtained using analysis of HapMap data (Figure 1A–C). Polymorphisms rs10483639, rs841, and rs3783641 belong to the first haplotype block while polymorphisms rs10137071 and rs8007267 belong to the second haplotype block.

GCH1 genetic polymorphisms and vascular outcome variables

We next studied the associations between each of the 5 genotyped SNPs, as well as each of the 2 haplotype blocks formed by these SNPs, with outcome variables (Table 2). Polymorphism rs841 was associated with endothelial function measured as maximal FMD (Figure 2A), while no association was found with control NMD (Figure 2B). Three polymorphisms belonging to the same haplotype block (rs10483639, rs841, and rs3783641) were associated with vWF concentration, a plasma biomarker of endothelial function - (Figure 3A and B). In the case of the last polymorphism, rs3783641, for the genotype mean value of vWF concentration we observed no progression from Aa to aa genotypes. This may suggest either a non-additive model of association or simply reflect the fact that there were only 6 people with the aa genotype in our study. Interestingly, 4 polymorphisms (rs10483639, rs841, rs3783641, and rs8007267) were also associated with plasma MDA concentration, a systemic oxidative stress marker (Figure 4A and B).

Table 1. Clinical characteristics of the studied T2DM patients.

Clinical feature	Value in 182 patients *
Female sex (%)	50
Age at examination (years)	56.5 [37–72]
Characteristics of T2DM	
Use of oral antidiabetic drugs (%)	63.2 **
Use of insulin (%)	52.8 **
Any form of retinopathy (%)	39
Nephropathy (%)	16.5
Neuropathy (%)	34.1
Age at diagnosis (years)	47 [26–68]
Duration of diabetes (years)	9 [1–31]
Current blood glucose (mmol/L)	9.2 [4.3–34]
Hemoglobin A1c (%)	7.6 [5.1–14.2]
Peptide C (ng/mL)	3 [0.15–11.5]
Serum creatinine (μmol/L)	75.3 [47–386.4]
Renal dysfunction; serum creatinine>155 μmol/L (%)	5.0
ALAT (IU/L)	20 [8–90]
Risk factors for atherosclerosis	
Hypertension (%)	88.5
Ever smoking status (%)	59.1
Current smoking status (%)	21.6
Overweight/Obesity (%)	Overweight –29.7; Obese –59.9
BMI (kg/m^2)	31.4 [21–56.4]
Total cholesterol (mmol/L)	5.1 [2.7–19.6]
LDL cholesterol (mmol/L)	2.9 [0.5–7.3]
HDL cholesterol (mmol/L)	1.1 [0.4–2.5]
Triglycerides (mmol/L)	1.9 [0.6–14.1]
Atherosclerosis and CAD	
Ischaemic heart disease (%)	47.8
CCS classification (%)	0–50; 1–24.7; 2–17.6; 3–7.7
PTCA performed in the past (%)	11.5
Myocardial infarction in the past (%)	12.1
Presence of atherosclerotic plaque (%)	60.4
Medications	
ACE inhibitors (%)	76.9
diuretics (%)	50
beta – blockers (%)	37
calcium blockers (%)	23.6
alpha – blockers (%)	7.7
nitrates (%)	14.8
aspirin (%)	43.4
statins (%)	49.7
Studied vascular endpoints	
IMT (mm, average of 12 measurements)	0.84 [0.55–1.1]
IMT (mm, maximum of 12 measurements)	1 [0.7–1.5]
FMD (ratio to baseline at 5 minutes)	1.03 [1–1.24]
NMD (ratio to baseline at 5 minutes)	1.12 [1–1.31]
MDA (μmol/L)	3.32 [0.16–22.3]
vWF (% of normal population)	101.3 [37.5–144.1]

* Frequency of occurrence among patients for categorical variables or median [minimum; maximum] value for continuous variables.
** At the time of examination 42 T2DM patients use both insulin and oral hypoglycemic drugs, 54 use only insulin, 73 use only oral hypoglycemic drugs, 13 use neither insulin nor oral hypoglycemic drugs (diet and physical exercises only).

Table 2. Association of individual GCH1 gene polymorphisms with outcome variables.

Outcome variable	SNP	P value
FMD (max)	Rs10483639	0.056
	Rs841	**0.01**
	Rs3783641	0.09
	Rs10137071	0.63
	Rs8007267	0.47
NMD (max)	Rs10483639	0.24
	Rs841	0.25
	Rs3783641	0.19
	Rs10137071	0.29
	Rs8007267	0.07
IMT (mean)	Rs10483639	0.15
	Rs841	0.22
	Rs3783641	0.08
	Rs10137071	0.28
	Rs8007267	0.11
IMT (max)	Rs10483639	0.21
	Rs841	0.09
	Rs3783641	0.06
	Rs10137071	0.40
	Rs8007267	0.13
MDA	Rs10483639	**0.012**
	Rs841	**0.0015**
	Rs3783641	**0.003**
	Rs10137071	0.51
	Rs8007267	**0.006**
vWF	Rs10483639	**0.016**
	Rs841	**0.03**
	Rs3783641	**0.045**
	Rs10137071	0.75
	Rs8007267	0.055

Association of haplotypes with outcome variables

Association of each of the two described above haplotype blocks with studied outcome variables was determined using omnibus haplotype association tests with studied variables (Table 3).

Haplotype analysis showed that MDA concentration was associated with both haplotype blocks while vWF concentration was associated only with the first haplotype block. This is in line with the analysis of associations of individual polymorphisms with outcome variables. In addition, we observed that association of both haplotype blocks with MDA concentration was less significant than the ones of individual polymorphisms. However, in case the of vWF concentration, the association of the first haplotype block was more significant than that of any individual polymorphism. There was no significant association between the haplotype blocks and FMD values.

Clinical variables as potential confounders of GCH1 polymorphisms associations

In addition to single polymorphism analyses and haplotype block analyses, we have also tested whether clinical covariates, described in the Statistical Analysis paragraph of the Materials and Methods section, changed the association between GCH1 polymorphisms and the outcome variables – FMD as well as MDA and vWF concentrations. The only covariate that significantly associated on its own with the outcome variables was current smoking status. However, we also forced in kidney dysfunction (defined as creatinine concentration above 155 ml/L) and duration of diabetes into the multivariate models, as these are known to particularly affect endothelial function in diabetes (Table 4). The relationships between polymorphisms and outcome variables were independent of the confounding variable of current smoking status. Changes in beta coefficients of association for any studied SNP were less than 10% upon addition of current smoking as a covariate in the model. Thus, covariates did not confound this relationship.

Discussion

In the present study we have found that polymorphisms in the GCH1 gene, that can affect tetrahydrobiopterin synthesis, are associated with markers of endothelial dysfunction and oxidative

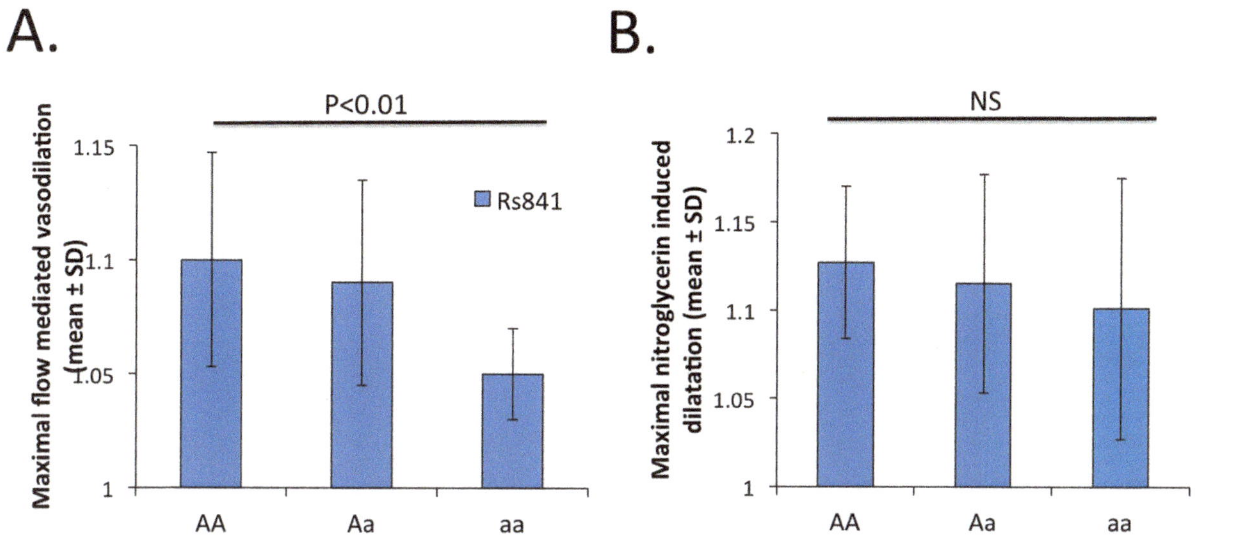

Figure 2. Relationship between rs841 polymorphism in the 3′-UTR of GCH1 gene and vascular function measured as endothelium dependent FMD (panel A) and endothelium independent NMD) (panel B). AA indicates frequent homozygote, Aa - heterozygote, aa - rare homozygote.

stress. This is important, as both endothelial dysfunction and oxidative stress in T2DM patients are the major mechanisms for the development of both micro- and macro-angiopathy. Further studies are required to determine if the same association of polymorphisms is true for patients with type 1 diabetes. Expanding this study to include a group of healthy, non-diabetic control subjects could also verify whether the described associations of polymorphisms with endothelial dysfunction and oxidative stress also remain significant during normoglycemia or are specific to diabetic patients only.

Functional effects of polymorphisms located in the *GCH1* gene locus have been initially shown in relation to the role of BH4 in catecholamine and serotonin synthesis [23]. Rare mutations in *GCH1* lead to hyperphenylalaninemia [24] or DOPA-responsive dystonia [25]. However, the association of sequence differences in this gene with NO biology have been quickly established. For example, the GCH1 haplotype with population frequency of 15.4% has been linked to lower pain sensitivity due to decreased NO production [15]. Although this association has not been replicated [26], recent interest has focused on the relationship with cardiovascular disease. Importantly, Lotsch et al. [27] demonstrated that the pain-protective haplotype can be inferred by genotyping just three polymorphisms, which we have included in our analysis.

A number of studies have looked at cardiovascular disease in relation to the GCH1 genetic variation. Zhang et al. [20] reported that a GCH1 polymorphism in the 3′-UTR is associated with cardiovascular risk, due to decreased NO production and higher

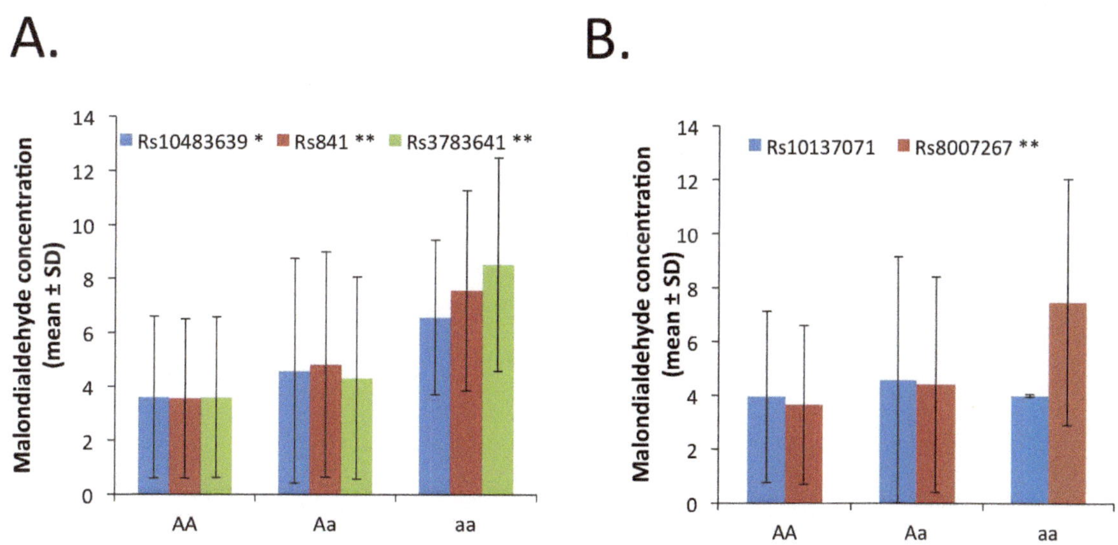

Figure 3. Relationship between studied polymorphisms and plasma vWF concentration. Relationship to polymorphisms forming haplotype block 1 (panel A) and haplotype block 2 (panel B) is demonstrated. Statistical significance of linear regression: * $p<0.05$.

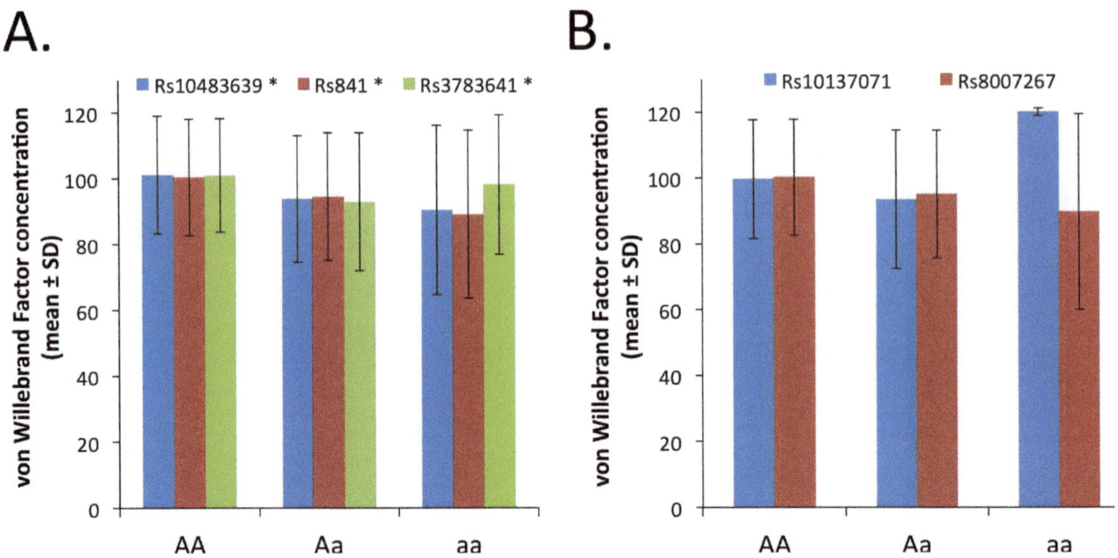

Figure 4. Relationship between studied polymorphisms and plasma MDA concentration measured by mass-spec analysis. Relationship to polymorphisms forming haplotype block 1 (panel A) and haplotype block 2 (panel B) is demonstrated. Statistical significance of linear regression: * $p<0.05$; ** $p<0.01$.

blood pressure in carriers of one of the alleles. Subsequently, Doehring et al. [21] showed that this 3′-UTR polymorphism is in complete LD with the pain-modulating haplotype. Polymorphisms rs1049255 and rs841 were independently associated with coronary artery disease [28]. According to this study, epistatic interactions with other polymorphisms of the NO biosynthesis pathway contribute additionally to the risk of coronary artery disease. The first direct link of genetic variation with BH4 levels was described by Antoniades et al. [16]. They observed lower BH4 levels in carriers of the deleterious GCH1 haplotype, which results in increased production of vascular superoxide and decreased acetylcholine mediated vasodilation in saphenous vein fragments. Considering this evidence and the role BH4 plays in diabetic vascular disease, the importance of genetic variation of the GCH1 gene in T2DM patients is particularly interesting. Polymorphism rs841, which forms a part of the first haplotype block, has been implicated in macrovascular disease in the Chinese cohort of T2DM patients [29]. In this earlier study, carriers of the deleterious genotype were characterized by lower plasma NOx concentrations and lower FMD but higher MDA level and IMT.

In the present project, we have studied 5 polymorphisms spread throughout the gene, which has allowed us to look at variation in the GCH1 gene. Careful examination of the structure of LD in the Polish cohort of T2DM patients showed that these polymorphisms belong to two separate haplotype blocks, in agreement with our analysis of HapMap data. A previous study reported the existence of various numbers of haplotype blocks in the GCH1 locus, depending on the population studied [15]. Two earlier papers suggested tight LD across the whole GCH1 locus [16,21]. However, Zhang and et al. [20], who performed a resequencing

Table 3. Association of two GCH1 gene haplotype blocks, formed by 5 studied polymorphisms with outcome variables.

Studied variable	Haplotype block *	P value for association
FMD max	1	0.27
	2	0.72
NMD	1	0.6
	2	0.16
IMT (average)	1	0.5
	2	0.1
IMT (max)	1	0.44
	2	0.16
MDA	1	**0.0253**
	2	**0.0145**
vWF	1	**0.00285**
	2	0.12

* Haplotype block 1 consists of the following SNPs: Rs10483639, Rs841, Rs3783641 (estimated haplotype frequencies: GAT 79.9%; CGA 15.4%; GAA 2%; CGT 2%. Haplotype block 2 consists of the following SNPs: Rs10137071, Rs8007267 (estimated haplotype frequencies: AC 75.5%; AT 16.8%; GC 7.7%).

Table 4. Models of association of GCH1 gene polymorphisms with outcome variables, accounting for current smoking, kidney dysfunction* and diabetes duration covariates.

Outcome variable	Model including single SNP	Model including SNP and covariates	Beta coefficient	P value
FMD max	rs841		−0.018	0.01
		rs841	−0.017	0.015
		Current smoking	−0.011	0.2
		Renal dysfunction	−0.0009	0.17
		Diabetes duration	−0.0022	0.93
MDA	rs10483639		1.216	0.01
		rs10483639	1.042	0.03
		Current smoking	−0.84	0.15
		Renal dysfunction	0.06	0.23
		Diabetes duration	−0.8	0.42
	rs841		1.583	0.001
		rs841	−0.755	0.19
		Current smoking	0.04	0.35
		Renal dysfunction	−1.341	0.44
		Diabetes duration	1.431	0.005
	rs3783641		1.457	0.003
		rs3783641	1.298	0.01
		Current smoking	−0.931	0.10
		Renal dysfunction	0.0412	0.35
		Diabetes duration	−1.068	0.50
	rs8007267		1.337	0.006
		rs8007267	1.136	0.024
		Current smoking	−0.862	0.14
		Renal dysfunction	0.05	0.28
		Diabetes duration	−1.243	0.44
vWF	rs10483639		−6.453	0.016
		rs10483639	−5.706	0.033
		Current smoking	−4.99	0.12
		Renal dysfunction	0.098	0.69
		Diabetes duration	16.91	0.03
	rs841		−5.839	0.031
		rs841	−5.371	0.047
		Current smoking	−4.546	0.13
		Renal dysfunction	−0.069	0.78
		Diabetes duration	15.47	0.065
	rs3783641		−5.445	0.045
		rs3783641	−4.728	0.081
		Current smoking	−4.486	0.15
		Renal dysfunction	−0.0389	0.87
		Diabetes duration	16.8	0.03

* Renal dysfunction is defined as patients having creatinine concentration above 155 μmol/L.

study, report two distinct haplotype blocks in subjects from Sub-Saharan Africa and a lack of LD of the 3′-end polymorphism with other areas of the gene in subjects of European ancestry. Therefore, our careful examination of the structure of LD in the Polish population in the context of HapMap data is of great interest.

We found that only one of the polymorphisms, rs841, was associated with impaired endothelium dependent vascular dilatation while no relationship was observed with non-endothelium dependent responses. This is in agreement with previous reports of the functional effects of this polymorphism on vascular function in T2DM. Subsequently, we found that three polymorphisms, which form the first haplotype block, were also associated with biomarker plasma vWF concentration, which clearly confirms the functional importance of the GCH1 gene variability in the regulation of vascular function in T2DM.

The major mechanism through which the GCH1 gene could affect endothelial function is eNOS uncoupling, which is directly linked to oxidative stress. Four polymorphisms, three constituting the first haplotype block and one from the second haplotype block, are associated with MDA plasma concentration. Moreover, the first haplotype block was even more strongly associated with this variable than any of the analyzed SNPs. This finding suggests that the first haplotype block may contain a non-genotyped polymorphism affecting MDA concentration. Therefore, this would be a stronger association than any of the polymorphisms previously genotyped by our group. An alternative explanation to this finding could be an epigenetic interaction between studied polymorphisms or other polymorphisms in haplotype block 1, modifying the presence of CpG islands in this locus, thereby affecting methylation pattern and expression of GCH1. Such a possibility was demonstrated at other loci [30]. In the case of vWF, association of the first haplotype block with this variable was less significant than with individual SNPs.

We also tested whether associations defined in this study could have been confounded by clinical factors. The only clinical variable associated with the outcome variables of MDA and vWF concentrations (but not with FMD), was the current smoking status. However, further statistical analysis has shown that the association of SNPs with outcome variables was not confounded by smoking, renal dysfunction, or diabetes duration. In summary, GCH1 polymorphisms or haplotype blocks are associated with FMD, malondialdehyde, and von Willebrand factor concentrations, independently of other clinical characteristics in Polish T2DM patients.

Interestingly, in our T2DM study group we did not observe an association between GCH1 genetic variation and IMT, which has been reported previously [29]. It is possible that our patients were younger and their IMT was overall not substantially increased (mean IMT below 0.9 mm). This could have implicated that we studied a population of T2DM patients at early stage of the development of atherosclerotic disease in whom an increase of IMT not yet developed. However, as discussed above, our data show that the functional polymorphisms, which may affect NO production, can also influence intermediate phenotypes of endothelial dysfunction and imbalanced redox homeostasis [31]. We cannot exclude an alternative explanation that slight interindividual differences in IMT, measured in fraction of millimeters are harder to associate with effects of polymorphism. Such a relationship would be easier to find in a larger population.

Macrovascular complications are responsible for mortality excess and lower quality of life in T2DM patients. Their occurrence may be accelerated and exacerbated by a deficiency in NO production [32]. While NO donors (such as nitrates) are widely used in some clinical situations, their protective efficacy in coronary artery disease has been questioned in numerous clinical trials [33]. Therefore, they do not constitute a first line treatment any longer. Correction of BH4 deficiency might be a better therapeutic option correcting not only NO deficiency but oxidative stress as well. For example, it has been postulated that in carriers of susceptibility GCH1 gene polymorphisms with elevated MDA, BH4 may be oxidized to BH2 and uncouple NO synthase, which leads to further production of reactive oxygen species by eNOS, rather than NO itself [34–36]. The findings of our study together with published evidence of the functional importance in GCH1 gene variation may in future form a basis for diagnostic screening tests to stratify the risk of early development of macrovascular complications in newly diagnosed T2DM patients. This also presents potential therapeutic implications that will need to be clinically tested. An interesting question would be whether supplementation of BH4 might improve the clinical course of T2DM macrovascular complications in relation to stratification based on GCH1 gene polymorphisms. Stratification of patients' therapy according to their genotype is an important aspect of personalized medicine, which becomes even more possible with the advent of new, genome-wide laboratory tools.

Apart from the correction of NO availability, another important strategy for preventing complications in diabetic patients could be to reverse endothelial progenitor cell dysfunction [37]. GCH1was demonstrated to effectively reverse such dysfunction and promote re-endothelization, which may be important for wound healing [37,38]. A group of patients who are particularly prone to complications due to endothelial dysfunction, and might therefore especially benefit from genotype-based BH4 correction, are patients with kidney-pancreas transplantation [39–41].

In summary, the results of our study indicate that functional polymorphisms of the GTP cyclohydrolase I gene, which directly affect tetrahydrobiopterin synthesis, are associated with endothelial dysfunction and oxidative stress in T2DM patients.

Acknowledgments

We acknowledge editorial assistance of Dr Kevin Luc.

Author Contributions

Conceived and designed the experiments: TG MM WKK. Performed the experiments: WKK PW AI GO GW BBG MK MWM. Analyzed the data: PW WKK TG GO. Contributed reagents/materials/analysis tools: DH TG MM. Wrote the paper: TG PW WKK MM RK.

References

1. Lozano R, Naghavi M, Foreman K, Lim S, Shibuya K, et al. (2012) Global and regional mortality from 235 causes of death for 20 age groups in 1990 and 2010: a systematic analysis for the Global Burden of Disease Study 2010. Lancet 380: 2095–2128.
2. Action to Control Cardiovascular Risk in Diabetes Study Group, Gerstein HC, Miller ME, Byington RP, Goff DC Jr, et al. (2008) Effects of intensive glucose lowering in type 2 diabetes. N Engl J Med 358: 2545–2559.
3. ADVANCE Collaborative Group, Patel A, MacMahon S, Chalmers J, Neal B, et al. (2008) Intensive blood glucose control and vascular outcomes in patients with type 2 diabetes. N Engl J Med 358: 2560–2572.
4. VADT Investigators, Duckworth W, Abraira C, Moritz T, Reda D, et al. (2009) Glucose control and vascular complications in veterans with type 2 diabetes. N Engl J Med 360: 129–139.
5. Flossmann E, Schulz UG, Rothwell PM (2005) Potential confounding by intermediate phenotypes in studies of the genetics of ischaemic stroke. Cerebrovasc Dis 19: 1–10.
6. Smith PG, Day NE (1984) The design of case-control studies: the influence of confounding and interaction effects. Int J Epidemiol 13: 356–365.
7. Watanabe T, Hirata M, Yoshikawa Y, Nagafuchi Y, Toyoshima H, et al. (1985) Role of macrophages in atherosclerosis. Sequential observations of cholesterol-induced rabbit aortic lesion by the immunoperoxidase technique using monoclonal antimacrophage antibody. Lab Invest 53: 80–90.
8. Werns SW, Walton JA, Hsia HH, Nabel EG, Sanz ML, et al. (1989) Evidence of endothelial dysfunction in angiographically normal coronary arteries of patients with coronary artery disease. Circulation 79: 287–291.
9. Guzik B, Sagan A, Ludew D, Mrowiecki W, Chwała M, et al. (2013) Mechanisms of oxidative stress in human aortic aneurysms—association with clinical risk factors for atherosclerosis and disease severity. Int J Cardiol 168: 2389–2396.
10. Hansson GK (1993) Immune and inflammatory mechanisms in the development of atherosclerosis. Br Heart J 69: S38–41.

11. Gotschy A, Bauer E, Schrodt C, Lykowsky G, Ye YX, et al. (2013) Local arterial stiffening assessed by MRI precedes atherosclerotic plaque formation. Circ Cardiovasc Imaging 6: 916–923.
12. Guzik TJ, Sadowski J, Kapelak B, Jopek A, Rudzinski P, et al. (2004) Systemic regulation of vascular NAD(P)H oxidase activity and nox isoform expression in human arteries and veins. Arterioscler Thromb Vasc Biol 24: 1614–1620.
13. Guzik TJ, Mussa S, Gastaldi D, Sadowski J, Ratnatunga C, et al. (2002) Mechanisms of increased vascular superoxide production in human diabetes mellitus: role of NAD(P)H oxidase and endothelial nitric oxide synthase. Circulation 105: 1656–1662.
14. Gesierich A, Niroomand F, Tiefenbacher CP (2003) Role of human GTP cyclohydrolase I and its regulatory protein in tetrahydrobiopterin metabolism. Basic Res Cardiol 98: 69–75.
15. Tegeder I, Costigan M, Griffin RS, Abele A, Belfer I, et al. (2006) GTP cyclohydrolase and tetrahydrobiopterin regulate pain sensitivity and persistence. Nat Med 12: 1269–1277.
16. Antoniades C, Shirodaria C, Van Assche T, Cunnington C, Tegeder I, et al. (2008) GCH1 haplotype determines vascular and plasma biopterin availability in coronary artery disease effects on vascular superoxide production and endothelial function. J Am Coll Cardiol 52: 158–165.
17. Malecki MT, Osmenda G, Walus-Miarka M, Skupien J, Cyganek K, et al. (2008) Retinopathy in type 2 diabetes mellitus is associated with increased intima-media thickness and endothelial dysfunction. Eur J Clin Invest 38: 925–930.
18. Wilk G, Osmenda G, Matusik P, Nowakowski D, Jasiewicz-Honkisz B, et al. (2013) Endothelial function assessment in atherosclerosis: comparison of brachial artery flow-mediated vasodilation and peripheral arterial tonometry. Pol Arch Med Wewn 123: 443–452.
19. Sim AS, Salonikas C, Naidoo D, Wilcken DE (2003) Improved method for plasma malondialdehyde measurement by high-performance liquid chromatography using methyl malondialdehyde as an internal standard. J Chromatogr - B Analyt Technol Biomed Life Sci 785: 337–344.
20. Zhang L, Rao F, Zhang K, Khandrika S, Das M, et al. (2007) Discovery of common human genetic variants of GTP cyclohydrolase 1 (GCH1) governing nitric oxide, autonomic activity, and cardiovascular risk. J Clin Invest 117: 2658–2671.
21. Doehring A, Antoniades C, Channon KM, Tegeder I, Lötsch J (2008) Clinical genetics of functionally mild non-coding GTP cyclohydrolase 1 (GCH1) polymorphisms modulating pain and cardiovascular risk. Mutat Res 659: 195–201.
22. International HapMap 3 Consortium, Altshuler DM, Gibbs RA, Peltonen L, Dermitzakis E, et al. (2010) Integrating common and rare genetic variation in diverse human populations. Nature 467: 52–58.
23. Kishi T, Ichinose H, Yoshimura R, Fukuo Y, Kitajima T, et al. (2012) GTP cyclohydrolase 1 gene haplotypes as predictors of SSRI response in Japanese patients with major depressive disorder. J Affect Disord 142: 315–22.
24. Thöny B, Blau N (1997) Mutations in the GTP cyclohydrolase I and 6-pyruvoyl-tetrahydropterin synthase genes. Hum Mutat 10: 11–20.
25. Steinberger D, Weber Y, Korinthenberg R, Deuschl G, Benecke R, et al. (1998) High penetrance and pronounced variation in expressivity of GCH1 mutations in five families with dopa-responsive dystonia. Ann Neurol 43: 634–639.
26. Kim H, Dionne RA (2007) Lack of influence of GTP cyclohydrolase gene (GCH1) variations on pain sensitivity in humans. Mol Pain 3: 6.
27. Lötsch J, Belfer I, Kirchhof A, Mishra BK, Max MB, et al. (2007) Reliable screening for a pain-protective haplotype in the GTP cyclohydrolase 1 gene (GCH1) through the use of 3 or fewer single nucleotide polymorphisms. Clin Chem 53: 1010–1015.
28. Tu YC, Ding H, Wang XJ, Xu YJ, Zhang L, et al. (2010) Exploring epistatic relationships of NO biosynthesis pathway genes in susceptibility to CHD. Acta Pharmacol Sin 31: 874–880
29. Liao YF, Zeng TS, Chen LL, Li YM, Yu F, et al. (2010) Association of a functional polymorphism (C59038T) in GTP cyclohydrolase 1 gene and Type 2 diabetic macrovascular disease in the Chinese population. J Diabetes Complications 24: 313–319.
30. Oertel BG, Doehring A, Roskam B, Kettner M, Hackmann N, et al. (2012) Genetic-epigenetic interaction modulates μ-opioid receptor regulation. Hum Mol Genet 21: 4751–60.
31. Channon KM, Guzik TJ (2002) Mechanisms of superoxide production in human blood vessels: relationship to endothelial dysfunction, clinical and genetic risk factors. J Physiol Pharmacol 53: 515–524.
32. Folli F, Corradi D, Fanti P, Davalli A, Paez A, et al. (2011) The role of oxidative stress in the pathogenesis of type 2 diabetes mellitus micro- and macrovascular complications: avenues for a mechanistic-based therapeutic approach. Curr Diabetes Rev 7: 313–324.
33. ISIS-4 (1995) a randomised factorial trial assessing early oral captopril, oral mononitrate, and intravenous magnesium sulphate in 58,050 patients with suspected acute myocardial infarction. ISIS-4 (Fourth International Study of Infarct Survival) Collaborative Group. Lancet 345: 669–685.
34. Werner ER, Blau N, Thöny B (2011) Tetrahydrobiopterin: biochemistry and pathophysiology. Biochem J 438: 397–414.
35. Kietadisorn R, Juni RP, Moens AL (2012) Tackling endothelial dysfunction by modulating NOS uncoupling: new insights into its pathogenesis and therapeutic possibilities. Am J Physiol Endocrinol Metab 302: E481–495.
36. Astorri E, Fiorina P, Gavaruzzi G, Astorri A, Magnati G (1997) Left ventricular function in insulin-dependent and in non-insulin-dependent diabetic patients: radionuclide assessment. Cardiology. 88: 152–5.
37. Petrelli A, Di Fenza R, Carvello, Gatti F, Secchi A, et al. (2012) Strategies to reverse endothelial progenitor cell dysfunction in diabetes Exp Diabetes Res 2012: 471823.
38. Tie L, Chen LY, Chen DD, Xie HH, Channon KM, et al. (2014) GTP cyclohydrolase I prevents diabetic-impaired endothelial progenitor cells and wound healing by suppressing oxidative stress/thrombospondin-1. Am J Physiol Endocrinol Metab 306: E1120–31.
39. De Cobelli F, Fiorina P, Perseghin G, Magnone M, Venturini M, et al. (2004) L-arginine-induced vasodilation of the renal vasculature is preserved in uremic type 1 diabetic patients after kidney and pancreas but not after kidney-alone transplantation. Diabetes Care 27: 947–54.
40. Fiorina P, La Rocca E, Venturini M, Minicucci F, Fermo I, et al. (2001) Effects of kidney-pancreas transplantation on atherosclerotic risk factors and endothelial function in patients with uremia and type 1 diabetes. Diabetes 50: 496–501.
41. Folli F, Guzzi V, Perego L, Coletta DK, Finzi G, et al. (2010) Proteomics reveals novel oxidative and glycolytic mechanisms in type 1 diabetic patients' skin which are normalized by kidney-pancreas transplantation. PLoS One 5: e9923.

12

Finding Needles in a Haystack: Application of Network Analysis and Target Enrichment Studies for the Identification of Potential Anti-Diabetic Phytochemicals

Shaik M. Fayaz, Valsala S. Suvanish Kumar, Krishnamurthy G. Rajanikant*

School of Biotechnology, National Institute of Technology Calicut, Calicut 673601, India

Abstract

Diabetes mellitus is a debilitating metabolic disorder and remains a significant threat to public health. Herbal medicines have been proven to be effective anti-diabetic agents compared to synthetic drugs in terms of side effects. However, the complexity in their chemical constituents and mechanism of action, hinder the effort to discover novel anti-diabetic drugs. Hence, understanding the biological and chemical basis of pharmacological action of phytochemicals is essential for the discovery of potential anti-diabetic drugs. Identifying important active compounds, their protein targets and the pathways involved in diabetes would serve this purpose. In this context, the present study was aimed at exploring the mechanism of action of anti-diabetic plants phytochemicals through network and chemical-based approaches. This study also involves a focused and constructive strategy for preparing new effective anti-diabetic formulations. Further, a protocol for target enrichment was proposed, to identify novel protein targets for important active compounds. Therefore, the successive use of network analysis combined with target enrichment studies would accelerate the discovery of potential anti-diabetic phytochemicals.

Editor: Muzamil Ahmad, Indian Institute of Integrative Medicine, India

Funding: This work was supported by the Kerala State Council for Science, Technology and Environment, Kerala Biotechnology Commission, Government of Kerala, Thiruvananthapuram, India (Grant number: 1051/2013/KSCSTE). The funders had no role in study design, data collection and analysis, decision to publish, or preparation of the manuscript.

Competing Interests: The authors have declared that no competing interests exist.

* Email: rajanikant@nitc.ac.in

Introduction

Diabetes mellitus is a major chronic metabolic disorder and an extremely serious condition from both clinical and public health standpoints. Nearly 5% of the world's population is affected by diabetes. According to the World Health Organisation (WHO) projections, the diabetic population is likely to increase to 300 million or more by the year 2025 [1]. Current studies in India indicate that there is an alarming rise in the prevalence of diabetes, which has gone beyond epidemic to pandemic proportions [2]. Diabetes imperils public health through various complications such as retinopathy, neuropathy, nephropathy, ischemic heart disease, stroke and peripheral vascular disease [3]. Despite the advances in medicinal science, diabetes remains a burning health issue worldwide. Even though the insulin therapy and oral hypoglycemic agents are the first line of treatment for the disease, they show side effects and fail to significantly alter the course of diabetic complications. Due to these reasons, there is a growing interest in herbal medicines [4].

Since time immemorial, herbal remedies have been the highly esteemed source of therapeutics for various diseases. These remedies show great value in treating and preventing diseases, and are currently becoming more mainstream in clinical practice. Herbal medicines are frequently considered to be less toxic and possess fewer side-effects than synthetic drugs [5]. India is sometimes referred to as the botanical garden of the world because it is the largest producer of medicinal herbs and is endowed with a wide diversity of agro-climatic conditions. In India, a number of plants are mentioned in the ancient literature of Ayurveda and Siddha for the treatment of diabetic conditions. Indigenous remedies have been used in India for the treatment of diabetes mellitus since the time of Charaka and Sushruta [6]. Many Indian plants have been investigated for their beneficial use in different types of diabetes [7]. A number of medicinal plants and their polyherbal formulations are being used for treating diabetes in Ayurveda, Siddha and ethnomedicinal practices [8–10]. In the traditional system of Indian medicinal plant formulations, combined extracts of plants are used as the drug of choice rather than individual plant extracts [11]. It is believed that the synergistic effect of combined extracts of many plants is more beneficial than extract of a single plant. The inherent anti-diabetic property of these plants is due to their phytochemicals.

Phytochemicals have been the single most prolific source of leads for the development of new drug entities from the dawn of drug discovery. They cover a wide range of therapeutic indications with a great diversity of chemical structures. A number of pure compounds from plant sources were reported to show a blood glucose lowering effect [12]. However, due to extreme complexity both in chemical components and mechanisms of action, the proper use of phytochemicals is still a challenging task and further hinders the effort to design novel anti-diabetic drugs, using the therapeutic principles of herbal medicines. Knowing the biological and chemical basis of pharmacological properties of phytochemicals is important for the identification of novel anti-diabetic drugs. Therefore, due to their extensive use and the therapeutic effects, there is an increasing interest and need to rigorously evaluate the mechanisms of action of herbal products.

This problem could be partially alleviated by the application of comprehensive and advanced computational tools, which might help us to understand the biological and chemical basis of the pharmacological action of phytomedicines. The biological basis of pharmacological action depends on the protein targets on which the phytochemicals act and the pathways involved. The chemical basis of pharmacological action depends on the structural scaffolds of the active compounds. Therefore, structure-based computational approach would help in understanding the critical components responsible for the anti-diabetic activity of the active compounds. Thus, sophisticated computational methods enable us to investigate the complex mechanism of action of drugs and circumvent the challenges associated with biological experiments.

In the present study, we have utilized an integrated network analysis approach of systems biology and chemical analysis approach of structural biology to predict the mechanism of action of anti-diabetic plants and their active compounds. This study would facilitate the understanding of two important aspects. The first one is that since a number of anti-diabetic plants are available, it becomes difficult to identify which among them are important for preparing effective anti-diabetic formulations. In this study, we have tried to address this issue through network analysis of anti-diabetic plants, active compounds, their protein targets and pathways. However, these plants contain a lot of active compounds and they in turn target many proteins and pathways. Therefore, identification of important anti-diabetic plants becomes a daunting task. In this regard, we are proposing the following hypotheses to identify the important anti-diabetic plants, active compounds and protein targets.

Hypothesis 1

The anti-diabetic plants with maximum number of active compounds would have good anti-diabetic property.

Hypothesis 2

The active compounds that are present in many anti-diabetic plants may be therapeutically important.

Hypothesis 3

The active compounds that target many proteins have therapeutic relevancy.

Hypothesis 4

The proteins that are targeted by many active compounds are important.

Hypothesis 5

The protein targets that are involved in multiple pathways related to diabetes are important.

The present study was designed to examine these hypotheses. In order to infer hypothesis 1 and 2, a network containing anti-diabetic plants and active compounds was built and analyzed. To infer hypothesis 3 and 4, a network containing active compounds and protein targets was built and analyzed. Further, to infer hypothesis 5, a network containing protein targets and pathways was built and analyzed. Therefore, through network analysis, inferences were made for these hypotheses. These inferences would assist in the identification of important active compounds and thus the anti-diabetic plants containing these compounds could be used for preparing anti-diabetic formulations. Further, by conceptualizing this entire analysis, a strategy for preparing new anti-diabetic formulations has been proposed in this study.

The second aspect is to identify the biological and chemical basis of pharmacological action of phytochemicals. This was achieved through network analysis of phytochemicals and their respective protein targets and pathways involved in diabetes. Further, pharmacophore analysis of the phytochemicals, combined with docking studies, provided insight in to their mechanism of action.

This entire study is conceptualized into three levels (Figure 1). The first level is the selection of anti-diabetic medicinal plants of Indian origin, identification of their active compounds, protein targets and pathways from the available literature and existing databases. The second level involves construction and analysis of meaningful networks from the collected data. In the third and the final level, target-enrichment was carried out to enhance the set of multi-targeting active compounds through pharmacophore feature analysis, structural similarity and docking studies. Pharmacological promiscuous bioactive compounds are gaining increased attention in the field of drug discovery. In this regard, the current target-enrichment approach would extend the path for the identification of novel multi-targeting bio-active molecules, deciding the fate of various diabetes-related pathways and thus would aid in the treatment of diabetes.

Materials and Methods

1. Data collection

An extensive literature survey was carried out in this regard. The anti-diabetic plants available in India were selected for this study (Table 1). Almost all the plants [except ADP14] are being used in Ayurvedic treatment (Table 1).

The active compounds present in these plants were identified through the review of published research articles from PubMed-NCBI and from the databases such as Dr. Duke's phytochemical and ethnobotanical database, Floridata, PhytoDiabCare, Plants for a Future database, DIACAN and DADMP (Table 2). During the literature survey, we collected only the compounds that were reported to be active compounds or that have shown anti-diabetic activity.

The proteins that are targeted by the active compounds were identified from research publications (PubMed-NCBI) and also from multiple online databases like DrugBank, Therapeutic Target Database (TTD), PharmGKB, STITCH and SuperTarget (Table 3). The protein target collection was focused on the mammalian system of biochemical processes, to suit the study. All the protein targets that are directly (through binding of active compound) or indirectly influenced by the active compounds were collected. This data was used to build networks. Further, the dataset was filtered on the basis of direct interaction between the active compound and the protein target and only these direct interactions were carried down for the target enrichment studies.

The biological pathways of the respective protein targets and the diseases in which they are involved were retrieved from databases such as BRENDA, KEGG, PDTD, Binding DB, Pathway Interaction Database, WikiPathways, GeneCards, SMPDB, Reactome, Pathway Linker and SPIKE (Table 4).

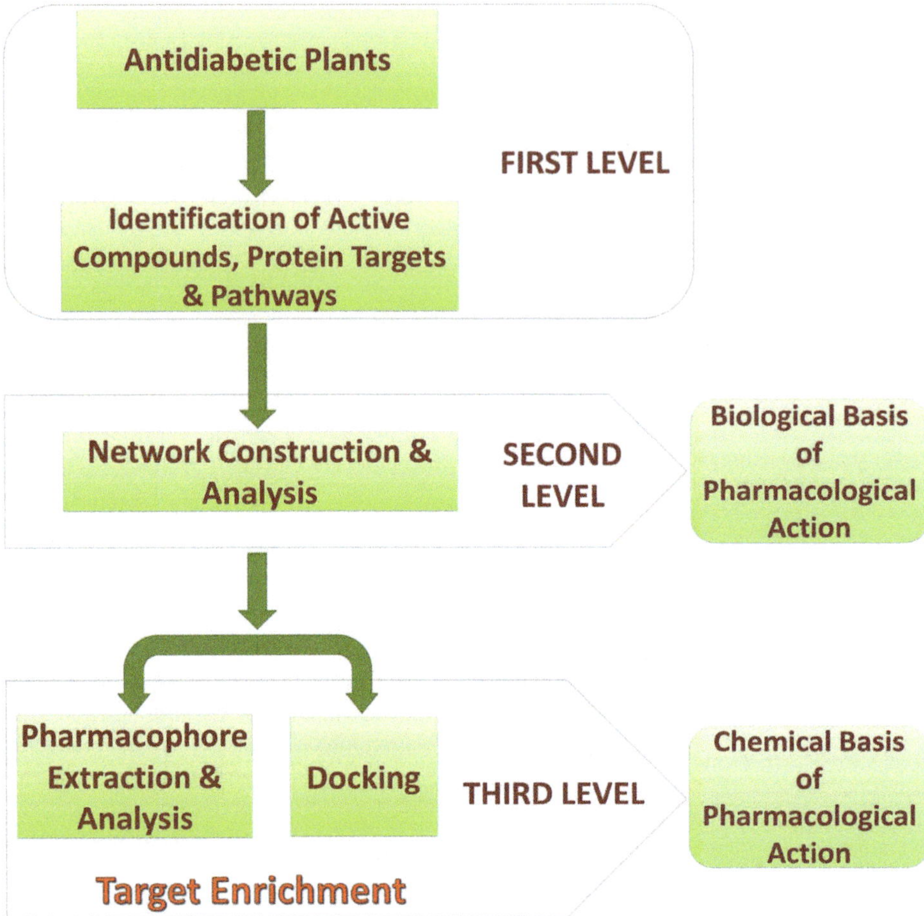

Figure 1. The three levels of methodology used in this study. First level involves identification of active compounds, protein targets and pathways. Second level involves network construction and analysis. This helps in the identification of the biological basis of pharmacological action of anti-diabetic plants. Third level involves target enrichment through pharmacophore analysis and docking studies. This helps in the identification of the chemical basis of pharmacological action of anti-diabetic plants.

2. Network construction and analysis

In order to find the biological means of pharmacological action of anti-diabetic plants, networks were constructed through Cytoscape v3 software [13]. Using alternative combinations of anti-diabetic plants (ADP), active compounds (AC), protein targets (PT), biochemical pathways (P) and diseases, the networks ADP-AC, AC-PT, PT-P and PT-Diseases were constructed, respectively. The networks thus created were analyzed for potential nodes and hubs.

3. Structures of proteins and active compounds

The information regarding these active compounds and their structures were collected from PubChem. The structure for each protein target was retrieved from protein data bank (PDB). If multiple protein structure entries were available in PDB, then the structure solved through X-ray diffraction and also with good resolution was considered.

4. ADME prediction

The ADME (absorption, distribution, metabolism, and excretion) properties of the active compounds were studied using the QikProp program in Schrodinger suite (Schrödinger LLC, New York, NY). QikProp efficiently predicts and evaluates physically significant descriptors and pharmaceutically relevant properties of molecules, making it an indispensable tool for applying ADME principles in lead discovery and optimization.

The properties of all the compounds were predicted by processing the program in normal mode. Principal descriptors and physiochemical properties with a detailed analysis of the log P (Octanol/Water) and % human oral absorption were predicted. The acceptability of the compounds based on Lipinski's rule of 5 [14], which predicts the drug likeliness essential for rational drug design, was also evaluated.

5. Structural alignment and pharmacophore extraction

The active compounds that have a common protein target were used for pharmacophore generation. The 3D structures of active compounds were prepared using the LigPrep module (Schrödinger LLC). In this step, all the possible conformations of the compounds were generated. The conformations of all the active compounds for a particular protein were aligned and the pharmacophores were extracted. The structural alignment of compounds and the pharmacophore extraction was carried out using the Phase module (Schrödinger LLC). The pharmacophores thus extracted contained six features: H-bond acceptor (A), H-bond donor (D), hydrophobic group (H), negatively ionizable (N), positively ionizable region (P), and aromatic ring (R). These

Table 1. Anti-diabetic plants (Scientific and Sanskrit names) and their respective codes.

SL No.	Anti-diabetic Plant [Sanskrit name]	Code	Reference	SL No.	Anti-diabetic Plant [Sanskrit name]	Code	Reference
1	*Citrus maxima* (Burm.) Merr. [Madhukarkati]	ADP1	[85]	16	*Phyllanthus niruri var. amarus* (Schumach. & Thonn.) Leandri [Bhumyamalaki]	ADP16	[98]
2	*Morus alba* L. [Tuda/Tooda]	ADP2	[86]	17	*Cullen corylifolium* (L.) Medik. [Bakuchi]	ADP17	[99]
3	*Abelmoschus moschatus* Medik. [latakasturikam]	ADP3	[87]	18	*Salacia oblonga* Wall. [Saptarangi]	ADP18	[100]
4	*Allium sativum* L. [Lasuna]	ADP4	[88]	19	*Sesamum orientale* L. [Snehaphala]	ADP19	[101]
5	*Cyamopsis tetragonoloba* (L.) Taub. [Bakuchi]	ADP5	[89]	20	*Swertia chirayita* (Roxb. ex Fleming) H. Karst [Anaryatikta]	ADP20	[91]
6	*Hydnocarpus wightiana* Blume. [Tuvaraka]	ADP6	[90]	21	*Syzygium cumini* (L.) Skeels [Jambu]	ADP21	[102]
7	*Salacia reticulate* Wight. [Vairi]	ADP7	[91]	22	*Vigna mungo var. silvestris* Lukoki, Maréchal & Otoul, E. [Mashaparni]	ADP22	[103]
8	*Tinospora malabarica* (Lam.) Hook. f. & Thomson [Gulvel sattva]	ADP8	[91]	23	*Zingiber officinale* Roscoe [Ardraka]	ADP23	[104]
9	*Zanthoxylum armatum* DC. [Tejasvini]	ADP9	[92]	24	*Trigonella foenum-graecum* L. [Medhika]	ADP24	[105]
10	*Achyranthes aspera* L. [Apamarga]	ADP10	[93]	25	*Eclipta prostrata* (L.) L. [Bhringaraj]	ADP25	[106]
11	*Cajanus cajan* (L.) Huth [Adhaki]	ADP11	[91]	26	*Aegle marmelos* (L.) Corrêa [Bilva]	ADP26	[107]
12	*Nelumbo nucifera* Gaertn. [Padma]	ADP12	[94]	27	*Syzygium cumini var. cumini* [Jambu]	ADP27	[91]
13	*Withania somnifera* (L.) Dunal [Ashwagandha]	ADP13	[95]	28	*Casearia esculenta* Roxb. [Saptchakra]	ADP28	[108]
14	*Perilla frutescens* (L.) Britton [Ajeka]	ADP14	[96]	29	*Avena sativa* L. [Jai/Yavika]	ADP29	[109]
15	*Phaseolus vulgaris* L. [Mudga]	ADP15	[97]				

Table 2. Active compounds and their respective codes.

SL No.	Active Compound	Code	SL No.	Active Compound	Code
1	Synephrine	AC1	30	Perilloside C	AC33
2	1-deoxynojirimycin	AC2	31	Beta estradiol	AC34
3	Betulinic acid	AC3	32	Kaempferol-3-o-glucoside	AC35
4	Beta sitosterol	AC4	33	Delphinidin	AC36
5	Oleanolic acid	AC5	34	Gallocatechin	AC37
6	Myricetin	AC6	35	Angelicin	AC38
7	Kaempferol	AC7	36	Bakuchicin	AC39
8	Apigenin	AC9	37	Corylifolin	AC40
9	Ferulic acid	AC10	38	Bakuchiol	AC41
10	Gallic acid	AC11	39	Diadzein	AC42
11	Ellagic acid	AC12	40	Stigmasterol	AC43
12	Astragalin	AC13	41	Pinoresinol	AC44
13	Quercetin	AC14	42	Arachidonic acid	AC45
14	Genistein	AC15	43	Folic acid	AC46
15	Luteolin	AC16	44	Guaiacol	AC47
16	Mangiferin	AC17	45	Oleic acid	AC48
17	Salacinol	AC18	46	Coniferin	AC49
18	Kotalanol	AC19	47	Palmitic acid	AC50
19	(−)-Epigallocatechin	AC20	48	Stearic acid	AC51
20	(−)-Epicatechin-(4beta−>8)-(−)-4′-O-methylepigallocatechin	AC21	49	Linolenic acid	AC52
21	(−)-Epicatechin	AC22	50	Pipecolic acid	AC53
22	3-beta dihydroxyolean-12-en-29-oic acid	AC23	51	Shogaol	AC54
23	22-beta dihydroxyolean-12-en-29-oic acid	AC24	52	Geraniol	AC55
24	Berberine	AC25	53	Isoquercitrin	AC56
25	Avenasterol	AC26	54	Diosgenin	AC57
26	Amyrin	AC27	55	Wedelolactone	AC58
27	Protocatechuic acid	AC30	56	Marmesin	AC59
28	osmarinic acid	AC31	57	Beta glucan	AC60
29	Perilloside A	AC32			

features are necessary for the active compounds to bind to their protein targets.

6. Docking studies

The protein structures extracted from PDB were initially prepared using the protein preparation wizard. In this step, the structures were treated to add missing hydrogens, assign proper bond orders and delete unwanted water molecules, ligands and protein chains. The H-bonds were optimized using sample orientations. Finally, the protein structures were minimized to the default Root Mean Square Deviation (RMSD) value of 0.30 A°. Glide energy grids were generated for each of the prepared proteins. A grid box of approximately 10 A° was around the binding site of the protein. The atoms were scaled by van der Waals radii of 1.0 A° with the partial atomic charge less than 0.25 defaults. No constraints were defined. These grids were employed in the docking studies.

Docking of active compounds to their respective protein targets was carried out using the Glide module (Schrödinger LLC) [15]. The XP (Extra-Precision) docking method in glide was used to dock the compounds in to the binding site of the protein, using OPLS 2005 force field. The default settings as available in the software package were used for the refinement and docking calculations. The van der Waals radii were scaled using a default scaling factor of 0.80 and default partial cut-off charge of 0.15 to decrease the penalties. The option to output Glide XP descriptor information was chosen, which deduces energy terms such as H-bond interactions, electrostatic interaction, hydrophobic enclosure, and π-π stacking interactions. The binding modes and interactions of active compounds with their respective protein targets were analyzed from the docking output.

Results

1. Anti-diabetic Plants (ADP) - Active Compounds (AC) network

The active compounds present in all the anti-diabetic plants were collected and a network was built from this data (Figure 2). The anti-diabetic plants ADP5, ADP7, ADP14, ADP17, ADP19, ADP22, ADP23 and ADP24 contain many active compounds. These plants cover nearly 70% of the entire active compounds. Since the anti-diabetic property of the plant is due to the plant's active compounds, it may be hypothesized that a plant with the

Table 3. Protein targets and their respective codes.

SL No.	Protein Target	Code	SL No.	Protein Target	Code
1	Mono amine oxidase	PT1	34	Phospholipase A2	PT41
2	Glucosidase	PT2	35	Glutamate dehydrogenase	PT42
3	Alpha glucosidase	PT3	36	Glutathione transferase	PT43
4	Glycogen debranching enzyme	PT5	37	Pyruvate dehydrogenase	PT44
5	Cytosolic beta glucosidase	PT6	38	Protein tyrosine phosphatase	PT45
6	Lactase glycosylceramidase	PT7	39	Thromboxane synthase	PT46
7	Glucosidase II beta subunit precursor	PT8	40	IKK beta	PT47
8	Diacylglycerol acyltransferase	PT9	41	Acetylcholine esterase	PT48
9	Nitric oxide synthase	PT10	42	IGF	PT49
10	5-alpha reductase	PT11	43	NADPH oxidase	PT50
11	Glycogen phosphorylase	PT12	44	Insulin receptor	PT51
12	Gaba transaminase	PT13	45	PI3K	PT52
13	Alpha amylase	PT14	46	Lipoxygenase	PT53
14	Xanthine oxidase	PT15	47	Maltase glucoamylase	PT54
15	Aldose reductase	PT16	48	Beta secretase1 (BACE1)	PT55
16	20-alpha hydroxysteroid dehydrogenase	PT21	49	NFK-beta	PT56
17	Carbonic anhydrase	PT22	50	PSORS1C2	PT57
18	Udp glucose dehydrogenase	PT23	51	Lysosomal alpha glucosidase precursor	PT58
19	Ribonucleotide reductase	PT24	52	Tyrosine phosphatase 1B	PT59
20	COX 1	PT25	53	LXR alpha	PT60
21	COX 2	PT26	54	DNA topoisomerase 1	PT61
22	Steroid-5-alpha reductase type II	PT27	55	Protein tyrosine phosphatase 1B	PT62
23	Pancreatic lipase	PT29	56	NA+/K+ -ATPase	PT63
24	Lipoprotein lipase	PT30	57	3-Beta hydroxysteroid dehydrogenase type II	PT64
25	AMPK	PT31	58	Quinone reductase 2	PT65
26	Caspase 3	PT32	59	CARM1	PT66
27	Catechol-o-methyltransferase	PT34	60	Protein tyrosine kinase	PT67
28	Estrogen receptor	PT35	61	IGFR	PT68
29	MAPK	PT36	62	Sucrase isomaltase n-terminal domains	PT69
30	Glyoxalase	PT37	63	7-Dehydrocholesterol reductase	PT70
31	DNA topoisomerase 2	PT38	64	Protein tyrosine kinase IIB	PT71
32	DNA Polymerase	PT39	65	FABP4	PT72
33	DNA Polymerase beta	PT40			

maximum number of active compounds would have good anti-diabetic property (Hypothesis 1).

The active compounds AC3, AC4, AC5, AC6, AC7, AC11, AC14, AC17, AC34, AC43 and AC48 are present in many anti-diabetic plants. Since these compounds are present in many plants, they may be important for anti-diabetic activity. Hence, it could be hypothesized that the active compounds that are present in many anti-diabetic plants may be therapeutically important (Hypothesis 2).

Presence of common active compounds in plants shows that the anti-diabetic activity of these plants might be due to common mechanisms. However, the mechanism of action of these active compounds that are involved in anti-diabetic activity need to be unravelled. This could be achieved by studying the proteins that are targeted by these compounds.

2. Active Compounds (AC) - Protein Targets (PT) network

The anti-diabetic property of plants depends on their active compounds, which in turn relies upon the proteins that are targeted by them. It means that the active compounds that target proteins involved in diabetes will have anti-diabetic activity. In this regard, we have collected all the proteins that are targeted by these active compounds. The network built from this data shows active compounds and their protein targets that either are or are not involved in diabetes (Figure 3). When the protein targets involved in diabetes are considered, the active compounds may be targeting them directly by binding to them, or indirectly by influencing other proteins.

Among the proteins that are targeted by the active compounds, most of them are involved in diabetes. The active compounds AC2, AC3, AC5, AC6 and AC11 target either directly or indirectly many proteins involved in diabetes. This proves the

Table 4. Diabetes-related pathways and their respective codes.

SL No.	Pathways	Code	SL No.	Pathways	Code
1	Aminoacid metabolism	P1	23	Aldosterone-regulated sodium reabsorption	P26
2	Glycogen degradation	P2	24	Pyruvate metabolism	P27
3	N-Glycan biosynthesis	P3	25	Cell cycle and DNA replication	P28
4	Starch and sucrose metabolism	P4	26	Alpha-linolenic acid metabolism	P29
5	Galactose metabolism	P5	27	Linoleic acid metabolism	P30
6	Glycerolipid metabolism	P6	28	Glutamine biosynthesis	P31
7	Apoptosis	P7	29	Glutathione metabolism	P32
8	Steroid hormone biosynthesis	P8	30	Metabolism of xenobiotics by CYP450	P33
9	Starch degradation-I	P9	31	Drug metabolism by CYP450	P34
10	Carbohydrate digestion and absorption	P10	32	Citrate cycle (TCA cycle)	P35
11	Pancreatic secretion	P11	33	JAK-STAT cascade in growth hormone signaling pathway	P36
12	Purine metabolism	P12	34	MAPK signaling pathway	P37
13	Fructose and mannose metabolism	P13	35	Chemokine signaling pathway	P38
14	Glycolysis/Gluconeogenesis	P14	36	NFKB activation	P40
15	Nitrogen metabolism	P18	37	Leukocyte endothelial migration	P41
16	Arachidonic acid metabolism	P19	38	Osteoclast differentiation	P42
17	Sucrose metabolic process	P20	39	ROS generation and oxidative stress	P43
18	Retinoid metabolism and transport	P21	40	Adherens junction	P44
19	PPAR signaling pathway	P22	41	Inositol phosphate metabolism	P45
20	Insulin signaling pathway	P23	42	Phosphatidylinositol signaling pathway	P46
21	BDNF signaling pathway	P24	43	JAG1-NOTCH pathway	P47
22	STAT3 signaling pathway	P25	44	Toll-like receptor signaling pathway	P48

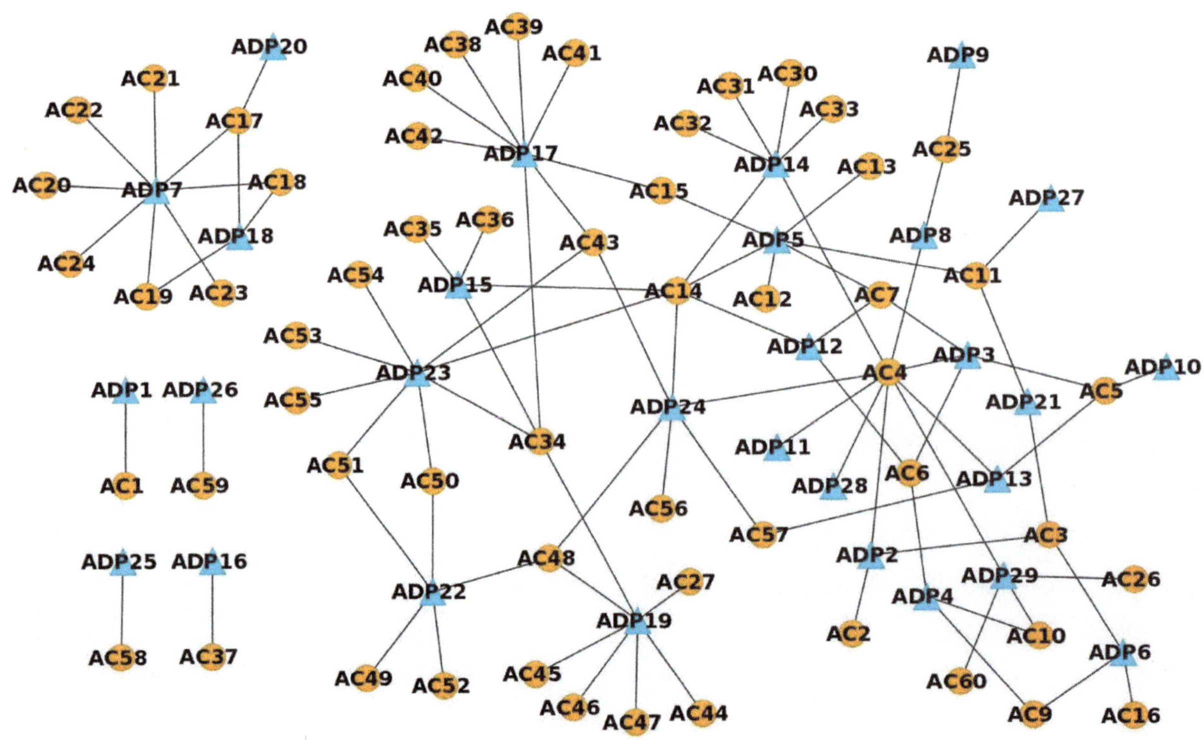

Figure 2. Network containing anti-diabetic plants and their respective active compounds.

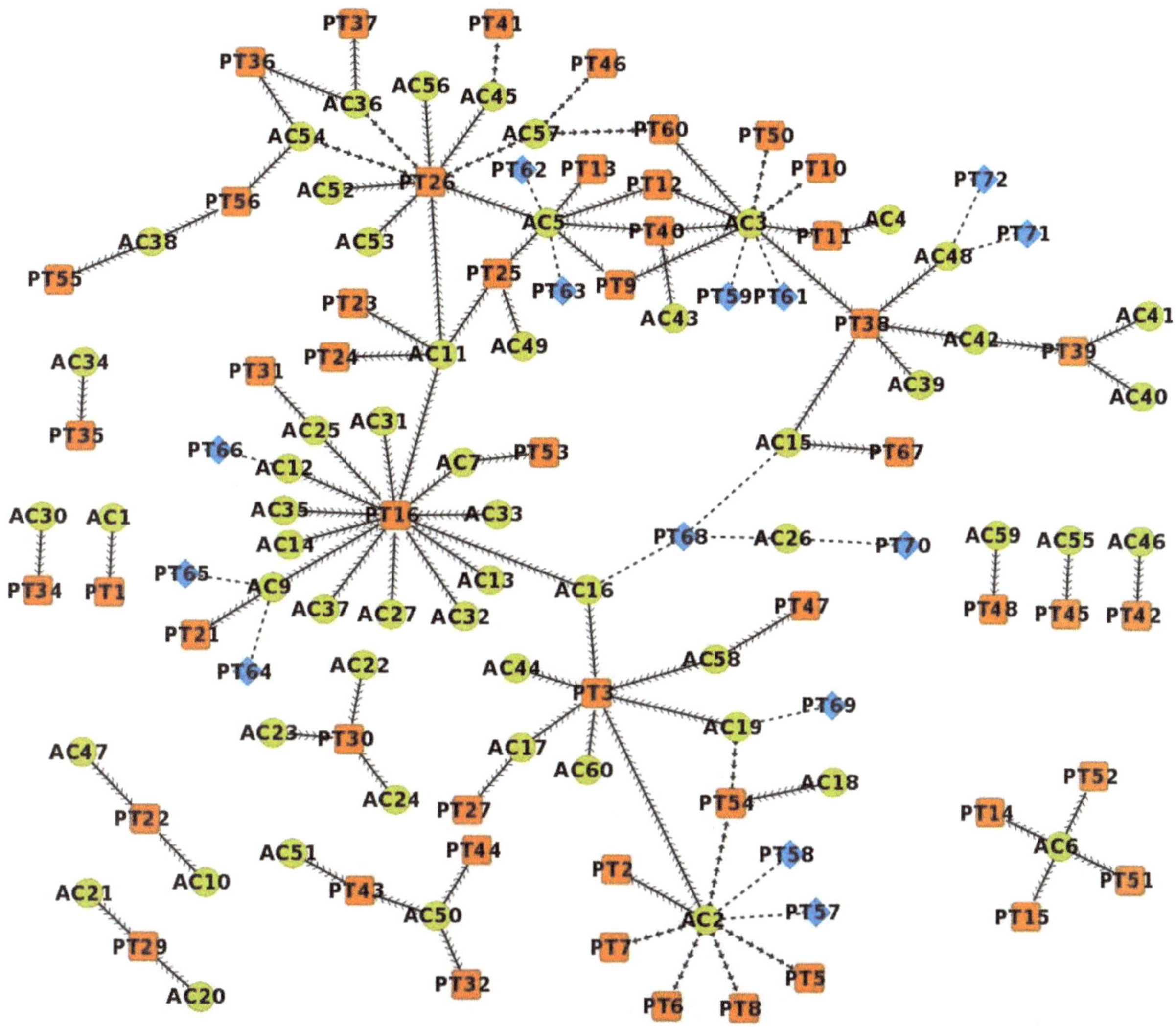

Figure 3. Network containing active compounds and their respective protein targets. Contiguous arrow – AC directly targets PT involved in diabetes, Separate arrow – AC indirectly targets PT involved in diabetes, Dash line – AC targets PT not involved in diabetes.

known fact that the action of phytochemicals is typically multi-targeted. A single active compound may target multiple proteins involved in a particular disease. Among the diabetes-related proteins that are targeted by these compounds, the majority are exclusive to them and are not shared by any other compound. Here, it may be hypothesized that the active compounds that target many proteins have therapeutic relevancy (Hypothesis 3). AC3, AC5, AC6 and AC11 are present in many anti-diabetic plants, as listed in the previous section, whereas AC2 is present only in ADP2.

The protein targets PT3, PT16, PT25, PT26, PT30, PT38, PT39, PT40, and PT54, which are involved in diabetes, are targeted by many active compounds. Hence, it may be hypothesized that these proteins are important since they are targeted by most of the active compounds (Hypothesis 4).

Interestingly, most of the proteins that are targeted by many compounds are covered by the active compounds that target many proteins. Presence of common active compounds in anti-diabetic plants and in turn the presence of common proteins that are targeted by most of the active compounds indicate that the plants and compounds share common mechanism of action, which imparts them anti-diabetic property.

3. Protein Targets (PT) – Pathways (P) Network

The pathways with which the protein targets related to diabetes are involved were collected and a network was constructed (Figure 4). The pathways P1, P4, P5, P6, P7, P12, P19 and P23 involve many protein targets. The protein targets PT14, PT47, PT52 and PT56 are involved in many pathways. These proteins are important since their modulation would alter multiple pathways related to diabetes. Interestingly, none of these protein targets match those that are targeted by many active compounds. Thus, it may be hypothesized that the proteins that are involved in multiple pathways related to diabetes are important (Hypothesis 5).

4. Protein Targets – Diseases Network

The data regarding different diseases in which the diabetes-related protein targets are involved was collected and a network was drawn from it (Figure 5). Here it can be seen that most of the proteins involved in diabetes are also involved in cancer. Diabetes

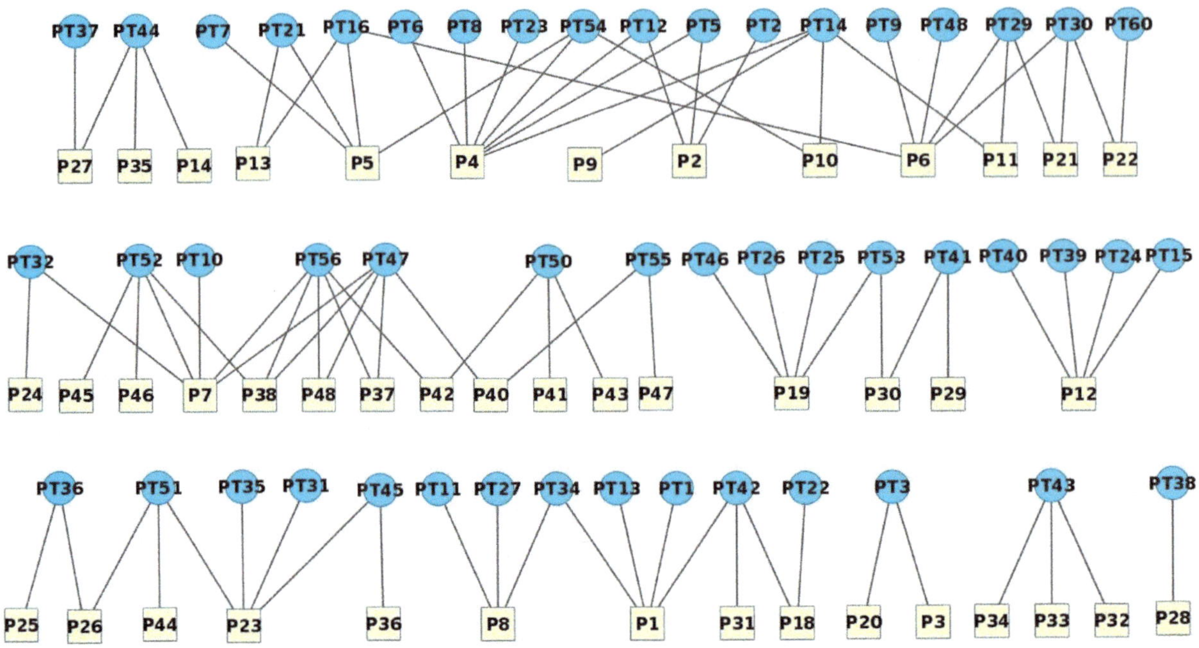

Figure 4. Network containing protein targets and their respective pathways.

and cancer are two heterogeneous, multifactorial, severe, and chronic diseases. Numerous studies have shown a contiguous association between diabetes and cancer. The American Diabetes Association and the American Cancer Society jointly stated that cancer incidence is associated with diabetes as well as certain diabetes risk factors and diabetes treatments [16]. The association between diabetes and cancer incidence or prognosis and existence of risk factors common to both the diseases has been reported [16]. Further, epidemiological studies have indicated that the risk of several types of cancer (including pancreas, liver, breast, colorectal, urinary tract, and female reproductive organs) has increased in diabetic patients [17].

Apart from cancer, many proteins are involved in other diseases like Parkinson's disease, Alzheimer's disease, ischemia, hepatitis and liver diseases. It was reported that type 2 diabetes (T2D) is associated with an increased risk of Parkinson's disease [18]. Numerous studies have shown that common pathophysiological mechanisms exist between Parkinson's disease and T2D [19]. Further, an integrative network analysis has unveiled convergent molecular pathways in Parkinson's disease and diabetes [20]. Mounting evidence also indicates the shared mechanisms of pathogenesis between T2D and Alzheimer's disease [21]. Alzheimer's disease represents a form of diabetes that selectively involves the brain. It also contains molecular and biochemical features that overlap with both T1D and T2D. Therefore, Alzheimer's disease was termed as type 3 diabetes [22]. Further, intranasal administration of insulin in patients with Alzheimer's disease exhibited neuroprotective effects [23,24]. In diabetic patients, cardiovascular disease remains the leading cause of death. Myocardial infarctions and ischemia tend to be more extensive and have a poorer survival rate compared to individuals without diabetes. Similarly, liver diseases were also reported to be very well associated with diabetes [25].

The relation between protein targets and different types of diabetes and its related complications has been studied and the network constructed from this data shows that the proteins are mainly involved in T1D, T2D, diabetic neuropathy, diabetic nephropathy, diabetic angiopathy, diabetic retinopathy and hyperglycemia (Figure 6). Most of the proteins involved in T1D are also involved in T2D and vice versa. This may be due to the similar pathophysiological mechanisms involved in both the types of diabetes. For instance, T1D and T2D are characterized by

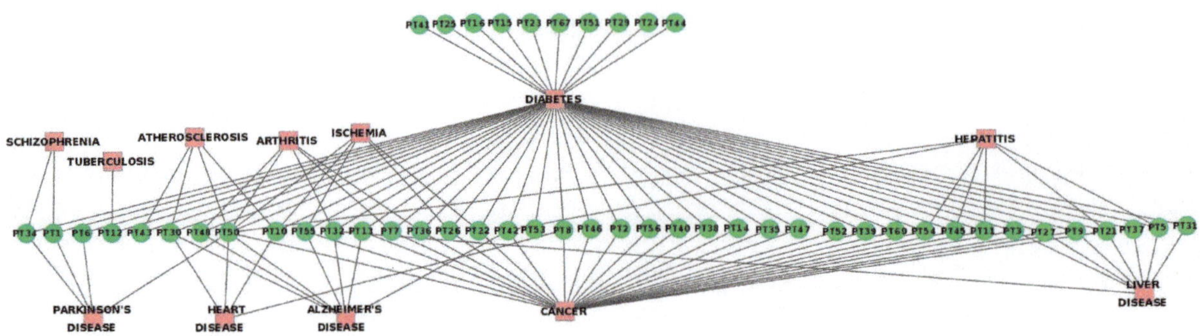

Figure 5. Network containing various diseases in which the protein targets are involved.

progressive beta-cell failure. Apoptosis is probably the main form of beta-cell death in both forms of the disease. The mechanisms leading to nutrient- and cytokine-induced beta-cell death in T2D and T1D, respectively, share the activation of a final common pathway involving interleukin IL-1beta, nuclear factor NF-kappaB, and Fas. All forms of diabetes increase the risk of long-term complications. The major long-term complications are related to the damage of blood vessels and are known as microvascular diseases. The primary microvascular complications of diabetes include damage to the eyes, kidneys, and nerves, known as diabetic retinopathy, diabetic nephropathy and diabetic neuropathy, respectively. From Figure 6, it is evident that these diabetic complications share similar protein targets and hence similar pathological mechanisms.

5. Hypotheses and inferences

In this study, different hypotheses were made at various stages (Figure 7). Inferences were made through careful observation of various networks.

Hypothesis 1. The anti-diabetic plants with the maximum number of active compounds would have good anti-diabetic property.

Inference. This might not be true. The anti-diabetic property of plants depends on the mechanism of action of their active compounds. The anti-diabetic plant that contains therapeutically relevant active compounds need to be considered important, rather than the one with maximum number of active compounds. For example, ADP7, ADP17 and ADP19 contain many active compounds (Figure 2). However, these compounds target very few proteins or pathways involved in diabetes (Figure 3). Hence, these plants might not exhibit comparatively good anti-diabetic property and thus need not be considered important for anti-diabetic treatment. Further, it was observed that most of the important active compounds, like AC2, AC3, AC6, AC11 and AC58 that target multiple proteins and pathways closely related to diabetes, are present in plants (ADP2, ADP21, ADP4, ADP21, ADP27 and ADP25 respectively) that do not contain many active compounds (Figure 2).

Hypothesis 2. The active compounds that are present in many anti-diabetic plants may be therapeutically important.

Inference. This might not be true. For example, AC4 present in the maximum number of anti-diabetic plants, targets only one protein target (PT11), which is involved in only one pathway (Figures 2–4). Similarly, the compounds AC7, AC14, AC17, AC34, AC43 and AC48 that are present in many anti-diabetic plants target very few proteins and pathways. On the contrary, the active compounds, AC2, AC54 and AC58 that target multiple proteins and pathways are present only in ADP2, ADP23, and ADP25, respectively (Figure 2). However, the active compounds AC3, AC5 and AC11 that also target multiple proteins and pathways are present in many plants. But the importance of the active compound depends only on its mechanism of action and not on the number of plants in which it is present.

Hypothesis 3. The active compounds that target many proteins have therapeutic relevancy.

Inference. This is true. Since proteins play a key role in the pathways and disease pathology, they need to be modulated. Diabetes is a multifactorial disease that involves various proteins, pathways and mechanisms. Targeting multiple disease-related proteins and pathways would be beneficial in such diseases. For instance, AC2, AC3, AC5, AC6 and AC11 target multiple proteins involved in diabetes (Figure 3). Hence, due to this polypharmacological effect, they might exhibit better anti-diabetic activity compared to other compounds. Therefore, active compounds that target multiple proteins involved in the disease-related mechanisms are important.

Hypothesis 4. The proteins that are targeted by many active compounds are important.

Inference. This might not be true. For instance, the proteins PT3, PT16 and PT26 are targeted by many active compounds (Figure 3). However, these targets are not involved in multiple pathways related to diabetes. Thus, the proteins with higher involvement in the disease pathology need to be considered important rather than those that are targeted by multiple active compounds.

Hypothesis 5. The protein targets that are involved in multiple pathways related to diabetes are important.

Inference. This is true. The protein targets that are involved in multiple pathways related to diabetes are the proteins with higher involvement in the disease pathology. Therefore, they need to be targeted for effective disease treatment. For instance, the proteins PT14 and PT47 are involved in multiple pathways related to diabetes (Figure 4). Hence, targeting these proteins would prove

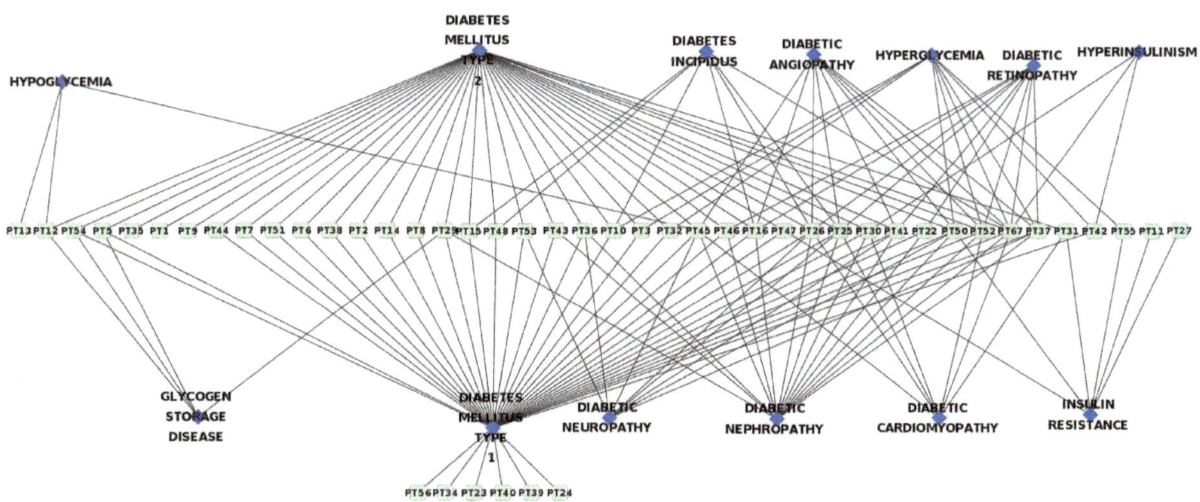

Figure 6. Network containing protein targets involved in different diabetic complications.

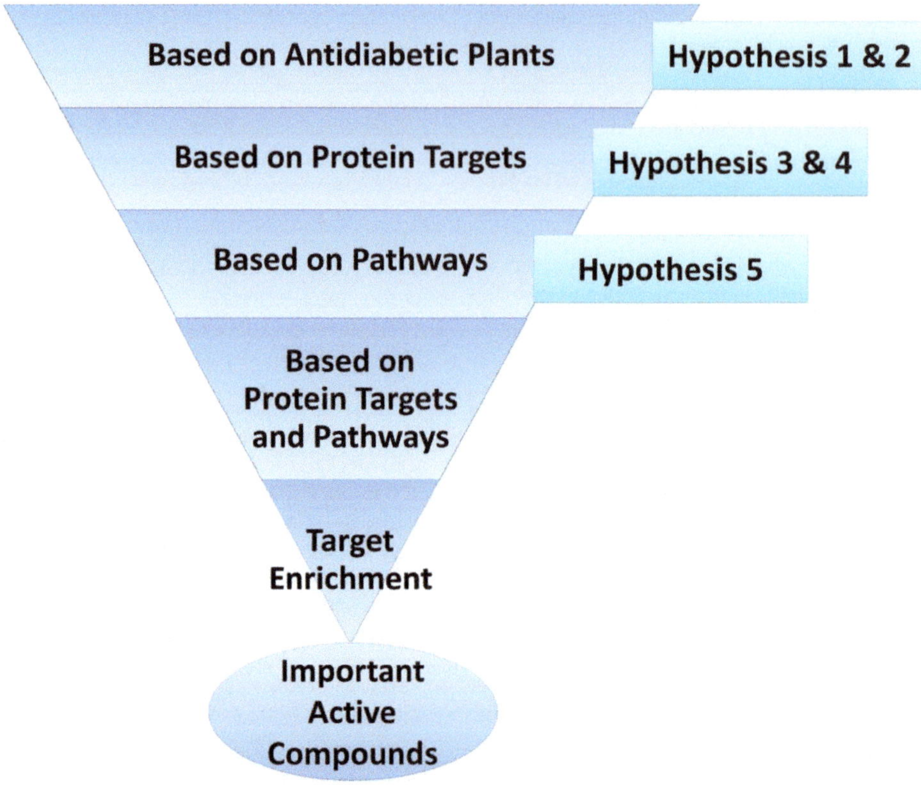

Figure 7. Step-wise representation of the discovery of important/potential active compounds that have been discovered, and the various hypotheses made during these stages.

to be beneficial rather than targeting any of the proteins involved in diabetes.

Thus, these hypotheses and inferences revealed the key phytochemicals and protein targets involved in diabetes. This would help in the preparation of effective anti-diabetic formulations that contain therapeutically important active compounds.

6. Strategy for formulations

Through network analysis, the active compounds present in anti-diabetic plants, their protein targets and the pathways involving these targets have been studied. This would provide an overall view of the mechanism of action of anti-diabetic plants. Further, this would help us to know which proteins need to be targeted and hence, which anti-diabetic plants or rather which active compounds need to be used to achieve this. Therefore, this type of study would assist us in preparing new effective anti-diabetic formulations. In fact, the present strategy could be used to prepare more focused and goal oriented formulations for any disease.

Polyherbal formulations with various active principles and properties have been used from ancient days to treat a whole range of human diseases. Generally, they are a collection of therapeutic recipes that are formulated and prepared on the basis of the healing properties of individual ingredients with respect to the condition of sickness. Such herbal constituents with diverse pharmacological actions principally work together in a dynamic way to produce maximum therapeutic efficacy with minimum side effects. Therefore, studying the biological means of action of various medicinal plants for a disease and then preparing the formulation based on this information would be a more constructive and focused approach. Here, considering plant extracts that contain active compounds that target multiple therapeutically relevant protein targets would be an ideal choice.

For anti-diabetic treatment, we need to consider and target most of the disease-related proteins and pathways. Therefore, a good or ideal formulation would contain active compounds that target multiple proteins as well as the proteins that are involved in multiple pathways related to diabetes. Based on the plants considered in this study, an ideal formulation would be the plant extract containing the active compounds AC2, AC3, AC5, AC6, AC11, AC54 and AC58. The plants containing such active compounds should be considered during anti-diabetic formulations.

$$\text{Ideal Formulation (IF)} = \text{Plant extracts}\left[\left(\begin{array}{c}\text{Active compounds that target}\\ \text{many proteins involved in diabetes}\end{array}\right)+\left(\begin{array}{c}\text{Active compounds that target}\\ \text{proteins which are involved in}\\ \text{many diabetes related pathways}\end{array}\right)\right]$$

$$AC_{PT} = \bigcup_{i=1}^{n}\left[AC_{PT(i)\ \text{with}\ x\geq 1}\right]$$

[AC_{PT} = Active compounds that target many proteins involved in diabetes, i.e., combination of all the active compounds with $x \geq 1$].

$$AC_{PT}(i) = \frac{\text{Degree of Active Compound (i) in AC-PT network}}{\text{Threshold Degree}} = x$$

i = 1 to n (n = number of active compounds).

Degree is an important feature in network analysis. The degree of a node 'N' is the number of nodes connecting it. If three nodes are connecting N, then the degree of this node is three. Threshold Degree is the minimum number of nodes an active compound should be targeting to consider it important. This is manually suggested by analyzing the minimum and maximum degree of active compounds. For example, in this study, the minimum and maximum degree of AC nodes in the AC-PT network are 1 and 8, respectively. If we consider an optimum value of 4 as threshold degree, then AC_{PT} of AC5 (i.e., i = 5) would be,

$$AC_{PT}(5) = \frac{6}{4} = 1.5 \text{ (here, } x > 1)$$

Similarly, when $AC_{PT}(i)$ is calculated for all the active compounds, then AC_{PT} would be,

$$AC_{PT} = AC2, AC3, AC5, AC6 \text{ and } AC11$$

AC_{PT} would help us identify the active compounds that target many proteins. In order to find the active compounds that target proteins which are involved in many pathways,

$$AC\{PT_P\} = \bigcup_{j=1}^{m} [AC\{PT_P(j)\} \text{ with } y \geq 1]$$

[$AC\{PT_P\}$ = Active compounds that target proteins which are involved in many pathways, i.e., combination of all the active compounds that target proteins with y≥1].

[$AC\{PT_P(j)\}$ = Active compound with highest degree among all the compounds that target $PT_P(j)$].

$$PT_P(j) = \frac{\text{Degree of Protein Target (j) in PT-P network}}{\text{Threshold Degree}} = y$$

j = 1 to m (m = number of protein targets).

In this study, if $AC\{PT_P\}$ is calculated with threshold degree 4, then it would be,

$$AC\{PT_P\} = AC6, AC54 \text{ and } AC58$$

Therefore, Ideal formulation (IF) would be,

$$IF = AC_{PT} \bigcup AC\{PT_P\}$$

Finally, from our study, IF would contain active compounds AC2, AC3, AC5, AC6, AC11, AC54 and AC58. Thus, they could be considered the important active compounds and the plants containing these compounds might be used for anti-diabetic formulations.

The IF proposed in this study is based on the fact that targeting multiple proteins involved in diabetes is essential for better anti-diabetic activity. However, the active compounds present in the IF might not target all the important proteins involved in diabetes. In order to cover these important proteins, we might have to include additional active compounds other than those reported in the IF. This might ultimately result in a huge list of compounds and their respective plants. However, this number could be reduced by increasing/enriching the protein targets of the active compounds present in IF. This could be achieved by predicting whether these active compounds could bind to additional proteins, other than those reported in the literature, through structural and pharmacophore studies. In this context, we are proposing a novel methodology named target enrichment to predict additional protein targets of the active compounds. This would help in deciding the active compounds that may target all the important proteins and would make them an ideal choice for formulations.

7. Target enrichment

Since most of the phytochemicals act on multiple targets and exhibit diverse effects, the active compounds that bind to multiple protein targets would be beneficial. Hence, it would be advantageous if we could add new targets to the known active compounds. Target enrichment acts here precisely by predicting novel protein targets. We have employed target enrichment to further increase or enrich the protein targets of active compounds so that it would help us predict which compound would finally bind to a higher number of proteins. This would in turn help in developing effective anti-diabetic polyherbal formulations.

Target enrichment was performed through pharmacophore analysis and docking studies. A pharmacophore is an abstract description of molecular features, which are necessary for molecular recognition of a ligand by a biological macromolecule like protein. The features such as H-bond acceptor, H-bond donor, aromatic ring and hydrophobic group are represented in a pharmacophore. A pharmacophore model explains how structurally diverse ligands can bind to a common receptor site. Numerous studies have shown that the compounds that share similar pharmacophoric features bind to similar proteins [26–28]. This concept has been adopted in our target enrichment study. Since pharmacophore of an active compound represents its binding to a protein target, the target enrichment would only involve active compounds and their 'directly' targeted proteins.

In this study, the pharmacophore analysis showed that the compounds that have similar pharmacophoric features bind to the same target. For example, the active compounds that bind to their respective protein targets like aldose reductase, DNA polymerase, DNA polymerase β and alpha glucosidase have similar pharmacophoric features (Figures 8–11). All the compounds that bind to aldose reductase share similar pharmacophoric features (Figure 8). It can be seen that the benzene rings on the left harbours pharmacophoric features that are common to all of them. The compounds that target DNA polymerase also share similar pharmacophoric features (Figure 9). They contain an aromatic benzene ring to which an H-bond acceptor and a donor group are attached. Similarly, all the compounds of DNA polymerase β share similar pharmacophoric features (Figure 10). On their left side, they contain an H-bond acceptor and a donor group. The compounds of alpha glucosidase do not have similar structures. However, they share few common pharmacophoric features, due to which, all of them might be binding to alpha glucosidase (Figure 11).

Since the compounds with similar structures and pharmacophoric features bind to similar protein targets, during target enrichment, we would consider active compounds that have similar pharmacophoric features and then append the protein targets of each compound to all of them. However, though structurally similar compounds bind to similar targets, the inverse is not always true. That is, all the compounds that bind to a particular target might not have similar structures and pharmacophoric features. For example, compounds that bind to Cyclooxygenase-1 (COX-1), Cyclooxygenase-2 (COX-2) and DNA topoisomerase 2, respectively, do not have similar structures and pharmacophoric features. Among the compounds of DNA topoisomerase 2, only diadzein is similar to genistein (Figure 12). In the case of COX-1, only coniferin and gallic acid have little structural similarity (Figure 13). This may be due to the fact that the binding of compounds to a protein not only depends on their pharmacophoric features but also on the binding site conformations. All the compounds that have similar pharmacophoric features might bind to the same protein conformation, whereas the compounds with different pharmacophoric features might bind to the different conformations of the same protein. Therefore, the compounds that have similar structures and pharmacophoric features may bind to the same protein target, whereas compounds that bind to a particular protein may not have similar structures and pharmacophoric features. Hence, two compounds binding to a protein target might or might not have similar structures or pharmacophoric features.

During target enrichment, addition of targets to compounds cannot be done merely by checking whether these compounds have common targets. For instance, though bakuchicin and betulinic acid bind to DNA topoisomerase 2, it should not be simply assumed that they might have similar pharmacophoric features and thus bakuchicin may bind to the other targets of betulinic acid. This may not be true because these compounds have different pharmacophoric features. Therefore, pharmacophore analysis and docking studies are necessary and they play a key role in target enrichment.

Since we need active compounds that target multiple proteins, it would be ideal to consider the already discovered active compounds that directly target multiple proteins and then apply target enrichment methodology to further increase their protein targets. For instance, diadzein (AC42) may not be an ideal choice in anti-diabetic formulation since it targets only two proteins, namely DNA polymerase and DNA topoisomerase 2. We could check for alternate compounds that might target many other proteins apart from these two. It turns out that no other compound binds to these two targets. However, betulinic acid (AC3) that targets multiple proteins also binds to DNA topoisomerase 2, a common target for both AC3 and AC42. Therefore, by applying target enrichment studies we could check whether these compounds share similar pharmacophoric features. In case they do, we could hypothesize that since AC3 and AC42 have similar pharmacophore features and similar protein targets, AC3 may bind to DNA polymerase also. This could be verified through docking studies. If AC3 is binding to DNA polymerase, then we could enrich the targets of AC3 by adding this protein. Therefore, in the anti-diabetic formulations, instead of AC42 we could use AC3 that targets multiple proteins. This would further reduce the usage of therapeutically insignificant plants in anti-diabetic formulations.

In this study, betulinic acid, oleanolic acid, gallic acid and myricetin have high number of direct protein targets (Table S1). Therefore, target enrichment was carried out on them. For target enrichment of these compounds, we need to check for other compounds that share at least one of their protein targets.

In the case of betulinic acid, the active compound, diadzein, shares the protein target DNA topoisomerase 2 and oleanolic acid shares the protein targets, namely, glycogen phosphorylase, diacylglycerol acyltransferase and DNA polymerase beta. Betulinic acid and diadzein do not have similar pharmacophoric features. Therefore, betulinic acid might not bind to the other targets of diadzein. This was further confirmed through docking of betulinic acid and diadzein to DNA topoisomerase 2. Both these compounds bind to this protein with different features (Figure 14). During pharmacophore analysis, it was observed that among the compounds that bind to DNA topoisomerase 2, diadzein and genistein have similar pharmacophoric features. When these compounds were docked to this protein, it was found that they bind with similar features. This further supports the fact that if two compounds have similar pharmacophoric features, they bind to a common protein target, which could be proved through docking studies.

Betulinic acid and oleanolic acid have similar pharmacophoric features. These compounds were docked to their common target, DNA polymerase beta (Figure 15). It was observed that they bind similarly to this protein. Since compounds with similar pharmacophore features bind similarly to their protein targets and also might bind to similar protein targets as well, betulinic acid may bind to the other targets of oleanolic acid and vice versa. Thus, Gamma-Aminobutyric acid (GABA) transaminase, COX-1 and COX-2 could be added to the protein targets list of betulinic acid.

Oleanolic acid shares the targets diacylglycerol acyltransferase, glycogen phosphorylase and DNA polymerase beta with betulinic acid. It also shares COX-1 and COX-2 with gallic acid. The compounds oleanolic acid and gallic acid appear to have very few similar pharmacophoric features. Therefore, oleanolic acid might not be binding to the other proteins of gallic acid. Their mode of binding with these proteins could not be studied through docking, since these protein structures are not available. It has been observed that oleanolic acid and betulinic acid have similar pharmacophoric features and also bind similarly to DNA polymerase beta (Figure 15). So, oleanolic acid might bind to the other targets of betulinic acid. To verify this, oleanolic acid was docked to DNA topoisomerase 2. It was observed that it binds to this protein similar to betulinic acid (Figure 14). Thus, DNA topoisomerase 2, 5-alpha reductase and Liver X receptor alpha (LXR alpha) could be added to the protein targets list of oleanolic acid.

In the case of gallic acid, it shares aldose reductase with kaempferol, apigenin and luteolin. It shares COX-1 and COX-2 with oleanolic acid. During pharmacophore analysis, it was observed that all the compounds that bind to aldose reductase have similar pharmacophoric features (Figure 8). Therefore, all of them might share similar protein targets. To verify this, all these compounds were docked to aldose reductase. It was observed that they bind to it with similar features. (Figure 16). Therefore, gallic acid may bind to the other protein targets of these compounds. Thus, lipoxygenase, 20-alpha hydroxysteroid dehydrogenase and alpha glucosidase could be added to the protein targets list of gallic acid. Hence, during anti-diabetic formulations, the plants containing gallic acid could be considered instead of the plants containing kaempferol, apigenin and luteolin, since gallic acid binds to the protein targets of kaempferol, apigenin and luteolin and might exhibit effects similar to them.

Though oleanolic acid and gallic acid have COX-1 and COX-2 as common targets, they do not have very similar pharmacophoric features (Figure 13). Only a part of them is similar. This shows that

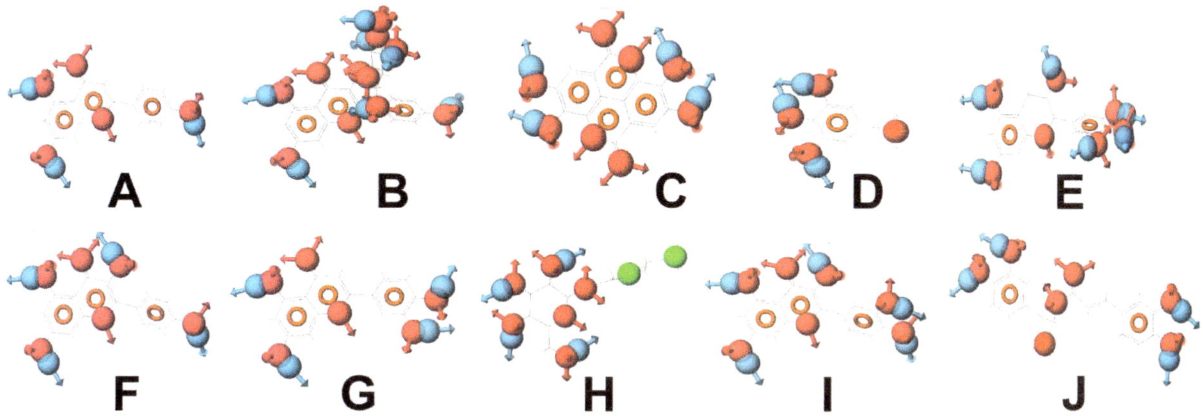

Figure 8. Compounds (with their pharmacophoric features) that target aldose reductase. (A) Apigenin, (B) Astragalin, (C) Ellagic acid, (D) Gallic acid, (E) Gallocatechin, (F) Kaempferol, (G) Luteolin, (H) Perilloside A, (I) Quercetin and (J) Rosmarinic acid. These compounds show similar pharmacophoric features.

they might not bind to all the protein targets commonly. Oleanolic acid may bind to very few or no protein targets of gallic acid and vice versa. To study this, gallic acid was docked to DNA polymerase beta, which is a target of oleanolic acid. It was observed that gallic acid binds well to DNA polymerase beta. It binds to the amino acid residues of DNA polymerase beta, similar to oleanolic acid and betulinic acid (Figure 15). However, when oleanolic acid and betulinic acid were docked to aldose reductase, which is a target of gallic acid, they were not able to bind properly. Gallic acid bound to a deep pocket whereas oleanolic acid and betulinic acid were not able to enter the pocket of aldose reductase (Figure 17). This might be due to the fact that the binding pocket of DNA polymerase beta is large so that it could accommodate the large oleanolic acid and betulinic acid molecules as well as the small gallic acid molecule. However, the binding pocket of aldose reductase is small; therefore, it could only accommodate gallic acid but not oleanolic acid and betulinic acid (Figure 17). This indicates that when compounds are partly similar, although they share a similar protein target, they may not share all the targets of each other. Thus, target enrichment might depend on the degree of structural and feature similarity of the compounds. The higher the similarity, higher may be their protein targets being shared.

Myricetin does not share its protein targets with any other active compounds. The protein targets of myricetin are exclusive to this compound only; therefore, target enrichment could not be applied on myricetin. This should be considered one of the most important compounds.

8. Predicted ADME properties

The ADME and pharmacokinetic properties of compounds are very important. We analyzed physically significant descriptors and pharmaceutically relevant properties of all the active compounds (Table S2). The number of stars, which represent the number of property or descriptor values that fall outside the 95% range of similar values for known drugs, were within the recommended range of 0–5 for almost all the compounds. Molecules with a large number of stars suggest that they are less drug-like than those with few stars. The molecular weight of all the compounds is within the recommended range of 130–725. The octanol/water partition coefficient (QP logPo/w) and aqueous solubility (QP logS), which

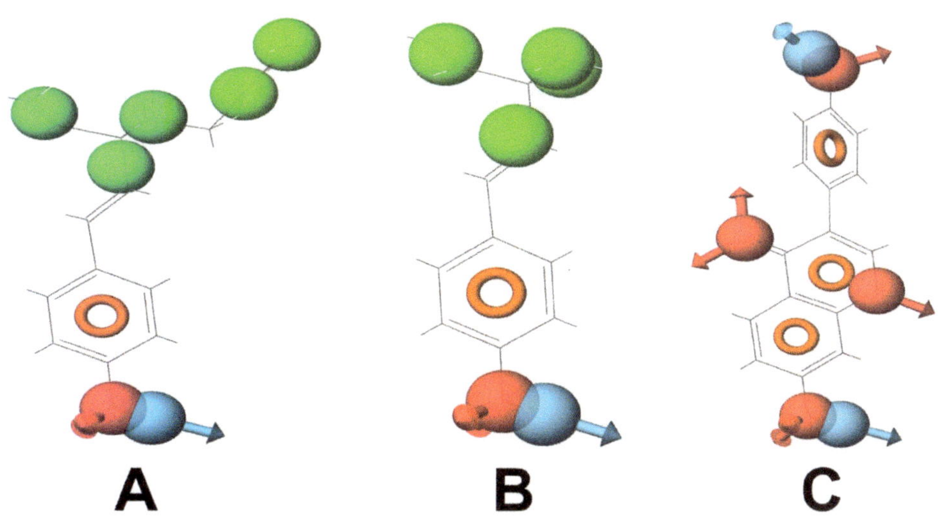

Figure 9. Compounds (with their pharmacophoric features) that target DNA polymerase. (A) Bakuchiol, (B) Corylifolin and (C) Diadzein. These compounds show similar pharmacophoric features.

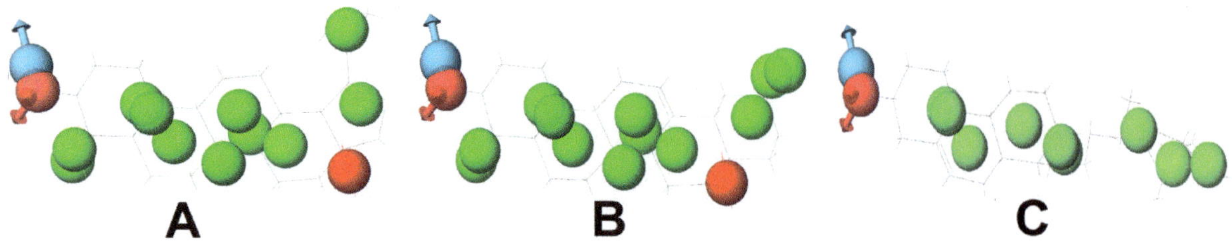

Figure 10. Compounds (with their pharmacophoric features) that target DNA polymerase beta. (A) Betulinic acid, (B) Oleanolic acid and (C) Stgmasterol. These compounds show similar pharmacophoric features.

are essential in the estimation of absorption and distribution of drugs within the body, ranged between −5.814 to 7.396 and −8.947 to 0.306, respectively. Most of the compounds were within the acceptable range of −2.0–6.5 for QP logPo/w and −6.5–0.5 for QP logS. The key factors, namely QPPCaco, which governs the drug metabolism and its access to biological membranes, and QPPMDCK, which predicts the cell permeability of the drugs, were within the recommended range for most of the compounds (values <25 are poor and >500 are good). The % human oral absorption for most of the compounds was within the range of 25–80 (<25% is poor and >80% is high). Further, all the compounds were violating Lipinski's rule of five in the range of 0–2 (maximum number of violations acceptable are 4). Thus, most of the pharmacokinetic parameters of the compounds are within the acceptable range for human use.

Discussion

Through network analysis, we have attempted to show the biological means of pharmacological action of anti-diabetic plants. It was observed that most of the active compounds present in anti-diabetic plants act on multiple protein targets. These proteins in turn are involved in multiple pathways related to diabetes and their complications. Network analysis revealed important information like 1) the anti-diabetic plants that contain many active compounds, 2) the active compounds that are present in most of the anti-diabetic plants, 3) the active compounds that target most of the proteins, 4) proteins that are targeted by most of the active compounds, 5) proteins that are involved in multiple pathways, 6) pathways that involve most of the proteins, 7) proteins that are involved in different diabetes-related complications and 8) the proteins that are involved in various other diseases. It was observed that these diseases share similar pathophysiological mechanisms with diabetes. This study provided an overview of the proteins and the pathways involved in diabetes. Thus, the mechanism of action of anti-diabetic plants and their active compounds was deduced by analyzing their protein targets and respective pathways. For instance, gallic acid was reported to have anti-lipid peroxidative and anti-lipidemic effects in diabeteic rats [29,30]. In this study, we have shown that gallic acid binds to protein targets PT16, PT23, PT24, PT25 and PT26. The protein PT16 is involved in glycerolipid metabolism pathway, P6. The proteins PT24 and PT25 are involved in the metabolism of a fatty acid namely arachidonic acid. The involvement of protein targets in lipid metabolism pathways explains the role of gallic acid in anti-lipid peroxidative and anti-lipidemic effects.

Pharmacophore analysis has revealed the chemical basis of pharmacological action of anti-diabetic plants. It was observed that the anti-diabetic plants that show similar mechanisms of action contain active compounds with similar pharmacophoric features. These active compounds in turn bind to similar protein targets and thus show similar pharmacological action. Further, through pharmacophore analysis and docking studies, we have introduced a target enrichment protocol to discover novel protein targets for the important active compounds. The step-by-step methodology used in this study is represented in the form of a flow chart, which also reflects the decision making at various stages (Figure 18).

In this study we have proposed various hypotheses that have been derived from network analysis. Observations made from them revealed that the active compounds that target multiple proteins and also that target proteins which are involved in multiple pathways are important for effective anti-diabetic activity. Taking this in to consideration, we have proposed a strategy that could be used in the preparation of new effective anti-diabetic formulations.

From this study, it could be deduced that an anti-diabetic formulation containing active compounds AC2, AC3, AC5, AC6, AC11, AC54 and AC58, which are present in the anti-diabetic plants ADP2, ADP3, ADP5, ADP23 and ADP25, might have better anti-diabetic activity. The significance of these compounds

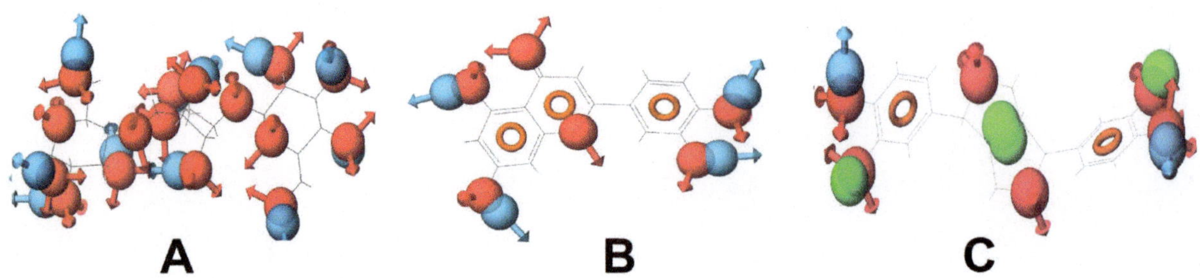

Figure 11. Compounds (with their pharmacophoric features) that target alpha glucosidase. (A) Beta Glucan, (B) Luteolin and (C) Pinoresinol. These compounds show similar pharmacophoric features.

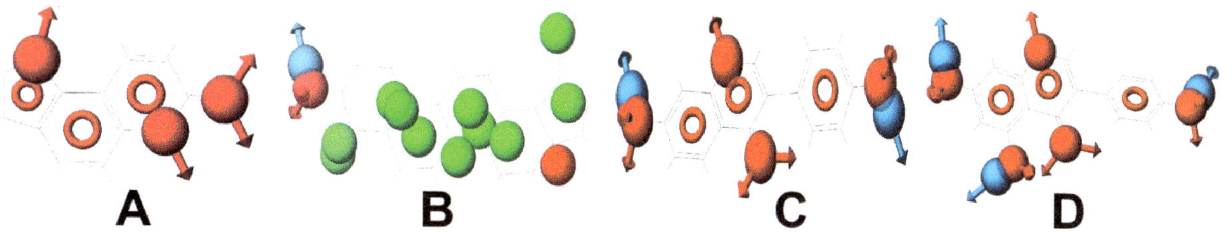

Figure 12. Compounds (with their pharmacophoric features) that target DNA topoisomerase 2. (A) Bakuchicin, (B) Betulinic acid, (C) Diadzein and (D) Genistein. These compounds do not show similar pharmacophoric features. Only diadzein is similar to genistein.

and their possible mechanism of action against diabetes are as follows.

AC2 (1-deoxynojirimycin)

AC2 was reported as an alpha-glucosidase inhibitor, but little or no information is available regarding its anti-diabetic activity. It is structurally similar to known FDA approved alpha-glucosidase inhibitors, Miglustat and Miglitol (Figure S1). Miglustat (N-butyl-deoxynojirimycin) is used primarily to treat Type-1 Gaucher disease (GD1). It is an imino sugar, a synthetic analogue of D-glucose. Miglitol is an oral anti-diabetic drug that acts by inhibiting the ability of the patient to break down complex carbohydrates into glucose. It is primarily used in T2D for establishing greater glycemic control by preventing the digestion of carbohydrates (such as disaccharides, oligosaccharides, and polysaccharides) into monosaccharides, which can be absorbed by the body. Miglustat and Miglitol inhibits alpha-glucosidases. Since AC2 also inhibits alpha-glucosidases, its mechanism of action might be similar to these drugs.

AC2 targets alpha glucosidases directly. Alpha glucosidase is a carbohydrate-hydrolase that breaks down starch and disaccharides to glucose. It is involved in N-glycan biosynthesis (P3) and sucrose metabolism (P20) pathways. Alpha glucosidases are very well known enzymes involved in diabetes and their inhibitors were reported to show good anti-diabetic effects. Alpha glucosidase inhibitors could inhibit the absorption of carbohydrates from the gut and are used in the treatment of patients with T2D or impaired glucose tolerance. It was reported that inhibition of intestinal alpha-glucosidases reduced the rate of glucose absorption by delaying the carbohydrate digestion and prolonging the overall carbohydrate digestion time [31]. Further, the postprandial rise in blood glucose was dose-dependently decreased, and glucose-induced insulin secretion was also attenuated. Thus, alpha glucosidase inhibition was proved to have potential in delaying and possibly preventing the development of diabetic complications [31]. AC2 was reported to strongly inhibit alpha glucosidases [32]. Therefore, inhibition of alpha glucosidases might be an important reason behind the anti-diabetic activity of AC2.

AC2 targets glycogen debranching enzyme, cytosolic beta glucosidase, lactase-glycosylceramidase and glucosidase II beta subunit precursor enzyme indirectly through glucosidases. Glycogen debranching enzyme is involved in glycogenolysis. Conversion of glycogen to glucose-1-phosphate occurs in glycogenolysis that leads to the increase in blood glucose levels. The role of cytosolic beta glucosidase in diabetes is not reported in the literature. But, from our data analysis, it can be seen that cytosolic beta glucosidase is involved in starch and sucrose metabolism, which is an important pathway related to diabetes. Similarly, the role of glycosylceramidase in diabetes is also not known. The substrates of this enzyme are glycosyl-N-acylsphingosine and H_2O, whereas its two products are N-acylsphingosine and sugar. Further, it is involved in galactose metabolism pathway. Therefore, glycosylceramidase may lead to an increase in sugar levels, which is targeted by AC2.

AC3 (Betulinic acid)

AC3 is a naturally occurring pentacyclic triterpenoid, having anti-retroviral, anti-malarial and anti-inflammatory properties. Recently, it has been discovered as a potential anti-cancer agent [33]. Since it functions as both a hypolipidemic and a hypoglycemic agent, it was proposed that AC3 may have therapeutic potential in combating T2D and obesity, by effectively modulating the various enzymes and hormones involved in the absorption and metabolism of carbohydrates and lipids [34]. Betulinic acid and oleanolic acid, both pentacyclic triterpenoids, have shown multiple biological activities with apparent effects on glucose absorption, glucose uptake, insulin secretion, diabetic vascular dysfunction, retinopathy and nephropathy. The versatility of the pentacyclic triterpenes provides a promising approach for diabetes management [35].

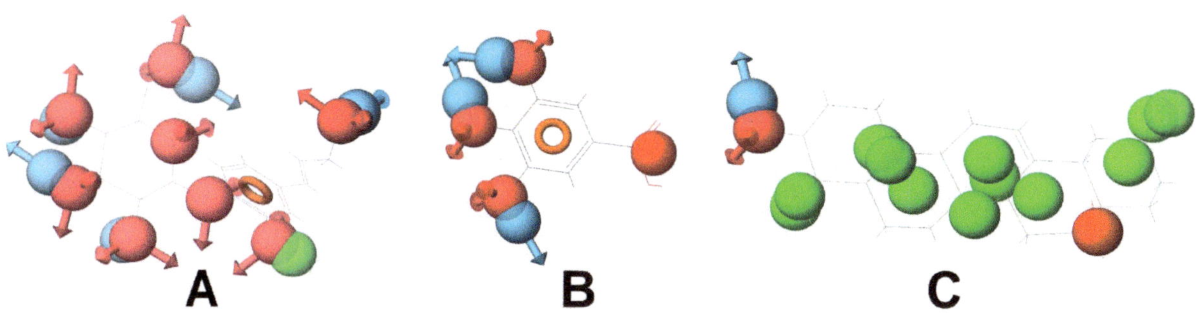

Figure 13. Compounds (with their pharmacophoric features) that target COX-1. (A) Coniferin, (B) Gallic acid and (C) Oleanolic acid. These compounds do not show similar pharmacophoric features. Only coniferin and gallic acid have little structural similarity.

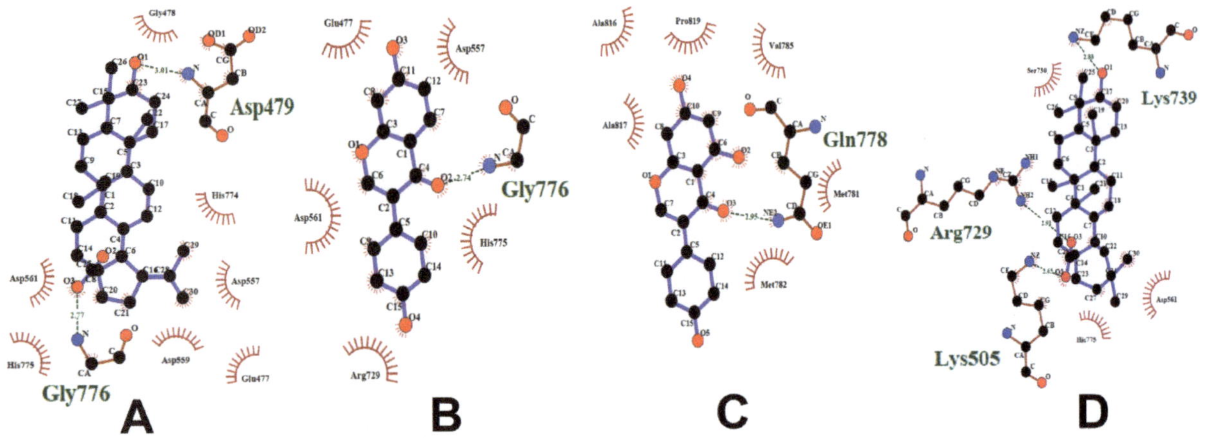

Figure 14. Compounds docked to DNA topoisomerase 2. (A) Betulinic acid, (B) Diadzein, (C) Genistein and (D) Oleanolic acid. Betulinic acid and diadzein bind to this protein with different features. Diadzein and genistein bind with similar features. Oleanolic acid and betulinic acid also bind with similar features.

AC3 directly targets six proteins: diacylglycerol acyltransferase, 5-alpha reductase, glycogen phosphorylase, DNA topoisomerase 2, DNA polymerase beta and LXR alpha. The first enzyme, diacylglycerol acyltransferase, catalyzes the final step in triglyceride synthesis. Pharmacological studies suggest that inhibition of this enzyme is a promising strategy for the treatment of T2D [36]. It was reported that the mice with hepatic overexpression of diacylglycerol acyltransferase showed hepatic insulin resistance [36]. This enzyme is also involved in glycerolipid metabolism. The second enzyme, 5-alpha reductase, is involved in steroid metabolism. It converts testosterone to 5α-dihydrotestosterone (DHT) in peripheral tissues. The role of this enzyme in diabetes is not well known. It is involved in steroid hormone biosynthesis pathway. The natural mechanism of 5-alpha reductase inhibition involves the binding of nicotinamide adenine dinucleotide phosphate (NADPH) to the enzyme followed by the substrate. The structure of AC3 is similar to the known synthetic drugs of 5-alpha reductase, namely, finasteride and dutasteride (Figure S2). These drugs are mainly used for the treatment of benign prostatic hyperplasia (BPH) and male pattern baldness (MPB).

The third enzyme targeted by AC3, glycogen phosphorylase, catalyzes the rate-limiting step in glycogenolysis. It breaks up glycogen into glucose subunits. It was reported that inhibition of hepatic glycogen phosphorylase is a promising treatment strategy for attenuating hyperglycemia in T2D [37]. The regulation of the hepatic glucose output through glycogenolysis is an important target for T2D therapy. This mechanism of action of AC3 is similar to AC2, which also targets glycogenolysis through glycogen debranching enzyme. The fourth enzyme, DNA topoisomerase 2, cut the strands of the DNA helix in order to manage DNA tangles and supercoils. It was reported that chronically elevated levels of glucose increases the mitochondrial DNA damage and thus contributes to mitochondrial dysfunction [38]. Mitochondria-dependent DNA cleavage was significantly exacerbated and mitochondrial topoisomerase function was significantly altered in the presence of hydrogen peroxide (H_2O_2). Further, when mitochondria were chronically exposed to elevated glucose, significant increase in topoisomerase-linked DNA cleavage was observed [38]. Therefore, inhibition of this topoisomerase by compounds like AC3 might have beneficial effects in the case of diabetes. DNA polymerase beta is another enzyme involved in the maintenance of DNA, during DNA damage, through base excision repair. The sixth protein, LXR alpha, is a sensor of cholesterol metabolism and lipid biosynthesis. It is an important regulator of cholesterol, triglyceride and glucose homeostasis. It has been reported that LXR is a highly interesting target for drug development for treating diabetes [39].

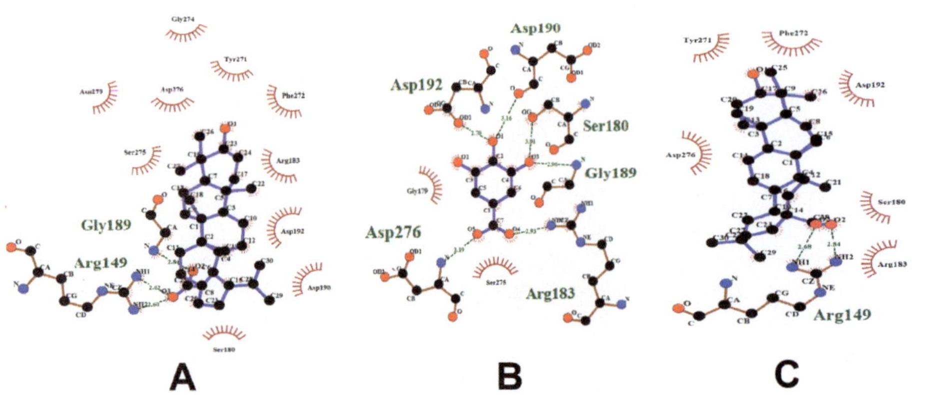

Figure 15. Compounds docked to DNA polymerase beta. (A) Betulinic acid, (B) Gallic acid and (C) Oleanolic acid. Betulinic acid and oleanolic bind similarly to this protein.

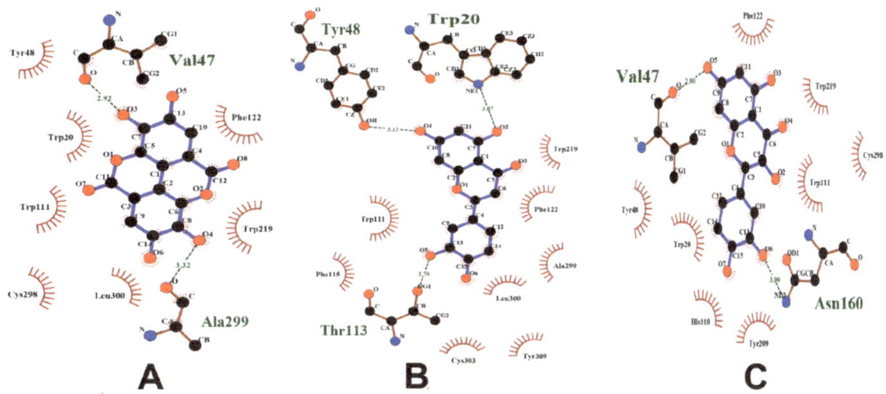

Figure 16. Compounds docked to aldose reductase. (A) Ellagic acid, (B) Luteolin and (C) Quercetin. All these compounds bind to this protein with similar features.

AC3 indirectly targets nitric oxide synthase (NOS) and NADPH oxidase. Impaired NOS pathway was seen in diabetes mellitus. It was reported that endothelial nitric oxide synthase (eNOS) deficiency produced accelerated nephropathy in diabetic mice [40]. Similarly, eNOS knockout in diabetic mice developed advanced diabetic nephropathy [41]. Therefore, a higher level of NOS is desirable to reduce diabetic complications. AC3 was reported to up-regulate eNOS. AC3-treated endothelial cells showed an increased production of bioactive nitric oxide [42]. NADPH oxidase is an important protein involved in diabetes. It catalyzes the conversion of NADPH to NADP, thereby producing superoxide free radicals. These free radicals in turn are involved in DNA damage and in the impairment of the function of DNA repairing enzymes such as DNA topoisomerase 2 and DNA polymerase beta. AC3 downregulates the NADPH oxidase levels [42]. As it was mentioned previously that the natural mechanism of inhibition of 5-alpha reductase involves the binding of NADPH to that enzyme, presence of NADPH oxidase may lower the concentration of NADPH and thus decreases 5α reductase inhibition. However, inhibition of NADPH oxidase not only reduces the formation of free radicals but also increases the levels of NADPH. Therefore, AC3 may inhibit 5α reductase both directly through binding to it and indirectly by inhibiting NADPH oxidase.

AC5 (Oleanolic acid)

AC5 is a naturally occurring triterpenoid, widely distributed in food and medicinal plants. It is relatively non-toxic, hepatoprotective, and exhibits anti-tumor and anti-viral properties [43]. AC5 directly targets diacylglycerol acyltransferase, glycogen phosphorylase, GABA transaminase, cyclooxygenase-1 (COX-1), cyclooxygenase-2 (COX-2) and DNA polymerase beta. The proteins diacylglycerol acyltransferase, glycogen phosphorylase and DNA polymerase beta have been discussed with respect to AC3 since they share common targets. Thus, AC5, by targeting these proteins, may show mechanism of action similar to AC3. Among the remaining proteins, GABA transaminase is exclusively targeted by AC5. This enzyme is involved in amino acid metabolism pathways and catalyzes the conversion of 4-aminobutanoate to amino acids such as alanine, glycine and glutamate. It was reported that alterations in the alanine cycle and increase in the levels of serum alanine aminotransferase (ALT) is linked to the development of T2D. Further, elevated level of ALT increases the risk of developing T2D [44]. Inhibition of GABA transaminase would in turn inhibit alanine formation. This enzyme also forms glutamate whose abnormal homeostasis is commonly observed in diabetes. Abnormal glutamate homeostasis might contribute to diabetes pathogenesis and excessive glutamate consumption might cause insulin resistance [45]. Further, high extracellular glutamate

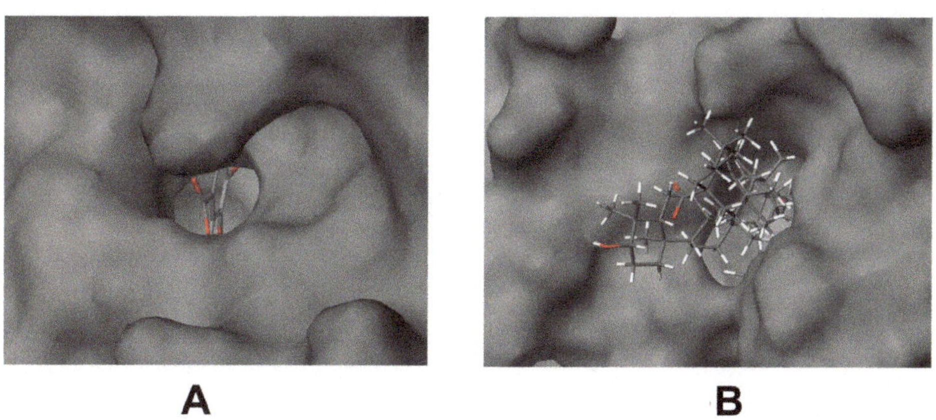

Figure 17. Compounds docked to aldose reductase. (A) Gallic acid, (B) Oleanolic acid and Betulinic acid. The binding pocket of aldose reductase is small. Gallic acid bound to a deep pocket whereas oleanolic acid and betulinic acid were not able to enter the pocket. Therefore, it could only accommodate gallic acid but not oleanolic acid and betulinic acid.

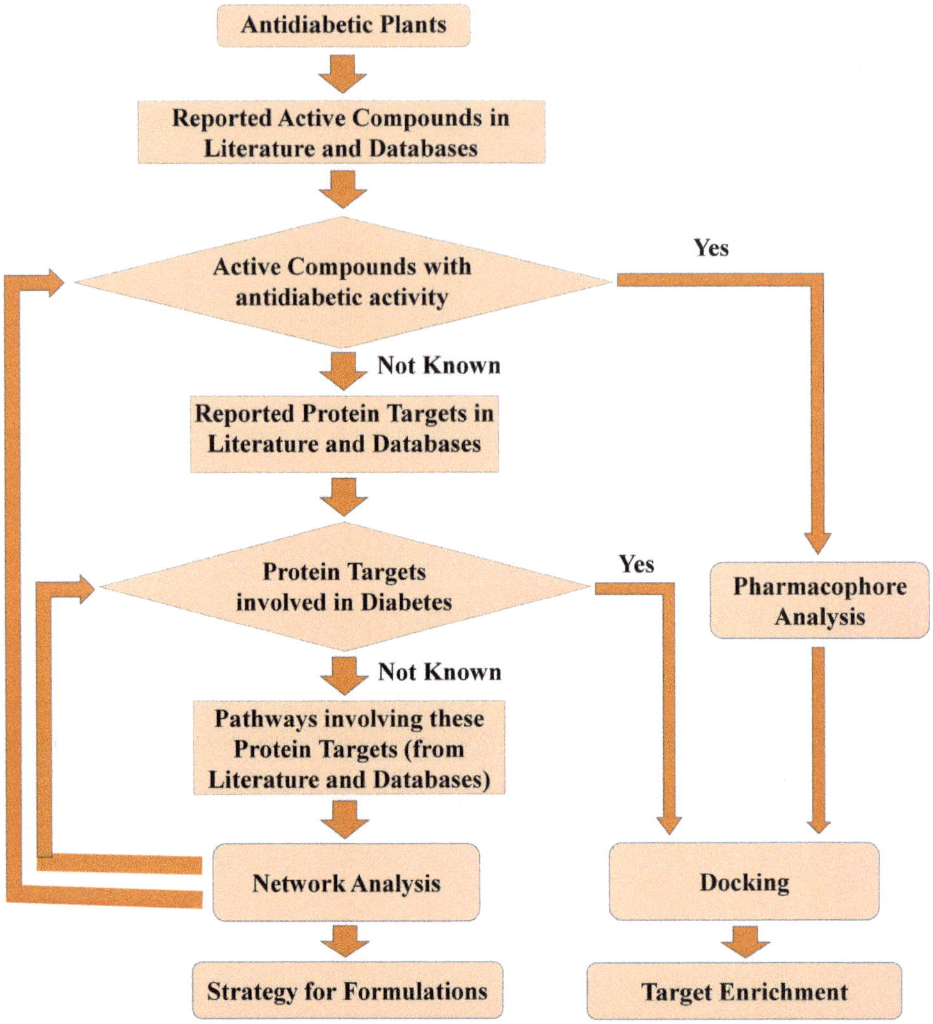

Figure 18. The step-by-step methodology used in this study. The active compounds of anti-diabetic plants, their protein targets, and the pathways in which these proteins are involved were retrieved from literature and databases. If the anti-diabetic activity of the active compounds is not reported/known, then it is identified through network analysis by analyzing whether their protein targets and respective pathways are involved in diabetes. The target enrichment of active compounds with anti-diabetic activity was carried out through pharmacophore analysis and docking. If the involvement of protein targets in diabetes is not known, then it is identified through network analysis by analyzing whether their respective pathways are involved in diabetes. The protein targets involved in diabetes were employed in docking for target enrichment.

levels exert direct and indirect effects that might participate in the progressive loss of beta-cells occurring in both T1D and T2D [45]. Therefore, inhibition of GABA transaminase by AC5 might reduce the formation of glutamate and its diabetic complications.

Glycine is formed from the reaction between 4-aminobutanoate and glyoxylate, catalyzed by GABA transaminase. Theoretically, inhibition of GABA transaminase would inhibit this reaction and thereby reduces the formation of glycine. Interestingly, glycine shows anti-diabetic effects. Patients with uncontrolled T2D have severely deficient synthesis of glutathione (GSH). Dietary supplementation with glycine restored GSH synthesis and lowered oxidative stress and oxidant damage in the face of persistent hyperglycemia [46]. Further, glycine reduced the alterations induced by hyperglycemia in streptozotocin-induced diabetic rats [47]. Moreover, glyoxylate, one of the substrates in the above mentioned GABA transaminase catalyzed reaction was reported to be at significantly higher levels in diabetes patients. It was proposed that glyoxylate could be used as a potential novel marker for early detection of T2D [48]. Therefore, a higher level of GABA transaminase is needed to produce glycine through glyoxylate-based reaction. Hence, inhibition of this enzyme by AC5 is not desirable. However, the relation between GABA transaminase, glyoxylate and glycine has not been practically studied. Since the role of GABA transaminase in diabetes is not clearly known, this would be an interesting study to understand the mechanism of action of this enzyme. The enzymes COX-1 and COX-2 are responsible for the conversion of arachidonic acid to prostanoids. COX-1 is the rate-limiting enzyme in the control of prostanoid metabolism. Altered prostanoid metabolism is seen in the pathogenesis of diabetic complications. Therefore, targeting of COX-1 and COX-2 enzymes might be one of the reasons behind the anti-diabetic activity of AC5. These enzymes are involved in arachidonic acid metabolism pathway. It was reported that inhibitors of these enzymes would have a dual protective role in diabetes, by minimizing beta-cell dysfunction and by maintaining insulin secretion through enhancing endogenous arachidonic acid levels [49].

AC6 (Myricetin)

AC6 is a natural bioflavonoid whose occurrence in nature is widespread among plants. It has been demonstrated to possess both antioxidative and prooxidative properties. It is a potent anti-carcinogen and anti-mutagen. It has therapeutic potential and benefits in cardiovascular diseases and diabetes mellitus [50]. AC6 provided protection against oxidative stress in T2D erythrocytes [51]. It had beneficial effect on renal functions in streptozotocin-induced diabetes and thus, it was suggested that AC6 could be of therapeutic potential in diabetic nephropathy [52].

AC6 targets alpha-amylase, xanthine oxidase, insulin receptor and phosphoinositide 3-kinase (PI3K). These proteins are exclusively targeted by this active compound. Alpha-amylase plays an important role in the digestion of starch and glycogen. This enzyme is involved in pancreatic secretion, starch and sucrose metabolism pathways. One of the therapeutic strategies for the treatment of T2D includes the inhibition of degradation of oligo and disaccharides. Phytochemicals as inhibitors of alpha-amylase has been proposed as a possibility to treat diabetes mellitus [53]. Further, significant reduction in the post-prandial increase of blood glucose was proposed as an important strategy in the management of blood glucose level in T2D [54]. Reactive oxygen species (ROS), such as superoxide, hydroxyl radical, and hydrogen peroxide arise from many cellular sources in response to hyperglycemia and diabetes. These sources include oxidative phosphorylation, glucose autoxidation, NADPH oxidase, and other enzymes such as xanthine oxidase. The role of NADPH oxidase in diabetes has been described in the earlier paragraphs and it was also mentioned that one of the reasons behind the anti-diabetic activity of AC3 is the down regulation of NADPH oxidase levels. Xanthine oxidase catalyzes the oxidation of hypoxanthine to xanthine and further catalyzes the oxidation of xanthine to uric acid. Superoxide, hydrogen peroxide, and hydroxyl radicals are produced as byproducts of the xanthine oxidase reaction. Treatment with allopurinol, a xanthine oxidase inhibitor, decreased oxidative stress in T1D patients [55]. Inhibition of xanthine oxidase was reported to attenuate the development of diabetic cardiomyopathy [56]. Further, inhibition of xanthine oxidase reduced hyperglycemia-induced oxidative stress and improved mitochondrial alterations in skeletal muscle of diabetic mice [57]. Therefore, inhibition of these proteins might attribute anti-diabetic effect to AC6.

Another enzyme that is targeted by AC6 is the insulin receptor. The insulin receptor (IR) is activated by insulin and plays a key role in the regulation of glucose homeostasis. Activation of the insulin receptor induces glucose uptake. A decrease in insulin receptor signaling or insulin insensitivity leads to T2D. In this case, the cells would be unable to take up glucose and would result in hyperglycemia. AC6 was found to ameliorate defective post-receptor insulin signaling through the enhancement of β-endorphin secretion [58]. AC6 attenuated hyperinsulinemia-induced insulin resistance in skeletal muscle cells. It also ameliorated insulin resistance induced by a high-fructose diet in rats. AC6 improved insulin sensitivity through the enhancement of insulin action on insulin receptor substrate-1 (IRS-1) associated phosphoinositide 3-kinase (PI3-kinase) and glucose transporter type 4 (GLUT4) activities in the muscles of animals exhibiting insulin resistance [59].

AC11 (Gallic acid)

AC11 exhibited anti-hyperglycemic, anti-lipid peroxidative, antioxidant, and anti-lipidemic effects in streptozotocin-induced type 2 diabetic rats [60]. It could provide a beneficial effect on diabetes by decreasing oxidative stress-related diabetic complications [61]. It was proposed that a diet containing gallic acid might be beneficial to T2D patients [60]. Cardioprotective effects of AC11 were observed in diabetes-induced myocardial dysfunction in rats. Thus, it was suggested that AC11 could be beneficial for the treatment of myocardial damage associated with T1D [62]. AC11 targets aldose reductase, UDP glucose dehydrogenase, ribonucleotide reductase, COX-1 and COX-2. Aldose reductase (AR) is widely expressed aldehyde-metabolizing enzyme. Aldose reductase catalyzes the reduction of a variety of aldehydes and carbonyls. It primarily catalyzes the reduction of glucose to sorbitol, the first step in polyol pathway of glucose metabolism. The reduction of glucose by the AR-catalyzed polyol pathway has been linked to the development of secondary diabetic complications. Glucose concentrations are often elevated in diabetics and AR was believed to be responsible for many diabetic complications. AR is involved in fructose, mannose, galactose and glycerolipid metabolism pathways. A study on the role of AR and the polyol pathway in diabetic nephropathy in a transgenic rat model showed that AR may both exacerbate and alleviate the production of metabolites that lead to hyperglycemia-induced cellular impairment [63]. Elevated level of AR expression was induced by hyperglycemia in patients with diabetic nephropathy [64]. Fidarestat, an AR inhibitor prevented diabetes-associated cataract formation, retinal oxidative-nitrosative stress, glial activation and apoptosis in streptozotocin induced diabetic rats [65]. AC11 was found to inhibit AR effectively [66] and this might be one of the reasons behind the effective anti-diabetic property of the plants containing this compound.

UDP glucose dehydrogenase is involved in starch and sucrose metabolism pathways. 40–50% increase in the expression of this enzyme was observed in streptozotocin-induced diabetic rats [67]. AC11 was reported to be an effective inhibitor of UDP glucose dehydrogenase [68]. Ribonucleotide reductase (RNR) catalyzes the formation of deoxyribonucleotides from ribonucleotides. RNR plays a critical role in DNA synthesis and repair. A high frequency of mitochondrial DNA (mtDNA) mutations is seen in T2D. During high DNA damage, similar to DNA topoisomerase 2 and DNA polymerase beta, the function of RNR gets impaired and leads to diabetic complications [69]. AC11 could significantly inhibit RNR [70]. The role of COX-1 and COX-2 in diabetes has been discussed previously. It was reported that AC11 could effectively inhibit COX-1 and COX-2 enzymes [70]. Taken together, AC11 might be exhibiting anti-diabetic activity by targeting these proteins.

AC54 (Shogaol)

AC54 is a pungent constituent of ginger (*Zingiber officinale*), similar in chemical structure to gingerol. AC54 targets nuclear factor kappa B (NF-kB), COX-2 and mitogen-activated protein kinase (MAPK). NF-kB mainly controls the transcription of DNA. A study involving NF-kB activation and overexpression of its regulated genes in patients with T2D revealed that the activation of NF-kB and the transcription of certain pro-inflammatory chemokines in tubular epithelial cells are markers of progressive diabetic nephropathy [71]. Apoptotic beta-cell death is the basic reason behind the pathogenesis of T1D and also in the islet graft rejection. It was reported that cell-death might be mediated by the activation of the NF-kB pathway. Use of NF-kB inhibitor significantly reduced apoptosis [72]. Beta-cell-specific activation of NF-kB was found to be a key event in the progressive loss of beta-cells in diabetes. Inhibition of this process was suggested as a potential effective strategy for beta-cell protection [72]. Administration of the antioxidants to the alloxan diabetic rats repressed the activation of NF-kB. *In vitro* studies showed that high glucose activates NF-kB and elevates NO and lipid peroxides in both retinal endothelial cells and pericytes. Inhibition of NF-kB and its downstream pathways had beneficial effects on the development of diabetic retinopathy [73]. Therefore, inhibition of NF-kB by AC54 might impart it anti-diabetic activity.

MAPK is another protein targeted by AC54. It is an important mediator of the extracellular stimuli, implicated in the pathogenesis of early diabetes mellitus. Elevated MAPK activity was observed in streptozotocin-induced diabetes mellitus rats [74]. The proteins p38 kinase (p38) and c-Jun NH2-terminal kinase (JNK) belong to the family of MAPK and are activated in response to hyperglycemia, oxidative stress, and proinflammtory cytokines. Increased activation of p38 and JNK have been reported as a fundamental mechanism responsible for cardiovascular dysfunction in diabetes [75,76]. Inhibition of p38/JNK improved nitric oxide–mediated vasodilatation and reduced inflammation in hypercholesterolemic patients [77]. MAPKs were implicated in the etiology of diabetic neuropathy both *via* direct effects of glucose and indirectly through glucose-induced oxidative stress [78]. It was reported that p38 MAPK inhibition reduced diabetes-induced impairment of wound healing. This was achieved by p38 MAPK inhibitors which demonstrated anti-inflammatory effects, primarily by inhibiting the expression of inflammatory cytokines and regulating cellular traffic into the wounds. It was suggested that chronic wounds associated with diabetes could be managed by means of p38 MAPK inhibitors [79]. p38 MAPK also plays an important role in diabetes-induced inflammation in the retina. Streptozotocin-induced insulin-deficient diabetic control rats exhibited significant increases in retinal superoxide, nitric oxide (NO), COX-2, and leukostasis within retinal microvessels. All these abnormalities were significantly inhibited by a p38 MAPK inhibitor [80]. It was suggested that inhibition of p38 MAPK would offer a novel therapeutic approach to inhibiting the development of early stages of diabetic retinopathy and other complications of diabetes. AC54 significantly inhibited the function of NF-kB and also the expression of COX-2 and MAPK [81]. The role of COX-2 in diabetes has been discussed previously. Therefore, the anti-diabetic activity of AC54 might be due to its inhibition of NF-kB, COX-2 and MAPK, and this might have attributed the anti-diabetic property to the plants containing this compound.

AC58 (Wedelolactone)

AC58 targets alpha glucosidase and inhibitor of NF-kB kinase subunit beta (IKK-beta). AC58 inhibited adipogenesis through the IKK-beta and the ERK pathway in human adipose tissue-derived mesenchymal stem cells [82]. The metabolic disorders of insulin resistance and T2D are mainly caused due to inflammation. IKK-beta was found to be a central coordinator of inflammatory response through the activation of NF-kB. IKK-beta acted locally on liver and systemically on myeloid cells, where NF-kB activation induced inflammatory mediators caused insulin resistance in mice [83]. Therefore, IKK-beta was thought to link inflammation to obesity-induced insulin resistance. It was suggested that inhibition of IKK-beta might be used to treat insulin resistance [83]. The role of alpha glucosidase in diabetes has been discussed previously at AC2. One of the effective therapeutic approaches in the treatment of diabetes mellitus is decreasing the postprandial hyperglycemia through the inhibition of alpha glucosidase. AC58 exhibited intensive inhibitory effect on alpha glucosidase [84]. Oral administration of AC58 could significantly decrease blood glucose after maltose loading in the diabetic rats in a dose-dependent manner. Thus, it was proposed that AC58 might reduce the postprandial glucose level and exert an anti-diabetic effect by suppressing carbohydrate absorption from the intestine [84]. Thus, inhibition of alpha glucosidase and IKK-beta might be the reason behind the anti-diabetic activity of AC58 and also for the anti-diabetic property of the plants containing AC58.

Network analysis and pharmacophore-based studies would help us in understanding the biological and chemical basis of pharmacological action of anti-diabetic plants. Further, this study also provides the framework for synthetic modification of bioactive phytochemicals, as well as delineates possible modifications of the active compounds to increase potency or selectivity, since some of the active compounds have been already structurally modified to produce effective synthetic drugs (Figures S1 and S2). Thus, an integrated approach of network analysis combined with pharmacophore analysis and docking studies could be used to discover potential active compounds. The combined use of these compounds either in the form of plant formulations or pharmaceutical drugs might show synergistic effect against multiple mechanisms involved in diabetes and its complications.

Supporting Information

Figure S1 Alpha-glucosidase inhibitors. (A) AC2 (1-deoxynojirimycin), (B) Miglustat and (C) Miglitol. The synthetic drugs, miglustat and miglitol, are structurally similar to and derived from the anti-diabetic plant compound AC2.

Figure S2 5α reductase inhibitors. (A) Betulinic acid, (B) Finasteride and (C) Dutasteride. The synthetic drugs, finasteride and dutasteride, are structurally similar to and derived from the anti-diabetic plant compound betulinic acid.

Table S1 Active compounds that directly target multiple proteins.

Table S2 ADME properties of active compounds.

Author Contributions

Conceived and designed the experiments: KGR SMF. Performed the experiments: SMF VSSK. Analyzed the data: KGR SMF VSSK. Contributed to the writing of the manuscript: KGR SMF VSSK.

References

1. King H, Aubert RE, Herman WH (1998) Global burden of diabetes, 1995–2025: prevalence, numerical estimates, and projections. Diabetes Care 21: 1414–1431.
2. Gupta OP, Phathak S (2003) Pandemic trends in prevalence of diabetes mellitus and associated coronary heart disease in India-Their causes and prevention. Int J Diab Dev Ctries 23: 37–49.
3. Bjerre M (2013) Osteoprotegerin (OPG) as a biomarker for diabetic cardiovascular complications. Springerplus 2: 658–664.
4. Saxena A, Vikram NK (2004) Role of selected Indian plants in management of type 2 diabetes: a review. J Altern Complement Med 10: 369–378.
5. Pari L, Umamaheswari J (2000) Anti-hyperglycaemic activity of *Musa sapientum* flowers. Effect of lipid peroxidation in alloxan diabetic rats. Phytother Res 14: 1–3.
6. Babu PA, Suneetha G, Boddepalli R, Lakshmi VV, Rani TS, et al. (2006) A database of 389 medicinal plants for diabetes. Bioinformation 1: 130–171.
7. Mukherjee PK, Maiti K, Mukherjee K, Houghton PJ (2006) Leads from Indian medicinal plants with hypoglycemic potentials. J Ethnopharmacol 106: 1–28.
8. Modak M, Dixit P, Londhe J, Ghaskadbi S, Devasagayam TP (2007) Indian herbs and herbal drugs used for the treatment of diabetes. J Clin Biochem Nutr 40: 163–173.

9. Yeh GY, Eisenberg DM, Kaptchuk TJ, Phillips RS (2003) Systematic review of herbs and dietary supplements for glycemic control in diabetes. Diabetes Care 26: 1277–1294.
10. Dhanbal SP (2004) Evaluation of therapeutic activity and development of quality control profiles for some anti-diabetic herbal drugs. Ind J Pharm Edu 8: 163–165.
11. SanthoshKumari KS, Devi KS (1993) Effect of indigenous drugs on glucuronoglycan metabolism in diabetic hypertensive rabbits. Ind J Exp Biol 31: 595–599.
12. Jung M, Park M, Lee HC, Kang YH, Kang ES, et al. (2006) Anti-diabetic agents from medicinal plants. Curr Med Chem 13: 1203–1218.
13. Shannon P1, Markiel A, Ozier O, Baliga NS, Wang JT, et al. (2003) Cytoscape: a software environment for integrated models of biomolecular interaction networks. Genome Res 13: 2498–2504.
14. Lipinski CA1, Lombardo F, Dominy BW, Feeney PJ (2001) Experimental and computational approaches to estimate solubility and permeability in drug discovery and development settings. Adv Drug Deliv Rev 46: 3–26.
15. Friesner RA, Banks JL, Murphy RB, Halgren TA, Klicic JJ, et al. (2004) Glide: a new approach for rapid, accurate docking and scoring. 1. method and assessment of docking accuracy. J Med Chem 47: 1739–1749.
16. Giovannucci E1, Harlan DM, Archer MC, Bergenstal RM, Gapstur SM, et al. (2010) Diabetes and cancer: a consensus report. CA Cancer J Clin 60: 207–221.
17. Vigneri P, Frasca F, Sciacca L, Pandini G, Vigneri R (2009) Diabetes and cancer. Endocr Relat Cancer 16: 1103–1123.
18. Hu G, Jousilahti P, Bidel S, Antikainen R, Tuomilehto J (2007) Type 2 diabetes and the risk of Parkinson's disease. Diabetes Care 30: 842–847.
19. Lima MMS, Targa ADS, Noseda ACD, Rodrigues LS, Delattre AM, et al. (2014) Does Parkinson's disease and type 2 diabetes mellitus present common pathophysiological mechanisms and treatments? CNS Neurol Disord Drug Targets 13: 418–428.
20. Santiago JA, Potashkin JA (2013) Integrative network analysis unveils convergent molecular pathways in Parkinson's disease and diabetes. PLoS One 8: e83940.
21. Ferreira ST, Clarke JR, Bomfim TR, De Felice FG (2014) Inflammation, defective insulin signaling, and neuronal dysfunction in Alzheimer's disease. Alzheimers Dement 10: S76–S83.
22. de la Monte SM, Wands JR (2008) Alzheimer's disease is type 3 diabetes-evidence reviewed. J Diabetes Sci Technol 2: 1101–1113.
23. Freiherr J, Hallschmid M, Frey WH, Brünner YF, Chapman CD, et al. (2013) Intranasal insulin as a treatment for Alzheimer's disease: a review of basic research and clinical evidence. CNS Drugs 27: 505–514.
24. Hölscher C (2014) First clinical data of the neuroprotective effects of nasal insulin application in patients with Alzheimer's disease. Alzheimers Dement 10: S33–S37.
25. Tolman KG, Fonseca V, Dalpiaz A, Tan MH (2007) Spectrum of liver disease in type 2 diabetes and management of patients with diabetes and liver disease. Diabetes Care 30: 734–743.
26. Nair SB, Teli MK, Pradeep H, Rajanikant GK (2012) Computational identification of novel histone deacetylase inhibitors by docking based QSAR. Comput Biol Med 42: 697–705.
27. Teli MK, Rajanikant GK (2012) Identification of novel potential HIF-prolyl hydroxylase inhibitors by *in silico* screening. Mol Divers 16: 193–202.
28. Nair SB, Fayaz SM, Rajanikant GK (2013) A novel multi-target drug screening strategy directed against key proteins of DAPk family. Comb Chem High Throughput Screen 16: 449–457.
29. Punithavathi VR, Prince PS, Kumar R, Selvakumari J (2011) Anti-hyperglycaemic, anti-lipidperoxidative and antioxidant effects of gallic acid on streptozotocin induced diabetic Wistar rats. Eur J Pharmacol 650: 465–471.
30. Punithavathi VR, StanelyMainzen Prince P, Kumar MR, Selvakumari CJ (2011) Protective effects of gallic acid on hepatic lipid peroxide metabolism, glycoprotein components and lipids in streptozotocin-induced type 2 diabetic wistar rats. J Biochem Mol Toxicol 25: 68–76.
31. Bischoff H (1995) The mechanism of alpha-glucosidase inhibition in the management of diabetes. Clin Invest Med 18: 303–311.
32. He H, Lu YH (2013) Comparison of inhibitory activities and mechanisms of five mulberry plant bioactive components against α-glucosidase. J Agric Food Chem 61: 8110–8119.
33. Chowdhury AR, Mandal S, Mittra B, Sharma S, Mukhopadhyay S, et al. (2002) Betulinic acid, a potent inhibitor of eukaryotic topoisomerase I: identification of the inhibitory step, the major functional group responsible and development of more potent derivatives. Med Sci Monit 8: 254–265.
34. de Melo CL, Queiroz MG, ArrudaFilho AC, Rodrigues AM, de Sousa DF, et al. (2009) Betulinic acid, a natural pentacyclic triterpenoid, prevents abdominal fat accumulation in mice fed a high-fat diet. J Agric Food Chem 57: 8776–8781.
35. Alqahtani A, Hamid K, Kam A, Wong KH, Abdelhak Z, et al. (2013) The pentacyclic triterpenoids in herbal medicines and their pharmacological activities in diabetes and diabetic complications. Curr Med Chem 20: 908–931.
36. Jornayvaz FR1, Birkenfeld AL, Jurczak MJ, Kanda S, GuigniBA, et al. (2011) Hepatic insulin resistance in mice with hepatic overexpression of diacylglycerol acyltransferase 2. Proc Natl Acad Sci U S A 108: 5748–5752.
37. Baker DJ, Timmons JA, Greenhaff PL (2005) Glycogen phosphorylase inhibition in type 2 diabetes therapy: a systematic evaluation of metabolic and functional effects in rat skeletal muscle. Diabetes 54: 2453–2459.
38. Medikayala S, Piteo B, Zhao X, Edwards JG (2011) Chronically elevated glucose compromises myocardial mitochondrial DNA integrity by alteration of mitochondrial topoisomerase function. Am J Physiol Cell Physiol 300: C338–348.
39. Steffensen KR, Gustafsson JA (2004) Putative metabolic effects of the liver X receptor (LXR). Diabetes 53: S36–S42.
40. Zhao HJ, Wang S, Cheng H, Zhang MZ, Takahashi T, et al. (2006) Endothelial nitric oxide synthase deficiency produces accelerated nephropathy in diabetic mice. J Am Soc Nephrol 17: 2664–2669.
41. Nakagawa T, Sato W, Glushakova O, Heinig M, Clarke T, et al. (2007) Diabetic endothelial nitric oxide synthase knockout mice develop advanced diabetic nephropathy. J Am Soc Nephrol 18: 539–550.
42. Steinkamp-Fenske K, Bollinger L, Xu H, Yao Y, Horke S, et al. (2007) Reciprocal regulation of endothelial nitric-oxide synthase and NADPH oxidase by betulinic acid in human endothelial cells. J Pharmacol Exp Ther 322: 836–842.
43. Liu J (1995) Pharmacology of oleanolic acid and ursolic acid. J Ethnopharmacol 49: 57–68.
44. Vozarova B, Stefan N, Lindsay RS, Saremi A, Pratley RE, et al. (2002) High alanine aminotransferase is associated with decreased hepatic insulin sensitivity and predicts the development of type 2 diabetes. Diabetes 51: 1889–1895.
45. Davalli AM, Perego C, Folli FB (2012) The potential role of glutamate in the current diabetes epidemic. Acta Diabetol 49: 167–183.
46. Sekhar RV, McKay SV, Patel SG, Guthikonda AP, Reddy VT, et al. (2011) Glutathione synthesis is diminished in patients with uncontrolled diabetes and restored by dietary supplementation with cysteine and glycine. Diabetes Care 34: 162–167.
47. Alvarado-Vásquez N, Zamudio P, Cerón E, Vanda B, Zenteno E, et al. (2003) Effect of glycine in streptozotocin-induced diabetic rats. Comp Biochem Physiol C Toxicol Pharmacol 134: 521–527.
48. Padberg I, Peter E, González-Maldonado S, Witt H, Mueller M, et al. (2014) A new metabolomic signature in type 2 diabetes mellitus and its pathophysiology. PLoS One 9: e85082.
49. Persaud SJ, Muller D, Belin VD, Kitsou-Mylona I, Asare-Anane H, et al. (2007) The role of arachidonic acid and its metabolites in insulin secretion from human islets of langerhans. Diabetes 56: 197–203.
50. Ong KC, Khoo HE (1997) Biological effects of myricetin. Gen Pharmacol 29: 121–126.
51. Pandey KB, Mishra N, Rizvi SI (2009) Myricetin may provide protection against oxidative stress in type 2 diabetic erythrocytes. Z Naturforsch C 64: 626–630.
52. Ozcan F, Ozmen A, Akkaya B, Aliciguzel Y, Aslan M (2012) Beneficial effect of myricetin on renal functions in streptozotocin-induced diabetes. Clin Exp Med 12: 265–272.
53. Melzig MF, Funke I (2007) Inhibitors of alpha-amylase from plants -a possibility to treat diabetes mellitus type II by phytotherapy? Wien Med Wochenschr 157: 320–324.
54. Tundis R, Loizzo MR, Menichini F (2010) Natural products as alpha-amylase and alpha-glucosidase inhibitors and their hypoglycaemic potential in the treatment of diabetes: an update. Mini Rev Med Chem 10: 315–331.
55. Desco MC, Asensi M, Márquez R, Martínez-Valls J, Vento M, et al. (2002) Xanthine oxidase is involved in free radical production in type 1 diabetes: protection by allopurinol. Diabetes 51: 1118–1124.
56. Rajesh M, Mukhopadhyay P, Bátkai S, Mukhopadhyay B, Patel V, et al. (2009) Xanthine oxidase inhibitor allopurinol attenuates the development of diabetic cardiomyopathy. J Cell Mol Med 13: 2330–2341.
57. Bravard A, Bonnard C, Durand A, Chauvin MA, Favier R, et al. (2011) Inhibition of xanthine oxidase reduces hyperglycemia-induced oxidative stress and improves mitochondrial alterations in skeletal muscle of diabetic mice. Am J Physiol Endocrinol Metab 300: E581–591.
58. Tzeng TF, Liou SS, Liu IM (2011) Myricetin Ameliorates defective post-receptor insulin signaling via β-endorphin signaling in the skeletal muscles of fructose-fed rats. Evid Based Complement Alternat Med 2011: 150752–150761.
59. Liu IM, Tzeng TF, Liou SS, Lan TW (2007) Myricetin, a naturally occurring flavonol, ameliorates insulin resistance induced by a high-fructose diet in rats. Life Sci 81: 1479–1488.
60. Punithavathi VR, StanelyMainzen Prince P, Kumar MR, Selvakumari CJ (2011) Protective effects of gallic acid on hepatic lipid peroxide metabolism, glycoprotein components and lipids in streptozotocin-induced type 2 diabetic wistar rats. J Biochem Mol Toxicol 25: 68–76.
61. Ramkumar K, Vijayakumar R, Vanitha P, Suganya N, Manjula C, et al. (2013) Protective effect of gallic acid on alloxan-induced oxidative stress and osmotic fragility in rats. Hum Exp Toxicol 33: 638–649.
62. Patel SS, Goyal RK (2011) Cardioprotective effects of gallic acid in diabetes-induced myocardial dysfunction in rats. Pharmacognosy Res 3: 239–245.
63. Dunlop M (2000) Aldose reductase and the role of the polyol pathway in diabetic nephropathy. Kidney Int 77: S3–S12.
64. Hodgkinson AD, Søndergaard KL, Yang B, Cross DF, Millward BA, et al. (2001) Aldose reductase expression is induced by hyperglycemia in diabetic nephropathy. Kidney Int 60: 211–218.

65. Drel VR, Pacher P, Ali TK, Shin J, Julius U, et al. (2008) Aldose reductase inhibitor fidarestat counteracts diabetes-associated cataract formation, retinal oxidative-nitrosative stress, glial activation, and apoptosis. Int J Mol Med 21: 667–676.
66. Chethan S, Dharmesh SM, Malleshi NG (2008) Inhibition of aldose reductase from cataracted eye lenses by finger millet (Eleusinecoracana) polyphenols. Bioorg Med Chem 16: 10085–10090.
67. Sochor M, Kunjara S, Greenbaum AL, McLean P (1986) Renal hypertrophy in experimental diabetes. Effect of diabetes on the pathways of glucose metabolism: differential response in adult and immature rats. Biochem J 234: 573–577.
68. Hwang EY, Huh JW, Choi MM, Choi SY, Hong HN, et al. (2008) Inhibitory effects of gallic acid and quercetin on UDP-glucose dehydrogenase activity. FEBS Lett 582: 3793–3797.
69. Todorov IN, Todorov GI (2009) Multifactorial nature of high frequency of mitochondrial DNA mutations in somatic mammalian cells. Biochemistry (Mosc) 74: 962–970.
70. Madlener S, Illmer C, Horvath Z, Saiko P, Losert A, et al. (2007) Gallic acid inhibits ribonucleotide reductase and cyclooxygenases in human HL-60 promyelocytic leukemia cells. Cancer Lett 245: 156–162.
71. Mezzano S, Aros C, Droguett A, Burgos ME, Ardiles L, et al. (2004) NF-kappaB activation and overexpression of regulated genes in human diabetic nephropathy. Nephrol Dial Transplant 19: 2505–2512.
72. Melloul D (2008) Role of NF-kappaB in beta-cell death. Biochem Soc Trans 36: 334–339.
73. Kowluru RA, Koppolu P, Chakrabarti S, Chen S (2003) Diabetes-induced activation of nuclear transcriptional factor in the retina, and its inhibition by antioxidants. Free Radic Res 37: 1169–1180.
74. Awazu M, Ishikura K, Hida M, Hoshiya M (1999) Mechanisms of mitogen-activated protein kinase activation in experimental diabetes. J Am Soc Nephrol 10: 738–745.
75. Evans JL, Goldfine ID, Maddux BA, Grodsky GM (2002) Oxidative stress and stress-activated signaling pathways: a unifying hypothesis of type 2 diabetes. Endocr Rev 23: 599–622.
76. Liu Z, Cao W (2009) p38 mitogen-activated protein kinase: a critical node linking insulin resistance and cardiovascular diseases in type 2 diabetes mellitus. Endocr Metab Immune Disord Drug Targets 9: 38–46.
77. Cheriyan J, Webb AJ, Sarov-Blat L, Elkhawad M, Wallace SM, et al. (2011) Inhibition of p38 mitogen-activated protein kinase improves nitric oxide-mediated vasodilatation and reduces inflammation in hypercholesterolemia. Circulation 123: 515–523.
78. Purves T, Middlemas A, Agthong S, Jude EB, Boulton AJ, et al. (2001) A role for mitogen-activated protein kinases in the etiology of diabetic neuropathy. FASEB J 15: 2508–2514.
79. Medicherla S, Wadsworth S, Cullen B, Silcock D, Ma JY, et al. (2009) p38 MAPK inhibition reduces diabetes-induced impairment of wound healing. Diabetes Metab Syndr Obes 2: 91–100.
80. Du Y, Tang J, Li G, Berti-Mattera L, Lee CA, et al. (2010) Effects of p38 MAPK inhibition on early stages of diabetic retinopathy and sensory nerve function. Invest Ophthalmol Vis Sci 51: 2158–2164.
81. Pan MH, Hsieh MC, Hsu PC, Ho SY, Lai CS, et al. (2008) 6-Shogaol suppressed lipopolysaccharide-induced up-expression of iNOS and COX-2 in murine macrophages. Mol Nutr Food Res 52: 1467–1477.
82. Lim S, Jang HJ, Park EH, Kim JK, Kim JM, et al. (2012) Wedelolactone inhibits adipogenesis through the ERK pathway in human adipose tissue-derived mesenchymal stem cells. J Cell Biochem 113: 3436–3445.
83. Arkan MC, Hevener AL, Greten FR, Maeda S, Li ZW, et al. (2005) IKK-beta links inflammation to obesity-induced insulin resistance. Nat Med 11: 191–198.
84. Prajapati H, Patel MB (2012) Potent α-glucosidase inhibitor and anti-glycemic agent from Eclipta alba. Chemistry & Biology Interface 2: 38–47.
85. Aswini K, Mangesh K, Kailash V, Pratibha C, Mahavir G (2012) Pharmacognostic investigation on leaves of *Citrus maxima* (Burm.) Merr. (Rutaceae). Int J Pharm Sci Res 3: 4913–4918.
86. Zinjarde SS, Bhargava SY, Kumar AR (2011) Potent α-amylase inhibitory activity of Indian Ayurvedic medicinal plants. BMC Complement Altern Med 11: 5 15.
87. Kapoor LD (2000) Handbook of Ayurvedic medicinal plants: Herbal Reference Library. Taylor & Francis. 416p.
88. Tiwari S, Sirohi B, Shukla A, Bigoniya P (2012) Phytochemical screening and diuretic activity of *Allium sativum* steroidal and triterpenoid saponin fraction. Int J Pharm Sci Res 3: 3354–3361.
89. Lakshmi CM (2003) Scientific basis for Ayurvedic therapies. CRC Press. 656p.
90. Reddy SV, Tiwari AK, Kumar US, Rao RJ, Rao JM (2005) Free radical scavenging, enzyme inhibitory constituents from anti-diabetic Ayurvedic medicinal plant *Hydnocarpus wightiana* Blume. Phytother Res 19: 277–281.
91. Grover JK, Yadav S, Vats V (2002) Medicinal plants of India with anti-diabetic potential. J Ethnopharmacol 81: 81–100.
92. Bhatia H, Sharma YP, Manhas RK, Kumar K (2014) Ethnomedicinal plants used by the villagers of district Udhampur, J&K, India. J Ethnopharmacol 151: 1005–1018.
93. Talukder FZ, Khan KA, Uddin R, Jahan N, Alam MA (2012) *In vitro* free radical scavenging and anti-hyperglycemic activities of *Achyranthes aspera* extract in alloxan-induced diabetic mice. Drug Discov Ther 6: 298–305.
94. Mathew M, Subramanian S (2014) *In vitro* screening for anti-cholinesterase and antioxidant activity of methanolic extracts of Ayurvedic medicinal plants used for cognitive disorders. PLoS One 9: e86804.
95. Asthana R, Raina MK (1989) Pharmacology of *Withania somnifera* (L.) Dunal: a review. Indian drugs 26: 199–205.
96. Paek JH, Shin KH, Kang YH, Lee JY, Lim SS (2013) Rapid identification of aldose reductase inhibitory compounds from *Perilla frutescens*. Biomed Res Int 2013: 679463–679471.
97. Pari L, Venkateswaran S (2003) Effect of an aqueous extract of *Phaseolus vulgaris* on the properties of tail tendon collagen of rats with streptozotocin-induced diabetes. Braz J Med Biol Res 36: 861–870.
98. Patel JR, Tripathi P, Sharma V, Chauhan NS, Dixit VK (2011) *Phyllanthus amarus*: ethnomedicinal uses, phytochemistry and pharmacology: a review. J Ethnopharmacol 138: 286–313.
99. Prashant MT, Sunita NB, Chandrasekar N, Shrikant AJ, Abhay SJ (2011) Evaluation of wound healing properties of *Psoreliya corolifolia* Linn in diabetic rats. Pharmacol online 1: 282–288.
100. He L, Qi Y, Rong X, Jiang J, Yang Q, et al. (2011) The Ayurvedic medicine *Salacia oblonga* attenuates diabetic renal fibrosis in rats: Suppression of angiotensin II/AT1 signaling. Evid Based Complement Alternat Med 2011: 807451–807463.
101. Bhuvaneswari P, Krishnakumari S (2012) Nephroprotective effects of ethanolic extract of *Sesamum indicum* seeds (Linn.) in streptozotocin induced diabetic male albino rats. Int J Green Pharm 6: 330–335.
102. Ayyanar M, Subash-Babu P (2012) Syzygium cumini (L.) Skeels: A review of its phytochemical constituents and traditional uses. Asian Pac J Trop Biomed 2: 240–246.
103. Meenu J, Sharma S, Kumar M (2011) Ameliorative potential of *Vigna mungo* seeds on hyperglycemia mediated oxidative stress and hyperlipidemia in STZ diabetic rats. Int J Green Pharm 5: 266–272.
104. Al-Amin ZM, Thomson M, Al-Qattan KK, Peltonen-Shalaby R, Ali M (2006) Anti-diabetic and hypolipidaemic properties of ginger (*Zingiber officinale*) in streptozotocin-induced diabetic rats. Br J Nutr 96: 660–666.
105. Saxena A, Vikram NK (2004) Role of selected Indian plants in management of type 2 diabetes: a review. J Altern Complement Med 10: 369–378.
106. Ananthi J, Prakasam A, Pugalendi KV (2003) Anti-hyperglycemic activity of *Eclipta alba* leaf on alloxan-induced diabetic rats. Yale J Biol Med 76: 97–102.
107. Sankeshi V, Kumar PA, Naik RR, Sridhar G, Kumar MP, et al. (2013) Inhibition of aldose reductase by *Aegle marmelos* and its protective role in diabetic cataract. J Ethnopharmacol 149: 215–221.
108. Prakasam A, Sethupathy S, Pugalendi KV (2003) Effect of *Casearia esculenta* root extract on blood glucose and plasma antioxidant status in streptozotocin diabetic rats. Pol J Pharmacol 55: 43–49.
109. Tapola N, Karvonen H, Niskanen L, Mikola M, Sarkkinen E (2005) Glycemic responses of oat bran products in type 2 diabetic patients. Nutr Metab Cardiovasc Dis 15: 255–261.

The Effects of Comorbidity on the Benefits and Harms of Treatment for Chronic Disease

Terri R. Fried[1,2]*, John O'Leary[1,3], Virginia Towle[3], Mary K. Goldstein[4,5], Mark Trentelange[3], Deanna K. Martin[1,3]

1 Clinical Epidemiology Research Center, VA Connecticut Healthcare System, West Haven, Connecticut, United States of America, 2 Department of Medicine, Yale School of Medicine, New Haven, Connecticut, United States of America, 3 Program on Aging, Yale School of Medicine, New Haven, Connecticut, United States of America, 4 Palo Alto Geriatrics Research Education and Clinical Center (GRECC), VA Palo Alto Health Care System, Palo Alto, Connecticut, 94304, United States of America, 5 Center for Primary Care and Outcomes Research, Stanford University School of Medicine, Stanford, California, 94305, United States of America

Abstract

Background: There are concerns about the potential for unintentional harms when clinical practice guidelines are applied to patients with multimorbidity. The objective was to summarize the evidence regarding the effect(s) of comorbidity on the outcomes of medication for an index chronic condition.

Methods: A systematic review was conducted of studies published in MEDLINE and Cochrane Trials before May 2012. The search strategy was constructed to identify articles indexed with "comorbidity" or a related term or by a given condition and one or more additional specified comorbid conditions. The search yielded 3252 articles, of which 37 passed the title/abstract screening process, and 22 were included after full-text review. An additional 23 articles were identified by screening the reference lists for included articles. Information was extracted on study design; population; therapy; comparison groups; outcome(s); main findings.

Findings: Indexing of articles was inconsistent, with no term for "multimorbidity," and rare use of "comorbidity". Only one article examined the effects of comorbidity *per se*, finding no benefit of tight control of DM among persons with high comorbidity, defined using a comorbidity index. The remainder examined pairs of conditions, the majority of which were post-hoc analyses of randomized controlled trials and which found no difference in outcomes according to whether a comorbid condition was present. Several demonstrated no difference or an increased risk of adverse outcome among persons with DM and tight control of HTN as compared to usual control. Several demonstrated lack of benefit of statins among persons with end-stage renal disease.

Conclusions: There is limited evidence regarding the effects of multiple comorbidities on treatment outcomes. The majority of studies demonstrated no effect of a single comorbid condition on outcomes. Additional studies examining a broad range of comorbidity are required, along with clear and consistent indexing to allow for improved synthesis of the evidence.

Editor: Olaf M. Dekkers, Leiden University Medical Centre, Netherlands

Funding: This project was supported by grant DF11-303 from the Donaghue Foundation (www.donaghue.org) and by grant P30 AG021342 from the NIH/NIA (www.nih.nia.gov). The funders had no role in study design, data collection and analysis, decision to publish, or preparation of the manuscript.

Competing Interests: The authors have declared that no competing interests exist.

* Email: terri.fried@yale.edu

Introduction

Multimorbidity, or the co-existence of multiple diseases, is the most common chronic condition among adults. [1] There is increasing concern about the appropriateness of disease-based clinical practice guidelines to the care of the patient with multimorbidity. When applied to a theoretical patient, the many medications recommended by these guidelines result in the potential for adverse drug-drug and drug-disease interactions. [2] The likelihood of adverse drug events increases with the number of medications, [3] leading to questions about altered benefit/harm ratios associated with the prescription of multiple medications for patients with multimorbidity. [4] In addition, evidence about the benefits and harms of interventions from randomized controlled trials (RCTs) may not be generalizable to patients with multimorbidity. These patients are frequently excluded from the trials that form the evidence base for practice guidelines, and the trials have incomplete ascertainment of harms [4].

We sought to determine the extent of the evidence regarding the treatment of persons with multimorbidity by performing a systematic literature review. Although RCTs are generally considered to provide the highest quality evidence regarding treatment benefits, we elected to include both RCTs and observational studies because of the limitations of RCTs as applied to this population of patients and because of evidence that rigorously conducted observational studies provide accurate estimates of treatment effects [5].

Materials and Methods

Data Sources and Searches

Because "multimorbidity" is not a MeSH terms, the search was constructed around the concept of "comorbidity" to address the following question: "Among persons age 65 years and older, what effect does the presence of comorbid conditions have on the benefits and/or harms of medical treatment for a specific index chronic condition?" The following databases were searched for relevant studies: MEDLINE (OvidSP 1946–May Week 5 2012, April 13, 2012); MEDLINE In-Process & Other Non-Indexed Citations (OvidSP, April 13, 2012); Cochrane Trials (Wiley, April 11, 2012). While there are medical subject headings (MeSH) for comorbidity, when we examined four key articles, we found that only one of the four articles was indexed using these terms. We therefore had to create search strategies to capture the concept of comorbidity. We did this by using search terms that consisted of a given condition and at least one other of a list of additional conditions (heart failure [HF], coronary artery disease [CAD], angina pectoris, stable angina, hypertension [HTN], chronic obstructive pulmonary disease, osteoarthritis, hyperlipidemias, chronic kidney disease [CKD], diabetes mellitus [DM]). We repeated this process, with each condition becoming the index condition, and the rest considered together as comorbid conditions, using controlled vocabulary terms and synonymous free text words. The search strategy was limited to cohort studies, randomized controlled trials, or decision support techniques (Appendix S1). We specified older age in our question because of the increasing prevalence of multimorbidity with age, [6] with the goal of identifying study populations with the broadest possible range of comorbid conditions.

Because of the large number of references resulting from this search, the first 100 abstracts were reviewed to determine whether the search strategy could be made more specific. We found that we had captured a large number of studies that examined appropriateness of a given therapy, with appropriateness determined according to whether the patient had a given condition rather than according to the outcome of therapy. We therefore reran the analysis excluding these studies. Because of our interest in medical therapies, we also excluded studies that focused on surgical interventions. The full strategy is shown in appendix S1.

Study Selection

We included articles that examined the outcomes of treatment for an index condition in the presence and absence of comorbidity. We also included articles that examined the outcomes associated with different intensity of treatment of an index condition in the presence of comorbidity, regardless of whether the treatment was explicitly defined. For example, we included articles examining outcomes according to different HgbA1C levels, regardless of whether the diabetic treatment was specified. We included articles that examined only the effect of a treatment for a given condition in the presence of comorbidity (e.g. there were no participants without the comorbid condition) when the effect of the treatment in the absence of the comorbidity is well established.

We excluded articles that examined surrogate outcomes, such as lab values. This exclusion was based on evidence that surrogate outcomes are frequently not accurate markers for clinically relevant outcomes and that studies examining surrogate outcomes may not capture relevant harms. [7] We did not exclude any clinically relevant outcomes, and planned to include studies examining quality of life outcomes, such as symptoms and function. In addition, it became apparent that the search strategy resulted in many articles with persons under the age of 65. Articles were therefore included if the study population included persons age 65 years or older, even if they also included younger persons. A total of 50 titles and/or abstracts were reviewed independently by three of the investigators (TRF, JRO, VT) to confirm uniformity in the process of excluding articles. The titles and/or abstracts of the remaining references were initially reviewed by one of two investigators (JRO, VT), and articles that were not excluded were re-reviewed by a third investigator (TRF) to achieve consensus regarding inclusion. Full text review was performed for these articles. The reference lists for the final set of articles identified by this search were also examined to identify additional articles meeting inclusion criterion.

Data Extraction and Quality Assessment

For each of the included studies, we extracted the following data elements: 1) study design; 2) study population, including index condition; 3) intervention; 4) comparison groups; 5) outcome; 6) main findings.

We did not perform quality assessments for the articles based on two considerations. First, for the reasons provided above, we included both RCTs and observational studies. This posed a challenge for doing quality assessment, since, on the one hand, observational studies are generally considered to provide lower quality evidence than are randomized controlled trials, [8] but, as discussed above, in the case of multimorbidity, randomized controlled trials may not enroll patients with representative comorbidity burden. It is therefore difficult to apply metrics across the two types of study design that reflect their relative quality as specifically related to the study question. Second, many studies consisted of post-hoc analyses of RCTs, so that the initial randomization no longer applied, and there are no established criteria to evaluate the extent to which this affects the quality of the study. Given these considerations, we concluded that the best representation of study quality was a description of the study design, as extracted from each of the studies.

Data Synthesis and Analysis

Because the large majority of studies examined treatment for an index condition among persons with or without a single comorbid condition, we organized studies according to the pairs of conditions being examined. Even within these groups, the heterogeneity in design, population, and interventions precluded combining the results in a meta-analysis.

Results

Identification of Articles

The literature search yielded 3252 articles. A total of 38 articles passed the title/abstract screening process. Full-text review resulted in the exclusion of 16 articles. Review of the reference lists for the remaining 22 articles resulted in the identification of an addition 23 articles, for a total of 45 (Figure 1).

Types of Studies Identified

Table 1 provides a description of the types of studies identified in the systematic review, including the approach to the analysis of comorbidity, conditions and outcomes examined, and study design. Only one of the studies examined the effect of comorbidity *per se*. [9] This study examined the cardiovascular outcomes associated with tight diabetic control among persons with different levels of comorbidity. The remaining 44 studies examined the

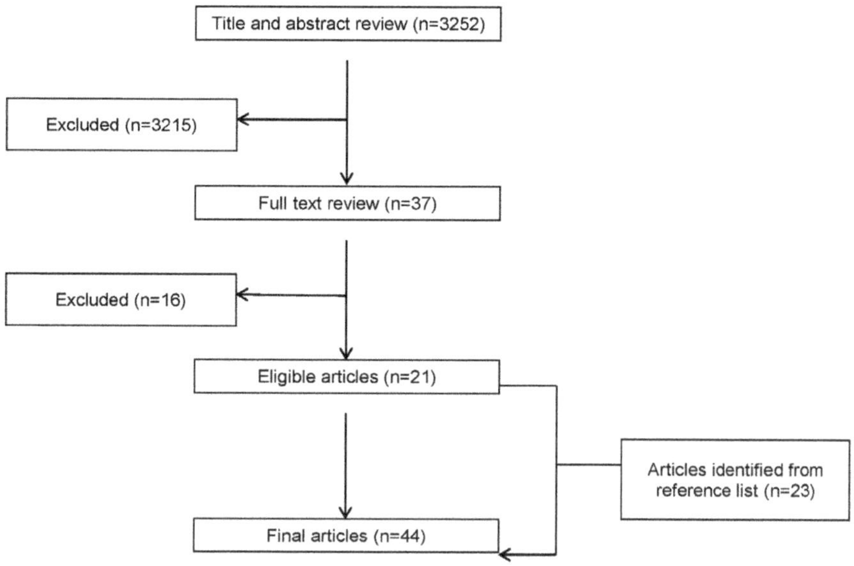

Figure 1. Summary of literature search and selection.

effects of treating an index condition in the presence or absence of a single other condition. The vast majority of these studies included DM as either the index or comorbid condition. The most common combinations of conditions examined were HF and DM (10 studies), [10–19] HTN and DM (9 studies), [20–28] and DM and CKD (10 studies) [29–38]. The studies examining HF and DM focused primarily on all-cause mortality among patients with HF who received treatment with beta blockers according to the presence or absence of DM. The majority of studies examining HTN and DM compared outcomes according to different intensities of HTN treatment, measured as the desired or achieved systolic and/or diastolic blood pressure. The studies examining CKD and DM primarily compared outcomes according to different intensities of diabetes treatment, measured as the achieved HgbA1C. An additional 5 studies examined DM and cardiovascular disease other than HF; these studies varied in terms of which was considered the index condition and which the comorbidity, the interventions, and outcomes [39–43].

A total of eight studies examined cardiovascular disease (HF, ischemic heart disease, or hyperlipidemia) and CKD [14,44–50]. A total of four studies examined a variety of miscellaneous disease combinations [41,51–53].

Across the different disease combinations, over one-half (55%) were conducted as post-hoc analyses of randomized controlled trials, in which patients with and without the comorbid condition were identified after study randomization, and the effect of the treatment was compared in these two groups. There were two studies that included only patients with both the index condition of hyperlipidemia or high cardiovascular disease risk and the comorbidity of CKD. These were randomized controlled trials in which patients were assigned to treatment with a statin versus a placebo. These studies assumed a well-established benefit of statins among patients with the index condition who did not have CKD. Only two studies examined differences in the likelihood of harm according to whether a comorbid condition was present; the remainder of the studies examined the likelihood of benefit. Of the studies examining benefit, only one examined functional outcomes; the remainder examined reduction in risk of mortality, hospitalization, or disease-specific outcomes, such as cardiovascular events.

Study Findings

The majority of studies found no effect of comorbidity on the benefits or harms of therapy for an index condition. Of the 25 studies examining the benefit of therapy for a given condition according to whether comorbidity was present or absent, 23 found no difference or a greater benefit in the presence of the comorbidity (Table 2). The two studies examining the harm of therapy according to whether comorbidity was present or absent found no difference in harms. Results were more mixed for the 15 studies examining the benefit of tighter versus less tight control of one condition in the presence of a second. Of these, seven found tighter control was more beneficial than less tight control, six found tighter control was of no greater benefit or was harmful compared to less tight control, one found a U-shaped relationship, and one had different findings for different outcomes.

Table 3 provides a detailed description of the study results according to the study population, study design, intervention(s) examined, and comparison groups. The single study examining comorbidity *per se* and its effects on the treatment of DM demonstrated that for persons with low to moderate comorbidity, measured with a validated comorbidity index, achieving a HgbA1C ≤6.5% was associated with a decreased risk of cardiovascular events, but for persons with high comorbidity, achieving this HgbA1C level was not associated with decreased risk [9].

All but two of the ten studies examining the effect of DM on the treatment of HF with beta blockers concluded that there were no differences in outcomes according to the presence or absence of DM or greater risk reduction among patient with DM [10–17,19]. Figure 2 provides a graphical summary of the results for those studies presenting their outcomes in terms of a form of relative risk. One study reported a significant benefit of beta-blockers on all-cause mortality and cardiovascular outcomes among patients without DM with a hazard ratio (HR) of.78 (95% confidence interval [CI].65, .93) but no benefit among patients with DM with a HR of 1.04 (.80, 1.35). [11] The second study concluding that

Table 1. Description of studies identified in systematic review.

Approach to analysis of comorbidity:	
Comorbidity index	1
Pairwise combinations of conditions	44
Combinations of conditions*:	
Heart failure and diabetes mellitus	10
Diabetes mellitus and hypertension	9
Cardiovascular disease and diabetes	5
Diabetes mellitus and renal disease	10
Cardiovascular disease and chronic kidney disease	8
Study design:	
Randomized controlled trial	6
Randomized controlled trial with post-hoc subgroup analysis	25
Observational cohort study	14
Miscellaneous combinations	5
Outcome(s) examined*:	
Mortality	35
Disease-specific outcome (e.g. stroke, cardiovascular event)	24
Hospitalization	5
Function/symptoms	1
Adverse effect	2

* Total >45 because some articles examined more than one combination of conditions and/or more than one outcome.

there was a difference in all-cause mortality reported a non-significant effect of beta-blockers among patients with DM with a hazard ratio (HR) of.79 (95% confidence interval [CI].50, 1.20) and a borderline significant effect among patients without DM with a HR of.60 (.35, 1.01). [18] While another study also showed a significant effect among patients without DM and a non-significant effect among patients with DM, it concluded that there was no difference in benefit because of a non-significant "heterogeneity test for interaction." [14].

Among the six studies examining intensity of HTN treatment in patients with DM, the definition of tight control changed over time, as did the study results. The United Kingdom Prospective

Table 2. Main study findings according to approach of article.

Examination of benefit of therapy in presence or absence of comorbidity (n = 25):	
No difference in benefit	19
Benefit greater in presence of comorbidity	4
Benefit smaller or absent in presence of comorbidity	2
Examination of harm of therapy in presence or absence of comorbidity (n = 2):	
No difference in harm	2
Harm smaller or absent in presence of comorbidity	0
Harm great in presence of comorbidity	0
Examination of benefit of tighter versus less tight control of one condition when second condition present (n = 15):	
Tighter control more beneficial versus less tight control	7
Tighter control of no greater benefit or harmful versus less tight control	6
U-shaped relationship, or different relationship for different outcomes	2
Examination of benefit of intervention established as standard of care when comorbidity absent in the presence of comorbidity (n = 3):	
Intervention beneficial	1
Intervention not beneficial	2

Table 3. Studies identified in systematic review.

Author, Year	Study Design & N	Population	Intervention/ Comparison Groups	Outcome/Main Findings (Differences between Groups)
Diseases: HEART FAILURE AND DIABETES MELLITUS				
Bobbio, 2003	Cohort N = 2,843	Italian patients w/HF, mean ages 63–66	Beta-blockers/with and w/o DM	All-cause mortality: no difference.
deBoer, 2010	Post-hoc RCT N = 2,128	Dutch patients ≥70 w/HF	Nebivolol (BB)/with and w/o DM	All-cause mortality and CV hospital admission: risk reduction greater in patients with DM.
Deedwania, 2005	Post-hoc RCT N = 3,991	European patients, ages 40–80 w/HF	Metoprolol CR/XL (BB)/with and w/o DM	All-cause mortality and hospitalization due to HF: no difference
Domanski, 2003	Post-hoc RCT N = 2,708	US patients, ages 19–93 w/HF	Bucindolol (BB)/with and w/o DM.	Death or HF hospitalizations: no difference.
Erdmann, 2001	Post-hoc RCT N = 2,647	European patients w/HF, mean age 61	Bisoprostol/with and w/o DM	All-cause mortality: no difference.
MacDonald, 2008	Post-hoc RCT N = 7,599	European patients w/HF, mean ages 65–67	Candesartan/with and w/o DM	All-cause mortality, CV morbidity and mortality: no difference.
Nodari, 2003	Cohort N = 193	Italian patients w/HF, mean ages 60 (w/DM) and 55 (w/o DM)	Carvedilol/with and w/o DM	NYHA functional class, exercise tests, and other hemodynamic parameters: no difference.
Ryden, 2000	Post-hoc RCT N = 3,164	International patients >55 w/HF	Lisinopril high vs. low dose/with and w/o DM	All-cause mortality: no difference.
Subramanian 2009	Cohort N = 412	Veterans w/HF, mean ages 66–70	Beta-blockers (cardioselective CSB)/with and w/o DM	All-cause mortality: no benefit for patients with DM; borderline significant benefit for patients without DM.
Torp-Pedersen, 2007	Post-hoc RCT N = 3,029	European patients w/HF, mean ages 61–64	Carvedilol vs. metoprolol/with and w/o DM	All-cause mortality: no difference.
Diseases: DIABETES AND HYPERTENSION				
ACCORD, 2010 (Cushman)	Factorial RCT N = 4,733	DM pts ≥40 w/CVD or ≥55 w/atherosclerosis, albuminuria, LVH, or ≥2 risk factors for CVD	BP therapy/tight (<120 SBP) vs less tight (<140 SBP) BP control	Major cardiovascular event: no difference. All-cause or cardiovascular mortality: no difference Significantly higher rate SAE (3.3% vs. 1.29%, p<.001), hyperkalemia, and elevated Cr in tight control group vs less tight group.
Berl, 2005	Post-hoc RCT N = 1,715	US patients, ages 30–70 w/DM, HTN, proteinuria	BP therapy/observed SBP≤120 vs >120; DBP 10 mm Hg increments	All-cause mortality: increased risk with SBP<120. MI: increased risk with lower DBP. Stroke: decreased risk with lower DBP.
Cooper-DeHoff, 2010	Post-hoc RCT N = 6,400	US patients, ≥50 w/stable CAD and DM	BP control/observed tight (SBP<130), usual (SBP 130–139), uncontrolled (≥140)	All-cause mortality: no difference during study f/u. 5-yr mortality: higher in tight control.
Curb, 1996	Post-hoc RCT N = 4,736	US patients, ≥60 w/HTN	Chlorthalidone (+atenolol or reserpine as needed)/with and w/o DM	All-cause mortality, non-fatal plus fatal stroke, nonfatal MI plus fatal CHD, major CHD events, major CVD events: risk reduction as great if not greater for persons with DM (no formal test for interaction)
Estacio, 2000	RCT N = 470	US patients, ages 40–74 w/DM	Stepped BP therapy/DBP≤70 vs. DBP 80–89	CrCl, retinopathy, neuropathy: no difference. All-cause mortality: lower in tight control.
Hansson, 1998	Stratified RCT N = 1,501	European patients, ages 50–80 w/DM	Stepped BP therapy/DBP≤90 vs. ≤85 vs. ≤80	Major CV events: lower in tight control (significant difference ≤80 vs. ≤90).
Tuomilehto, 1999	Post-hoc RCT N = 4,695	European patients, ≥60 with HTN	Nitrendipine (+others as needed)/with and w/o DM	All-cause mortality, mortality from cardiovascular disease, all cardiovascular events: greater risk reduction in patients with DM
UKPDS, 1998	RCT N = 1,148	UK patients, ages 25–65 w/HTN & DM	BP therapy/tight (<150 SBP) vs. less tight (<180 SBP) BP control	All-cause mortality, MI: no difference. Any DM-related endpoints, DM-related deaths, stroke, microvascular disease: lower in tight control.
Wang, 2000	Post-hoc RCT N = 2,394	Chinese patients, ≥60 w/HTN	Nitrendipine (+others as needed)/with and w/o DM	All-cause mortality, CV mortality, stroke, all cardiovascular events: no difference
Diseases: CARDIOVASCULAR DISEASE AND DIABETES				
Berthet, 2004	Post-hoc RCT N = 6,105	International patients w/hx of CVA or TIA, mean ages 63–64	ACE-inhibitor (+indapamide as needed)/with and w/o DM	Recurrent stroke: no difference.
Collins, 2003	Post-hoc RCT N = 20,536	UK patients, ages 40–80 w/CAD, PAD, or HTN.	Simvastatin/with and w/o DM	Coronary events and vascular events: no difference.
Komajda, 2010	Post-hoc RCT N = 4,447	International patients w/DM	Rosiglitazone/with and w/o CVD	Heart failure: no difference

Table 3. Cont.

Author, Year	Study Design & N	Population	Intervention/ Comparison Groups	Outcome/Main Findings (Differences between Groups)
Shinohara, 2008	Post-hoc RCT N = 1,095	Japanese patients w/prior CVA or TIA	Cilostazol/with and w/o DM, HTN	Recurrent stroke: no difference.
Wernicke, 2009	Post-hoc RCTs (pooled analysis) N = 1,024	US patients ≥18 with diabetic peripheral neuropathy	Duloxetine/with and w/o CVD	Adverse events: no difference.
Diseases: DIABETES AND RENAL DISEASE				
Hayashino, 2007	Cohort N = 1,569	Japanese patients w/ESRD on HD, mean ages 58–64	Glycemic control during stable, regular HD/Quintile of HgbA1C	All-cause mortality: top quintile of HgbA1C assoc w/increased risk compared to lowest quintile.
Kalantar-Zadeh, 2007	Cohort N = 23,618	US patients w/ESRD on HD, mean ages 60–63	Glycemic control during stable regular HD/HgbA1C level	All-cause mortality: unadjusted analysis demonstrated lower HR with higher HgbA1C; adjustment resulted in higher HR as HgbA1c increased.
Lambers Heerspink, 2010	Post-hoc RCT N = 10,640	European patients with DM, mean age 65–68	Perindopril-indapamide/w/o CKD and w/3 stages of CKD	Macrovascular events, cardiovascular death, all-cause mortality, cerebrovascular events, new or worsening nephropathy, renal death: no difference.
Mann, 2001	Post-hoc RCT N = 980	International patients >55 w/DM and cardiac risk factor	Ramipril/with and w/o CRI	CV death, MI or CVA (combined outcome): no difference. CV mortality, all-cause mortality, heart failure-related hospitalization: risk reduction greater in patients with CRI.
Morioka, 2001	Cohort N = 150	Japanese patients w/ESRD on HD, ages 29–85, mean age 60.5	Glycemic control prior to start of dialysis/HgbA1C level	1, 3, and 5-year mortality: Risk increased with higher HgbA1C.
Okada, 2007	Cohort N = 78	Japanese patients w/type 2 DM and ESRD, age ≥20, mean age 58	Glycemic control prior to start of dialysis and during dialysis/HgbA1C level	All-cause mortality: no difference.
Oomichi, 2006	Cohort N = 114	Japanese patients w/ESRD on HD, ages 33–80, mean age 60.8	Glycemic control during stable, regular dialysis/Good, fair, poor HgbA1C	5-year mortalty: Higher in those w/poor HgbA1C (≥8) than in those with fair (6.5–8) or good (<6.5) HgbA1C.
Shurraw, 2010	Cohort N = 1,484	Canadian patients receiving hemodialysis, mean age 66	Glycemic control/HgbA1C level	All-cause mortality: no difference.
Shurraw, 2011	Cohort N = 23,296	Canadian patients w/DM and CKD, mean age 65–73	Glycemic control/HgbA1C level	All-cause mortality: U-shaped association: increased risk with <6.5% and >8.0%.
Williams, 2006	Cohort N = 24,744	US patients w/ESRD on HD, mean age 63.7	Glycemic control during stable, regular dialysis/HgbA1C level	All-cause mortality: no difference.
Diseases: CARDIOVASCULAR DISEASE AND CHRONIC KIDNEY DISEASE				
Baigent, 2011	RCT N = 9,270	European patients, ≥40 with moderate-severe CKD	Simvastatin+ezetimibe vs. placebo*	17% decrease in major CVD events with treatment; no difference in effect comparing patients with ESRD on dialysis and those with less severe CKD
Cohen-Solal, 2009	Post-hoc RCT (prespecified group) N = 2,112	European patients, >70 w/HF	Nebivolol/Tertiles of eGFR	All-cause mortality and CV hospitalizations: no difference.
Erdmann, 2001	Post-hoc RCT N = 2,647	European patients w/HF, mean age 61	Bisoprostol/with and w/o CKD.	All-cause mortality: no difference.
Fellström, 2009	RCT N = 2,776	European patients, ages 50–80 w/ESRD on HD	Rosuvastatin vs. placebo*	CV death, non-fatal MI, or non-fatal stroke: no risk reduction with rosuvastatin
McAlister, 2004	Cohort N = 754	Canadian patients w/HF, median age 69	ACE-inhibitors and beta-blockers/with and w/o CKD (GFR <60)	All-cause mortality: no difference
Nakamura, 2009	Post-hoc RCT N = 7,195	Japanese patients, ages 40–70 w/HL	Pravastatin/with and w/o moderate CKD	CHD, stroke, CVD, all-cause mortality: risk reduction greater in moderate CKD than without moderate CKD.
Tonelli, 2004	Post-hoc RCT N = 19,700	International patients w/CAD or at high risk for CAD, mean ages 50–65	Pravastatin/with and w/o moderate CKD	MI, coronary death, PTCA/surgical revascularization: no difference.
Wanner, 2005	RCT N = 1,255	European patients, ages 18–80 w/Type II DM w/ESRD on HD	Atorvastatin vs. placebo*	Composite of cardiac death, nonfatal MI, and stroke: no risk reduction with atorvastatin
MISCELLANEOUS DISEASE COMBINATIONS				
Bavry, 2010	Post-hoc RCT N = 22,576	International patients, ≥50 w/HTN and stable CAD	BP lowering/with and w/o PAD	All-cause mortality, nonfatal MI and nonfatal CVA: more pronounced J-shaped curve for relationship of HTN and outcome among PAD compared to no PAD.

Table 3. Cont.

Author, Year	Study Design & N	Population	Intervention/ Comparison Groups	Outcome/Main Findings (Differences between Groups)
Du, 2009	Post-hoc RCT N = 11,140	International patients, ≥55 w/DM and 1 additional CV risk	Perindopril+indapamide/with and w/o AF	All-cause mortality, CV deaths, major coronary events, major cerebrovascular events, HF: no difference.
Greenfield, 2009	Cohort N = 2,613	UK patients w/DM, mean ages 61–64	Glycemic control/w/low-to-mod comorbidity (TIBI <12) vs. high comorbidity (TIBI ≥12)	CV events: HbA1c ≤6.5 associated with reduced risk in low CM but not mod-high CM.
Shinohara, 2008	Post-hoc RCT N = 1,095	Japanese patients w/prior CVA or TIA	Cilostazol/with and w/o HTN	Recurrent stroke: no difference.
Sin, 2002	Cohort N = 11,942	Canadian patients ≥65 w/HF	Beta-blockers/With and w/o IHD	All-cause mortality: no difference.

RCT = randomized controlled trial.
w/o = without.
HF = heart failure.
DM = diabetes mellitus.
CV = cardiovascular.
NYHA = New York Heart Association.
LVH = left ventricular hypertrophy.
CVD = cardiovascular disease.
BP = blood pressure.
HTN = hypertension.
SBP = systolic blood pressure.
SAE = serious adverse event.
DBP = diastolic blood pressure.
MI = myocardial infarction.
CAD = coronary artery disease.
CHD = coronary heart disease.
CrCl = creatinine clearance.
UK = United Kingdom.
ACE = angiotensin converting enzyme.
PAD = peripheral arterial disease.
CVA = cerebrovascular accident.
AF = atrial fibrillation.
IHD = ischemic heart disease.
ESRD = end = stage renal disease.
HD = hemodialysis.
CKD = chronic kidney disease.
PTCA = percutaneous transluminal coronary angioplasty.
TIBI = Total Illness Burden Index.
*No inclusion of patients without CKD and therefore no comparison between patients with and without CKD; study assumed established benefit of therapy in the absence of CKD.

Diabetes study (UKPDS), defining tight control as a systolic blood pressure (SBP) of <150 mmHg, versus less tight control as SBP< 180 mmHg, demonstrated no difference in overall mortality associated with tight control but a decrease in any DM-related endpoints, DM-related deaths, stroke, or microvascular disease. [27] Later studies defining tight control as SBP<130 or < 120 mmHg demonstrated either no difference in outcome or an increased risk of adverse outcome associated with tight control. [20,21,23] The results were less consistent when tight control was defined on the basis of diastolic blood pressure (DBP). Two studies defining tight control as DBP<80 mmHg and as <70 mmHg demonstrated benefits in terms of lower all-cause mortality and major cardiovascular events, [24,25] whereas a third study examining DBP in 10 mm increments demonstrated a decreased risk of stroke but increased risk of myocardial infarction associated with tighter control [20].

Of the five studies examining patients with cardiovascular disease and diabetes, three examined the effects of medications to reduce risk of vascular outcomes (ACE-inhibitor, simvastatin, and cilostazol) and found no differences according to the presence or absence of DM [39–41]. The remaining two studies examined the likelihood of harm associated with medication use among persons with DM with and without cardiovascular disease. These studies found no difference in adverse effects associated with duloxetine and no difference in the likelihood of heart failure associated with rosiglitazone.

The eight studies examining outcomes in patients with renal disease according to control of blood sugar in DM showed conflicting results. A total of three studies demonstrated an increased risk of mortality associated with higher HgbA1C levels, [29,33,35] whereas three other studies demonstrated no difference in survival, [34,37,38] and one study demonstrated a U-shaped association. [36] In one study, the unadjusted analysis demonstrated a lower risk of mortality with higher HgbA1C levels but the adjusted analysis demonstrated a higher risk, suggesting that HgbA1C levels may be a marker of underlying health status. [30] The two studies examining the effects of ACE-inhibitors on cardiovascular outcomes among patients with DM demonstrated either no differences according to the presence or absence of CKD [31] or greater risk reduction among patients with renal disease [32].

Of the five studies examining a variety of medications among patients with cardiovascular disease, four demonstrated no difference in outcomes according to the presence or absence of

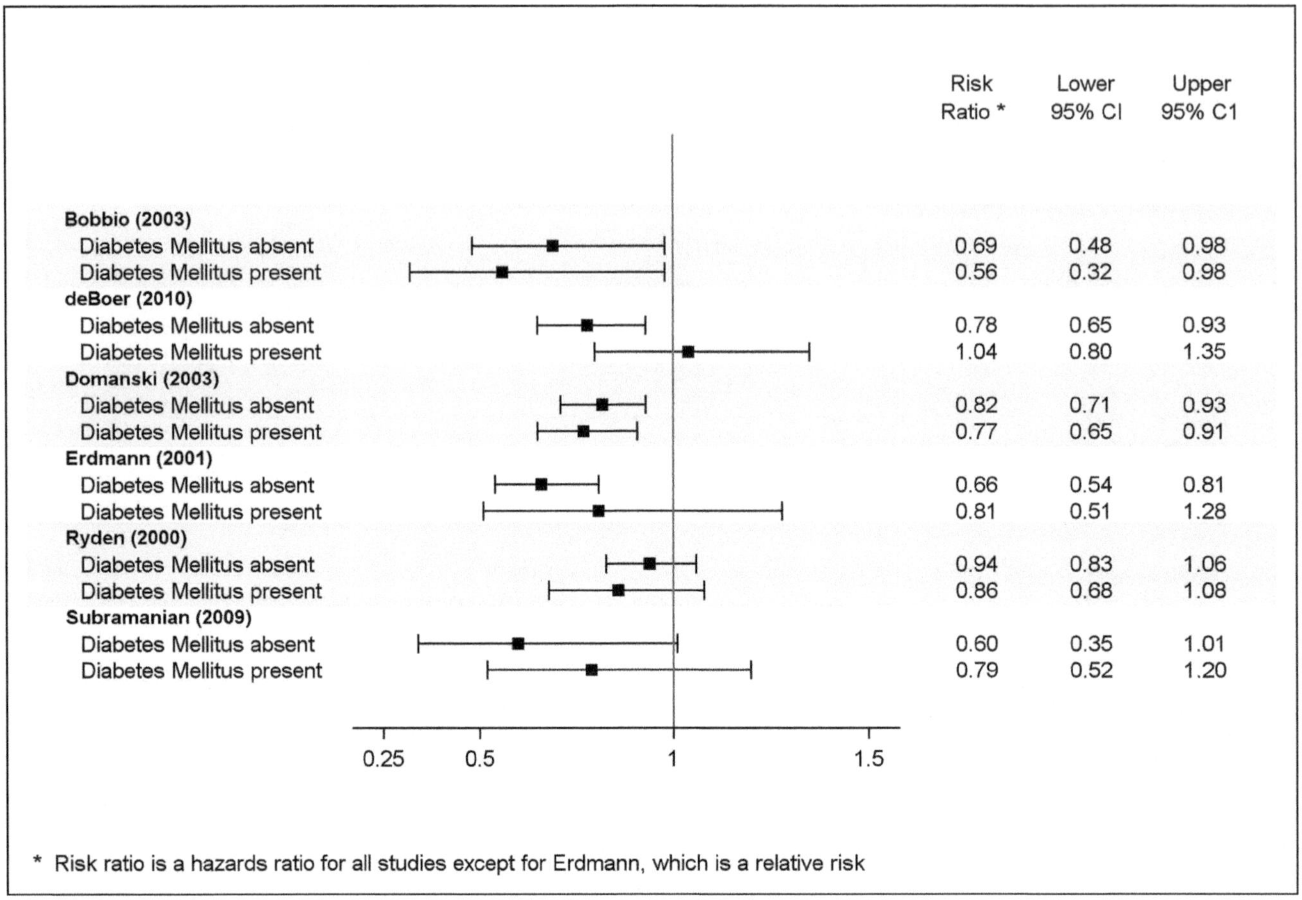

Figure 2. Risk Reduction Associated with Medication for Treatment of Heart Failure.

CKD. [14,45,47,49] The fifth, a study of pravastatin, demonstrated a decreased risk of a number of different outcomes among persons with moderate CKD but no decreased risk among persons with normal renal function or mild CKD, suggesting increased efficacy of the medication in the presence of CKD. [48] (Figure 3). Of the three studies examining the efficacy of statins among persons with CKD without a comparison group of persons without CKD, one demonstrated a decreased risk of major cardiac events with treatment and found no difference when comparing patients with end-stage renal disease (ESRD) and those with less severe CKD. [44] The two other studies demonstrated no decreased risk of major cardio/cerebrovascular events with treatment among patients with ESRD receiving hemodialysis [46,50].

Of the four studies examining miscellaneous combinations of conditions, three demonstrated no difference in the efficacy of treatment according to the presence or absence of the comorbid condition. This included the use of perindopril-indapamide among persons with DM and one additional cardiovascular risk factor in the presence or absence of AF, [52] the use of cilostazol in persons with prior cerebrovascular accident or transient ischemic attack in the presence or absence of HTN, [41] and the use of beta blockers in persons with HF in the presence or absence of ischemic heart disease. [53] The final study examined the effect of the intensity of treatment of HTN in persons with CAD in the presence or absence of PAD. This study found a J-shaped relationship between blood pressure and outcomes among persons with PAD, such that lower blood pressure was associated with increased risk, but no such relationship among persons without PAD [51].

Discussion

This systematic review was undertaken to address the question of how the presence of comorbid conditions affects the benefits and harms of medical treatment for an index chronic condition. The process of the review revealed that there is virtually no evidence regarding the effect of comorbidity *per se*, as the review identified only one study that characterized patients according to their burden of comorbid illnesses. Instead, the evidence consists of studies of pairs of conditions, in which investigators examine the effect of therapy in the presence or absence of a single comorbid condition. There is also little evidence regarding harms of treatment, as the vast majority of studies focused on examining benefit only. In addition, benefit was narrowly defined in terms of reducing the risk of mortality and other major disease-specific outcomes. Studies focused on a limited range of pairs, consisting of a combination of cardiovascular disease (HF and HTN), DM, and CKD. Few studies were originally designed to address the question of the effect of comorbidity on treatment of an index condition. The majority of studies demonstrated that the presence of a comorbid condition did not reduce the benefits associated with treatment of the index condition. The exceptions to this were the findings that patients with a high burden of comorbidity do not derive the same benefit from tight diabetic control as patients with a lower comorbidity burden, that patients with DM do not benefit

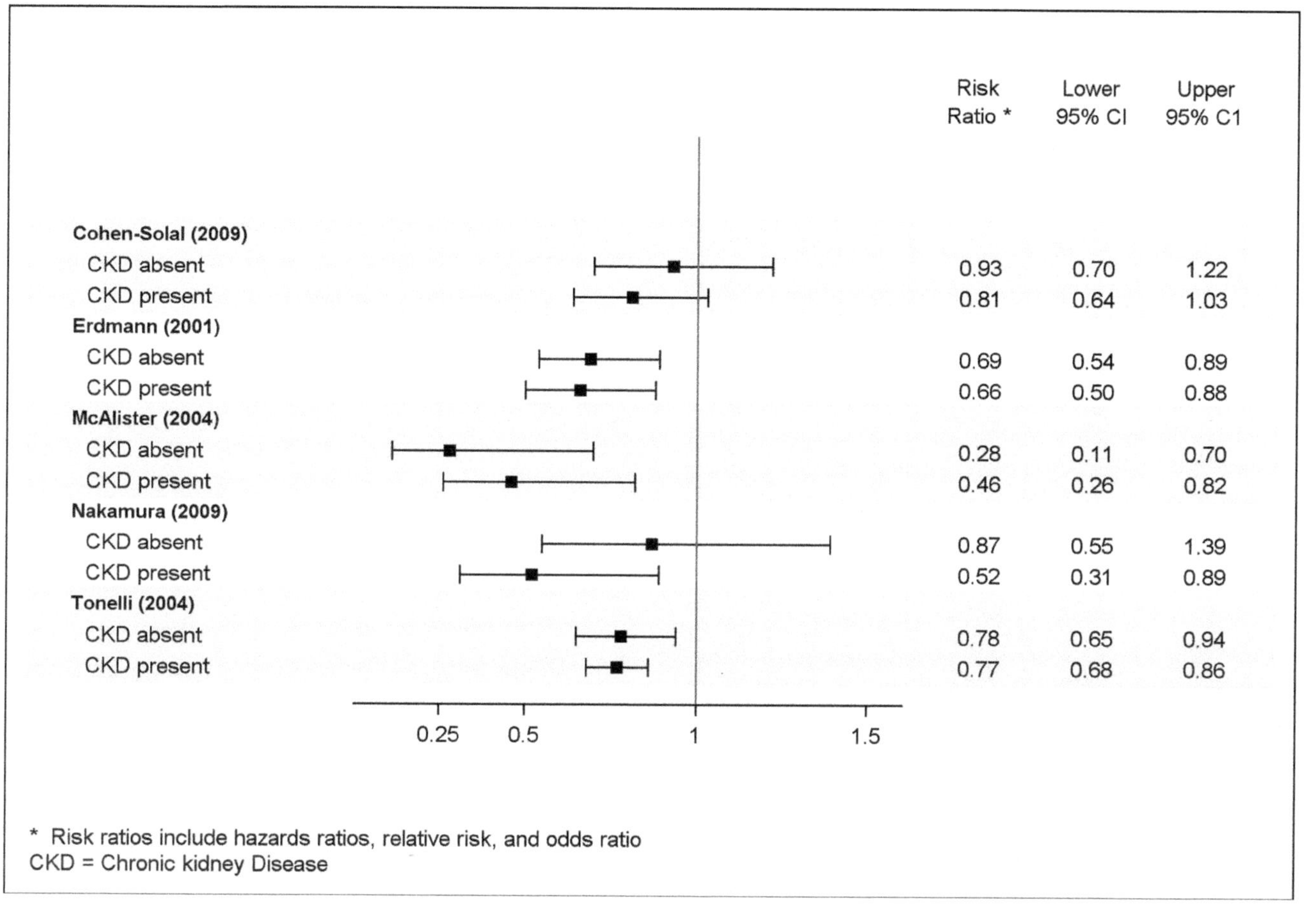

Figure 3. Risk Reduction Associated with Medication for Treatment of Cardiovascular Disease.

from tight control of HTN, and that patients with ESRD do not derive the same benefit from treatment with statin therapy as patients without ESRD.

This systematic review was motivated by concern raised in the literature about the unintended adverse consequences of treating patients with multimorbidity. This concern arises from the finding that treating patients with multimorbidity according to current disease-specific guidelines can result in polypharmacy with the potential for numerous drug-drug and drug-disease interactions. [2] Moreover, polypharmacy itself has been associated with adverse outcomes, including falls, [54] weight loss and balance impairment, [55] and hospitalization. [56] However, the existing literature does not address this patient population. Despite an extensive search, we found only one study that examined burden of comorbidity as a potential modifier of the effect of treatment. "Multimorbidity" is not an indexing term, and, while "comorbidity" is a term, it was infrequently used, so that it proved difficult to construct a search addressing our question of interest. With the growing attention being paid to the study of multiple medical conditions, there is a need for a clear and consistent approach to indexing future studies in order to facilitate the ability to synthesize evidence as it becomes available.

The great majority of studies examined either mortality or disease-specific outcomes, such as cardiovascular events. Disease-specific outcomes cannot be applied across individual diseases to facilitate treatment decision making that takes into account the net effect of an intervention on the health of a patient with multimorbidity, and universal outcomes that are applicable across diseases such as quality of life, physical function, or symptom reduction may be more important to these patients. [57,58] Moreover, studies did not examine time to benefit, a parameter particularly important for patients with multimorbidity because of their competing mortality risks [57].

The studies conducted as post-hoc analyses of randomized controlled trials are subject to the same limitations of their patient population as the original studies. The patients eligible for and participating in cardiovascular intervention studies are generally healthier and with fewer comorbid conditions than are patients who do not enroll in these studies. [59,60] There is evidence that these differences influence the benefits and harms of therapies. For example, the RALES RCT demonstrating the effectiveness of spironolactone in reducing hospitalization and mortality among patients with advanced HF had very low rates of adverse events. [61] The publication of the trial was followed by a marked increase in the use of spironolactone, and, among older persons who were taking ACE-inhibitors, this increase was accompanied by a substantial rise in the rates of hospitalization and mortality from hyperkalemia [62].

Because of the lack of studies examining comorbidity, our review ended up addressing the question of whether, among a limited spectrum of diseases, the presence of a second condition affects the benefits or harms of treatment for a first. While, for many pairs of conditions (DM and HF, DM and CKD, DM and CVD), the answer to this question appears to be "no," there was some evidence to suggest that the presence of a second condition can alter the outcomes of therapy. The finding of an increased risk of adverse outcome among patients with DM receiving tight blood pressure control illustrates an evolution in the approach to the treatment of HTN among diabetic patients. Recommendations published in 2003 included the statement that "there is no threshold value for blood pressure, and risk continues to decrease well into the normal range," [63] suggesting the lower the blood pressure, the better the outcomes. Recommendations published in 2013 call for treatment to a systolic blood pressure of <140, reserving treatment to lower targets for select populations, such as younger patients. [64] While these recommendations appear to be supported by the results of this systematic review, it is also worth noting that many disease management guidelines for DM also recommend different targets for HgbA1C according to comorbidities, ranging from 7% to 8%. Aside from the one study demonstrating a lack of benefit for patients with high comorbidity burden achieving a HgbA1C of <6.5%, our review did not identify any studies supporting these recommendations.

Our review has several limitations. First, because of the difficulty in constructing an effective search strategy, we found a relatively large proportion of our studies through review of the reference lists of articles identified in the search. This suggests that we may have missed relevant articles. Second data to inform our study question may exist that was not available in the articles we reviewed. For example, we identified two meta-analyses of studies examining the effect of DM on the treatment of HF. In our review of the articles referenced in the meta-analyses, we failed to find any subgroup analysis examining outcomes according to the presence or absence of DM. This suggests that the authors of the meta-analyses obtained additional data from the investigators of the original studies.

The conduct of this systematic review designed to address the question of how comorbid conditions affect the benefits and harms of treatment for an index chronic disease demonstrated that the evidence was difficult to find because of a lack of clear indexing. Moreover, few studies were designed to answer this question optimally. There was little evidence examining comorbidity *per se*, but rather studies examining pairs of conditions. Because many studies were derived from RCTs, their participants may not have had the full range of comorbidities present in unselected patient populations. While the majority of studies did not demonstrate an effect of the comorbid condition on outcomes, there is some evidence to support the notion that "less is more" [65] when treating patients with multiple chronic conditions. However, more evidence is needed to inform the care of these patients.

Supporting Information

Appendix S1.

Checklist S1 PRISMA checklist.

Acknowledgments

We would like to thank Janis Glover, MLS, for her assistance in designing and conducting the Medline search.

Views expressed are those of the authors and not necessarily those of the Department of Veterans Affairs.

Author Contributions

Conceived and designed the experiments: TRF. Performed the experiments: TRF JRO VT. Analyzed the data: TRF MG MT DKM. Contributed to the writing of the manuscript: TRF MG DKM.

References

1. Tinetti ME, Fried TR, Boyd CM (2012) Designing health care for the most common chronic condition-multimorbidity. JAMA 307: 2493–2494.
2. Boyd CM, Darer J, Boult C, Fried LP, Boult L, et al. (2005) Clinical practice guidelines and quality of care for older patients with multiple comorbid diseases: implications for pay for performance. JAMA 294: 716–724.
3. Gandhi TK, Weingart SN, Borus J, Seger AC, Peterson J, et al. (2003) Adverse drug events in ambulatory care. N Engl J Med 348: 1556–1564.
4. Tinetti ME, Bogardus ST Jr, Agostini JV (2004) Potential pitfalls of disease-specific guidelines for patients with multiple conditions. N Engl J Med 351: 2870–2874.
5. Concato J, Shah N, Horwitz RI (2000) Randomized, controlled trials, observational studies, and the hierarchy of research designs. N Engl J Med 342: 1887–1892.
6. Vogeli C, Shields A, Lee T, Gibson T, Marder W, et al. (2007) Multiple chronic conditions: prevalence, health consequences, and implications for quality, care management, and costs. J Gen Intern Med 22: 391–395.
7. D'Agostino RB (2000) Debate: The slippery slope of surrogate outcomes. Curr Control Trials Cardiovasc Med 1: 76–79.
8. Guyatt GH, Oxman AD, Vist GE, Kunz R, Falck-Ytter Y, et al. (2008) GRADE: an emerging consensus on rating quality of evidence and strength of recommendations. BMJ 336: 924–926.
9. Greenfield S, Billimek J, Pellegrini F, Franciosi M, De Berardis G, et al. (2009) Comorbidity affects the relationship between glycemic control and cardiovascular outcomes in diabetes: a cohort study. Ann Intern Med 151: 854–860.
10. Bobbio M, Ferrua S, Opasich C, Porcu M, Lucci D, et al. (2003) Survival and hospitalization in heart failure patients with or without diabetes treated with beta-blockers. J Card Fail 9: 192–202.
11. de Boer RA, Doehner W, van der Horst ICC, Anker SD, Babalis D, et al. (2010) Influence of diabetes mellitus and hyperglycemia on prognosis in patients> or = 70 years old with heart failure and effects of nebivolol (data from the Study of Effects of Nebivolol Intervention on Outcomes and Rehospitalization in Seniors with heart failure [SENIORS]). Am J Cardiol 106: 78–86.e71.
12. Deedwania PC, Giles TD, Klibaner M, Ghali JK, Herlitz J, et al. (2005) Efficacy, safety and tolerability of metoprolol CR/XL in patients with diabetes and chronic heart failure: experiences from MERIT-HF. Am Heart J 149: 159–167.
13. Domanski M, Krause-Steinrauf H, Deedwania P, Follmann D, Ghali JK, et al. (2003) The effect of diabetes on outcomes of patients with advanced heart failure in the BEST trial. J Am Coll Cardiol 42: 914–922.
14. Erdmann E, Lechat P, Verkenne P, Wiemann H (2001) Results from post-hoc analyses of the CIBIS II trial: effect of bisoprolol in high-risk patient groups with chronic heart failure. Eur J Heart Fail 3: 469–479.
15. MacDonald MR, Petrie MC, Varyani F, Östergren J, Michelson EL, et al. (2008) Impact of diabetes on outcomes in patients with low and preserved ejection fraction heart failure An analysis of the Candesartan in Heart failure: Assessment of reduction in mortality and morbidity (CHARM) programme. Eur Heart J 29: 1377–1385.
16. Nodari S, Metra M, Dei Cas A, Dei Cas L (2003) Efficacy and tolerability of the long-term administration of carvedilol in patients with chronic heart failure with and without concomitant diabetes mellitus. Eur J Heart Fail 5: 803–809.
17. Ryden L, Armstrong PW, Cleland J, Horowitz JD, Massie B, et al. (2000) Efficacy and safety of high-dose lisinopril in chronic heart failure patients at high cardiovascular risk, including those with diabetes mellitus. Results from the ATLAS trial. Eur Heart J 1 21: 1967–1978.
18. Subramanian U, Kamalesh M, Temkit Mh, Eckert GJ, Sawada S (2009) Do cardioselective beta-adrenoceptor antagonists reduce mortality in diabetic patients with congestive heart failure? Am J Cardiovasc Drugs 9: 231–240.
19. Torp-Pedersen C, Metra M, Charlesworth A, Spark P, Lukas MA, et al. (2007) Effects of metoprolol and carvedilol on pre-existing and new onset diabetes in patients with chronic heart failure: data from the Carvedilol Or Metoprolol European Trial (COMET). Heart 93: 968–973.
20. Berl T, Hunsicker LG, Lewis JB, Pfeffer MA, Porush JG, et al. (2005) Impact of achieved blood pressure on cardiovascular outcomes in the irbesartan diabetic nephropathy trial. J Am Soc Nephrol 16: 2170–2179.
21. Cooper-DeHoff RM, Gong Y, Handberg EM, Bavry AA, Denardo SJ, et al. (2010) Tight blood pressure control and cardiovascular outcomes among hypertensive patients with diabetes and coronary artery disease. JAMA 304: 61–68.
22. Curb JD, Pressel SL, Cutler JA, Savage PJ, Applegate WB, et al. (1996) Effect of diuretic-based antihypertensive treatment on cardiovascular disease risk in older diabetic patients with isolated systolic hypertension. Systolic Hypertension in the Elderly Program Cooperative Research Group. JAMA 276: 1886–1892.
23. Cushman WC (2010) Effects of Intensive blood-pressure control in type 2 diabetes mellitus. New Engl J Med 362: 1575–1585.

24. Estacio RO, Jeffers BW, Gifford N, Schrier RW (2000) Effect of blood pressure control on diabetic microvascular complications in patients with hypertension and type 2 diabetes. Diabetes Care 23 Suppl 2: B54–64.
25. Hansson L, Zanchetti A, Carruthers SG, Dahlöf B, Elmfeldt D, et al. (1998) Effects of intensive blood-pressure lowering and low-dose aspirin in patients with hypertension: principal results of the Hypertension Optimal Treatment (HOT) randomised trial. The Lancet 351: 1755–1762.
26. Tuomilehto J, Rastenyte D, Birkenhager WH, Thijs L, Antikainen R, et al. (1999) Effects of calcium-channel blockade in older patients with diabetes and systolic hypertension. Systolic Hypertension in Europe Trial Investigators. N Engl J Med 340: 677–684.
27. U. K. Prospective Diabetes Study Group (1998) Tight blood pressure control and risk of macrovascular and microvascular complications in type 2 diabetes: UKPDS 38. BMJ 317: 703–713.
28. Wang JG, Staessen JA, Gong L, Liu L (2000) Chinese trial on isolated systolic hypertension in the elderly. Systolic Hypertension in China (SYST-CHINA) Collaborative Group. Arch Intern Med 160: 211–220.
29. Hayashino Y, Fukuhara S, Akiba T, Akizawa T, Asano Y, et al. (2007) Diabetes, glycaemic control and mortality risk in patients on haemodialysis: the Japan Dialysis Outcomes and Practice Pattern Study. Diabetologia 50: 1170–1177.
30. Kalantar-Zadeh K, Kopple JD, Regidor DL, Jing J, Shinaberger CS, et al. (2007) A1C and survival in maintenance hemodialysis patients. Diabetes Care 30: 1049–1055.
31. Lambers Heerspink HJ, Ninomiya T, Perkovic V, Woodward M, Zoungas S, et al. (2010) Effects of a fixed combination of perindopril and indapamide in patients with type 2 diabetes and chronic kidney disease. Eur Heart J 31: 2888–2896.
32. Mann JFEMD, Gerstein HCMD, Pogue JM, Bosch JMA, Yusuf SMD, et al. (2001) Renal insufficiency as a predictor of cardiovascular outcomes and the impact of ramipril: the HOPE randomized trial. Ann Intern Med 134: 629–636.
33. Morioka T, Emoto M, Tabata T, Shoji T, Tahara H, et al. (2001) Glycemic control is a predictor of survival for diabetic patients on hemodialysis. Diabetes Care 24: 909–913.
34. Okada T, Nakao T, Matsumoto H, Shino T, Nagaoka Y, et al. (2007) Association between markers of glycemic control, cardiovascular complications and survival in type 2 diabetic patients with end-stage renal disease. Intern Medicine 46: 807–814.
35. Oomichi T, Emoto M, Tabata T, Morioka T, Tsujimoto Y, et al. (2006) Impact of glycemic control on survival of diabetic patients on chronic regular hemodialysis: a 7-year observational study. Diabetes Care 29: 1496–1500.
36. Shurraw S, Hemmelgarn B, Lin M, Majumdar SR, Klarenbach S, et al. (2011) Association between glycemic control and adverse outcomes in people with diabetes mellitus and chronic kidney disease: a population-based cohort study. Arch Intern Med 171: 1920–1927.
37. Shurraw S, Majumdar SR, Thadhani R, Wiebe N, Tonelli M, et al. (2010) Glycemic control and the risk of death in 1,484 patients receiving maintenance hemodialysis. Am J Kidney Dis 55: 875–884.
38. Williams ME, Lacson E Jr, Teng M, Ofsthun N, Lazarus JM (2006) Hemodialyzed type I and type II diabetic patients in the US: Characteristics, glycemic control, and survival. Kidney Int 70: 1503–1509.
39. Berthet K, Neal BC, Chalmers JP, MacMahon SW, Bousser M-G, et al. (2004) Reductions in the risks of recurrent stroke in patients with and without diabetes: the PROGRESS Trial. Blood Press 13: 7–13.
40. Collins R, Armitage J, Parish S, Sleigh P, Peto R (2003) MRC/BHF Heart Protection Study of cholesterol-lowering with simvastatin in 5963 people with diabetes: a randomised placebo-controlled trial. Lancet 361: 2005.
41. Shinohara Y, Gotoh F, Tohgi H, Hirai S, Terashi A, et al. (2008) Antiplatelet cilostazol is beneficial in diabetic and/or hypertensive ischemic stroke patients. Subgroup analysis of the cilostazol stroke prevention study. Cerebrovasc Dis 26: 63–70.
42. Wernicke JF, Prakash A, Kajdasz DK, Houston J (2009) Safety and tolerability of duloxetine treatment of diabetic peripheral neuropathic pain between patients with and without cardiovascular conditions. J Diabetes Complications 23: 349–359.
43. Komajda M, McMurray JJV, Beck-Nielsen H, Gomis R, Hanefeld M, et al. (2010) Heart failure events with rosiglitazone in type 2 diabetes: data from the RECORD clinical trial. Eur Heart J 31: 824–831.
44. Baigent C, Landray MJ, Reith C, Emberson J, Wheeler DC, et al. (2011) The effects of lowering LDL cholesterol with simvastatin plus ezetimibe in patients with chronic kidney disease (Study of Heart and Renal Protection): a randomised placebo-controlled trial. Lancet 377: 2181–2192.
45. Cohen-Solal A, Kotecha D, van Veldhuisen DJ, Babalis D, Böhm M, et al. (2009) Efficacy and safety of nebivolol in elderly heart failure patients with impaired renal function: insights from the SENIORS trial. Eur J Heart Fail 11: 872–880.
46. Fellstrom BC, Jardine AG, Schmieder RE, Holdaas H, Bannister K, et al. (2009) Rosuvastatin and cardiovascular events in patients undergoing hemodialysis. N Engl J Med 360: 1395–1407.
47. McAlister FA, Ezekowitz J, Tonelli M, Armstrong PW (2004) Renal insufficiency and heart failure: prognostic and therapeutic implications from a prospective cohort study. Circulation 109: 1004–1009.
48. Nakamura H, Mizuno K, Ohashi Y, Yoshida T, Hirao K, et al. (2009) Pravastatin and cardiovascular risk in moderate chronic kidney disease. Atherosclerosis 206: 512–517.
49. Tonelli M, Isles C, Curhan GC, Tonkin A, Pfeffer MA, et al. (2004) Effect of pravastatin on cardiovascular events in people with chronic kidney disease. Circulation 110: 1557–1563.
50. Wanner C, Krane V, März W, Olschewski M, Mann JFE, et al. (2005) Atorvastatin in patients with type 2 diabetes mellitus undergoing hemodialysis. N Engl J Med 353: 238–248.
51. Bavry AA, Anderson RD, Gong Y, Denardo SJ, Cooper-Dehoff RM, et al. (2010) Outcomes Among hypertensive patients with concomitant peripheral and coronary artery disease: findings from the INternational VErapamil-SR/Trandolapril STudy. Hypertension 55: 48–53.
52. Du X, Ninomiya T, de Galan B, Abadir E, Chalmers J, et al. (2009) Risks of cardiovascular events and effects of routine blood pressure lowering among patients with type 2 diabetes and atrial fibrillation: results of the ADVANCE study. Eur Heart J 30: 1128–1135.
53. Sin DD, McAlister FA (2002) The effects of beta-blockers on morbidity and mortality in a population-based cohort of 11,942 elderly patients with heart failure. Am J Med 113: 650–656.
54. Tinetti ME (2003) Preventing falls in elderly persons. N Engl J Med 348: 42–49.
55. Agostini JV, Han L, Tinetti ME (2004) The relationship between number of medications and weight loss or impaired balance in older adults. J Am Geriatr Soc 52: 1719–1723.
56. Beer C, Hyde Z, Almeida OP, Norman P, Hankey GJ, et al. (2011) Quality use of medicines and health outcomes among a cohort of community dwelling older men: an observational study. Br J Clin Pharmacol 71: 592–599.
57. American Geriatrics Society Expert Panel on the Care of Older Adults with Multimorbidity (2012) Patient-Centered Care for Older Adults with Multiple Chronic Conditions: A Stepwise Approach from the American Geriatrics Society. J Am Geriatr Soc 60: 1957–1968.
58. Fried TR, Tinetti ME, Iannone L, O'Leary JR, Towle V, et al. (2011) Health outcome prioritization as a tool for decision making among older persons with multiple chronic conditions. Arch Intern Med 171: 1854–1856.
59. Bahit MC, Cannon CP, Antman EM, Murphy SA, Gibson CM, et al. (2003) Direct comparison of characteristics, treatment, and outcomes of patients enrolled versus patients not enrolled in a clinical trial at centers participating in the TIMI 9 Trial and TIMI 9 Registry. Am Heart J 145: 109–117.
60. Hordijk-Trion M, Lenzen M, Wijns W, de Jaegere P, Simoons ML, et al. (2006) Patients enrolled in coronary intervention trials are not representative of patients in clinical practice: results from the Euro Heart Survey on Coronary Revascularization. Eur Heart J 27: 671–678.
61. Pitt B, Zannad F, Remme WJ, Cody R, Castaigne A, et al. (1999) The effect of spironolactone on morbidity and mortality in patients with severe heart failure. N Engl J Med 341: 709–717.
62. Juurlink DN, Mamdani MM, Lee DS, Kopp A, Austin PC, et al. (2004) Rates of hyperkalemia after publication of the randomized aldactone evaluation study. N Engl J Med 351: 543–551.
63. (2003) Treatment of hypertension in adults with diabetes. Diabetes Care 26: s80–s82.
64. (2013) Executive Summary: Standards of medical care in diabetes–2013. Diabetes Care 36: S4–S10.
65. Grady D, Redberg RF (2010) Less is more: How less health care can result in better health. Arch Intern Med 170: 749–750.

Prediction of Glycated Hemoglobin Levels at 3 Months after Metabolic Surgery Based on the 7-Day Plasma Metabolic Profile

Hyuk Nam Kwon[1]¶, Yeon Ji Lee[2]¶, Ju-Hee Kang[3]¶, Ji-ho Choi[2], Yong Jin An[1], Sunmi Kang[1], Dae Hyun Lee[4], Young Ju Suh[5], Yoonseok Heo[6]*, Sunghyouk Park[1]*

1 College of Pharmacy, Natural Product Research Institute, Seoul National University, Sillim-dong, Gwanak-gu, Seoul, Korea, 151-742, **2** Department of Family Medicine, Obesity center, Inha University Hospital, Inha University School of Medicine, Shinheung-dong, Jung-Gu, Incheon, Korea, 400-712, **3** Department of Pharmacology and Hypoxia-related disease Research, Inha University Hospital, Inha University School of Medicine, Shinheung-dong, Jung-Gu, Incheon, Korea, 400-712, **4** Department of Medicine, Inha University Hospital, Inha University School of Medicine, Shinheung-dong, Jung-Gu, Incheon, Korea, 400-712, **5** Department of Biostatistics, Inha University Hospital, Inha University School of Medicine, Shinheung-dong, Jung-Gu, Incheon, Korea, 400-712, **6** Department of General Surgery, Inha University Hospital, Inha University School of Medicine, Shinheung-dong, Jung-Gu, Incheon, Korea, 400-712

Abstract

Metabolic surgery has been shown to provide better glycemic control for type 2 diabetes than conventional therapies. Still, the outcomes of the surgery are variable, and prognostic markers reflecting the metabolic changes by the surgery are yet to be established. NMR-based plasma metabolomics followed by multivariate regression was used to test the correlation between the metabolomic profile at 7-days after surgery and glycated hemoglobin (HbA1c) levels at 3-months (and up to 12 months with less patients), and to identify the relevant markers. Metabolomic profiles at 7-days could differentiate the patients according to the HbA1c improvement status at 3-months. The HbA1c values were predicted based on the metabolomics profile with partial least square regression, and found to be correlated with the observed values. Metabolite analysis suggested that 3-Hydroxybutyrate (3-HB) and glucose contributes to this prediction, and the [3-HB]/[glucose] exhibited a modest to good correlation with the HbA1c level at 3-months. The prediction of 3-month HbA1c using 7-day metabolomic profile and the suggested new criterion [3-HB]/[glucose] could augment current prognostic modalities and help clinicians decide if drug therapy is necessary.

Editor: Andrea Motta, National Research Council of Italy, Italy

Funding: This research was supported by the Basic Science Research Program through the National Research Foundation of Korea (NRF) funded by the Ministry of Education, Science and Technology (2012011362, 2014009392, and 2009-93144), and by a grant from the National R&D Program for Cancer Control, Ministry of Health & Welfare, Republic of Korea (1420290). The funders had no role in study design, data collection and analysis, decision to publish, or preparation of the manuscript.

Competing Interests: The authors have declared that no competing interests exist.

* Email: psh@snu.ac.kr (SP); gshur@inha.ac.kr (YH)

¶ These authors contributed equally to this work.

Introduction

Diabetes mellitus (DM) is a worldwide disease causing serious health burden with the incidence of approximately 366 million in 2011. [1] A primary risk factor for type 2 diabetes mellitus (T2DM) is obesity and 90% of T2DM patients are either overweight or obese, as defined by body mass index (BMI) of 25 kg/m^2 or 30 kg/m^2, respectively. [2] The relative risks of diabetes are 40 times higher when BMI increases above 35 kg/m.^{2} [3] However, obesity seems to be less prevalent in T2DM patients in Asia, [4] suggesting that obesity occurs differently according to population. The main therapeutic modality of T2DM is pharmacotherapy accompanying lifestyle modification, [5] but it is for the control of hyperglycemia, rather than the cure of DM. To date, the only treatment options that have been demonstrated to manage DM without medication are pancreatic transplantation for type 1 DM [6] and surgical treatment for T2DM [7].

Bariatric surgery such as Roux-en Y gastric bypass (RYGB), originally used as a treatment for morbid obesity (>40 kg/m^2), also showed profound effects on various comorbidities of obesity including DM, [8] hyperlipidemia, hypertension and obstructive sleep apnea. [9] Because bariatric surgery had effects on a variety of metabolic syndrome, it is also called metabolic surgery, [10] and includes several variants: RYGB, duodenojejunal bypass (DJB), [11] and ileal transposition. [12] Metabolic surgery can lead to diabetes resolution, defined by lower levels of glycated hemoglobin (HbA1c) and fasting plasma glucose, occurring within days to weeks after surgery. Although the success rate of DM resolution is variable and long-term follow-up data are limited, a meta-analysis showed that 79.3% of patients exhibited diabetic resolution after RYGB, with 98.9% of patients showing improvement. [13] In addition, recent studies show that the surgical treatments outperform the conventional medical therapies in managing overall diabetic manifestation. [7,14] Despite these merits, the mechanism of improvement of diabetes by metabolic surgery has been elusive. It has been argued that the improvement of diabetes was due to the reduction in body weight, [15] but diabetes resolution occurred before the improvement in obesity. [8] Studies also demonstrated that metabolic surgery can confer improved glycemic control not only on obese but also on non-obese (< 30 kg/m^2) patients. [16] Therefore, the metabolic surgery seems to improve diabetes in a weight loss-independent way, and the molecular studies related to the detailed mechanism are anticipated.

As DM is essentially a metabolic disease, proper approaches to follow the disease course or the prognosis of treatment options should involve the monitoring of metabolite molecules. In fact, recent applications of metabolomics on DM have discovered useful markers for the alteration of pathophysiologic factors, prognosis prediction or identification of risk factors of the disease. [17,18] For the metabolic surgeries, metabolomics studies have found that changes in serum aromatic or branched amino acid levels and gut microorganism-derived metabolites may contribute to the improvement of the glycemic control. [19] Still, these marker metabolites are yet to be tested in evaluating the outcomes of the metabolic surgery, and their mechanistic implications are not firmly established. At this point, it is desired to have metabolic markers relevant for the prognostication of the metabolic surgery, as the degree of diabetic improvement can vary significantly. As NMR-based metabolomics has been applied to developing new diagnostic techniques or to predicting the outcomes of drug treatment, [20,21] we applied it to discovering metabolites related to the different outcomes of metabolic surgery, to understanding the metabolic changes mechanistically related to diabetic improvement, and to providing an approach for the prognosis prediction of glycemic control after metabolic surgery.

Materials and Methods

Patients

We recruited 22 patients who were to undergo metabolic surgery for uncontrolled diabetes at the department of general surgery at Inha University Hospital, Incheon, Korea. All agreed with surgical treatment for weight loss or diabetic control, and the expected benefits and risks were explained thoroughly. Written informed consent was obtained from each study participant upon enrollment and prior to the start of the study. The study protocol conforms to the ethical guidelines of the 1975 Declaration of Helsinki, and was approved by the institutional review board at the Inha University Medical School and Hospital (2009-1473) and Seoul National University (1205/001-010). For patient criteria and surgical method, see Materials and Methods S1.

Sample preparation and NMR measurement

Whole blood was centrifuged at 2,000 g for 10 min at 4°C, and the plasma was collected and immediately stored at −80°C until the NMR experiment. Plasma samples were thawed at room temperature and 250 μL plasma was mixed with 250 μL of NMR buffer based on deuterium oxide (D2O). The final buffer concentration of the plasma sample contained 100 mM potassium phosphate (pH 7.0) and 1 mM 2,2-dimethyl-2-silapentane-5-sulfonate (DSS) as a chemical shift reference. [22] After the buffer mixing, the sample was centrifuged at 20,000 g for 5 min at 4°C, and 480 μL of the sample was transferred to a 5 mm NMR tube. Standard clinical laboratory tests were performed at Inha University hospital. 3-Hydroxybutyrate measurement was done separately using GC-MS after the metabolomics data analysis with the remaining plasma samples kept in a −80°C freezer.

The ^{1}H NMR spectra of the plasma samples were measured with a 500 MHz NMR spectrometer (Bruker Biospin, Avance 500) operating at a 500.13 MHz proton NMR frequency at 25°C using Carr-Purell-Meiboom-Gill (CPMG) pulse sequence (cpmgpr1d) with 400 μs of total spin echo delay (Korea Basic Science Institute, Ochang, Korea). The ^{1}H spectral FID was collected with 8K complex data points within 30 ppm spectral width during 128 number of scans. The spectra were processed with 0.3 Hz exponential line broadening and zero-filling followed by manual phase and baseline correction. All the spectra were referenced against the DSS signal. The metabolites were identified using Chenomx (Spectral database; Edmonton, Canada) and an in-house built metabolite library. The entire data set of the normalized spectra is given in Fig. S1.

Multivariate data analysis

All the obtained NMR spectra were Fourier transformed, phase corrected and baseline corrected manually and the resulting spectra were binned at 0.0147 ppm to reduce the signal complexity. After the spectral binning, the data were normalized against total integration values and 1 mmol/L DSS, and then converted into an ASCII text file. The binning, normalization and data conversion were done by an in-house Perl script. For multivariate statistical analysis, the water and EDTA regions were excluded. The converted text file was imported into SIMCA-P version 11.0 (Umetrics, Umeå, Sweden), OriginPro 8 (OriginLab Corporation, Northampton, USA) and R (The R Foundation for Statistical Computing, Vienna, Austria) for statistical analysis. The binned data were mean-centered with Pareto scaling, and orthogonal projections to latent structure-discriminant analysis (OPLS-DA) was performed with one predictive and two orthogonal components, as reported previously. [23] Prediction of improved and non-improved group was performed based on the NMR data obtained 7 days after surgery using both leave-one-out and leave-seven-out analyses. The partial least square (PLS) regression was performed to predict the HbA1c values based on the metabolic profile from the NMR data. The uses of each software are recapitulated as follows: Perl script: numeric data binning and normalization; SIMCA-P 11.0: data scaling, orthogonal projections to latent structure discriminant analysis (OPLS-DA), partial least square (PLS); OriginPro 8, R: regression modeling, correlation analysis and student's t-test.

Results

We summarized the basal characteristics and demographics in Table 1, and the changes of clinical parameters after metabolic surgery in Table 2. When we applied the HbA1c value of 7.0 as the cut-off value for the glucose control, [24] about half of the patients (n = 10) showed an improved glycemic control during the follow-up period (3 months), whereas the others (n = 12) did not. Therefore, we categorized the former group as the improved group, and the latter as the non-improved group. The decrease in BMI and AC after the surgery was significant in both groups, with the significance being larger in the non-improved group (P of $\sim 10^{-3}$ for the non-improved vs. 10^{-2} for the improved). Only the improved group showed normalized oral glucose tolerance test results at 3 months after surgery, even though both group had significant reduction in BMI and AC. Furthermore, one of the patients exhibited a large improvement in HbA1c value with essentially the same BMI at 3 months after surgery with basal BMI (HbA1c from 8.9% to 6% at 3 months; BMI from 23.5 to 23.2). In the other extreme, a patient with large BMI reduction (from 32.4 to 26.7 at 3 months) had a worsened HbA1c value at 3 months after surgery (from 7.7% to 8.7% at 3 months). Therefore, the different prognosis is unlikely dependent on the differential weight loss. Then, we postulated that the improvement might result from the early post-operative changes of individual "metabolic signature", since diabetes is essentially a metabolic disorder. There are several ways in describing the metabolic status of an individual, but serum metabolomics should be very relevant to this purpose with its comprehensive coverage of metabolites of whole body. Therefore we applied NMR-based metabolomics to these patients' plasma collected at seven days after surgery to see if we can correlate the midterm prognosis at 3 months with this earlier metabolic signature.

Fig. 1a and b show the NMR data from the two groups of patients which show apparently similar signal patterns. As the NMR data contain many signals coming from a large number of metabolites, we performed multivariate analysis to analyze the data more holistically. We chose OPLS-DA, as it can differentiate patient groups with adjustment of possible confounding variables (i.e. gender, pre-op OGTT and BMI etc.). The differentiation model was obtained with one orthogonal and two predictive components ($R^2 = 0.671$ and $Q^2 = 0.419$) (Fig. 1c). The analysis shows that the improved and non-improved groups could be separated based on the 7-day post-operative metabolite profiles. Therefore, it seemed that the patient's metabolic signatures at an earlier post-operative stage (7-days) may be correlated with the post-operative glycemic control in individual patients at 3 months after metabolic surgery.

To further explore this possibility and to get some quantitative relationship, we performed multivariate regression analysis. We built a PLS regression model using the NMR profile at 7-day time point, and the 3-month post-operative HbA1c values were predicted. Comparison of the predicted and observed HbA1c values, obtained with 2 PLS components, showed reasonably good correlation and predictability ($R = 0.758$, $R^2 = 0.574$, $P = 4.2\times10^{-5}$) (Fig. 2a). Next, we validated the prediction model by removing one sample at a time and predicting the HbA1c value of the removed sample with a prediction model built without the removed sample. This corresponds to a leave-one-out analysis and can give estimated prediction performance on blind samples. Fig. 2b shows that there is at least a modest correlation between the observed and predicted values for all the samples ($R = 0.517$, $R^2 = 0.26729$, $P = 9.6\times10^{-3}$). We also performed a 3 fold cross validation (leave-seven-out) which yielded comparable results ($R = 0.582$, $R^2 = 0.33859$, $P = 3.3\times10^{-3}$) (Fig. 2c). Notably, when we predicted the successful management of the blood glucose based on the predicted HbA1c values (a dichotomic decision: successful management of HbA1c≤7.0; unsuccessful management of HbA1c>7.0), the model correctly classified the management status in 17 out of 21 patients (81% correct) (Fig. 2c).

Then, we tried to identify the plasma metabolites at 7-day that contribute most to the difference between successful (improved group) vs. unsuccessful management (non-improved group) of glucose and to the prediction of HbA1c values at 3-month after surgery. To identify the metabolites, we built the S-plot from the OPLS-DA model and loading plot from the PLS-regression model (Fig. 3a and b). Both of these plot show that 3-HB is higher in the improved group, whereas glucose and lipids (LDL, VLDL) are higher in the non-improved group. As 3-HB is a ketone body that can be used as a fuel when glucose is limited, the two molecules are closely related. We tested if the ratio between 3-HB and glucose can be a useful clinical criterion for prognosis prediction of metabolic surgery. For this, we re-measured the 3-HB levels using

Table 1. Demographics and pre-operative baseline characteristics (N = 22).

Parameter	Total (N = 22)	Improved* (n = 10)	Non-Improved (n = 12)	P-value[6]
Age (years)	45.2±9.3	39.8±9.2	49.8±6.9	0.009
Sex				0.305#
Male (n (%))	9 (40.9)	3	6	
Female (n (%))	13 (59.1)	7	6	
Diabetes Duration (years)	7.4±4.5	5.1±4.1	9.4±3.9	0.019
Anti-hypertensive medication (n (%))	10 (45.5)	6	4	0.206#
BMI[1] (Kg/m²)	27.4±5.3	30.8±5.6	24.6±3.1	0.004
AC[2] (cm)	89.7±11.6	97.1±12.7	83.5±5.8	0.009
HbA1c[3] (%)	8.2±1.3	7.9±1.1	8.5±1.5	0.266
FBG[4] (mg/dl)	185.5±58.6	188.2±69.9	183.5±50.4	0.849
PP2[5] (mg/dl)	271.1±82.7	234.2±69.0	301.8±83.0	0.054
Operation (n (%))				0.0286#
Roux-en Y Gastric bypass	12 (54.5)	8 (80.0)	4 (33.3)	
Duodenojejunal bypass	10 (45.5)	2 (20.0)	8 (66.7)	

*Patients who had glycated hemoglobin percentage less than 7.0% without glucose-lowering agent at 3 months after metabolic operation.
[1]Body mass index; the individual's body mass divided by the square of his or her height.
[2]Abdominal circumference.
[3]Glycated hemoglobin percentage.
[4]Fasting blood glucose level.
[5]Blood glucose level in 2 hours after a meal.
[6]P-value for unpaired t-test or #chi-square test comparing improved group with non-improved group.

Table 2. Change of Anthropometric and Metabolic Parameters in improved and non-improved groups.

	Improved* Mean ± SD				Non-Improved Mean ± SD			
	Pre-OP (n = 10)	Post-OP 7 days (n = 10)	Post-OP 3 months (n = 9)	P-value[2]	Pre-OP (n = 12)	Post-OP 7 days (n = 12)	Post-OP 3 months (n = 10)	P-value
BMI (Kg/m^2)	30.8±5.6	n.a.[3]	27.2±3.0	0.024	24.6±3.1	n.a.	21.7±2.2	<0.001
AC (cm)	97.1±12.7	n.a.	92.4±12.3	0.018	83.5±5.8	n.a.	79.4±5.5	0.002
HbA1c	7.9±1.1	n.a.	5.86±0.38	0.002	8.5±1.5	n.a.	7.79±0.75	0.157
FBG (mg/dl)	188.2±69.9	110.1±29.2	106.1±12.4		183.5±50.4	137.0±22.8	148.2±27.8	
OGTT30[1] (mg/dl)	277.4±73.1	171.3±48.0	217.5±29.4		294.3±67.8	208.6±42.6	249.7±46.3	
OGTT60[1] (mg/dl)	326.9±77.3	228.8±49.8	226.7±49.3		371.5±100.8	254.1±54.8	292.2±59.7	
OGTT90[1](mg/dl)	336.4±83.2	244.8±47.2	164.6±60.3		424.0±82.6	274.8±60.6	277.1±88.1	
OGTT120[1] (mg/dl)	313.8±90.9	220.6±53.5	106.1±50.4		423.2±89.9	280.4±56.1	249.4±95.0	

*Patients who had glycated hemoglobin percentage less than 7.0% without glucose-lowering agent in 3 months after metabolic surgery.
[1]OGTT indicates oral glucose tolerance test at 30, 60, 90, or 120 min after 75 g glucose intake.
[2]paired t-test.
[3]Not available.

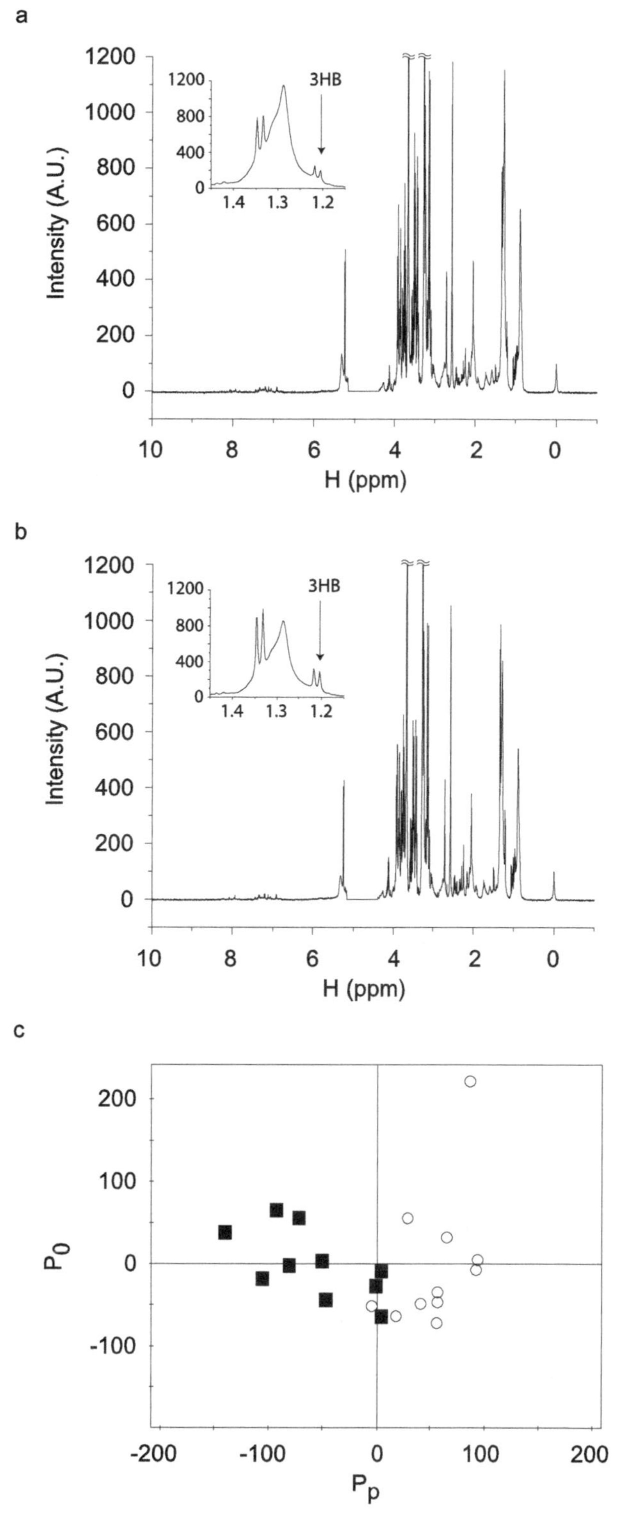

Figure 1. Representative ^{1}H NMR spectra of plasma samples and differentiation of improved and non-improved groups. The NMR spectra were taken for plasma samples at 500 MHz. The NMR sample contained final 100 mmol/L potassium phosphate (pH 7.0) and 1 mM DSS as a chemical shift reference. The insets show the 3-HB peak. ^{1}H NMR spectra of 7-day post-operative plasma samples from the improved group (a) and from the non-improved group (b). c. OPLS-DA scatter plot was obtained using one predictive and two orthogonal components with R^2 of 0.671 and Q^2 of 0.419. Pp and Po represent the

predictive component and the orthogonal component respectively. Black filled squares are for the improved group and red filled circles for the non-improved group.

GC-MS, as it is the standard method used in clinical laboratories. In comparison, NMR is yet to be generally used in clinics. The calculated [3-HB]/[glucose] ratio at 7 days were significantly different between the improved and non-improved groups ($P=4.2\times10^{-3}$) (Fig. 4a). The same ratio estimated with NMR data also gave similar trend (Fig. S2). Moreover, the ratio at 7 days showed at least a modest correlation with HbA1c level at 3 months ($R=-0.496$, $R^2=0.246$, $P=2.2\times10^{-2}$) (Fig. 4c). If we exclude those three distinctive outliers with exceptionally high 3-HB values (>1 mM; usual values of ~0.4 mM), the difference ($P=2.4\times10^{-5}$) (Fig. 4b) and the correlation would become much more robust ($R=-0.732$, $R^2=0.53599$, $P=3.3\times10^{-4}$) (Fig. 4d). These results suggest that the [3-HB]/[glucose] ratio may be a handy criterion for the prognostication after metabolic surgery, if proven in a larger study.

Encouraged by these results at 3 months, we applied the same procedure to the prediction of a longer term blood glucose control at 12 months post-operative time points. Unfortunately, the number of patients that were followed for 12 months was relatively small (n = 13), therefore, the statistical significance of PLS regression model is lower than that of 3 months. Nevertheless, we believe it is worth providing the results for future reference. Consistent with 3-month results, the PLS model showed a good correlation between predicted and observed HbA1c value at 12 months post-operative time ($R=0.846$, $R^2=0.71515$, $P=1.65\times10^{-4}$) (Fig. S3a), and the leave-one-out prediction test gave $R=0.572$, $R^2=0.32675$, and $P=2.4\times10^{-2}$ (Fig. S3b).

Discussion

Growing evidence has suggested that bariatric surgery is able to promote remission of T2DM, and to treat the morbid obesity as well. However, the glycemic control months after surgery within and across studies seems variable, and the indicators for the early decision of the improvement are not currently available. Here, we showed that the metabolic profiles in subjects with improved glycemic control could be differentiated from those without improvement as early as 7 days after metabolic surgery, and that the metabolic profile is correlated with HbA1c values at 3 months after surgery. Initial baseline (pre-operative) and post-operative results suggested that some general clinical parameters such as age, BMI, AC, and diabetes duration are also significantly different between the improved and non-improved groups (Table 1). Therefore, we performed correlation analysis with these possible confounding baseline characteristics against HbA1c level at 3 months. The resulting R values were 0.485 ($R^2=0.2348$), −0.623 ($R^2=0.3883$), 0.594 ($R^2=0.353$), and −0.548 ($R^2=0.3003$) for duration of diabetes, AC, age, and BMI, respectively (Fig. S4). The analysis also showed that the patients with less age, higher BMI, higher AC and lower diabetic duration are likely to have better prognosis. Compared to these, the correlation analysis using the metabolomic data to predict HbA1c level performed much better than these parameters ($R=0.758$, $R^2=0.574$; Fig. 2a). We believe our data warrant larger studies with more patients for longer follow-up period. If proven in these future studies, the blood metabolomic signature could be used to predict the long term diabetic prognosis with data obtained shortly after the metabolic surgery. As the metabolomic data represent the "individual metabolic signature" of a patient, the approach may be ultimately

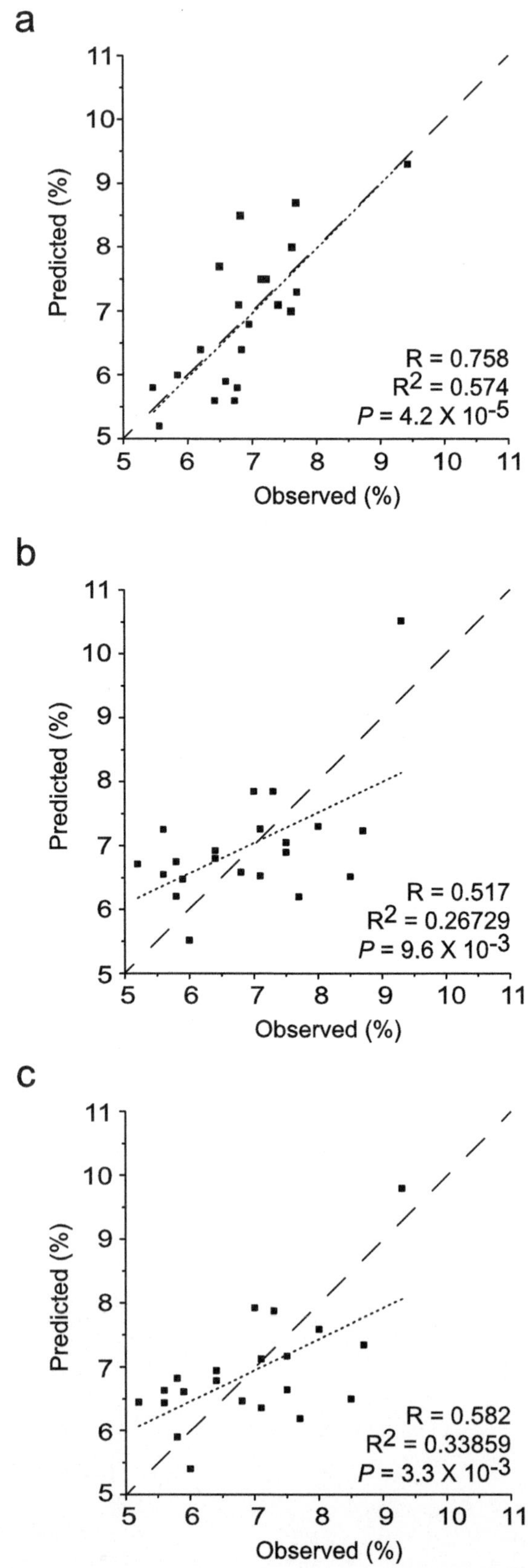

Figure 2. Prediction of HbA1c using PLS multivariate regression. PLS regression models were built with the NMR profile at 7-day time point and the 3-month post-operative HbA1c values. The observed

(X-axis) values are actually measured values and the predicted (Y-axis) values are from the PLS regression model obtained with two PLS components. The diagonal dashed line represents the theoretical perfect match, and the dotted line represents the least-square fitted line. Comparison between the observed and predicted values obtained from the training dataset (a), leave-one-out analysis (b), and three-fold cross validation (c). The predicted values in (a) do not represent true prediction since all the data were used in the model building. One (b) or seven (c) samples were left out at a time, and the predictions were made using the model built without the test data to be predicted until every sample was left out once.

applied to personalized diabetic management after metabolic surgery based on individual plasma molecular metabolic profiles.

Several studies provided evidence that improvement of T2DM is likely independent of the reduction of body weight by metabolic surgery. [25] Consistent with these, the significance of the post-operative BMI changes in the improved group is weaker than that in the non-improved group (Table 2). In addition, the mean ratio between the BMI change over 3 months by surgery and pre-operative basal BMI in the improved group (0.1169) was actually similar to the non-improved group (0.1179). To test the effects of BMI change in a more quantitative manner, we performed

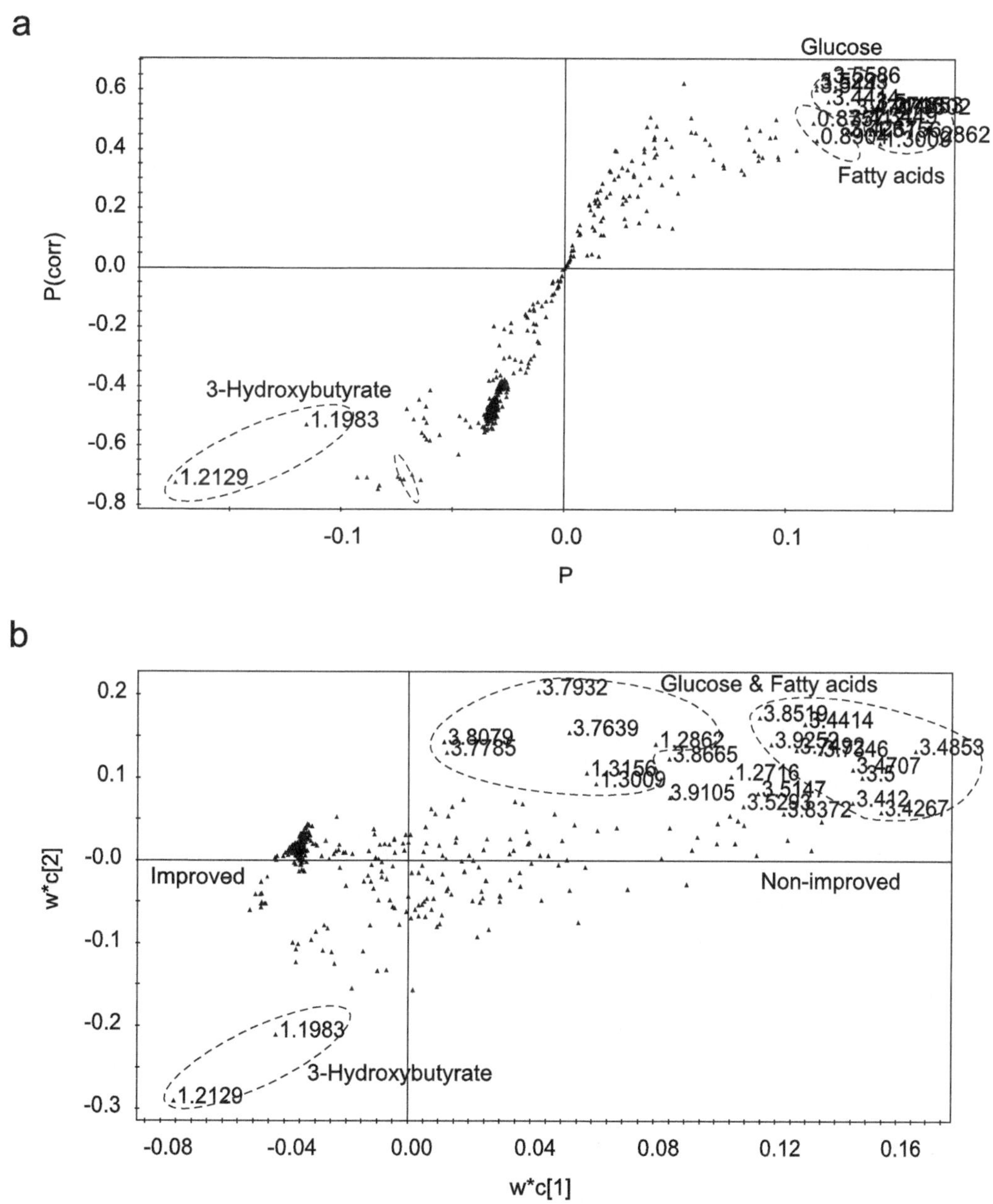

Figure 3. Metabolite marker signals contributing to the differentiation and prediction. a. S-plot analysis showing the correlation and covariation. Metabolites on the upper right corner contribute to the improved group and on the lower left corner contribute to the non-improved group. b. PLS loading plot showing the contribution to the prediction of the HbA1c. Metabolites signals were identified using Chenomx and in-house built metabolite libraries.

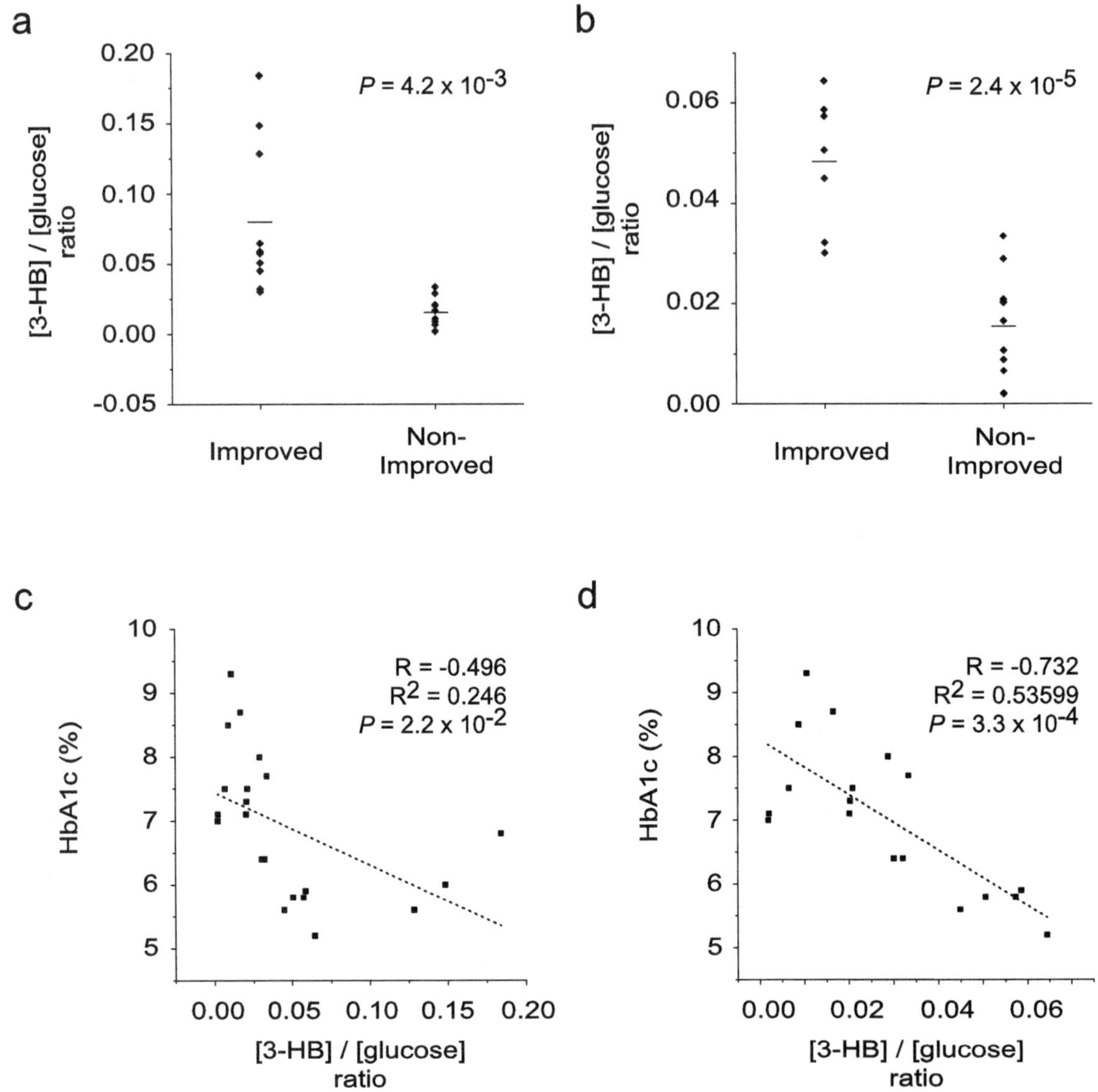

Figure 4. [3-HB]/[glucose] ratio as a criterion for the prognostication of metabolic surgery. 3-HB levels were measured using GC-MS, a standard approach in clinical laboratories. Both 3-HB and glucose levels were from the same plasma samples (7-day post-operative samples) from which the NMR data were obtained. The HbA1c values are from the 3-month post-operative samples. a. The comparison of [3-HB]/[glucose] ratio between the improved and non-improved groups with all the samples. b. The same analysis as (a) after removing the three distinctive outliers with exceptionally high 3-HB values (>1 mM; usual value of ~0.4 mM). c. Correlation analysis between HbA1c level and [3-HB]/[glucose] ratio with all the samples. d. The same analysis as (c) after removing the three distinctive outliers with exceptionally high 3-HB values (>1 mM; usual value of ~0.4 mM). The dotted line represents the least-square fitted line ((c) and (d)).

correlation analysis between the BMI changes and HbA1c at pre-operative, post-operative stages and their difference (Fig. S5). The R values from these analyses are all minimal (<0.2), indicating that post-op BMI changes may not have direct implication in diabetic improvement at least up to 3 months. These results are significant, since one of the key questions in this field is the involvement of BMI reduction in the diabetic improvement by metabolic surgery.

Another main finding of our study is that the most relevant metabolic features contributing to the correlation between the 7-day post-operative metabolic profile and 3-month HbA1c value are 3-HB and glucose concentrations. The patients with higher 3-HB and lower glucose concentrations at 7 days after surgery showed better glycemic control later (3 months). While lower glucose concentration may be easily accepted for its correlation with lower HbA1c value, 3-HB may deserve more discussion. 3-HB is a ketone body formed from acetyl CoA during fasting conditions for use in brain or other tissues as fuel. High levels of 3-HB can be present in diabetic ketoacidosis found usually in Type 1 DM or stress conditions after surgery. [26] It should be stressed that the increase in 3-HB in the improved group in our study is not simply due to the surgical stress or fasting, as the increase is relative to the non-improved group and both groups underwent surgery. Significant increases in 3-HB after bariatric surgery as compared to the pre-operative values have been also reported, but the 3-HB level was not implicated in the difference in the diabetic improvement months after the surgery. [25] As 3-HB is a marker of fatty acid oxidation, it is possible that the abrupt change of energy metabolism in T2DM patients by metabolic surgery may acutely reverse the insulin-resistant status. In fact, 3-HB is formed primarily when the energy source for the peripheral organs are shifted to lipid from glucose and, therefore, the early stage metabolic shifts by metabolic surgery may be a key factor for the success of the longer term post-operative glucose control. More mechanistically relevant for the current study are the reports on the direct effects of 3-HB on the insulin sensitivity shown in animal models. [27,28] Using partial pancreatectomized (Px) rats, a good model for non-obese T2DM, [29] Park et. al., showed that intraperitonial injection of 3-HB into the diabetic rats leads to decreased hepatic glucose output compared to the diabetic controls using hyperinsulinemic euglycemic clamp setting. [27] This improved glucose hometostasis by 3-HB was suggested to be due to the enhanced hepatic insulin signaling, as evidenced by the increased phosphorylation of IRS2 and AKT. In another study, [28] it was shown that intracranial injection of 3-HB into Px diabetic rats also leads to decreased hepatic glucose production and enhanced glucose tolerance through increased hepatic insulin signaling and decreased phosphoenolpyruvate carboxykinase (PEPCK) level, the rate-limiting enzyme for gluconeogenesis. These improved glycemic control by 3-HB was attributed to enhanced leptin and insulin signaling in the hypothalamus rather than increased insulin secretion. Therefore, higher levels of 3-HB at the early days after the bariatric surgery in the improved group in our study might have induced similar enhancement in insulin signaling leading to better glycemic control. With a recent report suggesting that early high levels of 3-HB after metabolic surgery return to normal levels after several months, [30] it seems that 3-HB values before, not after, significant weight loss might be mechanistically related to the diabetic improvement. With this mechanistic relevance and our data showing the correlation with the prognosis at 3 months, the [3-HB]/[glucose] ratio might be a useful prognostic marker for future glycemic control, if our results are reproduced in larger studies. These markers could help clinicians with deciding if early drug therapies are necessary shortly after metabolic surgery for individual patients, ultimately contributing to personalized treatment.

As with any other clinical studies, several limitations of our study should be noted. First, the number of subjects is relatively small, particularly for the subjects followed for 12 months. Therefore, our results could be stepping stones for future larger studies for confirming the clinical applicability. Second, the follow-up period (up to 12 months) was not enough to conclude the long-term (> years) effects of metabolic surgery on glycemic control in T2DM patients. Third, we measured the post-operative, not pre-operative, metabolic profiles to observe the correlation between metabolomics data and diabetic control. Therefore, to determine the baseline characteristics of metabolites affecting the post-operative prognosis, further study will be needed. Finally, we applied different surgical procedures according to clinical decision. However, the focus of this study was not the effects of different surgical procedure, but the discovery of metabolites related to the post-operative glycemic control. Therefore, future studies individually designed for different surgical procedures will be necessary to see the effects of the surgical procedure. Still, it should be noted that our prognosis prediction was obtained irrespective of the surgical procedures, and turned out to be significant.

In conclusion, the NMR-based metabolomics data obtained at 7 days after metabolic surgery could be correlated with the post-operative diabetic improvement according to the HbA1c level at post-op 3-months. The metabolomics data analysis showed that the higher level of [3-HB]/[glucose] ratio at 7 days after surgery can differentiate the patients with or without glycemic control at 3 months after surgery. These results provide evidence for the potential value of NMR-based metabolomics data to assess the heterogeneous results of metabolic surgery in T2DM, and suggest that 3-HB level may be related to the mechanism of the diabetic improvement effect of metabolic surgery. Our study warrants further studies with larger number of subjects followed for the longer term to confirm the mechanisms and/or clinical utility of the biomarkers.

Supporting Information

Figure S1 The entire normalized data set is presented as stacked spectra. The black data set represents the improved group and the red data set represents the non-improved group.

Figure S2 [3-HB]/[glucose] ratios of the improved and non-improved groups based on NMR spectral integration. The error bars represent the standard deviation.

Figure S3 Prediction of HbA1c using PLS multivariate regression: 12-month data. PLS regression models were built with the NMR profile at 7-day time point and the 12-month post-operative HbA1c values. The observed (X-axis) values are actually measured values and the predicted (Y-axis) values are from the PLS regression model obtained with two PLS components. The diagonal dashed line represents the theoretical perfect match, and the red dotted line represents the least-square fitted line (b). Comparison between the observed and predicted values obtained from the training dataset (a), leave-one-out analysis (b). The predicted values in (a) do not represent true prediction since all the data were used in the model building. One (b) sample was left out at a time, and the predictions were made using the model built without the test data to be predicted until every sample was left out once.

Figure S4 Correlation analysis between 3-month post-operative HbA1c values and possible confounding baseline characteristics. The dotted line was obtained with linear least square method. The correlation with HbA1c and duration of diabetes(a), AC(b), Age(c), and BMI(d) are presented.

Figure S5 Correlation. Correlation analysis between BMI changes and HbA1c at various times. HbA1c initial is for the pre-operative value (a), HbA1c 3-month for the 3-month value (b), and dHbA1c for the difference between the two (c). The dotted line was obtained with linear least square method. ΔBMI is for the BMI changes at the 3-month post-operative time point as compared to the pre-operative values.

Materials and Methods S1 Patients criteria and Surgical procedures.

Author Contributions

Conceived and designed the experiments: YJL JHC SP. Performed the experiments: HNK YJL JHC YJA SK DHL. Analyzed the data: HNK YJL YJA SK DHL. Contributed reagents/materials/analysis tools: HNK YJL

JHC YJA SK DHL YJS. Contributed to the writing of the manuscript: YJL JHK SP YH.

References

1. Federation ID (2011) IDF Diabetes Atlas. 5th ed. Brussels, Belgium: International Diabetes Federation.
2. Mokdad AH, Ford ES, Bowman BA, Dietz WH, Vinicor F, et al. (2003) Prevalence of Obesity, Diabetes, and Obesity-Related Health Risk Factors, 2001. JAMA: The Journal of the American Medical Association 289: 76–79.
3. Hu FB, Manson JAE, Stampfer MJ, Colditz G, Liu S, et al. (2001) Diet, lifestyle, and the risk of type 2 diabetes mellitus in women. New England Journal of Medicine 345: 790–797.
4. Yoon KH, Lee JH, Kim JW, Cho JH, Choi YH, et al. (2006) Epidemic obesity and type 2 diabetes in Asia. The Lancet 368: 1681–1688.
5. Nathan DM, Buse JB, Davidson MB, Ferrannini E, Holman RR, et al. (2009) Medical Management of Hyperglycemia in Type 2 Diabetes: A Consensus Algorithm for the Initiation and Adjustment of Therapy. Diabetes Care 32: 193–203.
6. Pirsch JD, Andrews C, Hricik DE, Josephson MA, Leichtman AB, et al. (1996) Pancreas Transplantation for Diabetes Mellitus. American Journal of Kidney Diseases 27: 444–450.
7. Mingrone G, Panunzi S, De Gaetano A, Guidone C, Iaconelli A, et al. (2012) Bariatric Surgery versus Conventional Medical Therapy for Type 2 Diabetes. N Engl J Med.
8. Pories WJ, Swanson MS, MacDonald KG, Long SB, Morris PG, et al. (1995) Who would have thought it? An operation proves to be the most effective therapy for adult-onset diabetes mellitus. Ann Surg 222: 339–350; discussion 350–332.
9. Buchwald H, Avidor Y, Braunwald E, Jensen MD, Pories W, et al. (2004) Bariatric surgery: a systematic review and meta-analysis. JAMA 292: 1724–1737.
10. Buchwald H, Varco, Richard Lynn (1978) Metabolic Surgery. New York: Grune & Stratton. 317 p.
11. de Moura EG, Orso IR, Martins Bda C, Lopes GS, de Oliveira SL, et al. (2011) Improvement of insulin resistance and reduction of cardiovascular risk among obese patients with type 2 diabetes with the duodenojejunal bypass liner. Obes Surg 21: 941–947.
12. DePaula AL, Macedo AL, Rassi N, Vencio S, Machado CA, et al. (2008) Laparoscopic treatment of metabolic syndrome in patients with type 2 diabetes mellitus. Surg Endosc 22: 2670–2678.
13. Buchwald H, Estok R, Fahrbach K, Banel D, Jensen MD, et al. (2009) Weight and type 2 diabetes after bariatric surgery: systematic review and meta-analysis. Am J Med 122: 248–256 e245.
14. Schauer PR, Kashyap SR, Wolski K, Brethauer SA, Kirwan JP, et al. (2012) Bariatric Surgery versus Intensive Medical Therapy in Obese Patients with Diabetes. N Engl J Med.
15. Halverson JD, Kramer J, Cave A, Permutt A, Santiago J (1982) Altered glucose tolerance, insulin response, and insulin sensitivity after massive weight reduction subsequent to gastric bypass. Surgery 92: 235–240.
16. Geloneze B, Geloneze SR, Chaim E, Hirsch FF, Felici AC, et al. (2012) Metabolic surgery for non-obese type 2 diabetes: incretins, adipocytokines, and insulin secretion/resistance changes in a 1-year interventional clinical controlled study. Ann Surg 256: 72–78.
17. Wang TJ, Larson MG, Vasan RS, Cheng S, Rhee EP, et al. (2011) Metabolite profiles and the risk of developing diabetes. Nat Med 17: 448–453.
18. Floegel A, Stefan N, Yu Z, Muhlenbruch K, Drogan D, et al. (2013) Identification of serum metabolites associated with risk of type 2 diabetes using a targeted metabolomic approach. Diabetes 62: 639–648.
19. Li JV, Ashrafian H, Bueter M, Kinross J, Sands C, et al. (2011) Metabolic surgery profoundly influences gut microbial-host metabolic cross-talk. Gut 60: 1214–1223.
20. Brindle JT, Antti H, Holmes E, Tranter G, Nicholson JK, et al. (2002) Rapid and noninvasive diagnosis of the presence and severity of coronary heart disease using 1H-NMR-based metabonomics. Nat Med 8: 1439–1444.
21. Clayton TA, Baker D, Lindon JC, Everett JR, Nicholson JK (2009) Pharmacometabonomic identification of a significant host-microbiome metabolic interaction affecting human drug metabolism. Proc Natl Acad Sci USA 106: 14728–14733.
22. Chikayama E, Sekiyama Y, Okamoto M, Nakanishi Y, Tsuboi Y, et al. (2010) Statistical indices for simultaneous large-scale metabolite detections for a single NMR spectrum. Anal Chem 82: 1653–1658.
23. Kang J, Choi MY, Kang S, Kwon HN, Wen H, et al. (2008) Application of a ^{1}H nuclear magnetic resonance (NMR) metabolomics approach combined with orthogonal projections to latent structure-discriminant analysis as an efficient tool for discriminating between Korean and Chinese herbal medicines. J Agric Food Chem 56: 11589–11595.
24. (2009) Executive summary: standards of medical care in diabetes–2009. Diabetes Care 32 Suppl 1: S6–12.
25. Laferrere B, Reilly D, Arias S, Swerdlow N, Gorroochurn P, et al. (2011) Differential metabolic impact of gastric bypass surgery versus dietary intervention in obese diabetic subjects despite identical weight loss. Sci Transl Med 3: 80–82.
26. Umpierrez GE, Kitabchi AE (2003) Diabetic ketoacidosis: risk factors and management strategies. Treat Endocrinol 2: 95–108.
27. Park S, Kim da S, Kang S, Daily JW, 3rd (2011) A ketogenic diet impairs energy and glucose homeostasis by the attenuation of hypothalamic leptin signaling and hepatic insulin signaling in a rat model of non-obese type 2 diabetes. Exp Biol Med (Maywood) 236: 194–204.
28. Park S, Kim da S, Daily JW (2011) Central infusion of ketone bodies modulates body weight and hepatic insulin sensitivity by modifying hypothalamic leptin and insulin signaling pathways in type 2 diabetic rats. Brain Research 1401: 95–103.
29. Hosokawa YA, Hosokawa H, Chen C, Leahy JL (1996) Mechanism of impaired glucose-potentiated insulin secretion in diabetic 90% pancreatectomy rats. Study using glucagonlike peptide-1 (7–37). J Clin Invest 97: 180–186.
30. Aberle J, Reining F, Dannheim V, Flitsch J, Klinge A, et al. (2012) Metformin after bariatric surgery–an acid problem. Experimental and Clinical Endocrinology and Diabetes 120: 152–153.

The Urinary Cytokine/Chemokine Signature of Renal Hyperfiltration in Adolescents with Type 1 Diabetes

Ron L. H. Har[1¶], Heather N. Reich[2¶], James W. Scholey[2¶], Denis Daneman[3], David B. Dunger[4], Rahim Moineddin[5], R. Neil Dalton[6], Laura Motran[3], Yesmino Elia[3], Livia Deda[3], Masha Ostrovsky[3], Etienne B. Sochett[3‡], Farid H. Mahmud[3‡], David Z. I. Cherney[1*‡]

1 Division of Nephrology, University Health Network - Toronto General Hospital, Banting and Best Diabetes Centre, University of Toronto, Toronto, Ontario, Canada, **2** Division of Nephrology, University Health Network - Toronto General Hospital, Toronto, Ontario, Canada, **3** Department of Pediatrics, Division of Endocrinology, Hospital for Sick Children, University of Toronto, Toronto, Ontario, Canada, **4** Department of Pediatrics, University of Cambridge, Cambridge, United Kingdom, **5** Family and Community Medicine, University of Toronto Toronto, Ontario, Canada, **6** WellChild Laboratory, Evelina Children's Hospital, St Thomas' Hospital, London, United Kingdom

Abstract

Objective: Urinary cytokine/chemokine levels are elevated in adults with type 1 diabetes (T1D) exhibiting renal hyperfiltration. Whether this observation extends to adolescents with T1D remains unknown. Our first objective was to determine the relationship between hyperfiltration and urinary cytokines/chemokines in normotensive, normoalbuminuric adolescents with T1D using $GFR_{cystatin}$. Our second aim was to determine the relationship between urine and plasma levels of inflammatory biomarkers, to clarify the origin of these factors.

Methods: Urine and serum cytokines/chemokines (Luminex platform) and $GFR_{cystatin}$ were measured in normofiltering ($n = 111$, T1D-N, $GFR < 135$ ml/min/1.73 m^2) and hyperfiltering ($n = 31$, T1D-H, $GFR \geq 135$ ml/min/1.73 m^2) adolescents with T1D (ages 10–16), and in age and sex matched healthy control subjects (HC, $n = 59$).

Results: We noted significant step-wise increases in urinary cytokine/chemokine excretion according to filtration status with highest levels in T1D-H, with parallel trends in serum analyte concentrations. After adjusting for serum glucose at the time of sampling, differences in urinary cytokine excretion were not statistically significant. Only serum IL-2 significantly differed between HC and T1D ($p = 0.0076$).

Conclusions: Hyperfiltration is associated with increased urinary cytokine/chemokine excretion in T1D adolescents, and parallel trends in serum cytokine concentration. The GFR-associated trends in cytokine excretion may be driven by the effects of ambient hyperglycemia. The relationship between hyperfiltration, glycemia, and variations in serum and urine cytokine expression and their impact on future renal and systemic vascular complications requires further study.

Editor: Juliet Spencer, University of San Francisco, United States of America

Funding: This work was supported by operating grants from the Juvenile Diabetes Research Foundation, Juvenile Diabetes Research Foundation - Canadian Clinical Trials Network (JDRF-CCTN), the Heart and Stroke Foundation of Canada and the Canadian Diabetes Association. RLH is supported by a Banting and Best Studentship and the Hilda and William Courtney Clayton Pediatric Research Fund. DZIC was also supported by a Kidney Foundation of Canada Scholarship and a Canadian Diabetes Association-KRESCENT Program Joint New Investigator Award and receives operating support from the Heart and Stroke Foundation of Canada and the Canadian Institutes of Health Research. The funders had no role in study design, data collection and analysis, decision to publish, or preparation of the manuscript.

Competing Interests: The authors have declared that no competing interests exist.

* Email: david.cherney@uhn.on.ca

¶ These authors are co-primary authors on this work.

‡ These authors are co-senior authors on this work.

Introduction

Diabetes mellitus is the most common cause of end-stage renal failure requiring renal placement therapy in the developed world. Unfortunately, despite the use of renin angiotensin aldosterone system (RAAS) blockers and intensive glycemic control, a significant proportion of patients continue to develop diabetic nephropathy. Furthermore, in type 1 diabetes (T1D), RAAS inhibition-based primary prevention of diabetic nephropathy, defined by changes on renal biopsy, has been unsuccessful [1]. The failure of current therapies may in part be due to a clinical inability to distinguish high-risk patients from those who may never develop complications. It is therefore critical to identify the role of additional factors that contribute to the initiation and progression of diabetic nephropathy to guide more targeted treatment strategies.

Hyperglycemia is necessary for the development of diabetic nephropathy in experimental models and in humans [2,3,4]. In young adult patients with T1D, acute clamped hyperglycemia increases the urinary excretion of pro-inflammatory and pro-fibrotic factors implicated in the pathogenesis of diabetic nephropathy, including eotaxin, fibroblast growth factor-2, granulocyte-monocyte colony stimulating factor (GM-CSF), interferon-α2, interleukin (IL)-12, IL-2, monocyte chemoattractant protein-3 (MCP-3), MCP-1, macrophage-derived chemokine (MDC), macrophage inflammatory proteins-1α (MIP-1α), platelet derived growth factor-BB (PDGF-AB/BB), tumour necrosis factor-β and sCD40 Ligand (sCD40L) [5]. We have further shown that renal hyperfiltration is associated with higher levels of urinary cytokines/chemokines compared with T1D patients with normal GFR values (T1D-N) and healthy controls (HC) [6]. Moreover, the increase in urinary cytokine/chemokine excretion induced by hyperglycemia is blunted by RAAS inhibition, and this effect is exaggerated in patients with T1D and renal hyperfiltration (T1D-H) [7]. However, GFR in this previous work was measured directly by inulin clearances under clamped glycemic conditions, and these techniques can only be used in controlled research laboratory setting. It is not known if renal hyperfiltration, defined with clinically applicable cystatin C-based methods, is also associated with increased urinary cytokine/chemokine excretion in an ambulatory setting [8].

The identification of urinary biomarkers of preclinical kidney disease that could be used clinically to distinguish adolescents with T1D at increased risk of developing renal disease is an important research goal for clinicians who take care of similar patients in the pediatric setting and as these patients transition to adult care [9]. Accordingly, our aim was to determine the relationship between GFR and urinary cytokines/chemokines in normotensive, normoalbuminuric adolescents with T1D and normal renal function. We hypothesized that in an adolescent cohort, urinary cytokines/chemokines would be elevated in patients with T1D-H compared to both T1D-N and a similar group of age and sex matched healthy control participants.

Research Design and Methods

Study Population and Ethnics Statement

Patients were recruited from the longitudinal, observational, non-interventional arm of the Adolescent Type 1 Diabetes Cardio-Renal Intervention Trial (AdDIT), from clinical sites in the Greater Toronto Area. In brief, the Non-Randomized Low-Risk arm of AdDIT is a 4-year observational/natural history study, following adolescents at low and middle risk of developing microalbuminuria (EudraCT Number: 2007-001039-72). High-risk adolescents are recruited into the AdDIT Interventional Study (http://www.clinicaltrials.gov/ct2/show/NCT01581476), which was designed to examine the effect of angiotensin converting enzyme inhibitors and statins on renal, retinal and cardiovascular endpoints. Our study did not include participants involved in the intervention trial, however, as an ancillary component of Non-Randomized Low-Risk arm of AdDIT we also included high-risk subjects who chose not to enter the AdDIT Intervention Study. All analyses in this manuscript were performed using biological specimens and data collected from subjects enrolled in the observational and ancillary arm of AdDIT, specifically baseline data from the study obtained at Greater Toronto Area sites.

T1D patients were recruited from endocrinology clinics at The Hospital for Sick Children, Credit Valley Hospital and Markham-Stouffville in the Greater Toronto Area (Ontario, Canada), while healthy controls were recruited through local advertisements. The Hospital for Sick Children was the primary site of recruitment and also coordinated recruitment at the secondary sites (REB#: 1000012240). The Hospital for Sick Children Research Ethics Board, Credit Valley Hospital Ethics Forum and Markham-Stouffville Research Ethics Board approved the protocol and the consent procedure. In accordance to the Declaration of Helsinki, written consent and informed consent was obtained from the legal guardian/next of kin/caretakers of minors aged 15 and younger, while the minors provided assent. All subjects, aged 16 and older with capacity to understand the study information, gave complete written and informed consent to participate in the study.

Normotensive, normoalbuminuric participants with T1D were recruited. T1D patients were analyzed based on whether GFR was in the normal range (n = 111, GFR 90–134 ml/min/1.73 m^2) or hyperfiltration range (n = 31, GFR≥135 ml/min/1.73 m^2) according to Larsson method, as we have previously published [8,10]. Fifty-nine healthy controls with normal renal function were also included for comparison.

Inclusion criteria for T1D patients were: age 10–16, duration of type 1 diabetes ≥1 year, no history of hypertension, proteinuria, renal disease or macrovascular disease. Two sets of 3 early morning urines were obtained and microalbuminuria was defined as an ACR>3.5 mg/mmol/l in males and >4.0 mg/mmol/l in females in 2 out of the 3 consecutive early morning urines [11]. In addition to those delineated in the AdDIT observational protocol, other exclusion criteria included chronic inflammatory disease, anti-inflammatory or corticosteroid medicines or medications that interfere with the renin angiotensin aldosterone system (RAAS) [12].

Sample Collection and Analytical Methods

Participants were asked to provide a first morning urine sample. This 50 ml mid-stream sterile urine specimen was used to measure levels of cytokines/chemokines using an established Cytokine/Chemokine Panel Luminex Assay urine creatinine concentration [5,9]. Immediately after collection, urine was centrifuged at 1500 g for 15 minutes to remove cells, then separated into 1 ml aliquots and frozen at −80°C. Urine was then thawed at 4°C one day prior to use. Due to the urine specimen handling protocol designed to avoid protein degradation, this analysis included spot urines and not the timed collections. Furthermore, *a priori* we only included selected analytes that either increase in response to hyperglycemia or renal hyperfiltration in our previous work in young adults [5,6]. Our analysis therefore included eotaxin, FGF-2, GM-CSF, IFNα2, IL-2, IL-12, MCP-3, MCP-1, MDC, MIP-1α, TNFβ, sCD40L, PDGF-AB/BB. We limited our analysis to these factors to maintain statistical power, to minimize false positive results, and to further elucidate mechanisms that may link high intraglomerular pressure with factors that promote initiation of renal disease. The accuracy and precision of the urinary cytokine/chemokine assay is available through the vendor at http://www.millipore.com/userguides/tech1/proto_mpxhcyto-60k. The detection limits of our assays have also been published previously [9]. The investigator performing data analysis was blinded to all study parameters.

Serum cystatin C was measured by a single operator using thawed samples by an immunoassay (Dade Behring Diagnostics, Newark, DE, USA) conducted on a BN Prospec System nephelometer. The between-assay coefficient of variation in samples from the lowest and highest quartiles of the cystatin C distribution was 6.2 and 0.9%, respectively. Cystatin C based GFR was derived using the body-surface area corrected Larsson formula, as described previously, which has superior operating characterstics compared with creatinine-based measurements in the hyperfiltration range using GFR_{INULIN} [10,13].

Urinary albumin to creatinine ratio was determined from a spot urine collection by immunoturbidimetry. Hemoglobin A1C (HbA1c) was measured by high-performance liquid chromatography [14].

Statistical analysis

All analyses in the manuscript were based on specimens and data collected at the baseline visit. Descriptive statistics were used to describe the sample. The baseline clinical and demographic characteristics were compared using appropriate test statistics. Between-group differences were determined by ANOVA, adjusted for multiple comparisons using Bonferroni's correction. The statistical package SAS 9.3 (SAS Institute, Cary, NC, USA) was used to analyze the data. Our sample size calculation was based on differences in urinary MCP-1 excretion due to the consistent relationship between this cytokine and renal disease. [5,6,15] Our previous data have shown that the SD for MCP-1 is 17 units [5,6,15]. To have an 80% power to detect a significant 25 unit between-group difference in MCP-1, for a two- sided test with $p = 0.01$, the sample size should be ≥ 16 per group. Participants with diabetes were analyzed on the basis of filtration status determined using cystatin C as described previously [8,10]. Filtration status was determined at the end of the study once cystatin C and creatinine assays were complete for the entire cohort. In the first analysis, *between-group* comparisons were adjusted for age, gender, ACR and HbA1c. In the second analysis, blood glucose at the time of the urine sample collection was included rather than HbA1c, since our previous work has demonstrated that acute, ambient glycemia increases urinary cytokine/chemokine excretion [5,7]. Additional statistical corrections for height and weight were not made because these parameters are already accounted for in eGFR equations. Serum levels of cytokines/chemokines were similarly analyzed using both dichotomous and continuous methods, except that ACR was not included.

Results

Baseline characteristics

For baseline demographic and biochemical parameters, the T1D-N had a higher proportion of males (56%) compared to HC (44%) and T1D-H (40%), and significant differences in age, weight and height were present (Table 1). The three groups had a heterogeneous composition of ethnicities. As expected, SBP tended to be higher in T1D groups compared to HC [16] and ACR within the normal range was higher in the T1D groups vs. HC, but the same in T1-N vs. T1D-H. For T1D-N and T1D-H, HbA1c and diabetes duration values were similar.

The effect of renal filtration status on urinary cytokine/chemokine excretion

After adjusting for baseline clinical characteristics including HbA1c and ACR, the first pattern observed was a step-wise increase from HC to T1D-N to T1D-H for urinary IL-12 (Figure 1, panel a, ANOVA $p = 0.0005$). Pair-wise comparisons were also significant except for HC vs. T1D-N ($p = 0.0518$). For IFNα2 (Figure 1, panel b, ANOVA $p = 0.0019$), pair-wise differences between HC vs. T1D-H and T1D-N vs. T1D-H were significant, while differences in HC vs. T1D-N were not. Finally, levels of IL-2 (ANOVA $p = 0.0002$), sCD40L (ANOVA $p = 0.001$), FGF-2 (ANOVA $p = 0.0038$) (Figure 1, panels c–e), generally increased from HC to T1D-N to T1D-H, but only pairwise differences for HC vs. T1D-N and HC vs. T1D-H reached significance. For TNF-β (ANOVA $p = 0.0097$) and MIP-1α (ANOVA $p = 0.0174$) (Figure 1, panel f–g), only HC and T1D-H group differences were significant. Similar trends for MDC, MCP-3 and GM-CSF did not reach significance. When ethnicity was added as a covariable to the regression model, *between-group* differences in urinary cytokine/chemokine excretion persisted.

After adjusting for the same baseline clinical characteristics including plasma glucose rather than HbA1c in a regression analysis, *between-group* differences for IL-12 and IFNα2 were no longer significant.

Correlation between urinary cytokines/chemokines and renal function, adjusted for age, gender, ACR and hemoglobin A1c

For HC, only PDGF-AB/BB ($\beta = 0.0433$, $p = 0.0019$) correlated with $GFR_{cystatin\ C}$. In the T1D group, $GFR_{cystatin\ C}$ correlated with MCP-1 ($\beta = 0.3189$, $p = 0.0162$) and PDGF-AB/BB ($\beta = 0.0231$, $p = 0.0331$).

Serum levels of cytokines/chemokines in HC and T1D Groups

For serum markers, *between-group* differences for IL-2 in HC vs. T1D-N and T1D-H reached significance (Figure 2), and the addition of ethnicity to the model had no effect. In the continuous analysis comparing serum analyte levels with GFR in the HC group, serum MIP-1α ($\beta = -0.2752$, $p = 0.0384$), MDC ($\beta = -12.702$, $p = 0.0061$), IL-12 ($\beta = -2.1089$, $p = 0.0237$) correlated with $GFR_{cystatin\ C}$. In the T1D cohort, correlations were also observed between serum IL-12 ($\beta = 4.0269$, $p = 0.0029$), IFNα2 ($\beta = 15.8123$, $p = 0.0015$), FGF-2 ($\beta = 2.1275$, $p = 0.0032$), TNF-β ($\beta = 21.7215$, $p = 0.0028$), MDC ($\beta = 20.3889$, $p = 0.0018$), GM-CSF ($\beta = 1.1626$, $p = 0.0029$), PDGF-AB/BB ($\beta = 20.0651$, $p = 0.0232$) and $GFR_{cystatin\ C}$.

Correlation between urine and serum levels of cytokines/chemokines in HC and T1D participants

In HC, none of the urine cytokines/chemokines correlated with corresponding cytokines/chemokines in serum. In the T1D group, correlations between urinary and plasma levels of eotaxin ($r = 0.20$, $p = 0.02$), sCD40L ($r = 0.22$, $p = 0.009$) and GM-CSF ($r = 0.23$, $p = 0.0062$) reached statistical significance.

Discussion

Albuminuria is an early clinical marker of diabetic nephropathy. Unfortunately, albuminuria is limited as a predictive biomarker because many patients exhibit stable levels of albuminuria and never develop impaired renal function, and spontaneous regression of albuminuria is also common [17]. Furthermore, progressive early GFR decline without albuminuria is common [18] and may reflect underlying vascular disease and tubulointerstitial inflammation rather than traditional diabetic glomerulosclerosis [19,20]. The identification of sensitive and specific early biomarkers to predict the development of nephropathy prior to the onset of albuminuria, such as urinary cytokines/chemokines, is therefore of the utmost importance.

Urinary cytokine/chemokine excretion is associated with factors that promote diabetic nephropathy, such as hyperglycemia, as well as hyperfiltration, a surrogate marker for high intraglomerular pressure leading to glomerulosclerosis [5,6]. Despite these promising pathophysiological rationale for the use of cytokines/chemokines as markers of early renal disease, the role of these

Table 1. Clinical Characteristics and Biochemistry in Healthy Controls and in Patients with Type 1 Diabetes Mellitus with Normofiltration or Hyperfiltration According to GFRcystatin C (mean ± SD).

	Healthy Controls(n = 59)	Normofiltration diabetic group (n = 111)	Hyperfiltration diabetic group (n = 31)	p-value
Clinical characteristics:				
Male/female	26/33	63/48	9/22	0.017
Ethnicity – n (%)				
White (Causcasian)	31 (52.5)	73 (65.8)	10 (32.3)	0.0005
Black (African, Caribbean)	3 (5.1)	7 (6.3)	4 (12.9)	0.395
South Asian	6 (10.2)	9 (8.1)	3 (9.7)	0.279
South East Asian	12 (20.3)	6 (5.4)	4 (12.9)	0.247
Aboriginal	0	0	0	-
Other	7 (11.9)	16 (14.1)	10 (32.2)	0.240
Age (years)	13.9±2.0	14.5±1.6	15.0±1.6	0.024
Diabetes duration (years)	N/A	7.4±3.1	7.3±3.3	0.890
Weight (kg)	54.2±13.0	62.2±14.1	60.4±16.13	0.017
Height (cm)	162±12	165±10	160±10	0.0008
Systolic blood pressure (mmHg)	111±10	116±11	114±7	0.683
Diastolic blood pressure (mmHg)	68±7	67±7	70±7	0.359
Pulse (beats per minute)	49±6.5	52±9	49±8	0.109
Biochemistry:				
Blood glucose (mmol/L)	4.7±0.7	9.3±4.5	11.5±3.4	<0.0001
HbA1c (%)	5.4±0.3	8.4±1.2	8.5±1.1	<0.0001
HbA1c (mmol/mol)	31±0.06	75±0.15	75±0.15	
Urine albumin/creatinine ratio (mg/mmol)	0.60±0.45	1.14±2.46	1.17±1.36	0.013
Serum LDL (mmol/L)	2.38±0.76	2.29±0.76	2.24±0.51	0.773
Serum triglyceride (mmol/L)	0.92±0.40	0.84±0.40	0.85±0.26	0.293

p-values provided for blood pressure are for z-scores; Blood glucose value obtained at the time of urine collection.

factors as markers of diabetic nephropathy prior to the onset of albuminuria remain unclear, especially in adolescents [21]. Our aim was therefore to determine the relationship between GFR and urinary cytokines/chemokines in a cohort of normotensive, normoalbuminuric adolescents with T1D analyzed on the basis of renal filtration status, since hyperfiltration may identify a group of individuals who are at an increased risk of developing clinical nephropathy in T1D and T2D [2,4].

Our first major finding was that renal hyperfiltration was associated with higher levels of urinary cytokines/chemokines in T1D adolescents prior to the development of microalbuminuria. There were also parallel trends in serum cytokine concentrations. This panel of biomarkers was selected due to associations between these factors with 1) renal hyperfiltration and acute responses to clamped hyperglycemia and 2) renal injury leading to diabetic nephropathy, including chemotaxis, inflammation and fibrosis [5,6] and 3) hyperglycemia-related increases in urinary excretion of cytokine/chemokines, including IFN, PDGF, TNF and MCP-1 [22,23,24], leading to chronic kidney disease [25,26,27,28,29]. In contrast with our previous work in adults using gold standard inulin clearance techniques to measure GFR under clamped euglycemic and hyperglycemic conditions, we used cystatin C-based measurements, since this estimate of GFR can be used clinically and has superior operating characteristics compared to creatinine-based estimates within the hyperfiltration range when compared to inulin clearances [8,10,30].

To account for the influence of ambient hyperglycemia at the time of GFR measurement on urinary cytokines/chemokines, we performed analyses with either HbA1c or plasma glucose as covariables [5]. Ambient plasma glucose concentration was an important determinant of urinary cytokine/chemokine excretion. On regression analysis, adjustment for serum glucose at the time of sampling mitigated the observed differences in cytokine excretion. This observation supports the hypothesis that ambient hyperglycemia is an independent determinant of urinary inflammatory biomarkers, and should be accounted for in future work. Chronic glycemic control, reflected by HbA1C, did not have the same confounding influence on cytokine excretion. This suggests that perhaps transient glycemia is more important than chronic glycemic status in determining acute variations in cytokine/chemokine production.

Renal hyperfiltration has been attributed to hyperglycemia-mediated activation of the RAAS causing efferent renal arteriolar vasoconstriction, and also to diabetes related increases in proximal tubular sodium-glucose cotransport, leading to altered tubuloglomerular feedback and afferent arteriolar vasodilatation [31,32]. Therefore, hyperglycemia may induce renal inflammation through direct mitogenic, angiotensin II-dependent pathways, and may also act indirectly through neurohormonal and tubular mechanisms that raise intraglomerular pressure and wall tension, leading to pro-inflammatory effects [33,34]. Regardless of the responsible mechanism, hyperfiltration is associated with the initiation and progression of nephropathy in T1D and T2D, and is present in

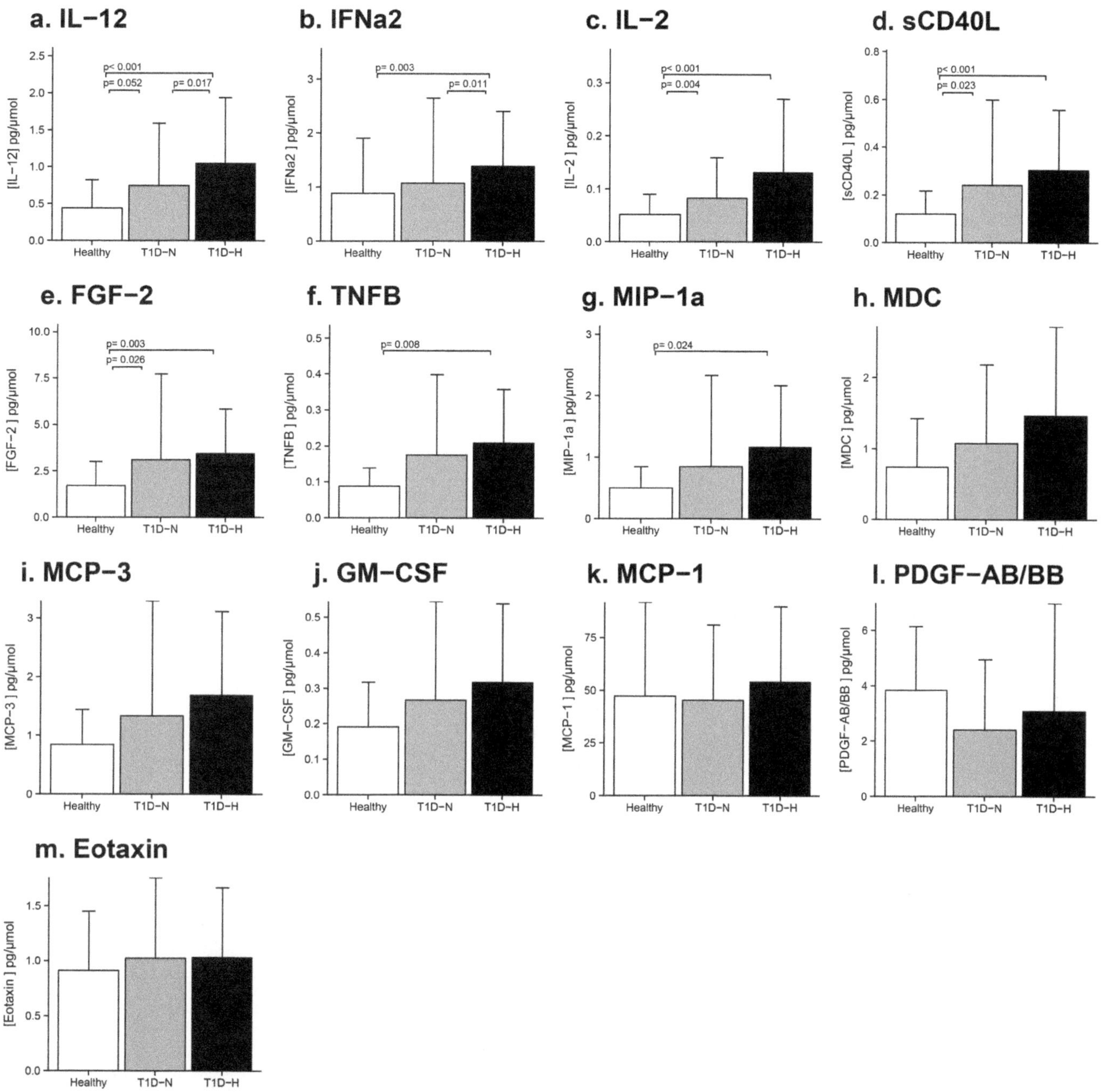

Figure 1. Urinary Excretion of Cytokine/Chemokines in Adolescents with Type 1 Diabetes According to Hyperfiltration Status vs Healthy Controls. Step-wise trends were observed for IL-12, IFNα2, IL-2, sCD40L, FGF-2, TNF-β, MIP-1α, MDC, MCP-3, GM-CSF, adjusted for age, gender, ACR and HbA1c. P-values show pair-wise comparisons with Bonferroni correction. After adjusting for plasma glucose at the time of collection, instead of HbA1c, pair-wise comparisons between normofilterers (T1D-N) and hyperfilterers (T1D-H) were no longer significant.

20–60% of young patients with T1D [2,4,35]. Mechanistically, high intraglomerular pressure is associated with hyperfiltration and increased wall tension in experimental diabetes, promoting renal parenchymal inflammation [36,37]. To determine if a similar relationship exists in humans, we previously compared urinary cytokine/chemokine excretion in adult patients with T1D with or without hyperfiltration defined by inulin-based clearances under controlled laboratory conditions [5,6]. We demonstrated that T1D-H exhibit higher urinary cytokines/chemokines levels vs. T1D-N and HC [6]. In a separate study we demonstrated that clamped hyperglycemia, a stimulus for hyperfiltration, also increases urinary cytokine/chemokine excretion [5]. To determine if hyperfiltration-related increases in urinary cytokines/chemokines are reversible, we examined the effect of RAAS blockade on these factors and demonstrated 1) a decline in many of these mediators and 2) that these effects were exaggerated hyperfilterers [7]. It was, however, unclear if these observations were applicable outside of a controlled laboratory setting, or if our observations would extend to an adolescent cohort. To our knowledge, the present study is the first to examine the interaction between renal

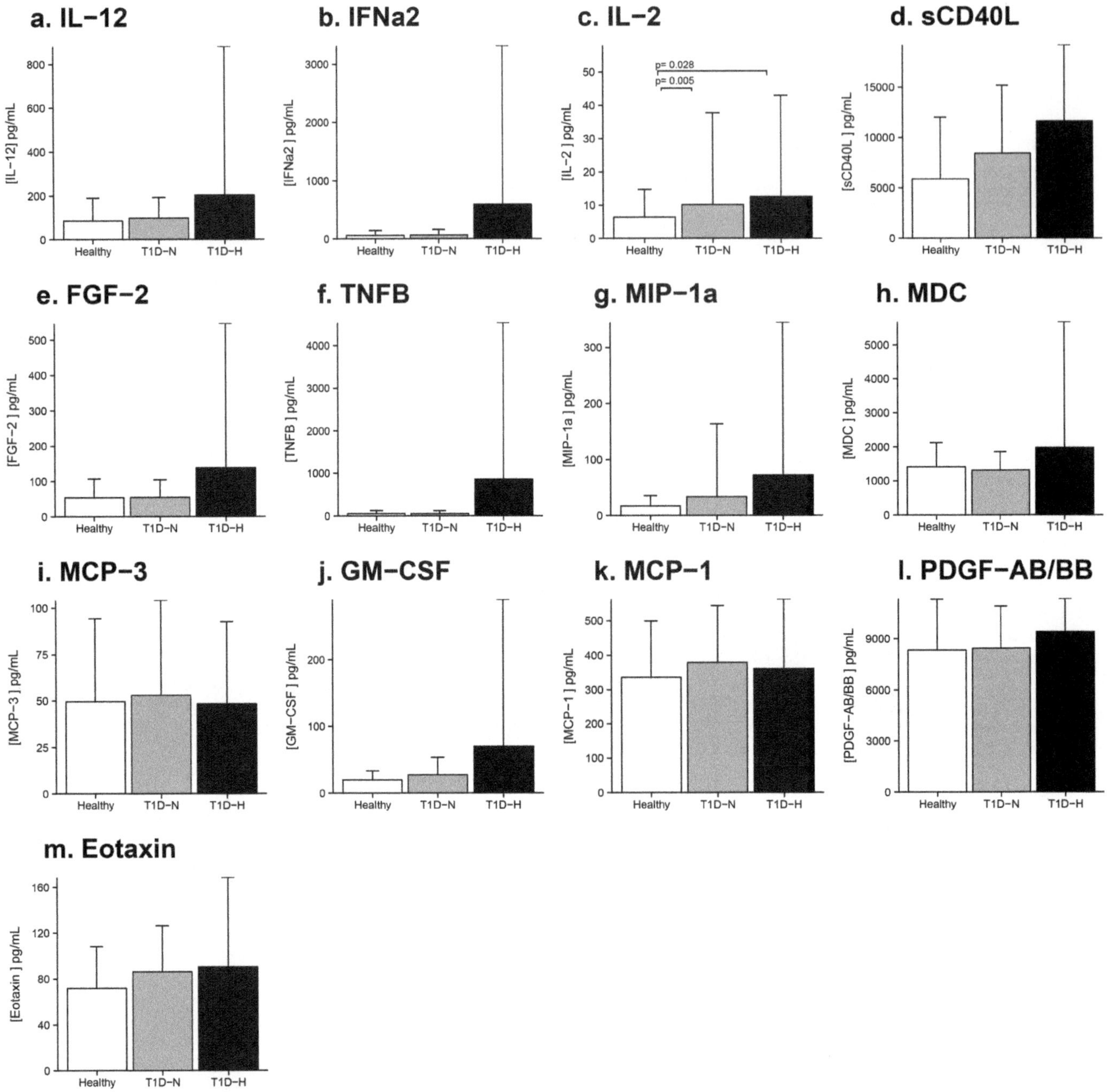

Figure 2. Serum Cytokine/Chemokine Signature in Adolescents with Type 1 Diabetes Based on Hyperfiltration Status and Healthy Controls. A parallel trend to urinary excretion of cytokine/chemokines was observed, although only IL-2 showed significance. P-values show pairwise comparisons with Bonferroni correction, adjusted for age, gender and HbA1c.

hyperfiltration, the earliest known hemodynamic abnormality related to the development of diabetic nephropathy, and urinary markers of inflammation in adolescents in a clinical setting. These results therefore confirm our previous work in adults with T1D, and suggest that inflammation associated with hyperfiltration begins much earlier in the natural history of the disease, potentially identifying an opportunity for future primary prevention strategies.

To determine whether the increase in urinary cytokines/chemokines in T1D-H patients is due to high systemic levels resulting in renal "overflow" or instead due to more local production, we also measured serum levels of each factor. Our second major finding was that in contrast with many *between-group* differences for urinary factors, serum levels of IL-2 differed between the three groups, with highest levels in T1D-H. Although by no means definitive, this observation suggests an interaction between systemic and renal levels of IL-2, possibly reflecting systemic production and consequent renal clearance. Interestingly, urinary levels of IL-12, IFNα2, FGF-2 and TNF-β tended to increase from HC to T1D-N to T1D-H, and serum levels of these factors correlated with GFR, again suggesting a relationship between systemic and renal levels of these factors. Even in the cases of MDC and GM-CSF where *between-group* differences for urinary levels were not significant, serum levels of these factors tended to follow the same trend, with a positive correlation between serum levels of GFR. We and others have previous observed systemic hemodynamic abnormalities in T1D-H patients, including endothelial dysfunction and higher blood pressure, suggesting that hyperfiltration reflects a generalized abnormality of the endothelium and vasculature rather than an isolated renal abnormality [16,38,39]. Therefore, our findings suggest that at least for IL-2, IL-12, IFNα2, FGF-2 and TNF-β higher urinary excretion rates in T1D-H may have been on the basis of increased clearance from the systemic circulation rather than renal production and subsequent urinary excretion.

In addition to increased risk of developing albuminuria and GFR loss in clinical trials [2,4], T1D patients with hyperfiltration including adolescents exhibit greater hemodynamic responses to ACE inhibition, reflected by declines in GFR toward the normal range [32]. We have also shown that T1D-H exhibit similar effects when tubuloglomerular feedback is activated using the sodium glucose cotransport inhibitor empagliflozin [40]. Finally, RAAS blockade results in greater urinary cytokine/chemokine suppression in T1D-H versus T1D-N [7]. Hyperfiltration therefore represents a distinct physiological state that identifies a subgroup of patients who may be at an increased risk of diabetic nephropathy, and who also exhibit greater hemodynamic and molecular responses to potential renal protective agents. Regardless of the source of cytokines/chemokines in the present study cohort, our results suggest that T1D-H patients generally exhibit higher levels of factors that have been linked with renal and cardiovascular injury. As such, patients with T1D-related hyperfiltration may therefore represent a high-risk group that should be targeted for earlier therapeutic interventions in future studies.

Our study has some important limitations. First, we were not able to study this large cohort under clamped glycemic conditions. We have demonstrated in previous work that strictly controlled physiologic environment that transient hyperglycemia significantly influences cytokine/chemokine levels. We therefore intentionally sought to study this in a more realistic clinical setting, and accounted for glycemia a priori with our analytic approach. A second limitation was the use of GFR based on estimating equations rather than direct GFR measures such as inulin. Nevertheless, use of $GFR_{cystatin\ C}$ to define hyperfiltration has provided important insights into how urinary cytokine/chemokine excretion rates may be translated into the clinical setting in future work [8]. Third, in this analysis, we hypothesized that *between-group* differences in urinary cytokines/chemokines were primarily on the basis of systemic overflow, and that increased renal production was also possible. We recognize, however, that children with T1D commonly exhibit evidence of proximal tubular dysfunction [41,42] and we have recently reported that proximal tubular function may be different in T1D-H vs. T1D-N [31]. As such, future work should determine if physiological differences in proximal tubule function, rather than activation of inflammatory pathways, contribute to abnormalities in urinary cytokine/chemokine handling, resulting in step-wise changes from HC to T1D-N to T1D-H observed in this study. Finally, it is important to recognize the cross-sectional nature of the data. As such, we were unable to assess changes in urinary cytokine/chemokine excretion over time, including the effect of intercurrent illness or changes in glycemic control on these factors.

In conclusion, hyperfiltration in adolescents with T1D is associated with higher levels of urinary cytokine/chemokine excretion, an effect that is in part dependent on ambient blood glucose levels. Future work is required to determine if high urinary cytokine/chemokine excretion rates are associated with early renal function decline or the onset of proteinuria. Future studies should also determine if suppression of urinary cytokines/chemokines with RAAS inhibition as observed in physiology studies can also be achieved in a clinical setting and if declines in these factors correlate with improved clinical outcomes [6].

Acknowledgments

Finally, the authors are grateful to the study participants whose time and effort are critical to the success of our research program. The results presented in this paper have not been published previously in whole or in part. These data were presented in abstract form to the American Society of Nephrology Meeting on November 9, 2013

Author Contributions

Conceived and designed the experiments: RLHH HNR JWS DD DBD RM RND LM YE LD MO EBS FHM DZIC. Performed the experiments: RLHH HNR JWS DD LM YE LD MO EBS FHM DZIC. Analyzed the data: RLHH HNR JWS DD RM LM YE LD MO EBS FHM DZIC. Contributed reagents/materials/analysis tools: RLHH HNR JWS DD DBD RM RND LM YE LD MO EBS FHM DZIC. Wrote the paper: RLHH HNR JWS DD DBD RM RND LM YE LD MO EBS FHM DZIC.

References

1. Mauer M, Zinman B, Gardiner R, Suissa S, Sinaiko A, et al. (2009) Renal and retinal effects of enalapril and losartan in type 1 diabetes. N Engl J Med 361: 40–51.
2. Magee GM, Bilous RW, Cardwell CR, Hunter SJ, Kee F, et al. (2009) Is hyperfiltration associated with the future risk of developing diabetic nephropathy? A meta-analysis. Diabetologia 52: 691–697.
3. Sasson AN, Cherney DZ (2012) Renal hyperfiltration related to diabetes mellitus and obesity in human disease. World J Diabetes 3: 1–6.
4. Ruggenenti P, Porrini EL, Gaspari F, Motterlini N, Cannata A, et al. (2012) Glomerular hyperfiltration and renal disease progression in type 2 diabetes. Diabetes Care 35: 2061–2068.
5. Cherney DZ, Scholey JW, Sochett E, Bradley TJ, Reich HN (2011) The acute effect of clamped hyperglycemia on the urinary excretion of inflammatory cytokines/chemokines in uncomplicated type 1 diabetes: a pilot study. Diabetes Care 34: 177–180.
6. Har R, Scholey JW, Daneman D, Mahmud FH, Dekker R, et al. (2013) The effect of renal hyperfiltration on urinary inflammatory cytokines/chemokines in patients with uncomplicated type 1 diabetes mellitus. Diabetologia 56: 1166–1173.
7. Cherney DZI, Reich HN, Scholey JW, Daneman D, Mahmud F, et al. (2013) The effect of aliskiren on urinary cytokine/chemokine responses to hyperglycemia in type 1 diabetes mellitus. Diabetologia epub July 28.
8. Cherney DZ, Sochett EB, Dekker MG, Perkins BA (2010) Ability of cystatin C to detect acute changes in glomerular filtration rate provoked by hyperglycaemia in uncomplicated Type 1 diabetes. Diabet Med 27: 1358–1365.
9. Cherney DZI, Scholey JW, Daneman D, Dunger DB, Dalton N, et al. (2012) Urinary markers of renal inflammation in subjects with type 1 diabetes and normoalbuminuria. Diabetic Medicine March 14.
10. Perkins BA, Sochett EB, Cherney DZ (2012) Ability of Cystatin C to detect changes in glomerular filtration rate after ACE inhibition in patients with uncomplicated type 1 diabetes. Clin Exp Hypertens 34: 606–611.
11. Group TDCaCTEoDIaCR (2000) Retinopathy and Nephropathy in Patients with Type 1 Diabetes Four Years after a Trial of Intensive Therapy. New England Journal of Medicine 342: 381–389.
12. AdDIT Study Group (2009) Adolescent type 1 Diabetes Cardio-renal Intervention Trial (AdDIT). BMC Pediatr 9: 79.
13. Bacchetta J, Cochat P, Rognant N, Ranchin B, Hadj-Aissa A, et al. (2011) Which creatinine and cystatin C equations can be reliably used in children? Clin J Am Soc Nephrol 6: 552–560.
14. Cherney DZ, Miller JA, Scholey JW, Nasrallah R, Hebert RL, et al. (2010) Renal hyperfiltration is a determinant of endothelial function responses to cyclooxygenase 2 inhibition in type 1 diabetes. Diabetes Care 33: 1344–1346.
15. Cherney DZ, Scholey JW, Daneman D, Dunger DB, Dalton RN, et al. (2012) Urinary markers of renal inflammation in adolescents with Type 1 diabetes mellitus and normoalbuminuria. Diabet Med 29: 1297–1302.

16. Yang GK, Maahs DM, Perkins B, Cherney DZI (2013) Renal Hyperfiltration and Systemic Blood Pressure in Patients with Uncomplicated Type 1 Diabetes Mellitus. PLoS One 8: e68908.
17. Perkins BA, Ficociello LH, Ostrander BE, Silva KH, Weinberg J, et al. (2007) Microalbuminuria and the risk for early progressive renal function decline in type 1 diabetes. J Am Soc Nephrol 18: 1353–1361.
18. Dwyer JP, Parving HH, Hunsicker LG, Ravid M, Remuzzi G, et al. (2012) Renal Dysfunction in the Presence of Normoalbuminuria in Type 2 Diabetes: Results from the DEMAND Study. Cardiorenal Med 2: 1–10.
19. Merchant ML, Perkins BA, Boratyn GM, Ficociello LH, Wilkey DW, et al. (2009) Urinary peptidome may predict renal function decline in type 1 diabetes and microalbuminuria. J Am Soc Nephrol 20: 2065–2074.
20. Perkins BA, Krolewski AS (2009) Early nephropathy in type 1 diabetes: the importance of early renal function decline. Curr Opin Nephrol Hypertens 18: 233–240.
21. Wolkow PP, Niewczas MA, Perkins B, Ficociello LH, Lipinski B, et al. (2008) Association of urinary inflammatory markers and renal decline in microalbuminuric type 1 diabetics. J Am Soc Nephrol 19: 789–797.
22. Morii T, Fujita H, Narita T, Shimotomai T, Fujishima H, et al. (2003) Association of monocyte chemoattractant protein-1 with renal tubular damage in diabetic nephropathy. J Diabetes Complications 17: 11–15.
23. Banba N, Nakamura T, Matsumura M, Kuroda H, Hattori Y, et al. (2000) Possible relationship of monocyte chemoattractant protein-1 with diabetic nephropathy. Kidney Int 58: 684–690.
24. Wada T, Furuichi K, Sakai N, Iwata Y, Yoshimoto K, et al. (2000) Up-regulation of monocyte chemoattractant protein-1 in tubulointerstitial lesions of human diabetic nephropathy. Kidney Int 58: 1492–1499.
25. Rao GN, Corson MA, Berk BC (1991) Uric acid stimulates vascular smooth muscle cell proliferation by increasing platelet-derived growth factor A-chain expression. J Biol Chem 266: 8604–8608.
26. Sanchez-Lozada LG, Nakagawa T, Kang DH, Feig DI, Franco M, et al. (2006) Hormonal and cytokine effects of uric acid. Curr Opin Nephrol Hypertens 15: 30–33.
27. Litwin M, Michalkiewicz J, Niemirska A, Gackowska L, Kubiszewska I, et al. (2010) Inflammatory activation in children with primary hypertension. Pediatr Nephrol 25: 1711–1718.
28. Tominaga M, Uno K, Yagi K, Fukui M, Hasegawa G, et al. (2010) Association between capacity of interferon-alpha production and metabolic parameters. J Interferon Cytokine Res 30: 451–454.
29. Mene P, Punzo G (2008) Uric acid: bystander or culprit in hypertension and progressive renal disease? J Hypertens 26: 2085–2092.
30. Odutayo A, Cherney D (2012) Cystatin C and acute changes in glomerular filtration rate. Clin Nephrol 78: 64–75.
31. Cherney DZI, Perkins BA, Soleymanlou N, Maione M, Lai V, et al. (2014) The Renal Hemodynamic Effect of SGLT2 Inhibition in Patients with Type 1 Diabetes. Circulation 129: 587–597.
32. Sochett EB, Cherney DZ, Curtis JR, Dekker MG, Scholey JW, et al. (2006) Impact of renin angiotensin system modulation on the hyperfiltration state in type 1 diabetes. J Am Soc Nephrol 17: 1703–1709.
33. Cherney DZ, Scholey JW, Miller JA (2008) Insights into the regulation of renal hemodynamic function in diabetic mellitus. Curr Diabetes Rev 4: 280–290.
34. Mezzano S, Droguett A, Burgos ME, Ardiles LG, Flores CA, et al. (2003) Renin-angiotensin system activation and interstitial inflammation in human diabetic nephropathy. Kidney Int Suppl: S64–70.
35. Moriya T, Tsuchiya A, Okizaki S, Hayashi A, Tanaka K, et al. (2012) Glomerular hyperfiltration and increased glomerular filtration surface are associated with renal function decline in normo- and microalbuminuric type 2 diabetes. Kidney Int 81: 486–493.
36. Riser BL, Cortes P, Heilig C, Grondin J, Ladson-Wofford S, et al. (1996) Cyclic stretching force selectively up-regulates transforming growth factor-beta isoforms in cultured rat mesangial cells. Am J Pathol 148: 1915–1923.
37. Riser BL, Cortes P, Zhao X, Bernstein J, Dumler F, et al. (1992) Intraglomerular pressure and mesangial stretching stimulate extracellular matrix formation in the rat. J Clin Invest 90: 1932–1943.
38. Pecis M, Azevedo MJ, Gross JL (1997) Glomerular hyperfiltration is associated with blood pressure abnormalities in normotensive normoalbuminuric IDDM patients. Diabetes Care 20: 1329–1333.
39. Cherney DZ, Reich HN, Jiang S, Har R, Nasrallah R, et al. (2012) Hyperfiltration and the effect of nitric oxide inhibition on renal and endothelial function in humans with uncomplicated type 1 diabetes mellitus. Am J Physiol Regul Integr Comp Physiol 303: R710–718.
40. Cherney DZI, Perkins BA, Soleymanlou N, Maione M, Lai V, et al. (2013) The Renal Hemodynamic Effect of SGLT2 Inhibition in Patients with Type 1 Diabetes. Circulation, in press.
41. Schultz CJ, Dalton RN, Neil HA, Konopelska-Bahu T, Dunger DB (2001) Markers of renal tubular dysfunction measured annually do not predict risk of microalbuminuria in the first few years after diagnosis of Type I diabetes. Diabetologia 44: 224–229.
42. Hourd P, Edge JA, Dunger DB, Dalton N, Edwards R (1991) Urinary growth hormone excretion during puberty in type 1 (insulin-dependent) diabetes mellitus. Diabet Med 8: 237–242.

16

Reduction of T Cell Receptor Diversity in NOD Mice Prevents Development of Type 1 Diabetes but Not Sjögren's Syndrome

Joanna Kern, Robert Drutel¤, Silvia Leanhart, Marek Bogacz, Rafal Pacholczyk*

Center for Biotechnology and Genomic Medicine, Georgia Regents University, Augusta, Georgia, United States of America

Abstract

Non-obese diabetic (NOD) mice are well-established models of independently developing spontaneous autoimmune diseases, Sjögren's syndrome (SS) and type 1 diabetes (T1D). The key determining factor for T1D is the strong association with particular MHCII molecule and recognition by diabetogenic T cell receptor (TCR) of an insulin peptide presented in the context of I-A^{g7} molecule. For SS the association with MHCII polymorphism is weaker and TCR diversity involved in the onset of the autoimmune phase of SS remains poorly understood. To compare the impact of TCR diversity reduction on the development of both diseases we generated two lines of TCR transgenic NOD mice. One line expresses transgenic TCRβ chain originated from a pathogenically irrelevant TCR, and the second line additionally expresses transgenic $TCR\alpha^{mini}$ locus. Analysis of TCR sequences on NOD background reveals lower TCR diversity on Treg cells not only in the thymus, but also in the periphery. This reduction in diversity does not affect conventional $CD4^+$ T cells, as compared to the TCR^{mini} repertoire on B6 background. Interestingly, neither transgenic TCRβ nor TCR^{mini} mice develop diabetes, which we show is due to lack of insulin B:9–23 specific T cells in the periphery. Conversely SS develops in both lines, with full glandular infiltration, production of autoantibodies and hyposalivation. It shows that SS development is not as sensitive to limited availability of TCR specificities as T1D, which suggests wider range of possible TCR/peptide/MHC interactions driving autoimmunity in SS.

Editor: John A. Chiorini, National Institute of Dental and Craniofacial Research, United States of America

Funding: This research was supported by grants from National Institute of Allergy and Infectious Diseases of the National Institutes of Health (R01AI081798) and Juvenile Diabetes Research Foundation (RP). The funders had no role in study design, data collection and analysis, decision to publish, or preparation of the manuscript.

Competing Interests: The authors have declared that no competing interests exist.

* Email: rpacholczyk@gru du

¤ Current address: Medical University of South Carolina, College of Medicine, Charleston, South Carolina, United States of America

Introduction

NOD mice serve as well-established models of independently developing autoimmune diseases, Type 1 Diabetes (T1D) and Sjögren's syndrome (SS) [1,2]. T1D is characterized by autoimmune attacks against the pancreatic beta-cells with T cells playing an essential role in the initiation and progression of the disease, leading to hyperglycemia and vascular complications [3,4]. SS is an autoimmune disease with local and systemic manifestations, characterized by mononuclear infiltrates into salivary and lacrimal glands leading to clinical symptoms of dry mouth and dry eyes [5,6]. Glandular infiltrates consist mostly of $CD4^+$ T cells with lesser amounts of $CD8^+$ T cells and B cells. Although factors like viral or bacterial infections, aberrant glandular development or cytokine production are important in the initial phase of the pathogenesis of SS, $CD4^+$ T cells are important players in the onset of autoimmunity and disease progression.

Autoimmunity in NOD mice is attributed to several different events occurring in the thymus and in the periphery. Studies in these mice showed a defect in negative selection [7], perturbed αβ/γδ lineage decision leading to a shift in selection niches [8], reduced relative diversity of thymic Treg cells [9], peripheral hyper-responsiveness of effector $CD4^+$ T cells [10], multiple binding registers of insulin B:9–23 peptide resulting in poor negative selection in the thymus [11,12], or peripheral post-translational modification of self-peptides/neo-antigens [13]. Despite genetic predispositions, the key component in the development of autoimmune diseases is the recognition of a particular antigen in the context of MHC Class II molecule by $CD4^+$ T cells. The development of diabetes in NOD mice is associated with the key I-A^{g7} molecule (HLA-DQ8 in humans) in the absence of a functional I-E molecule [14,15]. Co-expression of other MHC molecules with I-A^{g7} can prevent development of diabetes in a dominant fashion [14,15]. Replacement of I-A^{g7} with other MHC molecules, like I-A^b, I-A^p or I-A^q, does not promote the development of diabetes yet mice continue to develop autoimmune exocrinopathy and the severity of the SS and the profile of antibodies' specificities vary between congenic mice [16]. In large-scale association study of SS in humans, HLA was found to have the strongest linkage to the disease [17].

The strict dependence of T1D on the particular MHC allele correlates with its primary antigen requirement where insulin B:9–23 peptide has been identified as the epitope necessary for onset of the disease in NOD mice [18]. In SS, no key epitope(s) are identified, although several proteins have been implicated as a source of antigens: Ro/SSA 52 kDa, αFodrin, Muscarinic Acetylcholine 3 Receptor (M3R), α-amylase, islet cell autoantigen-69, kallikrein-13 [19–24]. Recently it has been shown that the transfer of T cells from M3R-immunized $M3R^{-/-}$ mice into $Rag^{-/-}$ mice leads to development of sialadenitis, showing pathogenic potential of M3R specific T cells [25].

Despite the strict requirement of the presence of the insulin B:9–23/I-A^{g7} combination, the development of T1D in NOD mice proceeds even when total TCR diversity and precursor frequency of diabetogenic TCRs is limited. The reduction of TCR diversity by use of TCRβ transgenic mice [26], or great reduction of precursor frequency relying on allelic exclusion escapees on NOD background does not prevent development of T1D [27], although not all endogenous TCRβ chains are permissive for the development of insulin B:9–23 specific TCRs [28]. In SS it is not clear as to what role diversity of interactions between TCRs and different peptide/MHCII complexes play in the onset and development of the disease. Previous studies in patients with SS found that TCR repertoire of infiltrating T cells is to some extent restricted with different dominant clonotypes of Vβ families [29–33]. Despite the lack of dominant Vα/Vβ families or dominant specificity in different patients these studies show clonal expansion of infiltrating T cells, which suggests that the number of epitopes participating in the autoimmunity of the disease is limited [34,35]. However, the weaker dependence of SS on MHC polymorphism suggests broad diversity of possible TCR/peptide/MHCII interactions participating in the pathogenesis of the disease. As the diversity of antigenic specificities and TCR repertoire on T cells involved in SS development is not well understood, we wanted to compare sensitivity of development of SS versus T1D to the diminishing diversities of TCRs in the presence of the same I-A^{g7} molecule in NOD mice. To reduce the diversity of TCRs in NOD mice we generated two types of transgenic strains, in which all T cells express either one transgenic TCRβ chain or additionally co-express TCRα chains from $TCR\alpha^{mini}$ locus [36]. Interestingly, these mice do not develop T1D but still develop SS with glandular infiltrations, autoantibody presence and hyposalivation. We investigated the reasons for the lack of T1D development and the role of reduced diversity on generated repertoires of TCRs on conventional and regulatory T cells in the thymus and periphery of NOD mice.

Materials and Methods

Ethics statement

All mice used in this study were housed in the animal care facility at the Georgia Regents University (GRU). All work involving animals was conducted under protocols approved by the Animal Care and Use Committee at the GRU (#2008–0231). All efforts were made to minimize suffering. Mice were euthanized by CO2 followed by cervical dislocation.

Mice

Production of $TCR\beta^{Tg}$ and $TCR\alpha^{mini}$ constructs and generation of transgenic mice on C57BL/6 (B6) background was described previously (Pacholczyk 2006). A similar strategy was used to microinject one or both DNA constructs into zygotes of NOD mice (Transgenic Mice Core Facility, GRU). To eliminate expression of endogenous TCRα chains, NOD.$TCR\beta^{Tg}$.$TCR\alpha^{mini}$ transgenic mice were crossed with NOD.$TCR\alpha^{-/-}$ (NOD.129P2(C)-Tcratm1Mjo/DoiJ) mice purchased from The Jackson Laboratory (Bar Harbor, ME). To facilitate identification of Treg cells both transgenic lines then were crossed with NOD.FoxP3GFP/cre mice (NOD/ShiLt-Tg(Foxp3-EGFP/cre)1Jbs/J) purchased from The Jackson Laboratory. The B6.Aec1Aec2 (B6.DC) mice were kindly provided by Dr. Ammon Peck [37].

Histology

Organs were removed from each mouse at the time of euthanasia, placed in 10% phosphate-buffered formalin for at least 24 h and then embedded in paraffin. Sections were taken at 5 µm of thickness 200 µm apart. The tissue sections were stained with hematoxylin and eosin (H&E) at the Histology Core Laboratory, GRU. One infiltrate was defined as a cluster of at least 50 nucleated cells, scoring described in figures.

Measurement of saliva flow

Mice were given an i.p. injection of 100 µl of pilocarpine (0.05 mg/ml in PBS) per 20 g of body weight. Saliva was collected for 10 min., starting 1 min. after injection of pilocarpine. The volume of saliva was measured and normalized to the mouse body weight.

Detection of auto-antibodies

Auto-antibodies and total IgG1 were measured using mouse serum with the following ELISA kits: αFodrin (American Research Products), ANA, ssDNA, dsDNA (Immuno-Biological Laboratories) and IgG1 (Immunology Consultants Laboratory). Assays were performed according to manufacturer's protocols with serum dilution 1:100 and 1:50,000 for IgG1. OD_{450} values of negative samples were subtracted from the OD_{450} of experimental samples.

Cell preparation, flow cytometry and cell sorting

Cells were isolated from peripheral lymph nodes (axillary, brachial and inguinal) and thymii by mechanical disruption through nylon mesh. Salivary mandibular and extraorbital lacrimal glands were first cut and digested using collagenase (1 ug/ml) for 30 min in 37°C. Cells were washed and counted (Countess, Invitrogen) and used for staining with monoclonal antibodies: CD4 (clone RM4-5), CD8α (53-6.7), B220 (RA3-6B2), TCRVα2 (B20.1), TCRVβ14 (14-2), TCRβ (H57-597), CD25 (PC61), CD45RB (16A), CD62L (MEL-14), all from BD Biosciences. Stained cells were either analyzed using FACS Canto (BD Biosciences) or sorted on MoFlo Sorter (Cytomation). Dead cells were excluded using forward vs side scatter dot plots and doublets discrimination was accomplished using forward scatter height vs width dot plots. Purities of all sorted populations were above 98%.

Immunization and generation of T cell hybridomas

Mice were immunized at the base of the tail with 50 µg of insulin B:9–23 peptide emulsified in Complete Freund's Adjuvant (Thermo Scientific). One week later lymphocytes were isolated from draining lymph nodes and cultured *in vitro* for 3–4 days with insulin B:9–23 peptide (50 µg/ml), followed by 3–4 days of expansion with murine recombinant IL-2 (20 U/ml, Peprotech). For generation of allo-specific T cell hybridomas, $CD4^+$ T cells sorted from un-immunized experimental mice were stimulated *in vitro* by co-culture with splenocytes from B6.$TCR\alpha^{-/-}$ mice, followed by expansion with IL-2. Activated T cells were fused to BW5147 TCRα-β- NFAT-EGFP cells as previously described [38]. BW NFAT-EGFP fusion partner expresses GFP protein under the minimal human IL-2 promoter, which contains NFAT-binding sites [39]. T cell hybridomas were selected using HAT

(Cellgro) selection media by limiting dilution method. For stimulation, cloned T cell hybridomas (10^5 cells) were co-cultured overnight with 5×10^5 splenocytes (from NOD.TCRα−/− or B6.TCRα−/− mice) with or without insulin B:9–23 peptide (50 μg/ml) or anti-CD3 antibody (1 μg/ml). Specific activation of the hybridomas was measured by detection of GFP-positive cells or by detection of IL-2 in culture supernatant using CBA Mouse IL-2 Flex Set (BD Biosciences).

MTT assay

The proliferation of the cells was measured using 3-(4,5-dimethythiazol-2-yl)-2,5-diphenyltetrazolium bromide (MTT; Sigma) assay. On the third day of *in vitro* stimulation 10 μl of MTT (5 mg/ml) was added to each well and incubated for 4 h. After discarding supernatant, the remaining formazan precipitates were dissolved in 150 ul of 70% isopropanol solution (70% isopropanol, 30% water, 0.02N hydrochloric acid) overnight. Absorbance was measured at 570 nm using Microplate Reader (Biotek Synergy HT).

Sequencing

Single cell sorting and sequencing was done as previously described [36]. High-throughput sequencing was done using Ion Torrent platform (Life Technologies) by Genomic Core Facility at GRU. Libraries of the TCRs were prepared according to protocol. Shortly, CDR3α regions were amplified using primers specific for Vα2 and Cα segments with integrated adapters and barcodes, provided by manufacturer. Before sequencing, consistency of samples was checked by 2D-F-SSCP analysis of PCR products from three aliquots of cDNA per each sample [36]. Only samples with three similar/identical profiles were considered without PCR bias and were used for further purification using Agencourt AMPure XP reagent (Beckman Coulter) and used for sequencing. FASTQ files with sequences were processed and analyzed using custom-written program in Pearl (ActivePearl, ActiveState Software Inc.). Sequences with quality score of CDR3α region above 27 were used for analysis. The length of CDR3α region was defined by counting from the third amino acid after the invariant C residue in all Vα regions (Y-L/F-C-A-X-first) to the amino acid immediately preceding common Jα motif (last-F-G-X-F-G-T).

Statistical analysis

The similarity, diversity and richness estimators were calculated using programs designed to measure biodiversity: EstimateS8.2 (Colwell, R. EstimateS: Biodiversity Estimation Software. Program and User's Guide at http://viceroy.eeb.uconn.edu/estimates) and SPADE (Chao, A. and Shen, T.-J. (2010) Program SPADE (Species Prediction And Diversity Estimation). Program and User's Guide published at http://chao.stat.nthu.edu.tw).

Results

Development of T cells in NOD$^{\beta Tg}$ and NOD^{mini} mice

We generated TCRβ transgenic mice, in which all T cells use the same TCRβ^{Tg} chain (Vβ14Dβ2Jβ2.6) and one of the endogenous TCRα chains. The TCRβ transgenic chain originated from I-A^b restricted TCR specific to Ep63 K peptide an analog of Eα 52–68 peptide in which the residue at position 63(I) was substituted with lysine [40]. To further reduce diversity of TCRs we used TCRα^{mini} transgenic construct, used previously to create TCR^{mini} mouse on B6 background (B6^{mini}) [36]. The TCRα^{mini} transgene allows a single Vα2.9 segment to rearrange to one of the two Jα (Jα26 and Jα2) segments. The generated transgenic mice were further crossed with TCR$\alpha^{-/-}$ mice to ensure that all developing T cells use transgenic TCRα^{mini} locus. To track CD4$^+$ Foxp3$^+$ regulatory T (Treg) cells we crossed transgenic mice with NOD.Foxp3.EGFP/cre mice as described in methods. Final characteristics of mice used in this paper were NOD^{mini} (NOD.TCRα^{mini}.TCRβ^{Tg}.TCR$\alpha^{-/-}$.Foxp3EGFP/cre), NOD$^{\beta Tg}$ (TCRβ^{Tg}.TCR$\alpha^{+/-}$.Foxp3EGFP/cre) and NOD (NOD.Foxp3EGFP/cre).

In NOD^{mini} and NOD$^{\beta Tg}$ transgenic mice thymic development of T cells proceeds normally, and selection of single positive (SP) thymocytes is very efficient with bias toward CD4$^+$ T cells in the thymus and in the periphery, similarly to a previously reported bias on B6 background (Fig. 1A, 1B) [36]. TCRβ transgenic mice are characterized by allelic exclusion, resulting in all T cells to express only one transgenic TCRβ chain. It has been proposed that allelic exclusion in NOD mice is less efficient [27]. In our mice all SP thymocytes and peripheral T cells have exclusive expression of transgenic TCRβ^{Tg} chain (TCRVβ14) in both types of transgenic mice and exclusive expression of TCRα^{mini} transgene (TCRVα2) in NOD^{mini} mice (Fig. 1A, 1B). Also we did not observe emergence of the cells bearing TCRs with Vβ segments other than Vβ14 even in older mice. Furthermore, we observed lower percentages of Treg cells in thymii and periphery of transgenic mice as compared to NOD mice and the percentages correlated with diversities of TCRs in analyzed mice (Fig. 1C, 1E). Nevertheless, the total numbers of peripheral Treg cells were similar in all of analyzed mice and reduced percentages of Treg cells were due to more efficient selection of CD4$^+$ T cells, rather than diversity of TCRs, as we observed this correlation on B6 background and in other types of mice that differ by efficiency of CD4$^+$ T cells selection (Fig. 1C, 1E) [36,41]. Finally, to check whether this particular TCRVβ14 transgenic chain can impose an unusual restriction on the TCRα repertoire, we evaluated the frequency of individual Vα families. We found no bias in TCR repertoire as the frequency of Vα families usage by CD4$^+$Vβ14$^+$ T cells was similar between NOD and NOD^{BTg} mice (Fig. 1D).

Lack of T cells specific to insulin B:9–23 in NOD transgenic mice

To test development of diabetes we measured blood glucose levels in experimental mice. Surprisingly, neither NOD$^{\beta Tg}$ nor NOD^{mini} transgenic mice develop diabetes (Fig. 2A). Evaluation of H&E stained pancreatic sections showed lack of lymphocytic infiltrates in 25 week old transgenic mice, with only insignificant infiltrates found in a few sections of NOD$^{\beta Tg}$ mice (Fig. 2B). As a control we used non-transgenic littermates of NOD$^{\beta Tg}$, NOD.TCR$\alpha^{+/-}$ mice. These mice developed diabetes and by 30 weeks of age more than 75% of females had high levels of blood glucose (Fig. 2A). One of the possibilities was that the lack of development of diabetes in transgenic mice is due to perturbed proportions of regulatory to effector T cell ratios, which could result in more efficient suppression of potentially diabetogenic T cells. We took advantage of cyclophosphamide treatment, which selectively affects numbers and function of Treg cells and accelerates development of diabetes in NOD mice [42,43]. This treatment however did not cause insulitis nor diabetes in transgenic mice indicating inability of effector T cells to initiate autoimmunity (unpublished data).

The onset of spontaneous diabetes in NOD mice is dependent upon presence of effector T cells specific to insulin B:9–23 antigen and lack of such specificity results in lack of early infiltrates into pancreatic islets [18]. As our mice did not develop islet-infiltrates, we tested their ability to respond to stimulation by insulin B:9–23 peptide (Fig. 3). CD4$^+$ T cells isolated from NOD^{mini}, NOD$^{\beta Tg}$ and NOD mice responded to stimulation by allogeneic spleno-

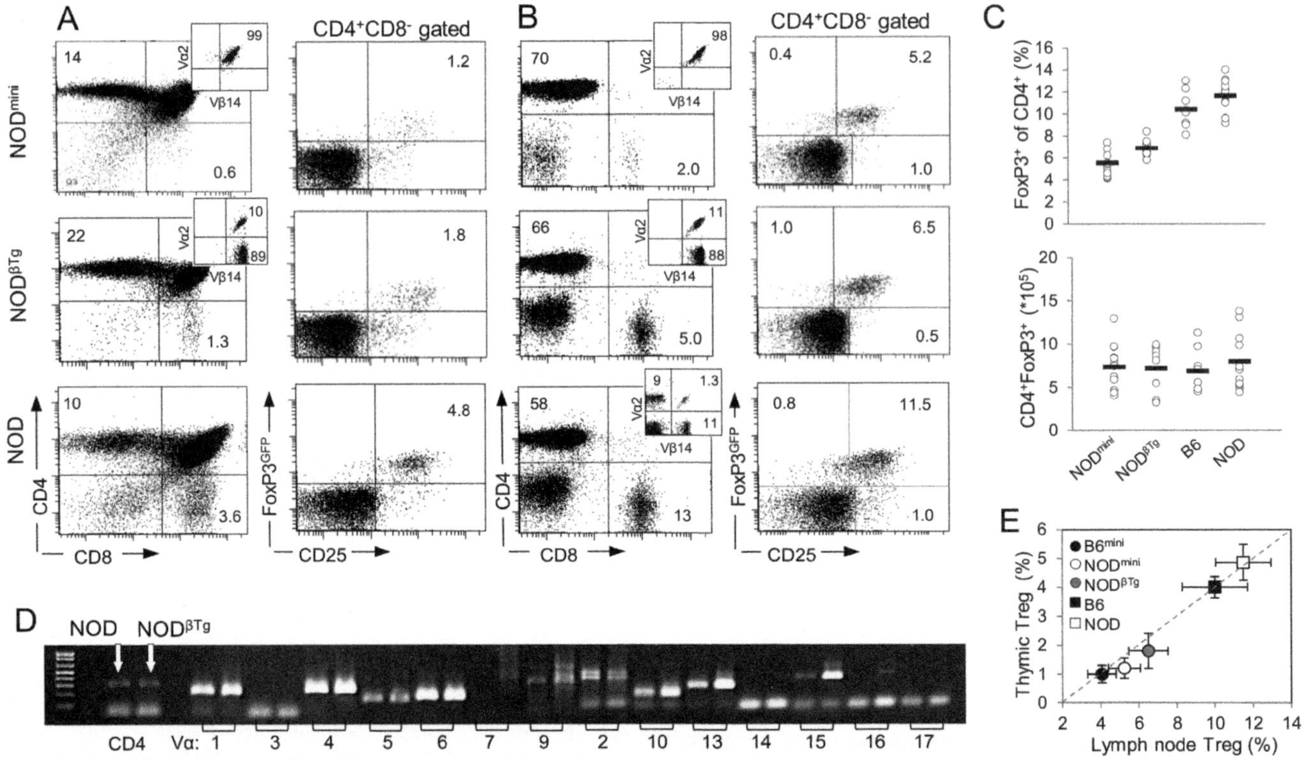

Figure 1. Efficient selection of CD4$^+$ T lymphocytes in NOD^{mini} and NOD$^{\beta Tg}$ mice. Lymphocytes isolated from thymii (A) and lymph nodes (B) of indicated mice were stained with monoclonal antibodies and analyzed by flow cytometry. Numbers in quadrants are representative percentages of at least six mice (6 week old) per group. The numbers of thymocytes and lymphocytes ± SD recovered from NOD^{mini}, NOD$^{\beta Tg}$ and NOD mice were: from thymii $78.5 \pm 16.7 \times 10^6$, $72.05 \pm 13.8 \times 10^6$ and $70.1 \pm 14.0 \times 10^6$, and from lymph nodes (axillary, brachial and inguinal) $17.2 \pm 5.8 \times 10^6$, $14.1 \pm 2.5 \times 10^6$, and $13.2 \pm 3.0 \times 10^6$, respectively. (C) Percentages (top) and total numbers (bottom) of CD4$^+$Foxp3$^+$ T cells in peripheral lymph nodes of 6 week old mice; each circle represents individual mouse. (D) Expression of mRNA of TCRVα genes in sorted CD4$^+$ T cells isolated from NOD and NOD$^{\beta Tg}$ mice. Analysis was done by RT-PCR using primers specific to indicated Vα segments and Cα region. (E) Comparison of CD4$^+$Foxp3$^+$ T (Treg) cells from thymii and peripheral lymph nodes of transgenic and wild type B6 and NOD mice. Mean percentage and SD of six young mice per group are shown.

cytes, however only CD4$^+$ T cells from immunized NOD mice were able to respond to B:9–23 peptide in the presence of syngeneic splenocytes (Fig. 3). As of note, B:9–23 peptide does not bind to I-A^b molecule and in the presence of B6 splenocytes does not lead to CD4 T cell response [44]. We were also unable to generate B:9–23 specific T cell hybridomas from immunized NOD^{mini} and NOD$^{\beta Tg}$ mice, however we had no problem generating allo-specific T cell hybridomas from transgenic mice. These results showed that changes introduced by transgenic chains to the TCR repertoire in NOD mice resulted in lack of peripheral specificity to the key antigen required for onset of T1D.

Development of SS in NOD$^{\beta Tg}$ and NOD^{mini} mice

The lack of T1D in transgenic mice prompted us to test whether reduced TCR diversity will affect development of Sjögren's syndrome – secondary autoimmune disease in NOD mice. It is characterized by lymphocytic infiltrates into salivary and lacrimal glands, production of auto-antibodies and the loss of saliva and tear production by 20 weeks of age [5,45]. Histological evaluation of tissue sections of submandibular salivary and extraorbital lacrimal glands showed focal lymphocytic infiltrates, in both transgenic NOD^{mini} and NOD$^{\beta Tg}$ and parental NOD mice (Fig. 4). Similarly to the NOD mice, males of both transgenic mice had milder infiltration of salivary glands than females, while the infiltration of lacrimal glands was more prominent in male NOD$^{\beta Tg}$ and NOD^{mini} mice. This infiltration is organ specific, as we did not detect infiltrates in lungs, kidney, liver, as well as sublingual and parotid salivary glands and harderian lacrimal glands of 20 week old transgenic mice, similarly to NOD mice (Fig. 4B). Of note, in some of 30 week old NOD^{mini} females, but not NOD$^{\beta Tg}$ mice, we noticed development of lymphoproliferation, manifested by enlarged lymph nodes and spleen and infiltration into multiple organs (unpublished data). FACS analysis of lymphocytic infiltrates in affected exocrine glands showed that all of the infiltrating CD4$^+$ T cells expressed transgenic Vβ14 chain in NOD$^{\beta Tg}$ mice and Vβ14/Vα2 transgenic chains in NOD^{mini} mice (Fig. 4C). This also showed the aforementioned stability of expression of transgenic TCRs in experimental mice.

Development of SS in humans is often correlated with presence of anti-nuclear antibodies (ANA), anti-Ro/SSA, anti-La/SSB, anti-dsDNA, anti-αFodrin and anti-M3R [5,22,46]. In the NOD mouse model of SS, anti-SSA and anti-SSB auto-antibodies are rarely present and they are found at the very low levels [47]. To determine the presence of auto-antibodies in experimental mice, we used ELISA-based assay. For negative control, we used sera from NOD.TCRα$^{-/-}$ mice, that do not have T cells. As shown in Fig. 5, transgenic and parental NOD mice from 14–17 week old group had elevated levels of antibodies against αFodrin, ssDNA, dsDNA and ANA. Additionally, we determined the staining pattern of ANA auto-antibodies using immunofluorescent staining of HEp-2 cells (Fig. 5B). The majority (>90%) of NOD^{mini} and

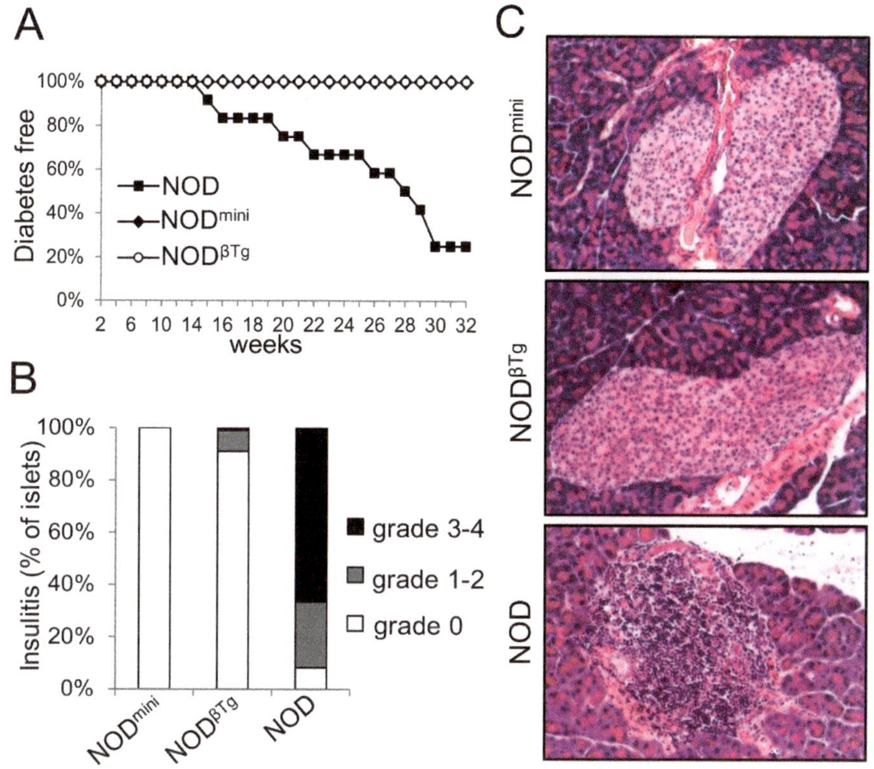

Figure 2. NOD$^{\beta Tg}$ and NOD^{mini} mice do not develop T1D. (A) Incidence of diabetes in mice shown as Kaplan–Meier survival curve. Mice with three consecutive measurements of blood glucose level above 250 mg/dL were considered diabetic. At least twelve mice per group were analyzed; $p<0.05$. (B) H&E staining of pancreatic tissue sections were analyzed for lymphocytic infiltrates and percentages of islets with grade of insulitis were counted. Insulitis was graded based on following criteria: no infiltrates – grade 0; peri-insulitis - grade 1; insulitis <25% - grade 2; insulitis <50% - grade 3; insulitis >50% - grade 4. At least six mice at 20 weeks of age were analyzed with the total number of 140 (NOD^{mini}), 155 (NOD$^{\beta Tg}$) and 160 (NOD) islets. (C) Example of H&E staining of pancreatic tissue sections of indicated mice at 20 weeks of age.

NOD$^{\beta Tg}$ mice tested had a speckled nuclear staining pattern, characteristic for SS development and found in parental NOD mice.

The onset of salivary gland dysfunction and presence of autoantibodies relies on B cells involvement and is dependent on IL-4 mediated IgM to IgG1 class switching [48–50]. Analysis of IgG1 concentration in sera of experimental mice revealed increased levels in older mice with the highest level in NOD^{mini} mice (Fig. 5C). This increase in IgG1 titer correlates with detection of auto-antibodies. Finally, to evaluate glandular dysfunction, we quantified secretion of saliva in 20 wks old mice. Both NOD$^{\beta Tg}$ and NOD^{mini} mice had reduced saliva flow as compared to healthy B6 mice and at the level of the reference parental NOD mice (Fig. 5D). Taken together, glandular infiltration, autoantibody production, and defective salivary secretion is diagnostic of Sjögren's syndrome in transgenic NOD$^{\beta Tg}$ and NOD^{mini} mice, similarly to the parental strain of NOD mice. Interestingly, the timing of infiltrates and levels of autoantibodies and total IgG1 production vary between analyzed mice, which differ only by TCR repertoire diversity.

Diversity of TCR repertoire on CD4$^+$ T cells in NOD^{mini} mice

Lack of certain specificities in NOD^{mini} TCR repertoire and the previously reported lower TCR diversity of thymic Treg cells on NOD background prompted us to take a closer look at the similarity and diversity of TCRα^{mini} repertoires. To determine the influence of TCR diversity reduction on the selection efficiency of TCRs in NOD mice we started with a single cell analysis to compare to a previously analyzed similar model of TCR^{mini} transgenic mice on "healthy" C57BL/6 background (B6^{mini}) [36]. We compared the similarity between TCR sequences from single cell sorted T_N (CD4$^+$Foxp3$^-$CD45RB$^+$CD62L$^+$) and Treg (CD4$^+$Foxp3$^+$) cells from thymii and peripheral lymph nodes of NOD^{mini} mice. As expected, based on the Morisita-Horn index, the highest similarity was observed between thymic and peripheral subsets of T_N or Treg cells, whereas comparison between populations of T_N and Treg cells showed mostly non-overlapping repertoires with values similar to those observed on B6 background (Fig. 6A and [36]). Previously we've shown that based on abundance coverage estimator (ACE), estimated richness (total unique CDR3α clonotypes in the population) of Treg cells in B6^{mini} mice significantly exceeded estimated richness of T_N cells [36]. Although ACE underestimates true richness at low sample size, it accounts for "unseen sequences" based on low abundance data and is suitable for comparative analyses. We combined thymic and peripheral sequences for each population and calculated the ACE index, based on 578 DNA sequences per subset. The ACE values for T_N and Treg cells were respectively 1187 and 994 for NOD^{mini} mice, and 1184 and 1815 for B6^{mini} mice. Interestingly, estimated ACE value for TCRs on T_N cells from NOD^{mini} mice was comparable to the ACE value for TCRs on T_N cells from B6^{mini} mice. However when we compared the ratio of ACE values for Treg cells between NOD^{mini} and B6^{mini}

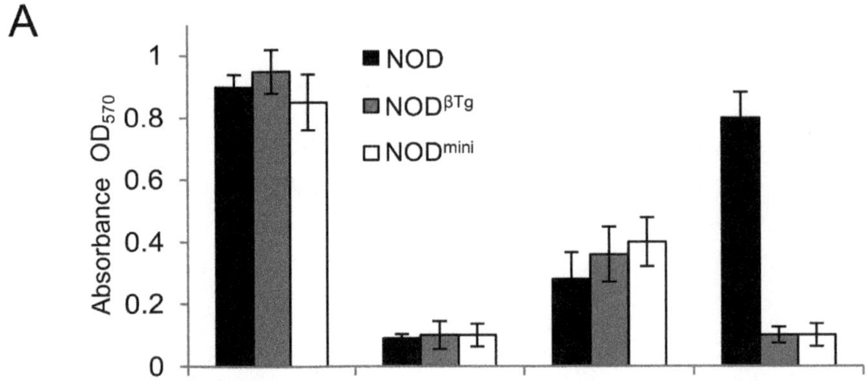

APC	A^{g7}	A^{g7}	A^b	A^{g7}
Ins B:9-23	-	-	-	+
anti-CD3	+	-	-	-

B

		Allo (A^b)	Ins B:9-23
Numbers of specific T-cell hybridomas	NOD	45/98	54/82
	$NOD^{\beta Tg}$	35/74	0/12
	NOD^{mini}	44/85	0/24

Figure 3. Lack of response to insulin B:9–23 peptide in transgenic NOD mice. (A) 5×10^4 of $CD4^+$ T cells sorted from lymph nodes of NOD, $NOD^{\beta Tg}$ and NOD^{mini} mice were cultured in the presence of 5×10^5 splenocytes from NOD.TCR$\alpha^{-/-}$ (A^{g7}) or B6.TCR$\alpha^{-/-}$ (A^b) mice and soluble anti-CD3 (1 μg/ml) or insulin B:9–23 peptide (50 μg/ml), as indicated. Proliferation of cells was measured after 3 days by MTT assay [38]. Experiments were done twice with 3 mice per group. (B) T-cell hybridomas specific to allo-antigens or insulin B:9–23 peptide were generated from indicated mice. For generation of B:9–23 specific hybridomas, mice were immunized with the peptide 7 days prior to isolation of lymph nodes for *in vitro* blasts generation [38]. Generated hybridomas were tested for their ability to respond to syngeneic (NOD.TCR$\alpha^{-/-}$) or allogeneic (B6.TCR$\alpha^{-/-}$) splenocytes with or without B:9–23 peptide or anti-CD3. Table shows numbers of identified hybridomas specific to indicated antigens and numbers of hybridomas responding to anti-CD3 stimulation. Table is representative of 3 independent experiments with two mice per group.

mice the number of possible unique TCRs on NOD background was reduced by almost 50% (Fig. 6B).

Previously it has been reported that based on analysis of two selected VJ (TCRα) or one VDJ (TVRβ) rearrangements in wild type mice, TCR repertoire of Treg cells in NOD mice was less diverse as compared to conventional T cells in the thymus, but also less diverse in the thymus of B6 mice [9]. These differences were observed based on calculation of Shannon entropy and normalization to the logarithm of unique sequences [9]. Such transformation is a measure of distribution of frequency of individual species and is a good measure of relative evenness of assemblage [51,52]. Together with richness, evenness is a descriptive measure of diversity not the diversity *per se* [51]. Therefore, as explained by Jost, to put the estimates in perspective, we converted Shannon entropy (diversity index) to "true diversity" by calculating "numbers equivalent" also called "effective number of species" (ENS), to preserve linear scale of comparison [51,53]. The ENS measure represents diversity of a particular sample, and the numeric value represents the theoretical number of equally common unique sequences in the assemblage. Comparison of "true diversity" between $B6^{mini}$ and NOD^{mini} mice showed almost reversal of ratios of diversities between TCRs on T_N and Treg cells, with the differences more profound in the thymus than in the periphery (Fig. 6C). These differences in NOD^{mini} mice were confirmed by high throughput sequencing, and were consistent regardless of total numbers of sequences analyzed (Fig. 6C, D). Lower diversity of Treg TCR repertoire was visualized empirically by plotting accumulation curves of observed sequences from peripheral T_N and Treg cells (Fig. 6E). These curves show that accumulation of unique CDR3 regions from the first 120 thousands of sequences for each population gives twice as many unique DNA clonotypes in T_N (9757) as compared to Treg cells (4968). This ratio is reversed in comparison to accumulation curves observed in $B6^{mini}$ mice [36]. Collectively our data show that although TCR diversity on Treg cells in NOD^{mini} mice is reduced, conventional T cells retain diverse TCR repertoire at least at the levels found on B6 background.

Discussion

In this study we investigated the impact of the reduction of TCR diversity on the development of two autoimmune diseases in NOD mice; T1D and SS. Previously it has been shown that T1D can develop despite use of transgenic TCRβ chains or reduction of precursor frequency of potentially diabetogenic T cell clones. In our model overall diversity of TCRs was reduced by allelic exclusion caused by use of transgenic TCRβ chain that was not only pathogenically irrelevant, but also was originally selected in B6 mice on I-A^b molecule. Despite normal distribution of Vα families in $NOD^{\beta Tg}$ mice, neither insulitis nor diabetes developed.

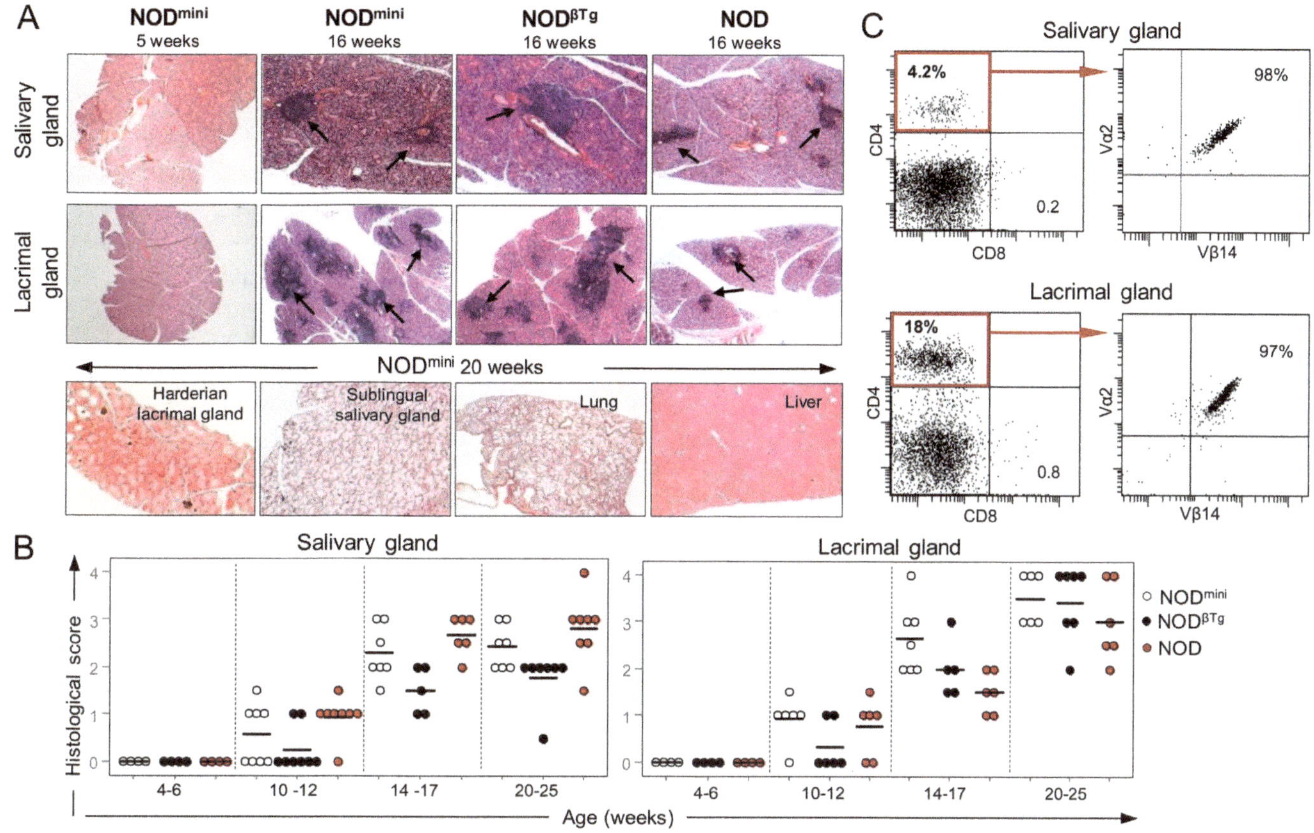

Figure 4. Lymphocytic infiltrates in mandibular salivary and extraorbital lacrimal glands. (A) H&E staining of tissue sections from indicated organs of analyzed mice, showing lymphocytic infiltrates indicated by arrows. (B) Histological score of infiltrated glands in indicated age groups. Scoring criteria: score 0, no infiltrates; score 1–1.5, 1–2 foci per section; 2–2.5, 3–5 foci per section; score 3, 6–10 foci per section; score 4, more than 10 foci per section. Infiltrate is considered as focus when number of infiltrating cells in continuous space is greater than 50. Three sections at different anatomical locations per organ were analyzed with at least 5 mice per age group. (C) FACS analysis of CD4 T cells infiltrating into salivary and lacrimal glands in 16 week old NOD^{mini} mice. Dot plots on the right show expression of transgenic TCR on CD4^{+} gated cells.

Conversely, these mice developed infiltrates in salivary and lacrimal glands, leading to autoantibody production and exocrine gland dysfunction. Further reduction of TCR diversity by generation of transgenic mice with TCR^{mini} repertoire, where one Vα segment is allowed to rearrange to only two Jα segments, did not prevent development of SS. Our results indicate that the difference between T1D and SS regarding the dependence on MHC polymorphism is directly correlated to the magnitude of possible TCR/peptide/MHCII interactions participating in the autoimmune phase of the disease.

We show that the lack of development of diabetes or even insulitis in our NOD$^{\beta Tg}$ or NOD^{mini} transgenic mice is due to lack of specificity to the key immunodominant insulin B:9–23 peptide, which is known to be instrumental for the onset of the T1D in NOD mice. The use of transgenic TCRVβ14 chain in our mice did not dramatically influence the ability of its binding to different TCRα chains, as T cells from NOD$^{\beta Tg}$ mice use all Vα families with frequencies found in NOD mice (Fig. 1). This includes efficient amplification of the Vα13 family which contains TRAV5D-4 chain (Vα13s1) that was shown to be sufficient to elicit anti-insulin autoimmunity without bias toward particular Vβ family of TCRβ chain partners [28,54]. Moreover, previous studies show that T cells using Vβ14 family were found on T cells specific to insulin antigen, T cells expanding in pancreatic lymph nodes or in T cells infiltrating pancreatic islets, showing that the Vβ14 family is not negatively influencing the development of diabetogenic TCRs [55–58]. One cannot exclude the possibility that this particular transgenic TCRVβ14 chain may be unable to pair with appropriate TCRα chain, preventing the ability of the expressed αβTCR to recognize the B:9–23 peptide. This selective requirement for a TCRβ chain would reinforce our observation that development of SS is less dependent than development of T1D on overall TCR diversity and a particular peptide/MHC combination.

Development of T1D relies on different insulin B:9–23 register recognition, allowing escape of specific T cells due to register shifting [11–13]. The lack of peripheral recognition of insulin B:9–23 in our transgenic mice can also be due to the impact of the limited TCR repertoire. Reduction of overall TCR diversity can influence (reduce) the precursor frequency of DP thymocytes bearing potentially autoreactive TCRs, resulting in more efficient negative selection in the thymus of NOD mice. It has been shown that early expression of transgenic αβTCR, due to ERK1/2 defect on NOD background results in greater commitment of the DN thymocytes to αβ lineage "overcrowding" DP compartment [8]. Our TCRα^{mini} transgene has natural timing of expression, similar to B6^{mini} and polyclonal NOD mice, where pre-TCR signaling is not perturbed by early expression of the transgene [36]. As suggested by Mingueneau et. al., in the polyclonal repertoire on the NOD background, the ERK1/2 defect increases the affinity threshold of positive selection, shifting the selection window of thymocytes toward self-reactivity, however not impacting the

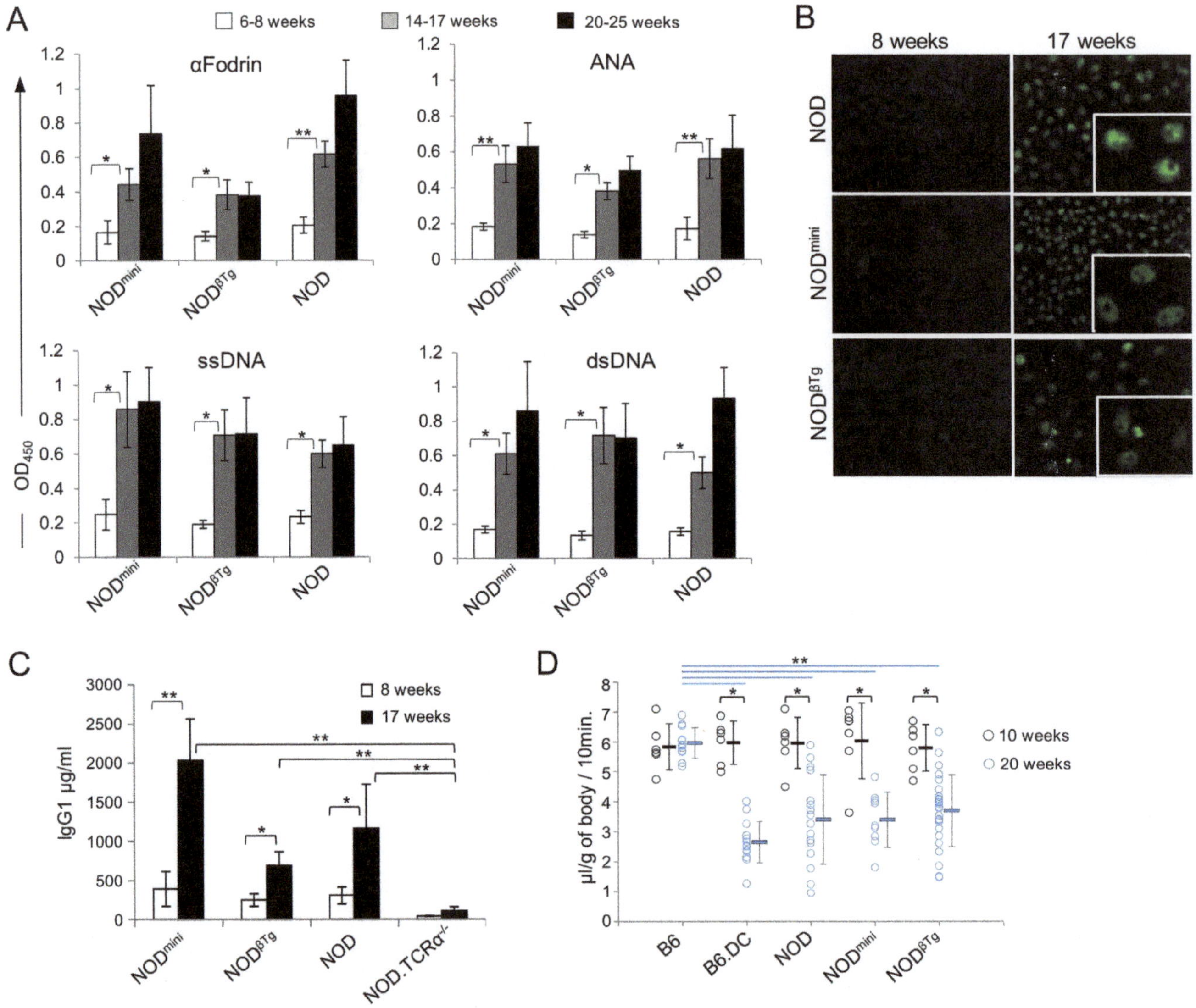

Figure 5. Detection of autoantibodies and hyposalivation in NOD^{mini} and NOD$^{\beta Tg}$ mice. (A) ELISA assay was performed using mouse serum (1:100) from indicated age groups. Each graph represents mean value of OD_{450} and standard deviation for indicated antigens. At least six mice were used per each group. *p<0.05, **p<0.005. (B) Detection of ANAs pattern using Hep-2 cell line. Sera from mice were diluted 1:40, incubated with HEp-2-fixed slides and evaluated under fluorescent microscope at x20 magnifications. Representative images are shown. (C) Quantitative ELISA analysis of IgG1 levels in sera (1:50,000) from indicated mice. Each bar represents mean value and standard deviation from six mice per experimental groups. (D) Salivary flow rates after pilocarpine injection in indicated mice at 10 and 20 wks of age. Double congenic B6.NODIdd3.NODIdd5 (B6.DC) mice, that develop SS on B6 genetic background, were used as a control. Saliva volume was measured and calculated in mg per mouse body mass. Each circle represents one mouse and horizontal lines indicate mean values of the experimental groups. T-test was used to calculate differences between groups. *p<0.002, **p<0.0002.

efficiency of negative selection. This results in higher overall self-reactivity of peripheral effector T cells and possibly explains lower diversity of thymic Treg cells on NOD background [8,9]. Considering partial overlap of specificities between Treg and autoreactive T cells, one could suggest similar effect of lower diversity on autoreactive population. However weak and unstable peptide-binding property of I-A^{g7} molecule does not favor the elimination or inactivation of autoreactive T cells [59]. This instability may have additional influence on "a leak" of autoreactive T cells, but also on inefficient generation of Treg population, which may require longer or stronger interactions with self MHC/peptide complexes [60,61]. Therefore the shift in selection window will not impact autoreactive T cells as much as it will impact Treg cells, after all, Treg development relies on recognition of self-peptide/MHCII complexes in the thymus, whereas thymic escape of autoreactive T cells relies on avoidance of such complexes during negative selection. It is possible that in our model, we reached the threshold of diversity required to generate autoreactive TCR repertoire without "holes" in specificities. Therefore despite reduced TCR diversity of Treg cells mice do not develop diabetes and we were unable to detect insulin B:9–23 specific T cells in the periphery. Similarly, the comparison of TCR^{mini} repertoires between B6 and NOD backgrounds shows minimal impact of the NOD genotype on TCR diversity of conventional CD4$^+$ T cells however it substantially reduces the TCR diversity on Treg cells in NOD mice.

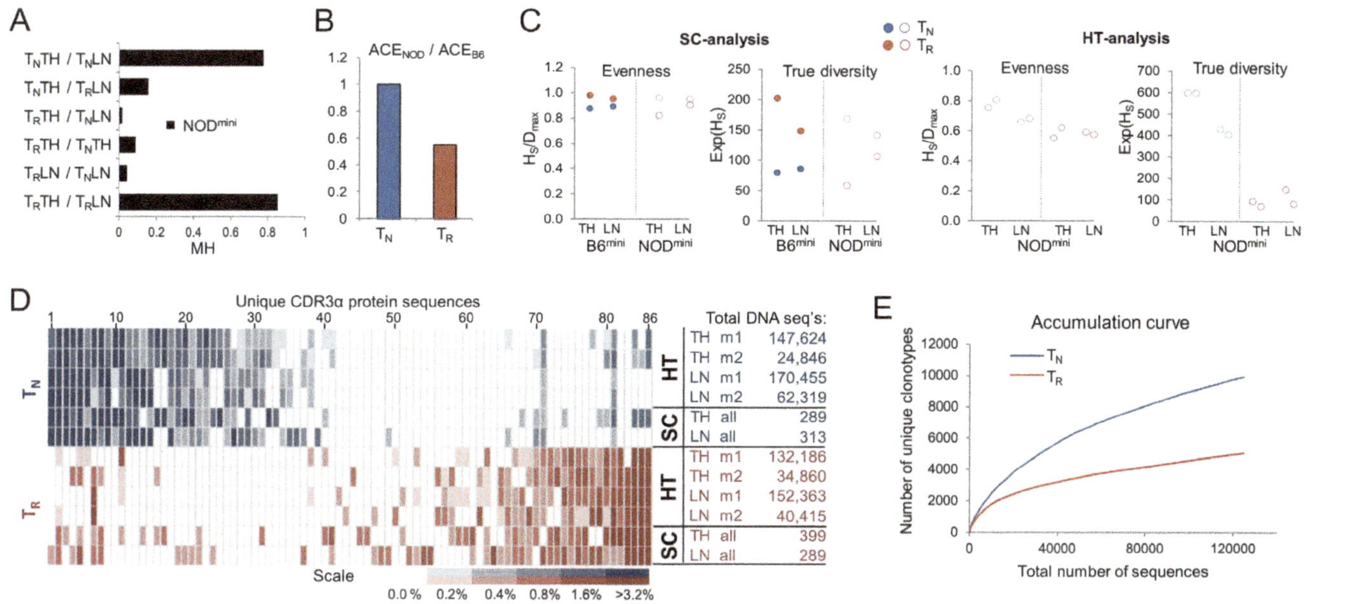

Figure 6. TCR repertoire of naïve and regulatory T cells in NOD^{mini} mice. (A) Similarity between indicated populations (first 289 single cell sequences per each population) was estimated based on Morisita-Horn index (MH). T_N - naïve CD4$^+$Foxp3$^-$CD45RB$^+$CD62L$^+$ T cells, T_R - regulatory CD4$^+$Foxp3$^+$ T cells, TH - thymus, LN - lymph nodes. (B) Ratio of richness of TCRs on T_N and T_R cells between NOD^{mini} and B6^{mini} mice. Abundance coverage estimator (ACE) was calculated based on 578 sequences for each population combined from thymus and peripheral lymph nodes. (C) Evenness and effective number of species (ENS) for analyzed TCR repertoires. Shannon evenness index was calculated as Shannon entropy (H_s) divided by maximum diversity D_{max}, where D_{max} equals natural logarithm of number of unique sequences in analyzed population. ENS (true diversity) was calculated as exponential of Shannon entropy. (D) Comparison of frequency of 20 most dominant unique protein CDR3 clonotypes found in each population indicated on the right of the heat map. Table indicates analyzed populations from lymph nodes and thymii by single cell analysis (SC) and high throughput sequencing (HT). Experimental mouse 1 and 2 are marked as m1 and m2. Numbers next to each population indicate total numbers of DNA sequences analyzed. All 86 unique CDR3α protein sequences in the heat map are shown in Table S1. (E) Accumulation curve of unique DNA clonotypes observed after accumulation of 124,730 sequences for T_N cells and 124,696 for T_R cells. (A–C) All indices were computed based on DNA sequences for each population using software SPADE and EstimateS8.2.

Development of SS in NOD^{mini} mice is especially interesting, since CD4$^+$ T cells are instrumental in immunopathogenesis and their recognition of self antigens is essential for the onset and progression of the disease [34,62]. It shows that the TCR^{mini} repertoire is diverse enough not only to drive glandular infiltration and activation of the CD4$^+$ T cells but also the repertoire is still diverse enough to support the full development of the disease with production of Th2-dependent IgG1 pathogenic autoantibodies (Fig. 5C) [50]. Moreover, we noticed differences in timing of infiltrates, levels of autoantibodies and total IgG1 production between transgenic mice and parental NOD mice, which indicates different frequencies of certain TCR specificities between mice. In congenic strains of NOD mice models of SS (NOD.B10-H2^b, NOD.H2^p, NOD.H2^q, NOD.H2^{h4}) replacement of I-A^{g7} with other MHC molecules does not prevent salivary and lacrimal gland infiltration and decreased saliva and tear production [16,48,63]. Interestingly, in NOD.H2^{h4}, contrary to the parental NOD strain, there is a high frequency of ANA with a high proportion of SSA/Ro and SSB/La observed [63]. Also, NOD.H2^q mice exhibit increased production of lupus-like types of autoantibodies and develop nephritis, as compared to NOD and NOD.H2^p mice [16]. This weak dependence of SS on a particular MHC haplotype in NOD mice correlates with our data that show development of SS despite limited TCR diversity. In human studies it was suggested that production profiles of certain autoantibodies were associated with HLA-DR haplotypes rather than with clinical manifestations [64], however studies of familial inheritance in patients with SS showed a linkage between particular HLA and disease susceptibility [65,66]. The most recent comprehensive analysis by Sjögren's Genetics Network showed that HLA has the strongest linkage to the SS, although it is not on the level of T1D [17]. Certain HLA haplotypes will influence binding diversity of self or environmental peptides and the nature of antigen presentation to T cells during thymic development or during immune responses in the periphery. Our results from the mouse model emphasize that SS may be less affected by requirement of a unique key antigen/MHCII combination but rather may be more influenced by a wider range of overall TCR/peptide/MHC interactions involved in the onset/progression of the disease. It can be due to a combination of cross-reactivity of the TCR repertoire on SS-specific T cells, wider range of antigens presented by MHCII molecules, higher peripheral self-reactivity of effector T cells, increased tissue expression of MHCII complexes on salivary epithelial cells and de novo expression or post-translational modification of self-antigens [67–69].

Supporting Information

Table S1 Protein sequences of unique CDR3α regions from the heat map of Fig. 6D.

Acknowledgments

Cell sorting was performed by Jeanene Pihkala in the GRU FACS Core, the sequencing was performed by John Nechtman in the GRU Genomic Core, and transgenic mice were generated by Gabriela Pacholczyk in the GRU Transgenic Core.

Author Contributions

Conceived and designed the experiments: JK RP. Performed the experiments: JK RD SL MB. Analyzed the data: JK RD SL MB RP. Contributed to the writing of the manuscript: JK RP.

References

1. Chaparro RJ, Dilorenzo TP (2010) An update on the use of NOD mice to study autoimmune (Type 1) diabetes. Expert Rev Clin Immunol 6: 939–955.
2. Lavoie TN, Lee BH, Nguyen CQ (2011) Current concepts: mouse models of Sjogren's syndrome. J Biomed Biotechnol 2011: 549107.
3. Anderson MS, Bluestone JA (2005) The NOD Mouse: A Model of Immune Dysregulation. Annu Rev Immunol 23: 447–485.
4. Mathis D, Vence L, Benoist C (2001) beta-Cell death during progression to diabetes. Nature 414: 792–798.
5. Nguyen CQ, Peck AB (2009) Unraveling the pathophysiology of Sjogren syndrome-associated dry eye disease. Ocul Surf 7: 11–27.
6. Fox RI (2005) Sjogren's syndrome. Lancet 366: 321–331.
7. Kishimoto H, Sprent J (2001) A defect in central tolerance in NOD mice. Nat Immunol 2: 1025–1031.
8. Mingueneau M, Jiang W, Feuerer M, Mathis D, Benoist C (2012) Thymic negative selection is functional in NOD mice. J Exp Med 209: 623–637.
9. Ferreira C, Singh Y, Furmanski AL, Wong FS, Garden OA, et al. (2009) Non-obese diabetic mice select a low-diversity repertoire of natural regulatory T cells. Proc Natl Acad Sci U S A 106: 8320–8325.
10. D'Alise AM, Auyeung V, Feuerer M, Nishio J, Fontenot J, et al. (2008) The defect in T-cell regulation in NOD mice is an effect on the T-cell effectors. Proceedings of the National Academy of Sciences 105: 19857–19862.
11. Stadinski BD, Zhang L, Crawford F, Marrack P, Eisenbarth GS, et al. (2010) Diabetogenic T cells recognize insulin bound to IAg7 in an unexpected, weakly binding register. Proceedings of the National Academy of Sciences 107: 10978–10983.
12. Mohan JF, Petzold SJ, Unanue ER (2011) Register shifting of an insulin peptide–MHC complex allows diabetogenic T cells to escape thymic deletion. J Exp Med 208: 2375–2383.
13. Marrack P, Kappler JW (2012) Do MHCII-Presented Neoantigens Drive Type 1 Diabetes and Other Autoimmune Diseases? Cold Spring Harbor Perspectives in Medicine 2.
14. Wicker LS, Appel MC, Dotta F, Pressey A, Miller BJ, et al. (1992) Autoimmune syndromes in major histocompatibility complex (MHC) congenic strains of nonobese diabetic (NOD) mice. The NOD MHC is dominant for insulitis and cyclophosphamide-induced diabetes. J Exp Med 176: 67–77.
15. Li X, Golden J, Faustman DL (1993) Faulty major histocompatibility complex class II I-E expression is associated with autoimmunity in diverse strains of mice. Autoantibodies, insulitis, and sialadenitis. Diabetes 42: 1166–1172.
16. Lindqvist AKB, Nakken B, Sundler M, Kjellen P, Jonsson R, et al. (2005) Influence on Spontaneous Tissue Inflammation by the Major Histocompatibility Complex Region in the Nonobese Diabetic Mouse. Scand J Immunol 61: 119–127.
17. Lessard CJ, Li H, Adrianto I, Ice JA, Rasmussen A, et al. (2013) Variants at multiple loci implicated in both innate and adaptive immune responses are associated with Sjogren's syndrome. Nat Genet 45: 1284–1292.
18. Nakayama M, Abiru N, Moriyama H, Babaya N, Liu E, et al. (2005) Prime role for an insulin epitope in the development of type[thinsp]1 diabetes in NOD mice. Nature 435: 220–223.
19. Arakaki R, Ishimaru N, Saito I, Kobayashi M, Yasui N, et al. (2003) Development of autoimmune exocrinopathy resembling Sjögren's syndrome in adoptively transferred mice with autoreactive CD4+ T cells. Arthritis Rheum 48: 3603–3609.
20. Takada K, Takiguchi M, Konno A, Inaba M (2005) Autoimmunity against a tissue kallikrein in IQI/Jic Mice: a model for Sjogren's syndrome. J Biol Chem 280: 3982–3988.
21. Winer S, Astsaturov I, Cheung R, Tsui H, Song A, et al. (2002) Primary Sjögren's syndrome and deficiency of ICA69. Lancet 360: 1063–1069.
22. Haneji N, Nakamura T, Takio K, Yanagi K, Higashiyama H, et al. (1997) Identification of alpha-fodrin as a candidate autoantigen in primary Sjogren's syndrome. Science 276: 604–607.
23. Naito Y, Matsumoto I, Wakamatsu E, Goto D, Ito S, et al. (2006) Altered peptide ligands regulate muscarinic acetylcholine receptor reactive T cells of patients with Sjogren's syndrome. Ann Rheum Dis 65: 269–271.
24. Matsumoto I, Maeda T, Takemoto Y, Hashimoto Y, Kimura F, et al. (1999) Alpha-amylase functions as a salivary gland-specific self T cell epitope in patients with Sjogren's syndrome. Int J Mol Med 3: 485–490.
25. Iizuka M, Wakamatsu E, Tsuboi H, Nakamura Y, Hayashi T, et al. (2010) Pathogenic role of immune response to M3 muscarinic acetylcholine receptor in Sjogren's syndrome-like sialoadenitis. J Autoimmun 35: 383–389.
26. Lipes MA, Rosenzweig A, Tan KN, Tanigawa G, Ladd D, et al. (1993) Progression to diabetes in nonobese diabetic (NOD) mice with transgenic T cell receptors. Science 259: 1165–1169.
27. Serreze DV, Johnson EA, Chapman HD, Graser RT, Marron MP, et al. (2001) Autoreactive diabetogenic T-cells in NOD mice can efficiently expand from a greatly reduced precursor pool. Diabetes 50: 1992–2000.
28. Zhang L, Jasinski JM, Kobayashi M, Davenport B, Johnson K, et al. (2009) Analysis of T cell receptor beta chains that combine with dominant conserved TRAV5D-4*04 anti-insulin B: 9–23 alpha chains. J Autoimmun 33: 42–49.
29. Dwyer E, Itescu S, Winchester R (1993) Characterization of the primary structure of T cell receptor beta chains in cells infiltrating the salivary gland in the sicca syndrome of HIV-1 infection. Evidence of antigen-driven clonal selection suggested by restricted combinations of V beta J beta gene segment usage and shared somatically encoded amino acid residues. J Clin Invest 92: 495–502.
30. Matsumoto I, Okada S, Kuroda K, Iwamoto I, Saito Y, et al. (1999) Single cell analysis of T cells infiltrating labial salivary glands from patients with Sjogren's syndrome. IntJ Mol Med 4: 519–527.
31. Pivetta B, De Vita S, Ferraccioli G, De RV, Gloghini A, et al. (1999) T cell receptor repertoire in B cell lymphoproliferative lesions in primary Sjogren's syndrome. J Rheumatol 26: 1101–1109.
32. Sumida T, Yonaha F, Maeda T, Tanabe E, Koike T, et al. (1992) T cell receptor repertoire of infiltrating T cells in lips of Sjogren's syndrome patients. J Clin Invest 89: 681–685.
33. Yonaha F, Sumida T, Maeda T, Tomioka H, Koike T, et al. (1992) Restricted junctional usage of T cell receptor V beta 2 and V beta 13 genes, which are overrepresented on infiltrating T cells in the lips of patients with Sjogren's syndrome. Arthritis Rheum 35: 1362–1367.
34. Singh N, Cohen PL (2012) The T cell in Sjogren's syndrome: Force majeure, not spectateur. J Autoimmun 39: 229–233.
35. Sumida T, Tsuboi H, Iizuka M, Hirota T, Asashima H, et al. (2014) The role of M3 muscarinic acetylcholine receptor reactive T cells in Sjögren's syndrome: A critical review. J Autoimmun.
36. Pacholczyk R, Ignatowicz H, Kraj P, Ignatowicz L (2006) Origin and T cell receptor diversity of Foxp3+CD4+CD25+ T cells. Immunity 25: 249–259.
37. Cha S, Nagashima H, Brown VB, Peck AB, Humphreys-Beher MG (2002) Two NOD Idd-associated intervals contribute synergistically to the development of autoimmune exocrinopathy (Sjogren's syndrome) on a healthy murine background. Arthritis Rheum 46: 1390–1398.
38. Pacholczyk R, Kern J, Singh N, Iwashima M, Kraj P, et al. (2007) Nonself-antigens are the cognate specificities of Foxp3+ regulatory T cells. Immunity 27: 493–504.
39. Kisielow J, Tortola L, Weber J, Karjalainen K, Kopf M (2011) Evidence for the divergence of innate and adaptive T-cell precursors before commitment to the alphabeta and gammadelta lineages. Blood 118: 6591–6600.
40. Kraj P, Pacholczyk R, Ignatowicz L (2001) Alpha beta TCRs differ in the degree of their specificity for the positively selecting MHC/peptide ligand. J Immunol 166: 2251–2259.
41. Pacholczyk R, Kraj P, Ignatowicz L (2002) Peptide specificity of thymic selection of CD4+CD25+ T cells. J Immunol 168: 613–620.
42. Lutsiak MEC, Semnani RT, De Pascalis R, Kashmiri SVS, Schlom J, et al. (2005) Inhibition of CD4+25+ T regulatory cell function implicated in enhanced immune response by low-dose cyclophosphamide. Blood 105: 2862–2868.
43. Harada M, Makino S (1984) Promotion of spontaneous diabetes in non-obese diabetes-prone mice by cyclophosphamide. Diabetologia 27: 604–606.
44. Michels AW, Ostrov DA, Zhang L, Nakayama M, Fuse M, et al. (2011) Structure-Based Selection of Small Molecules To Alter Allele-Specific MHC Class II Antigen Presentation. The Journal of Immunology 187: 5921–5930.
45. Cha S, Peck AB, Humphreys-Beher MG (2002) Progress in understanding autoimmune exocrinopathy using the non-obese diabetic mouse: an update. Crit RevOral BiolMed 13: 5–16.
46. Atkinson JC, Travis WD, Slocum L, Ebbs WL, Fox PC (1992) Serum anti-SS-B/La and IgA rheumatoid factor are markers of salivary gland disease activity in primary Sjogren's syndrome. Arthritis Rheum 35: 1368–1372.
47. Skarstein K, Wahren M, Zaura E, Hattori M, Jonsson R (1995) Characterization of T cell receptor repertoire and anti-Ro/SSA autoantibodies in relation to sialadenitis of NOD mice. Autoimmunity 22: 9–16.
48. Robinson CP, Yamachika S, Bounous DI, Brayer J, Jonsson R, et al. (1998) A novel NOD-derived murine model of primary Sjogren's syndrome. Arthritis Rheum 41: 150–156.
49. Brayer JB, Cha S, Nagashima H, Yasunari U, Lindberg A, et al. (2001) IL-4-dependent effector phase in autoimmune exocrinopathy as defined by the NOD.IL-4-gene knockout mouse model of Sjogren's syndrome. ScandJImmunol 54: 133–140.
50. Gao J, Killedar S, Cornelius JG, Nguyen C, Cha S, et al. (2006) Sjogren's syndrome in the NOD mouse model is an interleukin-4 time-dependent, antibody isotype-specific autoimmune disease. J Autoimmun 26: 90–103.
51. Jost L (2010) The Relation between Evenness and Diversity. Diversity 2: 207–232.
52. Pielou EC (1966) The measurement of diversity in different types of biological collections. J Theor Biol 13: 131–144.

53. Adelman MA (1969) Comment on the H Concentration Measure as a Numbers-Equivalent. The Review of Economics and Statistics 51: 99–101.
54. Nakayama M, Castoe T, Sosinowski T, He X, Johnson K, et al. (2012) Germline TRAV5D-4 T-Cell Receptor Sequence Targets a Primary Insulin Peptide of NOD Mice. Diabetes 61: 857–865.
55. Simone E, Daniel D, Schloot N, Gottlieb P, Babu S, et al. (1997) T cell receptor restriction of diabetogenic autoimmune NOD T cells. Proceedings of the National Academy of Sciences 94: 2518–2521.
56. Baker FJ, Lee M, Chien Y-h, Davis MM (2002) Restricted islet-cell reactive T cell repertoire of early pancreatic islet infiltrates in NOD mice. Proceedings of the National Academy of Sciences 99: 9374–9379.
57. Marrero I, Hamm DE, Davies JD (2013) High-Throughput Sequencing of Islet-Infiltrating Memory CD4$^+$ T Cells Reveals a Similar Pattern of TCR Vβ Usage in Prediabetic and Diabetic NOD Mice. PLoS ONE 8: e76546.
58. Petrovc Berglund J, Mariotti-Ferrandiz E, Rosmaraki E, Hall H, Cazenave P-A, et al. (2008) TCR repertoire dynamics in the pancreatic lymph nodes of non-obese diabetic (NOD) mice at the time of disease initiation. Mol Immunol 45: 3059–3064.
59. Carrasco-Marin E, Shimizu J, Kanagawa O, Unanue ER (1996) The class II MHC I-Ag7 molecules from non-obese diabetic mice are poor peptide binders. J Immunol 156: 450–458.
60. Aschenbrenner K, D'Cruz LM, Vollmann EH, Hinterberger M, Emmerich J, et al. (2007) Selection of Foxp3+ regulatory T cells specific for self antigen expressed and presented by Aire+ medullary thymic epithelial cells. Nat Immunol 8: 351–358.
61. Fontenot JD, Rasmussen JP, Williams LM, Dooley JL, Farr AG, et al. (2005) Regulatory T cell lineage specification by the forkhead transcription factor foxp3. Immunity 22: 329–341.
62. Sumida T, Tsuboi H, Iizuka M, Nakamura Y, Matsumoto I (2010) Functional role of M3 muscarinic acetylcholine receptor (M3R) reactive T cells and anti-M3R autoantibodies in patients with Sjögren's syndrome. Autoimmunity Reviews 9: 615–617.
63. Burek CL, Talor MV, Sharma RB, Rose NR (2007) The NOD.H2h4 mouse shows characteristics of human Sjogren's Syndrome. J Immunol 178: S232–S223d.
64. Gottenberg JE, Busson M, Loiseau P, Cohen-Solal J, Lepage V, et al. (2003) In primary Sjogren's syndrome, HLA class II is associated exclusively with autoantibody production and spreading of the autoimmune response. Arthritis Rheum 48: 2240–2245.
65. Fox RI, Kang HI (1992) Pathogenesis of Sjogren's syndrome. RheumDisClinNorth Am 18: 517–538.
66. Manoussakis MN, Georgopoulou C, Zintzaras E, Spyropoulou M, Stavropoulou A, et al. (2004) Sjogren's syndrome associated with systemic lupus erythematosus: clinical and laboratory profiles and comparison with primary Sjogren's syndrome. Arthritis Rheum 50: 882–891.
67. Anderton SM (2004) Post-translational modifications of self antigens: implications for autoimmunity. Curr Opin Immunol 16: 753–758.
68. Engelhard VH, Altrich-Vanlith M, Ostankovitch M, Zarling AL (2006) Post-translational modifications of naturally processed MHC-binding epitopes. Curr Opin Immunol 18: 92–97.
69. Moutsopoulos HM, Hooks JJ, Chan CC, Dalavanga YA, Skopouli FN, et al. (1986) HLA-DR expression by labial minor salivary gland tissues in Sjogren's syndrome. Ann Rheum Dis 45: 677–683.

Safety and Efficacy of Percutaneous Mitral Valve Repair Using the MitraClip® System in Patients with Diabetes Mellitus

Katharina Hellhammer[9], **Tobias Zeus**[9], **Jan Balzer, Silke van Hall, Christos Rammos, Rabea Wagstaff, Malte Kelm, Tienush Rassaf***

University Hospital Düsseldorf, Medical Faculty, Dept. of Medicine, Division of Cardiology, Pulmonology and Vascular Medicine, Düsseldorf, Germany

Abstract

Background: Patients with diabetes mellitus show a negative outcome in percutaneous coronary intervention, aortic valve replacement and cardiac surgery. The impact of diabetes on patients undergoing treatment of severe mitral regurgitation (MR) using the MitraClip system is not known. We therefore sought to assess whether percutaneous mitral valve repair with the MitraClip system is safe and effective in patients with diabetes mellitus.

Methods and Results: We included 58 patients with severe and moderate-to-severe MR in an open-label observational single-center study. Ninteen patients were under oral medication or insulin therapy for type II diabetes mellitus. MitraClip devices were successfully implanted in all patients with diabetes and in 97.4% (n = 38) of patients without diabetes (p = 0.672). Periprocedural major cardiac adverse and cerebrovascular events (MACCE) occurred in 5.1% (n = 2) of patients without diabetes whereas patients with diabetes did not show any MACCE (p = 0.448). 30-day mortality was 1.7% (n = 1) with no case of death in the diabetes group. Short-term follow up of three months showed a significant improvement of NYHA class and quality of life evaluated by the Minnesota Living with Heart Failure Questionnaire in both groups, with no changes in the 6-minute walk test.

Conclusions: Mitral valve repair with the MitraClip system is safe and effective in patients with type II diabetes mellitus.

Trial Registration: MitraClip Registry NCT02033811

Editor: Marc W. Merx, KRH Robert Koch Klinikum Gehrden, Germany

Funding: TR is a Heisenbergprofessor funded by the German Research Foundation (DFG RA969/7-2). This study was supported in part with a restricted grant from the federal state government of North Rhine-Westphalia and the European Union (EFRE-Program "Med in.NRW", support code 005-GW01-235A). The funders had no role in study design, data collection and analysis, decision to publish, or preparation of the manuscript.

Competing Interests: The authors have declared that no competing interests exist.

* Email: Tienush.Rassaf@med.uni-duesseldorf.de

[9] These authors contributed equally to this work.

Introduction

Mitral valve regurgitation (MR) is the second common valvular heart disease and severely affects morbidity and mortality [1–5]. Surgical treatment for many years used to be the first line treatment for patients with severe symptomatic MR [6]. Percutaneous mitral valve repair (PMVR) with the MitraClip system, however, has emerged to an effective therapeutic alternative for patients who can not undergo surgery due to high surgical risk [7]. Many of the high-risk patients present with diabetes mellitus, which is known to worsen outcome in patients referred to percutaneous coronary intervention (PCI) [8–12], cardiac surgery [13–15] or transcatheter aortic valve replacement (TAVI) [16,17]. The impact of diabetes on treatment of MR using the MitraClip system is not known. We therefore sought to assess whether percutaneous mitral valve repair with the MitraClip system is safe and effective in patients with diabetes mellitus.

Methods

The protocol for this trial and supporting CONSORT checklist are available as supporting information; see Checklist S1 and Protocol S1.

Patient selection and study design

A total of 58 Patients with symptomatic severe or moderate-to-severe MR evaluated by trans-thoracic and trans-esophageal echocardiography who underwent PMVR with the MitraClip System at the Heart Center Duesseldorf were included in the study (Figure 1). All patients were discussed in the institutional heart team and declined for surgical treatment due to high operative

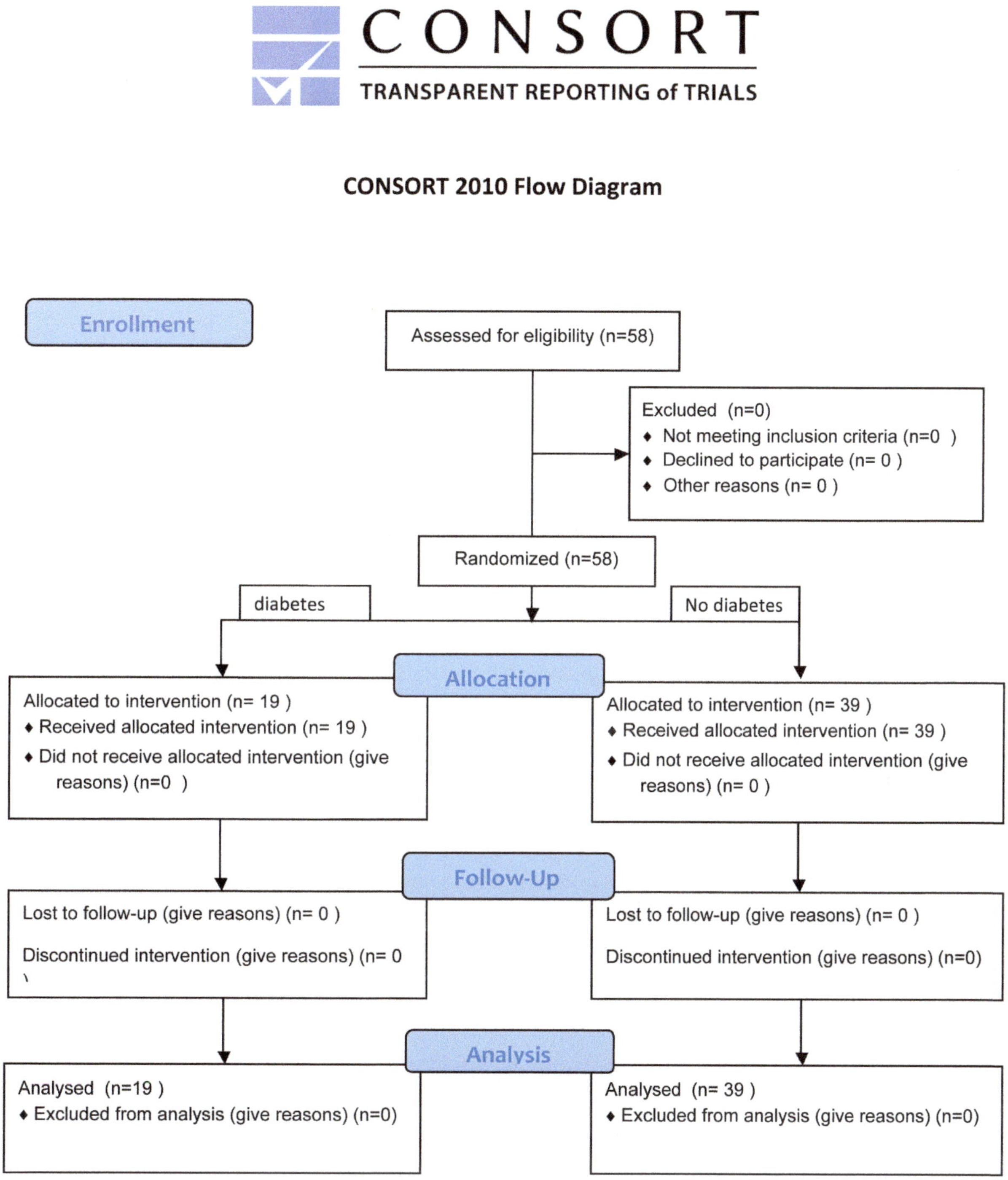

Figure 1. CONSORT flow chart.

risk. Patients were included into our registry after informed written consent was obtained. The registry is registered at clinical trials (NCT02033811). In a sub-analysis of this registry, patients were grouped according to the presence of type II diabetes mellitus (oral medication or on insulin therapy). The objective of the study was to evaluate the safety and efficacy of the MitraClip procedure in patients with diabetes mellitus with a follow-up after 3 months. Study procedures were in accordance with the Declaration of

Table 1. Baseline characteristics of patients undergoing MitraClip grouped according to the presence of diabetes mellitus type II.

	diabetes (n = 19)	no diabetes (n = 39)	p-value
Age, years ± SD	68±9.3	73±11.3	0.071
Male gender, n (%)	16 (84.2)	23 (59.0)	0.055
BMI, (kg/m^2) ± SD	28±4.5	26±4.6	0.175
Logistic EuroSCORE ± SD	18.7±15.5	18.6±17.6	0.975
CAD, n (%)	11 (57.9)	24 (61.5)	0.790
COPD, n (%)	5 (26.3)	9 (23.1)	0.787
Pulmonary hypertension, n (%)	11 (57.9)	26 (66.7)	0.514
Atrial fibrillation, n (%)	5 (26.3)	15 (38.5)	0.362
Hypertension, n (%)	19 (100)	36 (92.3)	0.214
Previous CABG, n (%)	5 (26.3)	11 (28.2)	0.880
Previous valve replacement, n (%)	2 (10.5)	8 (20.5)	0.472
Previous PCI (<3 month), n (%)	1 (5.3)	1 (2.6)	0.557
Previous myocardial infarction, n (5)	9 (47.4)	13 (33.3)	0.301
NYHA class III or IV, n (%)	17 (89.5)	35 (89.7)	0.649
Chronic kidney disease, n (%)	11 (57.9)	21 (53.8)	0.771
HbA1c, % ± SD	7.9±1.4	5.9±0.5	<0.01
Glucose, mg/dL ± SD	183±54	110±26	<0.01
GFR, mL/min ± SD	51±21	61±23	0.117
BNP, pg/mL ± SD	3315±4184	2918±2805	0.686
EF, % ± SD	37±13	45±16	0.062
LVEDD, mm ± SD	61±14	59±11	0.584
MR grade III, n (%)	18 (94.7)	30 (76.9)	0.142
MR type			
functional, n (%)	17 (89.5)	36 (92.3)	0.533
degenerative, n (%)	2 (10.5)	3 (7.7)	0.533
6-MWT, m ± SD	275±90	296±121	0.511
MLHF Q ± SD	44.7±14.9	43.4±12.3	0.734

SD = standard deviation; BMI = body mass index; CAD = coronary artery disease; COPD = chronic obstructive pulmonary disease; CABG = coronary artery bypass grafting; PCI = percutaneous coronary intervention; NYHA = New York Heart Association; BG = blood glucose; GFR = glomerular filtration rate; BNP = brain natriuretic peptide; EF = ejection fraction; LVEDD = left ventricular end-diastolic diameter; MR = mitral regurgitation; 6-MWT = 6-minute walk test; MLHF Q = Minnesota Living With Heart Failure Questionnaire.

Helsinki and the institutional Ethics Committee of the Heinrich-Heine University approved the study protocol.

Data collection and definitions

Collected data included patient characteristics, imaging findings, periprocedural in hospital data, laboratory results and follow up data up to three month after PMVR. Blood samples for biochemistry and hematology analysis results were taken before the procedure. Clinical outcome parameters for follow up after three months were NYHA classification, 6-minute walk test (6MWT), and quality of life measured by the Minnesota Living With Heart Failure Questionnaire (MLHF Q). Trans-thoracic echocardiography (TTE) was performed before the procedure and during follow up. Trans-esophageal echocardiography (TEE) was performed at baseline. Severity of mitral regurgitation was classified by TTE and TEE by measuring vena contracta (VC) and regurgitation volume. A severe mitral regurgitation was defined as a VC ≥0.7 cm and a regurgitation volume ≥60 ml [18,19].

In-hospital complications were reported for both groups. The definition of MACCE (major adverse cardiac and cerebrovascular event) included death, ST-elevation myocardial infarction, stroke and procedure related re-operation. A significant mitral stenosis after procedure was defined as a mean gradient >10 mmHg. Peripheral vascular complications were defined as minor vascular complication according to VARC II [38]. A major vascular complication was defined according to VARC II as overt bleeding either associated with a drop in hemoglobin level of at least 3.0 g/dL or requiring transfusion of two or three units of whole blood, or causing hospitalization, or permanent injury, or requiring surgery and does not meet criteria of life-threatening or disabling bleeding.

Procedure

The MitraClip procedure was performed either in general anesthesia or deep sedation using TEE and fluoroscopy for guidance. The procedure and the MitraClip System have previously been described in detail [20,21]. After a femoral venous access and transseptal puncture, the system is positioned in the left atrium. The arms of the clip are aligned perpendicular to the long axis of the leaflet edges and the clip is advanced into the left ventricle. After grasping the leaflets and checking the leaflet insertion the clip is deployed and the system removed.

Table 2. Periprocedural results of patients undergoing MitraClip grouped according to the presence of diabetes mellitus type II.

	diabetes (n = 19)	no diabetes (n = 39)	p-value
Successful clip implantation, n (%)	19 (100.0)	38 (97.4)	0.672
multiple clip implantation (>2), n (%)	0 (0.0)	0 (0.0)	
Procedure duration, min ± SD	121±43	120±37	0.895
Radiation time, min ± SD	30±12	27±11	0.388
Significant mitral stenosis, n (%)	0 (0.0)	1 (2.6)	0.672
Peripher vascular complication, n (%)	1 (5.3)	2 (5.1)	0.704
Stroke, n (%)	0 (0.0)	0 (0.0)	
MACCE, n (%)	0 (0.0)	2 (5.1)	0.448
Pacemaker damage, n (%)	0 (0.0)	1 (2.6)	0.672
Sepsis, n (%)	0 (0.0)	2 (5.1)	0.448
Ventilation>24 h, n (%)	0 (0.0)	1 (2.6)	0.672
Acute kidney injury stage III, n (%)	0 (0.0)	0 (0.0)	
Major bleeding, n (%)	0 (0.0)	1 (2.6)	0.672
Mitral valve surgery, n (%)	0 (0.0)	1 (2.6)	0.672
Death			
periprocedural (<72 hours), n (%)	0 (0.0)	0 (0.0)	
30-day mortality, n (%)	0 (0.0)	1 (2.6)	0.672

MACCE = major cardiac and cerebrovascular events.
Major bleeding was defined according to VARC II as overt bleeding either associated with a drop in hemoglobin level of at least 3.0 g/dL or requiring transfusion of two or three units of whole blood, or causing hospitalization, or permanent injury, or requiring surgery and does not meet criteria of life-threatening or disabling bleeding.

Statistical Analysis

Continuous data were expressed as mean ± standard deviation (SD) and compared with the unpaired student's t-test or Mann-Whitney U test if not normally distributed. Normality was checked with the Kolmogorov-Smirnov test. Categorical variables were evaluated as percentage and compared with the χ-square test or Fisher's exact test. Statistical analysis was performed with SPSS Statistics 22 (IBM) and Prism (GraphPad). A p-value <0.05 was considered to be significant.

Results

We enrolled 58 patients with symptomatic severe and moderate-to-severe MR. Nineteen patients (32.8%) presented with diabetes mellitus type II with either oral medication or insulin therapy. Groups did not differ except for HbA1c and blood glucose levels. Baseline characteristics are summarized in Table 1.

Primary endpoint – safety

The primary endpoint of this study was related to safety with regard to successful clip implantation, in-hospital complication rate, and 30-day mortality. MitraClips have been implanted successfully in all patients with diabetes, whereas one patient in the non-diabetic group had to undergo surgery for significant mitral stenosis. Complications were defined as MACCE (non-diabetes: 5.1% vs. diabetes: 0.0%), sepsis (non-diabetes: 5.1% vs. diabetes: 0.0%), ventilation >24 hours (non-diabetes: 2.6% vs. diabetes: 0.0%), peripheral vascular complications (non-diabetes: 5.1% vs. diabetes: 5.3%), acute kidney injury stage III (0.0% vs. 0.0%), pacemaker damage (non-diabetes: 2.6% vs. diabetes: 0.0%), stroke

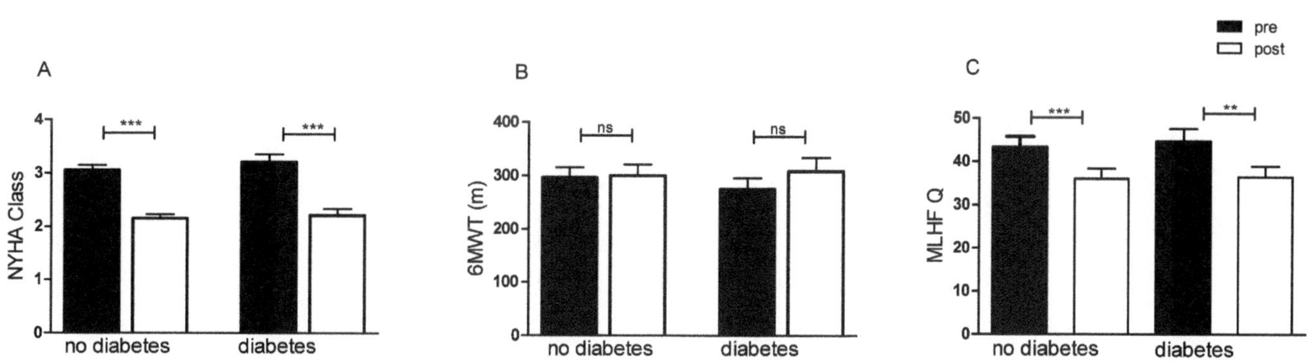

Figure 2. Changes in functional parameters after short-term follow up (3 months). A NYHA class before and 3 months after MitraClip. **B** 6-MWT before and 3 months after MitraClip. **C** Results of MLHF Q before and 3 months after MitraClip. NYHA = New York Heart Association; 6-MWT = 6-minute walk test; MLHF Q = Minnesota Living With Heart Failure Questionnaire. ns = non significant (p≥0.05). *** denotes p<0.0001, ** denotes p< 0.001.

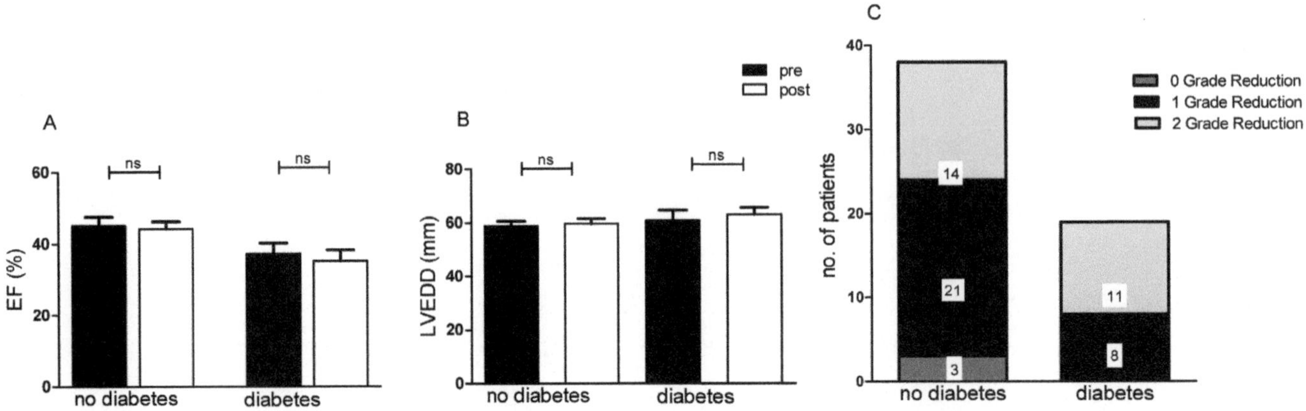

Figure 3. Changes in cardiac parameters after short-term follow up (3 month) in patients undergoing MitraClip. A Ejection fraction before and 3 months after MitraClip. **B** Left ventricular end-diastolic diameter before and 3 months after MitraClip. **C** Grade of reduction of mitral regurgitation 3 months after MitraClip. EF = ejection fraction; LVEDD = left ventricular end-diastolic diameter. ns = non significant ($p \geq 0.05$).

(0.0% vs. 0.0%) and major bleeding (non-diabetes: 2.6% vs. diabetes: 0.0%). Thirty-day mortality was 2.6% (n = 1) in non-diabetic patients due to a septic event. No patient died in the diabetes group. At the time of follow up overall survival was 98.3% (n = 57) with no death after discharge from hospital in both groups (Table 2).

Secondary endpoint – efficacy

The secondary endpoints were related to efficacy with regard to procedure duration (non-diabetes: 120±37 min vs. diabetes: 121±43 min; p >0.05), multiple clip implantation (0.0% vs. 0.0%) and radiation time (non-diabetes: 27±11 min vs. diabetes: 30±12 min; p >0.05).

At the time of follow up, significant improvement of NYHA class was seen in both groups from 3.1±0.6 to 2.2±0.5 (p<0.0001) in patients without diabetes and 3.2±0.6 to 2.2±0.5 (p<0.0001) in patients with diabetes. Quality of life measured by the MLHF Questionnaire was improved with a score reduction from 43±15 to 36±14 (p<0.0001) in non-diabetic patients and 45±12 to 36±11 (p<0.001) in patients with diabetes (Figure 2). 6-MWT (296±121.6 m to 300±130.8 m; p = 0.743), left ventricular ejection fraction (45±16% to 44±13%; p = 0.660), and left ventricular end-diastolic diameter (59±11 mm to 60±12 mm; p = 0.163) did not change in patients without diabetes. In patients with diabetes 6-MWT (275±90 m to 308±11 m; p = 0.057), ejection fraction (37±13% to 35±13%; p = 0.455) and left ventricular end-diastolic diameter (61±14 mm to 63±11 mm; p = 0.243) were also unaffected. MR reduction ≥1 grade was observed in 65.8% (n = 25) of patients without diabetes and in all patients with diabetes (Figure 3).

Discussion

The key findings of our study are: i) mitral valve repair with the MitraClip system is safe and effective in patients with diabetes mellitus. ii) This is associated with an improvement in functional status after three months follow up.

Patients with diabetes are at higher risk when undergoing PCI or cardiac surgery [8–15]. The underlying mechanisms are multifarious and involve an increased platelet activity, endothelial dysfunction [22,23], impaired wound healing, and a higher risk for infections caused by hyperglycemia [24,25]. Patients with diabetes moreover often present with comorbidities such as impaired renal function or coronary artery disease, which increase the surgical risk. PMVR with the MitraClip system has been shown to be safe and feasible and an alternative for surgical mitral valve repair in high-risk patients [7,20]. The role of diabetes in those patients, however, has not been investigated so far.

In our study population none of the diabetic patients died within 3 months follow-up. However, slightly higher mortality rates have been described [26–28]. These high mortality rates may reflect the morbidity of the patients who are referred to MitraClip procedure - sometimes as palliative therapy - and the importance of careful patient selection and risk stratification. Successful clip implantation was 100% in the diabetic group and 97.4% in the non-diabetic group. Overall complication rate was low in our study population, which has also been proved in other studies [29,30] and confirms the safety of the procedure. Diabetic patients did not present with a higher complication rate.

Previous studies have identified diabetes mellitus to be a risk factor for early and late mortality after surgical mitral valve repair [31,32,35]. Therefore it has been included in risk models like the Euroscore II or the STS score. Hospital mortality rates for mitral valve repair have been described from 1.5% to 6.5% [36,37]. Complications like deep sternal wound infection, stroke or acute renal failure after cardiac surgery are more likely in diabetic patients [33,34,35]. A less invasive treatment option like the MitraClip procedure in diabetic patients therefore seems to be an good alternative. Clinical outcome was improved after three months follow up in patients with diabetes and in non-diabetic patients. NYHA class was reduced and quality of life improved. These findings consist with other reports [26,28]. No improvement was observed in the 6-MWT in both groups, which may be due to the short-term follow up of three months in our study. In previous studies 6MWT was improved after 12 months [26,29]. Echocardiographic evaluation after three months showed a good result with an MR reduction ≥1 grade in 93.1% (n = 54) of the patients. All patients in the diabetes group did benefit from PMVR with an MR reduction ≥1 grade. There were no relevant changes in ejection fraction and LVEDD in our study population, which may be due to the short term period of follow up. Baseline ejection fraction was moderately to severely reduced in both groups and left ventricular end-diastolic diameter enlarged. Recovery might be seen after a longer period. In contrast, a previously published study reported a reduction of left ventricular end-diastolic volume after short-term follow up of 30 days and one year probably due to early reverse remodeling [28].

Our study has limitations. PMVR using the MitraClip system is safe and event rates are low. Therefore, a prospective randomized study with more patients and longer follow-up time is needed. Furthermore, patients should be classified concerning the duration of diabetes and diabetes-induced comorbidities.

Conclusion

We here show that the MitraClip procedure can be performed safely and effectively in patients with type II diabetes mellitus. Our short-term follow up shows an improvement in functional status in our patients with no negative influence on 3-month-mortality.

Supporting Information

Checklist S1 CONSORT Checklist.

Protocol S1 Trial Protocol.

Acknowledgments

All authors take responsibility for all aspects of the reliability and freedom from bias of the data presented and their discussed interpretation.

Author Contributions

Conceived and designed the experiments: TR MK TZ JB. Performed the experiments: KH RW CR SvH. Analyzed the data: CR RW KH SvH TR MK. Contributed reagents/materials/analysis tools: TR KH MK TZ JB. Wrote the paper: KH TZ JB CR SvH RW MK TR.

References

1. Iung B, Baron G, Butchart EG, Delahaye F, Gohlke-Bärwolf C, et al. (2003) A prospective survey of patients with valvular heart disease in Europe: The Euro Heart Survey on Valvular Heart Disease. Eur Heart J 24: 1231–43.
2. Nkomo VT, Gardin JM, Skelton TN, Gottdiener JS, Scott CG, et al. (2006) The burden of valvular heart diseases: a population-based study. Lancet 368: 1005–11.
3. Rossi A, Dini FL, Faggiano P, Agricola E, Cicoira M, et al. (2011) Independent prognostic value of functional mitral regurgitation in patients with heart failure. A quantitative analysis of 1256 patients with ischaemic and non-ischaemic dilated cardiomyopathy. Heart 97: 1675–80.
4. Trichon BH, Felker GM, Shaw LK, Cabell CH, O'Connor CM (2003) Relation of frequency and severity of mitral regurgitation to survival among patients with left ventricular systolic dysfunction and heart failure. Am J Cardiol 91: 538–43.
5. Patel JB, Borgeson DD, Barnes ME, Rihal CS, Daly RC, et al. (2004) Mitral regurgitation in patients with advanced systolic heart failure. J Card Fail 10: 285–91.
6. Bonow RO, Carabello BA, Chatterjee K, de Leon AC Jr, Faxon DP, et al. (2008) 2008 focused update incorporated into the ACC/AHA 2006 guidelines for the management of patients with valvular heart disease: a report of the American College of Cardiology/American Heart Association Task Force on Practice Guidelines. J Am Coll Cardiol 52: e1–142.
7. Feldman T, Foster E, Glower DD, Kar S, Rinaldi MJ, et al. (2011) Percutaneous repair or surgery for mitral regurgitation. N Engl J Med 364: 1395–406.
8. Ellis SG, Vandormael MG, Cowley MJ, DiSciascio G, Deligonul U, et al. (1990) The Multivessel Angioplasty Prognosis Study Group. Coronary morphologic and clinical determinants of procedural outcome with angioplasty for multivessel coronary disease: implications for patient selection. Circulation 82: 1193–1202.
9. Barsness GW, Peterson ED, Ohman EM, Nelson CL, DeLong ER, et al. (1997) Relationship between diabetes mellitus and long-term survival after coronary bypass and angioplasty. Circulation 96: 2551–6.
10. Cutlip DE, Chhabra AG, Baim DS, Chauhan MS, Marulkar S, et al. (2004) Beyond restenosis: five-year clinical outcomes from second-generation coronary stent trials. Circulation 110: 1226–30.
11. Malmberg K, Yusuf S, Gerstein HC, Brown J, Zhao F, et al. (2000) Impact of diabetes on long-term prognosis in patients with unstable angina and non-Q-wave myocardial infarction: results of the OASIS (Organization to Assess Strategies for Ischemic Syndromes) registry. Circulation 102: 1014–9.
12. Hillegass WB, Patel MR, Klein LW, Gurm HS, Brennan JM, et al. (2012) Long-term outcomes of older diabetic patients after percutaneous coronary stenting in the United States: a report from the National Cardiovascular Data Registry, 2004 to 2008. J Am Coll Cardiol 60: 2280–9.
13. Koch CG, Weng YS, Zhou SX, Savino JS, Mathew JP, et al. (2003) Prevalence of risk factors, and not gender per se, determines short- and long-term survival after coronary artery bypass surgery. J Cardiothorac Vasc Anesth 17: 585–93.
14. Olsen MA, Lock-Buckley P, Hopkins D, Polish LB, Sundt TM, et al. (2002) The risk factors for deep and superficial chest surgical-site infections after coronary artery bypass graft surgery are different. J Thorac Cardiovasc Surg 124: 136–45.
15. Halkos ME, Kilgo P, Lattouf OM, Puskas JD, Cooper WA, et al. (2010) The effect of diabetes mellitus on in-hospital and long-term outcomes after heart valve operations. Ann Thorac Surg 90: 124–130.
16. Conrotto F, D'Ascenzo F, Giordana F, Salizzoni S, Tamburino C, et al. (2014) Impact of diabetes mellitus on short-term and mid-term outcome after transcather aortic valve replacement (from a multicenter registry). Am J Cardiol 113: 529–534.
17. Pilgrim T, Stortecky S, Luterbacher F, Windecker S, Wenaweser P (2013) Transcatheter aortic valve implantation and bleeding: incidence, predictors and prognosis. J Thromb Thrombolysis 35: 456–462.
18. Bonow RO, Carabello BA, Chatterjee K, de Leon AC Jr, Faxon DP, et al. (2008) 2008 focused update incorporated into the ACC/AHA 2006 guidelines for the management of patients with valvular heart disease: a report of the American College of Cardiology/American Heart Association Task Force on Practice Guidelines (Writing Committee to revise the 1998 guidelines for the management of patients with valvular heart disease). Endorsed by the Society of Cardiovascular Anesthesiologists, Society for Cardiovascular Angiography and Interventions, and Society of Thoracic Surgeons. J Am Coll Cardiol 52: e1–142.
19. Zoghbi WA, Enriquez-Sarano M, Foster E, Grayburn PA, Kraft CD, et al. (2003) Recommendations for evaluation of the severity of native valvular regurgitation with two-dimensional and doppler echocardiography. J Am Soc Echocardiogr 16: 777–802.
20. Feldman T, Wasserman HS, Herrmann HC, Gray W, Block PC, et al. (2005) Percutaneous mitral valve repair using the edge-to edge technique: six-month results of the EVEREST Phase 1 Clinical Trial. J Am Coll Cardiol 46: 2134–2140.
21. Feldman T, Kar S, Rinaldi M, Fail P, Hermiller JT, et al. (2009) Percutaneous mitral repair with the MitraClip system: safety and midterm durability in the initial EVEREST (Endovascular Valve Edge-to-Edge REpair Study) cohort. J Am Coll Cardiol 54: 686–694.
22. Jain SK, Nagi DK, Slavin BM, Lumb PJ, Yudkin JS (1993) Insulin therapy in type 2 diabetic subjects suppresses plasminogen activator inhibitor (PAI-1) activity and proinsulin-like molecules independently of glycaemic control. Diabetes Med 10: 27–32.
23. Williams SB, Goldfine AB, Timimi FK, Ting HH, Roddy MA, et al. (1998) Acute hyperglycemia attenuates endothelium-dependent vasodilation in humans in vivo. Circulation 97: 1695–1701.
24. Bitkover CY, Gardlund B (1998) Mediastinitis after cardiovascular operations: a case-control study of risk factors. Ann Thorac Surg 65: 36–40.
25. Salomon NW, Page US, Okies JE, Stephens J, Krause AH, et al. (1983) Diabetes mellitus and coronary artery bypass: short-term risk and long-term prognosis. J Thorac Cardiovasc Surg 85: 264–271.
26. Taramasso M, Maisano F, Denti P, Latib A, La Canna G, et al. (2014) Percutaneous edge-to-edge repair in high-risk and elderly patients with degenerative mitral regurgitation: Midterm outcomes in a single-center experience. J Thorac Cardiovasc Surg DOI: 10.1016/j.jtcvs.2014.03.036. In press.
27. Reichenspurner H, Schillinger W, Baldus S, Hausleiter J, Butter C, et al. (2013) Clinical outcomes through 12 months in patients with degenerative mitral regurgitation treated with the MitraClip® device in the ACCESS-EUrope Phase I trial. Eur J Cardiothorac Surg 44: e280–8.
28. Whitlow PL, Feldman T, Pedersen WR, Lim DS, Kipperman R, et al. (2012) Acute and 12-month results with catheter-based mitral valve leaflet repair: the EVEREST II (Endovascular Valve Edge-to-Edge Repair) High Risk Study. J Am Coll Cardiol 59: 130–139.
29. Maisano F, Franzen O, Baldus S, Schäfer U, Hausleiter J, et al. (2013) Percutaneous mitral valve interventions in the real world: early and one year results from the ACCESS-EU, a prospective, multicenter, non-randomized post-approval study of the MitraClip® therapy in Europe. J Am Coll Cardiol 62: 1052–1061.
30. Bakker AL, Swaans MJ, van der Heyden JA, Eefting FD, Rensing BJ, et al. (2013) Complications during percutaneous edge-to-edge mitral valve repair. Herz 38: 484–9.
31. Crabtree TD, Bailey MS, Moon MR, Munfakh N, Pasque MK, et al. (2008) Recurrent mitral regurgitation and risk factors for early and late mortality after mitral valve repair for functional ischemic mitral regurgitation. Ann Thorac Surg 85: 1537–43.
32. Nowicki ER, Birkmeyer NJ, Weintraub RW, Leavitt BJ, Sanders JH, et al. (2004) Multivariable prediction of in-hospital mortality associated with aortic and mitral valve surgery in Northern New England. Ann Thorac Surg 77: 1966–77.

33. Parolari A, Pesce LL, Pacini D, Mazzanti V, Salis S, et al. (2012) Risk factors for perioperative acute kidney injury after adult cardiac surgery: role of perioperative management. Ann Thorac Surg 93: 584–91.
34. Ariyaratnam P, Bland M, Loubani M (2010) Risk factors and mortality associated with deep sternal wound infections following coronary bypass surgery with or without concomitant procedures in a UK population: A basis for a new risk model? Interact Cardiovasc Thorac Surg 11: 543–546.
35. Brown JR, Edwards FH, O'Connor GT, Ross CS, Furnary AP (2006) The diabetic disadvantage: historical outcomes measures in diabetic patients undergoing cardiac surgery — the pre-intravenous insulin era. Semin Thorac Cardiovasc Surg 18: 281–8.
36. Craver JM, Cohen C, Weintraub WS (1990) Case-matched comparison of mitral valve replacement and repair. Ann Thorac Surg 49: 964–9.
37. Fremes SE, Goldman BS, Ivanov J, Weisel RD, David TE, et al. (1989) Valvular surgery in the elderly. Circulation 80: I77–90.
38. Kappetein AP, Head SJ, Généreux P, Piazza N, van Mieghem NM, et al. (2013) Updated standardized endpoint definitions for transcatheter aortic valve implantation: the Valve Academic Research Consortium-2 consensus document. J Thorac Cardiovasc Surg 145: 6–23.

18

An Immunohistochemical Analysis to Validate the Rationale behind the Enhanced Immunogenicity of D-Ribosylated Low Density Lipo-Protein

Firoz Akhter[1,2], M. Salman Khan[2]*, Sarika Singh[3], Saheem Ahmad[2]*

1 Department of Bio-Engineering, Integral University, Lucknow, India, 2 Department of Bio-Sciences, Integral University, Lucknow, India, 3 Department Toxicology, Central Drug Research Institute (CDRI), Lucknow, India

Abstract

Advanced glycation end products (AGEs) are thought to contribute to the abnormal lipoprotein profiles and increased risk of cardiovascular disease in patients with diabetes and renal failure. D-ribose is one of the naturally occurring pentose monosaccharide present in all living cells and is a key component of numerous biomolecules involved in many important metabolic pathways. Formation of D-ribose derived glycated low density lipoprotein (LDL) has been previously demonstrated but no studies have been performed to assess the immune complex deposition in the kidney of rabbits immunized with glycated LDL. In this study, LDL was glycated with D-ribose, and it was further used as an immunogen for immunizing NZW female rabbits. The results showed that female rabbits immunized with D-ribose modified LDL induced antibodies as detected by direct binding and competitive ELISA. The modified LDL was found to be highly immunogenic eliciting high titer immunogen-specific antibodies, while the native forms were moderately immunogenic. The induced antibodies from modified LDL exhibited wide range of heterogeneity in recognizing various proteins and amino acids conformers. Furthermore, our histopathological results illustrated the deposits of immune complex in glomerular basement membrane in rabbits immunized with D-ribose-LDL.

Editor: Cordula M. Stover, University of Leicester, United Kingdom

Funding: The authors have no support or funding to report.

Competing Interests: The authors have declared that no competing interests exist.

* Email: ahmadsaheem@gmail.com (SA); contactskhan@gmail.com (MSK)

Introduction

Non-enzymatic glycation of proteins is a post-translational modification process [1], leading to the formation of fructosamine [2] and advanced glycation end products (AGEs) [3,4]. It has also been reported that there is the generation of oxygen free radicals in the formation of early and advanced glycation end-products [5]. Basically, glycation is a condensation of free carbonyl group of reducing sugars with a free amino group of DNA, proteins and LDL macromolecules. The reaction proceeds by nucleophilic addition reaction followed by dehydration, cyclization and rearrangement to form AGEs. The role of glucose in the glycation of proteins has been widely studied however the role of other reducing monosaccharides such as D-ribose in glycation and their resulting effects on animal model has received much less attention. AGEs are heterogeneous class of compounds containing a mixture of cyclic and open chain structures out of which large numbers of AGEs are not determined till date. However, few AGEs which are known like pentosidine, carboxymethyl-lysine (CML), carboxyethyl-lysine (CEL), fructosyl-lysine (FL), which plays an important role in atherosclerosis and nephropathy. The lipoprotein glycation process occurs both on the apoprotein B (apoB) and on phospholipid components of LDL. It leads both functional alterations in LDL clearance and increased susceptibility to oxidative modifications [6]. In addition, oxidative stress and other conditions causing oxidation of LDL stimulate the synthesis of nuclear polymers of adenosine diphosphate ribose (ADP-ribose), which in turn can release monomeric ADP-ribose. The bioavailability of D-ribose makes this carbonyl species quite reactive and damaging, therefore having direct implication in diabetes.

There are ample evidences which indicate the role of lipoprotein glycation in the inflammatory reactions in the vessel wall [7]. Various oxidative stresses of different proteins may be involved in proinflammatory immune mechanisms. These may involve innate immune signals, Toll-like receptors [8] and adaptive immunity signals which are both cell-mediated [9] and antibody-mediated [10]. There are ample of evidences supporting the pathogenic role of humoral response to modified lipoproteins [11–14]. This is mainly due to the fact that modified LDL and its corresponding antibodies form modified LDL immune complexes (mLDL-IC), which are able to activate phagocytic cells through engagement of Fc receptors [14]. Engagement of Fc receptors by mLDL-IC is particularly significant because it delivers stronger activating signals to phagocytic cells than the engagement of scavenger receptors by modified LDL [11]. Native LDL was found to be moderately immunogenic in experimental animals, while, modified form of LDL was found to be highly immunogenic [15].

This study was aimed to see the immunogenicity of native and glycated LDL. The cross reactivity experiments were performed to check the specificity of the raised antibodies using various glycated and non-glycated inhibitors including poly amino acids. Moreover, the immuno-histochemistry was performed to see the immune complex deposition in the kidney of immunized female rabbits.

Materials and Methods

Ethics statement

The immunization work was approved by Institutional Animal Ethical Committee of Integral University, Lucknow, India by approval No: IU/Biotech/Project/CPCSEA/12/20. The animals were treated with utmost care and treatments were done with minimum pain. The *in vivo* experiments on rabbits were performed according to the ARRIVE guidelines. After the end of experiment the rabbits were sacrificed by the over dosage of thiopentone sodium anesthesia by intra venous mode of injection (≥150 mg/kg).

Materials

D-ribose, Tris-HCl, EDTA, PTA, TBA, Protein A-Agarose column were obtained from Sigma, St. Louis, MO. Polystyrene plates obtained from Nunc (Roskilde, Denmark), HSA, Hb, IgG, Poly-L-lysine, Poly-L-arginine, Poly-L-histidine were obtained from MP Biomedicals and LDL, Anti rabbit IgG, pNPP were purchased from Calbiochem. All other chemicals used in this study were of highest analytical grade available in the country.

Glycation of LDL

LDL was modified by using different concentrations of D-ribose [16]. LDL (62.5 µg/ml) was thoroughly mixed with 80 mM of ribose sugar in 100 mM phosphate buffer saline (PBS), pH 7.4 and incubated at 37°C for three weeks, followed by extensive dialysis against phosphate buffer saline to remove unbound constituents. LDL alone was served as control [17].

Various proteins like HSA, Hb, IgG and Poly amino acids like Poly-L-lysine, Poly-L-arginine and Poly-L-histidine were also modified by using D-ribose with same concentration and with the same procedure [17].

Measurement of superoxide anion

To detect the presence of $O2^{\cdot -}$ anion in the LDL glycation mixture, a cytochrome-c reduction assay was performed. The reaction mixture contained D-ribose (80 mM) and 100 µM cytochrome-c in 20 mM phosphate buffer (pH 7.4). The reduction rate was determined as the increase in absorbance at 550 nm for 10 min at room temperature. Absorbance was taken at one min intervals [18].

Measurement of hydroxyl radical

Detection of hydroxyl radicals was carried out by measuring thiobarbituric acid (TBA) reactive 2-deoxy-D-ribose oxidation products. Reaction mixtures containing 80 mM D-ribose, and LDL (62.5 µg/ml) was incubated at 37°C for two weeks. The degradation of 2-deoxy-D-ribose was measured by adding 1 mL of 2.8% (w/v) trichloroacetic acid, 1 mL of 1% (w/v) thiobarbituric acid followed by heating at 100°C for 10 min. After cooling the absorbance was read at 532 nm [19].

Immunization Schedule

LDL (25 µg), its D-ribose modified counterpart and D-ribose (25 µg) were emulsified with complete Freund's adjuvant. The complex and 500 µl CFA were injected intramuscularly in the hind leg muscles of rabbits (three animals in each group). Subsequent injections were given in incomplete Freund's adjuvant until the period of study. Weekly injections of antigen (LDL/D-ribose modified LDL/D-ribose) were given for seven weeks and thus each animal received a total of 175 µg antigen during the course of immunization. One week after the last dose of immunogen, blood was collected and put it at 37°C for 2–3 hours. The serum separated and decomplemented by heating at 56°C for 30 min on the water bath. Preimmune blood was collected prior to immunization. The serum was stored in small aliquots at −80°C with sodium azide (0.1%) as preservative [20].

Estimation of Conjugate diene (CD) and Thiobarbituric acid reducing substance (TBARS) in plasma

The blood from each NZW female rabbit in a given group was collected in heparinized tubes, for 2–3 h, mixed gently by inversion 2–3 times and incubated at 40°C. Plasma was separated from blood by centrifugation at 2,500 rpm for 30 min, aliquoted and stored at −20°C.

For the extraction of Lipid contents from plasma, the method of Folch *et al.* [21] was employed. One volume of plasma was mixed with 5.0 volume of chloroform: methanol (2:1), followed by centrifugation at 1,000 rpm for 5 min to separate the phases. Most of the upper layer was removed; and 3.0 ml of the lower chloroform layer was recovered. The chloroform layer was placed in a test tube and incubated at 45°C till dryness. For the determination of conjugated diene (CD) in plasma, corresponding lipid residues were dissolved in 1.5 ml of cyclohexane and the absorbance was recorded at 234 nm against a cyclohexane blank in a Beckman DU 640 spectrophotometer. The concentration of conjugated diene formation was calculated by using a molar extinction coefficient of $2.52 \times 1\,0^4\ M^{-1}cm^{-1}$.

Lipid peroxide conteOnts in plasma were assayed by the method of Yagi [22]. Plasma (25 µl) was mixed with 4.0 ml of 0.083 N

Table 1. Effect of CFA, D-ribose, N-LDL and G-LDL on plasma TBARS and Conjugated Diene (CD) in control and treated NZW female rabbits.

S.No.	Sera	Conjugated diene (CD)	TBARS
1.	Preimmune sera	15.15 nM±0.041 nM	0.48 µM±0.044 µM
2.	CFA immunized sera	22.5 nM±0.17 nM	0.044 µM±0.006 µM
3.	D-ribose immunized sera	27.22 nM±0.73 nM	0.09 µM±0.03 µM
4.	N-LDL immunized sera	27.38 nM±0.13 nM	0.112 µM±0.042 µM
5.	G-LDL immunized sera	54.76 nM±0.088 nM	3.85 µM±0.057 µM

Each data represents average of three experiments. The values represent the mean ± SD.

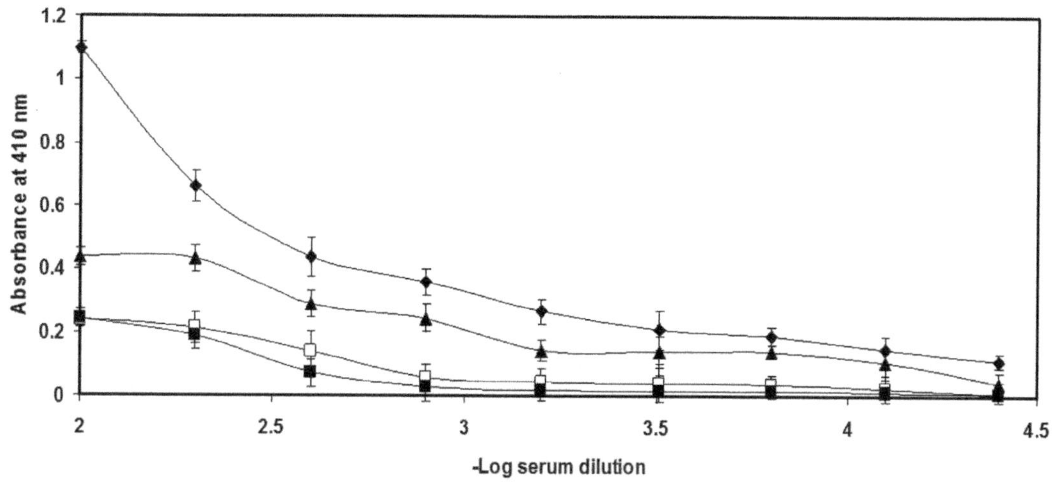

Figure 1. Level of induced antibodies against D-ribose-modified LDL. Direct binding ELISA of D-ribose antisera (□), N-LDL antisera (▲), G-LDL antisera (♦) and preimmune sera (■). The microtiter wells were coated with D-ribose, N-LDL and G-LDL (10 μg/ml) in direct binding ELISA of D-ribose antisera, native LDL antisera and G-LDL antisera respectively. Each data represents average of three experiments. The values represent the mean ± SD.

H_2SO_4 followed by the addition of 0.5 ml of 10% phosphotungstic acid. The samples were mixed and incubated for 5 min at room temperature and then centrifuged at 3,000 rpm for 10 min. The supernatant was discarded and the sediment was mixed with 2.0 ml of 0.083 N H_2SO_4 and 0.3 ml of 10% phosphotungstic acid. The mixture was centrifuged at 3,000 rpm for 10 min, the sediment was suspended in 4.0 ml of water and 1.0 ml of TBA reagent (a mixture containing equal volumes of 0.67% aqueous TBA solution and glacial acetic acid) was added. The reaction mixture was heated for 60 min at 95°C, cooled and the tubes were centrifuged at 3,000 rpm for 10 min. The absorbance of the supernatant was determined at 532 nm against a reagent blank in an Eppendorf Bio Spectrometer. The concentration of MDA was calculated by using a standard malondialdehyde [23].

Enzyme linked immunosorbent assay (ELISA)

ELISA was performed on polystyrene plates [24] with slight modification. Polystyrene polysorp immunoplates were coated with 100 μl of the D-ribose, native or glycated LDL (10 μg/ml) in 0.05 mol/l carbonate–bicarbonate buffer, pH 9.6. The plates were incubated for 2 hours at 37°C and overnight at 4°C. Each sample was coated in duplicate and half of the plate, devoid of antigen coating, served as control. Unbound antigen was washed three times with TBS-T (20 mmol/l Tris, 150 mmol/l NaCl, pH 7.4 containing 0.05% Tween-20), and unoccupied sites were blocked with 2% fat-free skimmed milk in TBS (10 mmol/l Tris, 150 mmol/l NaCl, pH 7.4) for 6 hours at 37°C. After incubation, the plates were washed again three times with TBS-T. Test serum was added to antigen-coated wells and reincubated for 2 hours at 37°C and overnight at 4°C. Bound antibodies were assayed with anti-rabbit IgG-alkaline phosphatase conjugate using *p*-nitrophenyl phosphate (pNPP) as substrate. Absorbance (A) of each well was monitored at 410 nm on an automatic microplate reader, and the mean of duplicate readings for each sample was recorded. Results have been expressed as a mean of A_{test}-$A_{control}$.

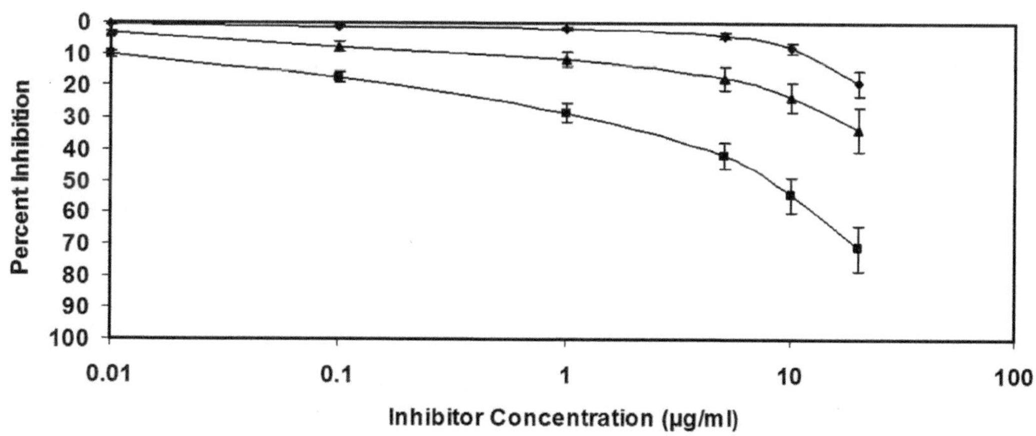

Figure 2. Inhibition of serum antibodies against N-LDL and G-LDL binding by D-ribose (♦), N-LDL (▲) and G-LDL (■) respectively. The microtiter plate was coated with D-ribose, N-LDL and G-LDL (10 μg/ml) respectively. Each data represents average of three experiments. The values represent the mean ± SD.

Table 2. Cross reaction of anti-D-ribose-modified LDL IgG.

S.No.	Inhibitors	Maximum % inhibition At 20 μg/ml	Concentration for 50% inhibition (μg/ml)	Percent relative affinity
1.	D-ribose-LDL	82.3±0.71	2.5±0.04	100±0.04
2.	Native LDL	33.4±0.15	---	---
3.	D-ribose-HSA	46.22±1.34	---	---
4.	Native HAS	32.15±1.03	---	---
5.	D-ribose-Hb	52.03±1.74	18.4±0.12	13.59±0.25
6.	Native Hb	24.21±0.78	---	---
7.	D-ribose-IgG	48.101±0.86	---	---
8.	Native IgG	23.17±0.23	---	---
9.	D-ribose-Poly-L-lysine	56.8±1.81	15.3±0.22	16.34±0.26
10.	Native Poly-L-lysine	27.27±0.32	---	---
11.	D-ribose-Poly-L-arginiine	58.312±1.32	13.7±0.11	18.25±0.28
12.	Native Poly-L- arginiine	18.27±0.21	---	---
13.	D-ribose-Poly-L-Histidine	39.78±0.42	---	---
14.	Native Poly-L- Histidine	26.022±0.32	---	---

Micro titer plates were coated with D-ribose-modified LDL (10.0 μg/mL). Each data represents average of three experiments. The values represent the mean ± SD.

Competitive ELISA/Cross reactivity

The antigen-binding specificity of the antibodies was evaluated by competitive ELISA and cross reactivity [25]. In direct binding ELISA D-ribose, N-LDL and G-LDL (0–20 μg/ml) were mixed with constant amount of induced respective sera. In cross reactivity varying amounts of inhibitors like native and D-ribose

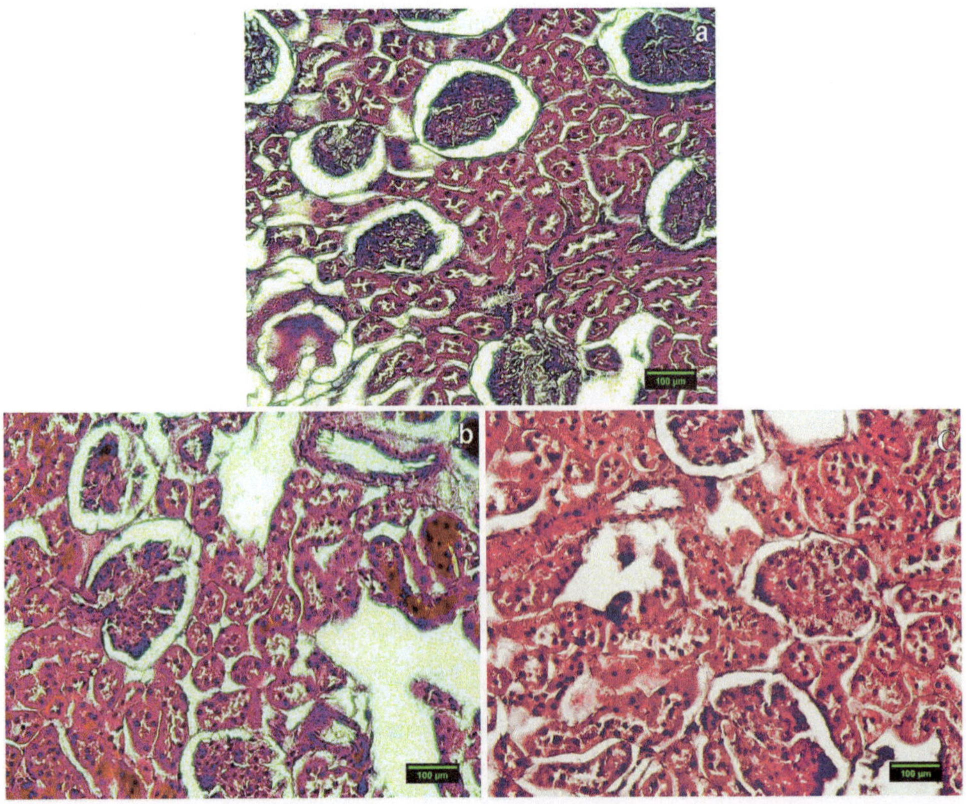

Figure 3. Kidney section from female rabbit immunized with native LDL showing normal morphology of glomeruli (a) (Magnification-60x); whereas, Kidney section from female rabbit immunized with D-ribose-modified LDL showing larger glomerular capillary tuft with increased number of nuclei showing proliferation of endothelium and mesenglial cells (b & c) (Magnification-60x). Scale bar 100 μm.

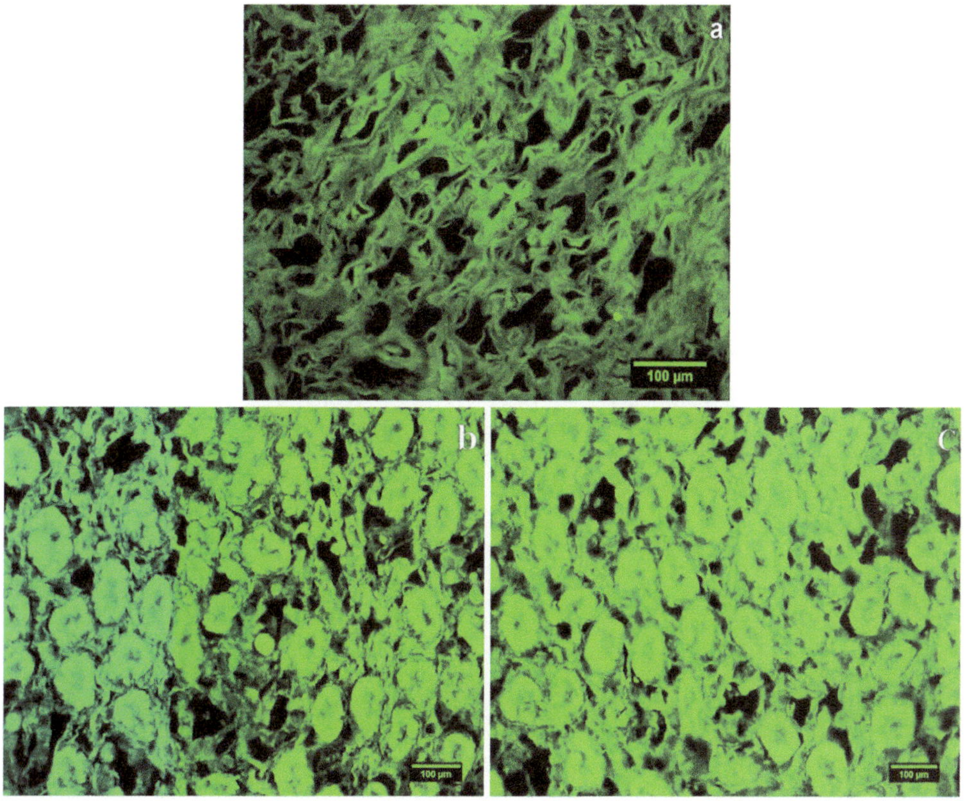

Figure 4. Immunofluorescence of kidney sections of rabbit immunized with native LDL (a); whereas Immunofluorescence of kidney sections of rabbit immunized with D-ribose-modified LDL showing immune complex deposition on GBM (b & c). Scale bar 100 µm.

modified proteins (LDL, HSA, Hb, IgG) and amino acids (Poly-L-lysine, Poly-L-arginine, Poly-L-histidine) (0–20 µg/ml) were mixed with a constant amount of IgG. The mixture was incubated at room temperature for 2 hours and overnight at 4°C. The immune complex thus formed was added to the wells, in place of serum. The remaining steps were same as in direct binding ELISA. Percent inhibition was calculated using the following formula:

Percent Inhibition $= 1-(A_{inhibited}/A_{uninhibited})\times 100$.

In order to perform the cross reactivity, firstly the IgG antibodies were isolated using protein-A-Agarose column, based on affinity chromatography.

Purification of Antibodies

Immunoglobulin G (IgG) was affinity purified from preimmune and immune sera on a protein A-Agarose column [26]. Serum (0.5 ml) diluted with equal volume of PBS (pH 7.4), was applied to the column (0.9×15 cm) pre-equilibrated with above buffer. The wash through was recycled 2–3 times. Unbound IgG was removed by extensive washing with PBS (pH 7.4). The bound IgG was eluted with 0.58% acetic acid in 0.85% sodium chloride [27]. Three milliliter fractions were collected in a measuring cylinder already containing 1 ml of 1 M Tris–HCl, pH 8.5, and absorbance was recorded. The IgG concentration was determined considering 1.4 $OD_{280} = 1.0$ mg mammalian IgG/ml. The isolated IgG was then dialyzed against PBS (pH 7.4) and stored at −80°C.

Histopathological study of Kidney Sections

Light Microscopic analysis. Slices of kidney from rabbits immunized with native and modified LDL was fixed in 10% formalin, dehydrated with increasing strength of ethanol, cleared in xylene, and wax impregnated. Paraffin blocks of the kidney pieces were fixed to block holder to cut 5-µm thick sections. Sections were dewaxed with xylene and hydrated using descending grades of alcohol. Hematoxylin (nuclei stain) and eosin (cytoplasmic stain) were used for staining. Again, the sections were dehydrated with ascending grades of alcohol and cleared with xylene before finally mounting in a mixture of distyrene, a plasticizer, and xylene (DPX) for microscopic observation [28].

Immunofluorescence analysis. 5 µm thick sections were cut with the help of a cryostat at −30°C. Sections were fixed with acetone on glass slides, incubated with anti-rabbit IgG fluorescein isothiocyanate conjugate (FITC) obtained from Sigma (St. Louis, MO) for 30 min. After three wash with phosphate buffer saline (PBS, pH 7.4), the sections were mounted with 50% glycerol and viewed under fluorescent microscope [28].

Results

Modification of LDL by D-ribose

We previously demonstrated that *in vitro* treatment of commercially available LDL with D-ribose results in biophysical and biochemical alterations in LDL to form LDL-AGEs [16].

Estimation of superoxide anion

Superoxide generation in the D-ribose modified human LDL was quantitated by a cytochrome c reduction experiment. During incubation of D-ribose with LDL, the formation of superoxide anion was gradually increased in time dependent manner. The incubation of D-ribose with LDL produced 30.5 nmol $O2^{\cdot -}$

ml^{-1} h^{-1} compared to 2.34 nmol $O2^{\cdot -}$ ml^{-1} h^{-1} with D-ribose alone. Superoxide dismutase (SOD) inhibited the superoxide radical generation. Upon, increasing concentration of SOD, the superoxide generation was gradually decreased.

Estimation of hydroxyl radicals

Incubation of 2-deoxy-D-ribose with D-ribose produced 14.2 nmol TBARS ml^{-1} however; reaction of LDL with D-ribose in the presence of Fe^{3+} enhanced it to 22.1 nmol TBARS ml^{-1}. Radical scavengers like mannitol, catalase and a metal ion chelator, desferrioxamine significantly inhibited the production of TBARS. TBARS generation was inhibited up to 58.3% when mannitol was used as a scavenger. However, catalase and desferrioxamine inhibited TBARS up to 52.4 and 60.2% respectively. The result suggests that D-ribose-mediated hydroxyl radical generation may be caused by traces of transition metals. Furthermore, it is also being suggested that the redox reactions of iron may facilitate the generation of hydroxyl radical by reaction of LDL and D-Ribose.

Estimation of CD and TBARS in plasma

CD in plasma was significantly increased in D-ribose glycated LDL induced plasma of NZW female rabbit in comparison preimmune plasma while moderately increased in D-ribose, CFA and N-LDL induced plasma (Table 1). TBARS in plasma was also significantly increased in D-ribose glycated LDL induced plasma in comparison to preimmune plasma while a very less or no change in D-ribose, CFA and N-LDL induced plasma (Table 1).

Immunogenicity of LDL and its D-ribose-modified form

In the present study, antigenicity of D-ribose, CFA, native and D-ribose-modified LDL was probed in New Zealand white (NZW) female rabbits. The result from direct binding ELISA D-ribose showed not significant binding, native LDL was moderately immunogenic eliciting average titer of antibodies, while its modified form i.e. glycated LDL was found to be much more immunogenic than its native form (Figure 1). CFA not showed significant binding with its induced sera (data not shown). Native LDL showed the titer value of >1:3200 while D-ribose glycated LDL antiserum showed high titer antibodies (>1:25,600) in direct binding ELISA. Binding of the preimmune serum was of low magnitude (Figure 1).

Furthermore, in the competitive inhibition ELISA we used D-ribose glycated LDL antiserum to explore its specificity against the immunogen i.e. D-ribose glycated LDL (Figure 2).

The purified IgG from protein A-Agarose column showed single homogenous band on denaturing SDS-PAGE (data not shown).

The IgG antibodies exhibited wide range of heterogeneity in recognizing varied inhibitors that included native and glycated analogues of LDL, HSA, Hb, IgG, poly L-lysine, poly L-arginine and poly L-histidine. A maximum of 82.3% inhibition of the D-ribose-LDL-IgG antibody was observed with the immunogen, when it was used as an inhibitor (Figure 2). The antibody was highly specific for the immunogen as only 2.5 μg/mL D-ribose modified-LDL caused 50% inhibition in the antiserum activity (Table 2). The IgG antibody showed considerably low recognition for native LDL, which caused a maximum inhibition of only 33.4%. The inhibition of D-ribose-LDL-IgG antibody by various competitors is given in Table 2. IgG concentration was kept constant (40 μg/ml) in all experiments. The cross reactivity observed with various amino acids (poly L-lysine, poly L-arginine, poly L-histidine) and protein (HSA, Hb, IgG) was due to the recognition of antigenic determinants. Reports show that D-ribose induces maximum modification at arginine and lysine residue in modified LDL case (Table 2), which explains that the higher cross reactivity of antiserum with D-ribose-arginine and D-ribose-lysine. This result is corroborated with the previously published reports [29].

In Histopathological study of NZW female rabbit's immunized with native LDL showing normal morphology of glomeruli (Figure 3a) while female rabbit's immunized with D-ribosylated LDL showing larger glomerular capillary tuft with increased number of nuclei (Figure 3b and 3c). In the fluorescence microscopic examination, low fluorescence signal was detected in FITC-labelled kidney sections of rabbits immunized with native LDL (Figure 4a) while D-ribosylated-LDL-immunized rabbit's kidney section showing GBM having a series of intense fluorescence points (Figure 4b and 4c).

Discussion

The LDL concentration used in these experiments for glycation is 62.5 μg/ml. The average level of LDL in normal individual is 1 mg/ml, However, the level of glycated LDL in diabetic subjects is 30 μg/ml. Therefore, to see the significant change in LDL macromolecule we used double the amount of glycated LDL in diabetic subjects which is 62.5 μg/ml.

Furthermore, a small spectrum of information like body weight, food consumption and illness were observed in phenotypic studies. In-life parameters we have monitored daily clinical observations, weekly body weights. Up to 3rd week of immunization there was no phenotypic changes were observed moreover no significant alterations were found in the total daily food consumption and weekly food consumption without any illness. We also observed that animals immunized with glycated LDL were more prone to reduction in body weight & food consumption as composed to native LDL.

Ribose is a naturally occurring pentose monosaccharide present in all living cells including the blood and is a key component of many important bio-molecules such as riboflavin, RNA and ATP [30]. Our study has shown that D-ribose causes structural perturbations in LDL molecule resulting in the generation of neo-antigenic epitopes which are recognized as non-self by the immune system, thus breaking the immune tolerance existing normally to self-antigens. Previously it has been shown that oxidized form of the LDL is highly immunogenic and shows potential recognition of auto-antibodies raised against modified LDL [31]. This is the first study in which we explored the immunogenicity of native and glycated LDL by D-ribose. Our results also point towards the possible involvement of this pentose sugar in the induction of antibody response in different diseases. Thus, it is reasonable to conclude that at present the exact pathophysiological role of glycation of apo B is still obscure and needs further study.

Vigorous humoral response in animals immunized with D-ribose-modified LDL suggests an alteration in the LDL structure, resulting in the generation of neo-epitopes, which are recognized as nonself by the immune system, leading to the robust production of antibodies.

The half-life of LDL in the circulation is in the order of 3–4 days. Some research groups experimentally showed in rabbits that *in vitro* glycated low density lipoprotein (glycated-LDL) was cleared at a slower rate than control LDL and thus stayed longer in the circulation (vascular mean residence time: 10 vs 8 h, p less than 0.001). The bodies mean residence time for glycated-LDL was 22 h vs 17 h for control LDL. In diabetic animals the catabolic parameters of both LDL preparations changed towards a faster clearance, the effect being greatest for glycated-LDL (total mean residence times of glycated-LDL pre-diabetic: 19 h, diabetic: 16 h; control LDL pre-diabetic and diabetic: 14 h). The difference in clearance between glycated and control LDL was thus strongly reduced. This suggests an increased activity of the non-receptor mediated pathway in diabetes mellitus, possibly co-responsible for an increased atherosclerotic risk [32].

Histological examination of kidney sections of rabbits immunized with native LDL showed a normal kidney morphology having normal glomerular, tubular, and vascular structure (Figure 3a). Whereas D-ribose-LDL immunized rabbits revealed hyper cellular and congested glomeruli with thickened basement membrane indicative of immune complex deposition (Figure 3b and 3c). In the fluorescence microscopic examination, low fluorescence signal was detected in FITC-labeled kidney sections of rabbits immunized with native LDL (Figure 4a). However, kidney sections of D-ribose-LDL-immunized rabbits showed GBM having a series of intense fluorescence points (Figure 4b and 4c). The deposition of immune complexes in the kidney points toward the possible involvement of D-ribose in glomerulonephritis.

Our research group and others too have shown that D-ribose causes structural perturbations in the LDL molecule [16] resulting in the metabolic abnormalities associated with glycation of LDL molecule that include diminished recognition of LDL by the classic LDL receptor; increased covalent binding of LDL in vessel walls; enhanced uptake of LDL by macrophages, thus stimulating foam cell formation; increased platelet aggregation; generation of neo-antigenic epitopes which are recognized as non-self by the immune system, thus breaking the immune tolerance existing normally to self-antigens. Formation of LDL-immune complexes; and generation of oxygen free radicals, resulting in oxidative damage to both the lipid and protein components of LDL and to any nearby macromolecules. We have also indicated its possible role in glomerulonephritis, an aspect that needs further probe. Our results would pave the way for further studies to evaluate the role of AGE-LDL in the progression and pathophysiology of diabetes-mediated atherosclerosis.

Recently, the presence of auto-antibodies in experimental and diabetes mellitus patients against the glycated DNA was investigated by our group [33–36]. There are also couple of recent reports for the presence of the auto-antibodies in the sera of the cancer patients which needs to be validated further [37]. Therefore the need of the hour is to stop this dreaded reaction using novel approach like nanoconjugation [38,39]. Our research group has recently shown some medicinal plants that have potent antioxidant property like *Phyllanthus virgatus*, *Ficus virens* and *Boerhaavia diffusa* [40–42]. Eventually, based on its antioxidant and antidiabetic characteristics, it is hypothesized that these plants might exhibit antiglycating properties as well. This is just a hypothesis to prove the same to get rid of the anomalies happening due to the glycation reaction as discussed above. We hope our findings would also help the way for the treatment of diabetes and its secondary complications like retinopathy, neuropathy and nephropathy.

Acknowledgments

The Authors are highly thankful to the Vice Chancellor of Integral University, Prof. Waseem Akhtar Sb. for the establishment of highly advanced research laboratories in the department of Bio-Sciences and Bio-Engineering.

Author Contributions

Conceived and designed the experiments: FA SA. Performed the experiments: FA SS. Analyzed the data: MSK SA. Contributed reagents/materials/analysis tools: MSK. Contributed to the writing of the manuscript: FA MSK SA.

References

1. Gillery P, Jenison S (2014) Post-translational modification derived products (PTMDPs): toxins in chronic diseases? Clin Chem Lab Med 52(1): 33–38.
2. Lapolla A, Traldi P, Fedele D (2005) Importance of measuring products of non-enzymatic glycation of proteins. Clin Biochem 38: 103–115.
3. Goldin A, Beckman JA, Schmidt AM, Creager MA (2006) Advanced Glycation End Products: Sparking the Development of Diabetic Vascular Injury. Circulation 114: 597–605.
4. Ahmad S, Shahab U, Baig MH, Khan MS, Khan MS, et al. (2013) Inhibitory effect of metformin and pyridoxamine in the formation of early, intermediate and advanced glycation end-products. PLoS One 8(9): e72128.
5. Azevedo M, Falcao J, Raposo J, Manso C (1988) Free Radic Res Commun 4: 331–335.
6. Mironova M, Virella G, Virella-Lowell I, Lopes-Virella MF (1997) Anti-modified LDL antibodies and LDL-containing immune complexes in IDDM patients and healthy controls. Clin Immunol Immunopath 85: 73–82.
7. Akanji AO, Abdella N, Mojiminiyi OA (2002) Determinants of glycated LDL levels in nondiabetic and diabetic hyperlipidaemic patients in Kuwait. Clin Chim Acta 317(1–2): 171–176.
8. Lundberg AM, Hansson GK (2010) Innate immune signals in atherosclerosis. Clin Immunol 134: 5–24.
9. Andersson J, Libby P, Hansson GK (2010) Adaptive immunity and atherosclerosis. Clin Immunol 134: 33–46.
10. Lopes-Virella MF, Virella G (2010) Clinical significance of the humoral immune response to modified LDL. Clin Immunol 134: 55–65.
11. Saad AF, Virella G, Chassereau C, Boackle RJ, Lopes-Virella MF (2006) OxLDL immune complexes activate complement and induce cytokine production by MonoMac 6 cells and human macrophages. J Lipid Res 47: 1975–1983.
12. Lopes-Virella MF, McHenry MB, Lipsitz S, Yim E, Wilson PF, et al. (2007) Immune complexes containing modified lipoproteins are related to the progression of internal carotid intima-media thickness in patients with type 1 diabetes. Atherosclerosis 190: 359–369.
13. Yishak AA, Costacou T, Virella G, Zgibor J, Fried L, et al. (2006) Novel predictors of overt nephropathy in subjects with type 1 diabetes. A nested case control study from the Pittsburgh Epidemiology of Diabetes Complications cohort. Nephrol Dial Transplant 21: 93–100.
14. Kummu O, Turunen SP, Wang C, Lehtimäki J, Veneskoski M (2013) Carbamyl adducts on low-density lipoprotein induce IgG response in LDLR −/− mice and bind plasma autoantibodies in humans under enhanced carbamylation. Antioxid Redox Signal 19(10): 1047–1062.
15. Steinberg D (2009) The LDL modification hypothesis of atherogenesis: an update. J Lipid Res 50: S376–S381.
16. Ahmad S, Akhter F, Moinuddin, Shahab U, Khan MS (2013) Studies on glycation of human low density lipoprotein: A functional insight into physico-chemical analysis. Int J Biol Macro 62: 167–171.
17. Akhter F, Khan MS, Shahab U, Ahmad S (2013) Bio-physical characterization of ribose induced glycation: A mechanistic study on DNA perturbations. Int J Biol Macromol 58: 206–210.
18. Beauchamp C, Fridovich I (1971) Superoxide dismutase: improved assays and an assay applicable to acrylamide gels. Anal Biochem 44: 276–287.
19. Halliwell B, Gutteridge JMC (1981) Formation of thiobarbituric acid-reactive substance from deoxyribose in the presence of iron salts: the role of superoxide and hydroxyl radicals. FEBS Lett 128: 347–352.
20. Moinuddin, Dixit K, Ahmad S, Shahab U, Habib S, et al. (2012) Human DNA damage by the synergistic action of 4-aminobiphenyl and nitric oxide: An immunochemical study. Environ Toxicol 29(5): 68–76.
21. Folch J, Lees M, Sloane Stanley GH (1957) A simple method for the isolation and purification of total lipides from animal tissues. J Biol Chem 226: 497–509.
22. Yagi K (1987) Lipid peroxides and human diseases. Chem Phus Lipids 45(2–4): 337–51.
23. Liu KT, Lesca P (1982) Pharmacological properties of Dibenzo[a, c]cyclooctene derivatives isolated from Fructus Schizandrae Chinensis III. Inhibitory effects on carbon tetrachloride-induced lipid peroxidation, metabolism and covalent binding of carbon tetra chloride to lipids. Chem Biol Interact 41(1): 39–47.
24. Shahab U, Ahmad S, Moinuddin, Dixit K, Habib S, et al. (2012) Hydroxyl Radical Modification of Collagen Type II Increases Its Arthritogenicity and Immunogenicity. PLoS ONE 7(2): e31199.
25. Shahab U, Moinuddin, Ahmad S, Dixit K, Habib S, et al. (2013) Genotoxic effect of N-hydroxy-4-acetylaminobiphenyl on human DNA: implications in bladder cancer. PLoS One 8(1): e53205.
26. Mustafa I, Ahmad S, Dixit K, Moinuddin, Ahmad J, et al. (2012) Glycated human DNA is a preferred antigen for anti-DNA antibodies in diabetic patients. Diabetes Res Clin Pract 95(1): 98–104.

27. Goding JW (1976) Use of staphylococcal protein-A as an immunological reagent. Immuol Methods 20: 241–253.
28. Shahab U, Moinuddin, Ahmad S, Dixit K, Abidi SMA, et al. (2012) Acquired Immunogenicity of Human DNA Damaged by N-Hydroxy-N-acetyl-4-amino-biphenyl. IUBMB Life 64(4): 340–345.
29. Cervantes-Laurean D, Minter DE, Jacobson EL, Jacobson MK (1993) Protein glycation by ADP-ribose: studies of model conjugates. Biochemistry 32(6): 1528–1534.
30. Kellar PJ, Kim SU, Bown DH, Chen HC, Kohnle A, et al. (1988) Biosynthesis of riboflavin: mechanism of formation of the ribitylamino linkage. Biochemistry 27: 1117–1120.
31. Lopes-Virella MF, Hunt KJ, Baker NL, Lachin J, Nathan DM, et al. (2011) Levels of Oxidized LDL and Advanced Glycation End Products-Modified LDL in Circulating Immune Complexes Are Strongly Associated With Increased Levels of Carotid Intima-Media Thickness and Its Progression in Type 1 Diabetes. Diabetes 60: 582–589.
32. Kortlandt W, Benschop C, van Rijn HJ, Erkelens DW (1992) Glycated low density lipoprotein catabolism is increased in rabbits with alloxan-induced diabetes mellitus. Diabetologia 35(3): 202–207.
33. Ahmad S, Moinuddin, Shahab U, Habib S, Salman Khan M, et al. (2014) Glycoxidative damage to human DNA: Neo-antigenic epitopes on DNA molecule could be a possible reason for autoimmune response in type 1 diabetes. Glycobiology 24(3): 281–291.
34. Ahmad S, Moinuddin, Habib S, Shahab U, Alam K, et al. (2014) Autoimmune response to AGE modified human DNA: Implications in type 1 Diabetes mellitus. J Clin. Trans. Endo. 1: 3; 66–72.
35. Ahmad S, Moinuddin, Dixit K, Shahab U, Alam K, et al. (2014) Genotoxicity and immunogenicity of DNA-advanced glycation end products formed by methylglyoxal and lysine in presence of Cu2+. Biochem Biophys Res Commun. 407(3): 568–574.
36. Shahab U, Tabrez S, Khan MS, Akhter F, Khan MS, et al. (2014) Immunogenicity of DNA-advanced glycation end product fashioned through glyoxal and arginine in the presence of Fe3+: its potential role in prompt recognition of diabetes mellitus auto-antibodies. Chemico Biol Int. 219; 229–240.
37. Ahmad MI, Ahmad S, Moinuddin (2011) preferential recognition of methylglyoxal modified calf thymus DNA by circulating autoantibodies in cancer patients. Ind Journal of Biochem and Biophys. 48: 290–296.
38. Rahim M, Iram S, Khan MS, Khan MS, Shukla AR, et al. (2013) Glycation-assisted synthesized gold nanoparticles inhibit growth of bone cancer cells. Colloids Surf B Biointerfaces 117: 473–479.
39. Ahmad S, Khan MS, Khan MS, Akhter F, Khan A, et al. (2014) Glycoxidation of biological macromolecules: A critical approach to halt the menace of glycation. Glycobiology 24: 979–990.
40. Iqbal D, Khan MS, Khan MS, Ahmad S, Srivastava AK (2013) An *In Vitro* and molecular informatics study to evaluate the antioxidative and β-hydroxy-β-methylglutaryl-CoA reductase inhibitory Property of *Ficus virens* Ait. Phytother Res doi:10.1002/ptr.5077.
41. Hashim A, Khan MS, Khan MS, Baig MH, Ahmad S (2013) Antioxidant and α-amylase inhibitory property of phyllanthus virgatus L.: an *in vitro* and molecular interaction study. Biomed Res Int doi:10.1155/2013/729393.
42. Akhter F, Hashim A, Khana MS, Ahmad S, Iqbal D, et al. (2013) Antioxidant, α-amylase inhibitory and oxidative DNA damage protective property of Boerhaavia diffusa (Linn.) root. S Afr J Biol 88: 265–272.

Diagnostic Criteria for Depression in Type 2 Diabetes: A Data-Driven Approach

Sergio E. Starkstein[2]*, Wendy A. Davis[1], Milan Dragovic[2], Violetta Cetrullo[1], Timothy M. E. Davis[1], David G. Bruce[1]

1 School of Medicine & Pharmacology, University of Western Australia, Crawley, Western Australia, Australia, **2** School of Psychiatry & Clinical Neuroscience, University of Western Australia, Crawley, Western Australia, Australia

Abstract

Background: While depression is a frequent psychiatric comorbid condition in diabetes and has significant clinical impact, the syndromal profile of depression and anxiety symptoms has not been examined in detail.

Aims: To determine the syndromal pattern of the depression and anxiety spectrum in a large series of patients with type 2 diabetes, as determined using a data-driven approach based on latent class analysis (LCA).

Method: Type 2 diabetes participants from the observational community-based Fremantle Diabetes Study Phase II underwent assessment of lifetime depression using the Brief Lifetime Depression Scale, the Patient Health Questionnaire 9-item version (PHQ-9) for current depression symptoms, and the Generalized Anxiety Disorder Scale that was specifically developed and validated for this study. The main outcome measure was classes of patients with a specific syndromal profile of depression and anxiety symptoms based on LCA.

Results: LCA identified four classes that were interpreted as "major anxious depression", "minor anxious depression", "subclinical anxiety", and "no anxious depression". All nine DSM-IV/5 diagnostic criteria for major depression identified a class with a high frequency of major depression. All symptoms of anxiety had similar high probabilities as symptoms of depression for the "major depression-anxiety" class. There were significant differences between classes in terms of history of depression and anxiety, use of psychoactive medication, and diabetes-related variables.

Conclusions: Patients with type 2 diabetes show specific profiles of depression and anxiety. Anxiety symptoms are an integral part of major depression in type 2 diabetes. The different classes identified here provide empirically validated phenotypes for future research.

Editor: Kenji Hashimoto, Chiba University Center for Forensic Mental Health, Japan

Funding: Funding was provided by National Health and Medical Research Council (Project Grant 513781). The funders had no role in study design, data collection and analysis, decision to publish, or preparation of the manuscript.

Competing Interests: The authors have declared that no competing interests exist.

* Email: ses@cyllene.uwa.edu.au

Introduction

Depression is one of the most frequent psychiatric disorders in patients with type 2 diabetes, with a lifetime prevalence of 24%–29% and a point prevalence of 10%-15% [1]. Depression in type 2 diabetes is significantly associated with poor glycaemic control [2], chronic complications [2], increased mortality [3], reduced physical and mental functioning [4], higher health costs and decreased adherence to diet and hypoglycaemic medications [5]. A recent epidemiological study demonstrated that individuals with diabetes and comorbid depression have a worse health-related quality of life and higher health service usage [6]. Collaborative care models for depression in diabetes demonstrated to significantly improve outcomes for depression and glycaemic control [7].

Depression may be underdiagnosed in diabetes. The limitations in diagnosing depression in diabetes include the lack of specific diagnostic criteria and the overlap of symptoms. Egede and Ellis [8] noted that poor management of diabetes is a barrier for early recognition of depressive symptoms, such as fatigue, changes in weight and appetite, sleep disturbances, and motor retardation. Furthermore, increased appetite is a cardinal diagnostic criterion for both major depression and diabetes, anhedonia may result from changes in lifestyle due to diabetes, loss of interest may be secondary to limitations to pursue usual free-time activities due to diabetes complications (e.g., visual problems, neuropathy), and loss of libido and reduced self-esteem may result from sexual dysfunction. Campayo and co-workers [9] suggested that depression in diabetic patients may be qualitatively different from depression observed among individuals without diabetes who have 'primary' (i.e. no organic cause) depression, but no supporting data were provided. A recent large prospective study showed that individuals with current depressive and/or anxiety disorders fad a 10-fold increased odds of diabetes incidence at two years, and the

Table 1. Generalized Anxiety Disorder Scale.

Over the <u>last 6 months</u>, how often have you been bothered by any of the following problems?	**Not at all**	**Several days**	**More than half the days**	**Nearly every day**
1. worrying excessively or being anxious about several things?	0	1	2	3
2. difficulty controlling the worries or found the worries interfering with your ability to focus on what you were doing?	0	1	2	3
3. feeling restless, keyed up or on edge?	0	1	2	3
4. feeling tense?	0	1	2	3
5. feeling tired, weak or exhausted easily?	0	1	2	3
6. difficulty concentrating or finding your mind going blank?	0	1	2	3
7. feeling irritable?	0	1	2	3
8. difficulty sleeping (falling asleep, waking in the middle of the night, early morning wakening, or sleeping excessively)?	0	1	2	3
9. the symptoms of anxiety caused you significant distress or impaired your ability to function at work, socially, or in some other important way?	0	1	2	3
10. Were you taking any drugs or medicines just before the symptoms began?				
☐ No ☐ Yes	If YES, which drugs/medicines? ____________			
11. 10b. Did you have any medical illness just before these symptoms began?				
☐ No ☐ Yes	If YES, what was the illness? ____________			

incidence was highest for those with comorbid depression and anxiety [10]. A valid and timely diagnosis of depression is of clinical relevance especially given that detection and treatment of depression improves glycaemic control [9].

Another potential confounder for a valid diagnosis of depression in diabetes is the potential comorbidity with anxiety. This is substantial in the general population, with 57% of individuals with major depression also meeting diagnostic criteria for an anxiety disorder [11]. Generalized anxiety disorder (GAD) is more frequent in diabetes than in age-comparable healthy controls [12], and is associated with poor health behaviours [13]. In the general population, comorbid depression and anxiety is highly prevalent [14]. Several studies examined the comorbidity between depression and anxiety in diabetes, but they were limited by important methodological shortcomings, such as a diagnosis of diabetes based only on self-report [13].

The aim of the present study was to examine the syndromal pattern of depression and anxiety in type 2 diabetes using a data-driven approach, as well as to examine the overlap with anxiety. We used baseline data from community-based participants of the Fremantle Diabetes Study Phase II (FDS2) [15], and used latent class analysis (LCA) to examine the homogeneity of depressive symptoms and the comorbidity between depression and anxiety. LCA assesses the symptom profile of individual patients and produces classes of patients in terms of their pattern of symptoms. Given that the classes thus identified do not overlap, individual patients can belong to only one group. Based on our experience with LCA in medical conditions, we expected to find three classes characterized by high, moderate and low probabilities for symptoms of depression, as well as a high comorbidity between depression and anxiety.

Methods

Patients

The FDS2 is a longitudinal observational study of known diabetes conducted in a postcode-defined geographical area surrounding the city of Fremantle (Western Australia) [15].

Details of FDS2 recruitment procedures, sample characteristics including classification of diabetes type and non-recruited patients have been published elsewhere [15]. Briefly, between 2008 and 2011, 4,667 diabetic patients were identified in the local population of 153,000 (crude diabetes prevalence 3%), of whom 1,668 (36%) were recruited to FDS2, in addition to 64 surviving FDS phase I participants who had moved out of the study area (1,732 participants altogether).

Ethics Statement

The Human Research Ethics Committee of the Southern Metropolitan Area Health Service specifically approved the study, and all subjects gave written informed consent.

Clinical and psychiatric assessment

Each participant underwent a baseline assessment that included a comprehensive clinical questionnaire, physical examination and fasting biochemical tests [15]. Diabetes type was assessed from treatment history, BMI, age at diagnosis, and nature of first presentation and/or self-identification. Non-insulin treated patients and those ≥60 years of age at diagnosis were usually considered to have type 2 diabetes, as were patients <60 years of age at diagnosis and taking insulin at the time of the study entry but whose first treatment was not insulin. In these cases, case records were consulted for evidence of ketonemia, as well as islet cell antibody, GAD antibodies, serum insulin and C-peptide levels, if available. Complications were ascertained using standard criteria [15,16].

All participants were assessed with the PHQ-9 [17], a brief and accurate assessment of depression that has been validated in patients with diabetes [16]. The PHQ-9 is a dual-purpose instrument that can establish depressive disorder diagnoses as well as ratings of depressive symptom severity [17]. Patients with type 2 diabetes have significant physical complaints that may artificially increase PHQ-9 scores on items that are not necessary symptoms of major depression. Using a PHQ-9 cut point rather than the diagnostic algorithm may increase the frequency of false-positive cases of depression [18]. Therefore, as suggested by the PHQ-9 authors [18], we used the instrument's diagnostic algorithm for making diagnoses of major and minor depression. Major depression was diagnosed when the first or second symptoms (i.e. depressed mood or loss of interest/anhedonia) were present more than half the days, and at least 5 of the 9 symptoms were present during the same period [19]. Minor depression was diagnosed whenever 2 to 4 symptoms (including depressed mood or loss of interest/anhedonia) were present for more than half the days. Lifetime history of depression was assessed with the Brief Lifetime Depression Scale (BLDS). This instrument was developed and validated by our group for use in diabetes [20]. The BLDS was modelled on the PHQ-9 and included similar items, general format and language, but the participants were asked whether they had ever had a period during their lives lasting for two weeks or more when they experienced any of the nine symptoms of depression listed in the DSM-IV/5.

For the study of anxiety in the FDS2, a specific questionnaire (the Generalized Anxiety Disorder Scale (GADS)) was devised by one of the authors (SES) with experience in developing psychiatric instruments to rate the severity of anxiety (Table 1). The GADS includes 9 items that correspond to all 9 DSM-IV criteria for GAD. Based on the PHQ-9, GADS items were rated as "not at all present", "present several days", "present more than half of the days", and "present nearly every day". As with the PHQ-9, a symptom was rated positive whenever the patient rated "more than half of the days" or "nearly every day". To make the instrument comparable to the DSM-IV criteria for GAD, the time criterion was the past 6 months. The validity of the GADS was examined by having a psychiatrist (SES) assess a convenience sample of 23 patients with the Structured Clinical Interview for the DSM-IV-Research Version (SCID)-Anxiety Disorders Module, blind to the GADS results. Kappa statistics showed a high diagnostic concordance for DSM-IV GAD diagnosis (kappa = 0.88). Six of the 23 patients received a diagnosis of GAD based on the SCID, as compared to 4 based on the GADS (McNemar's test, $P = 0.50$). Test-retest reliability was assessed in 25 patients, who completed the GADS twice, with an interval of (mean ± SD) 9±6 days. The intra-class correlation (ICC) was high (ICC = 0.88). The presence of cognitive deficits was based on the following algorithm (Bruce et al., 2008): patients scoring ≤26 on the MMSE were further assessed with the Clinical Dementia Rating (CDR) (Hughes et al., 1982) to establish the presence of dementia. This instrument generates ratings ranging from normal cognition (CDR 0) to severity levels of dementia (CDR 1–3) and

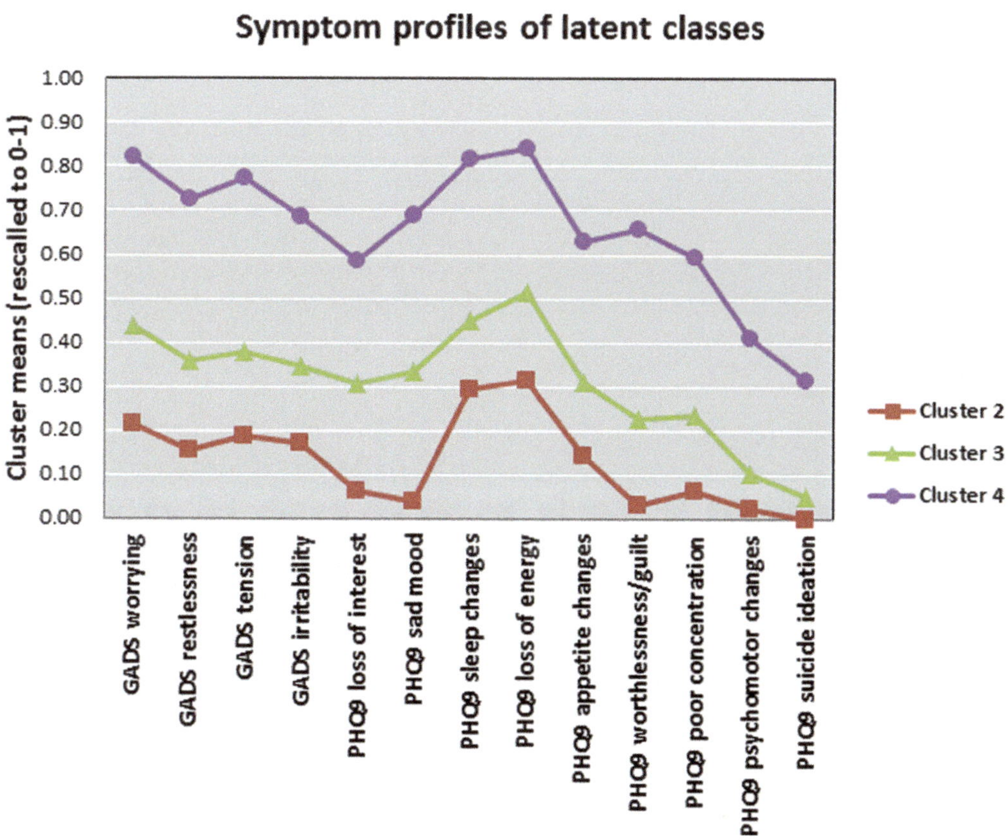

Figure 1. Symptom profile of the 4 (ordered) latent class model graph showing partial conditional probabilities for the 4-class model (LCA response profiles).

Table 2. Testing Six Subsequent Latent Class Analysis Models.

Number of classes	L^2	Reduction from baseline	Gain (%)	Classification error	BIC*	AWE*	CAIC
One class	17470.9	-		0.00	33396.3	33797.7	33435.3
Two classes	12744.7	27.1	27.1	0.04	28772.2	29555.7	28825.3
Three classes	11449.9	34.5	7.4	0.06	27579.6	28733.8	27646.6
Four classes	10988.6	37.8	2.6	0.10	27222.3	28785.1	27301.2
Five classes	10720.2	38.6	1.5	0.13	27053.9	28964.8	27148.9

* Information criteria evaluating the quality of latent class solution: L2 - The likelihood-ratio goodness-of-fit, BIC (Bayes Information Criterion), AWE (Approximate Weight of Evidence, similar to BIC but also takes classification performance into account), CAIC (Corrected Akaike Information Criterion).

an intermediate category defines very mild cognitive impairment or questionable dementia (CDR 0.5).

Statistical Analysis

To test for group differences, generalised linear modelling (GLM) was used. LCA (cluster procedure) was used to determine the latent structure of patients with diabetes and to categorize individuals based on their responses to the PHQ-9 and GADS. LCA was calculated using the software LatentGold version 4.0.4 [21]. LCA assumes that a 'class' explains the association among a set of symptoms. LCA computes latent class probabilities or prevalence, and conditional probabilities. The basic assumption of LCA is that a (presumably homogeneous) population of individuals is a mixture of distinct, but internally homogeneous subgroups [22]. LCA assesses the symptom profile of individual patients and produces classes of patients as suggested by their pattern of symptoms. Since the clusters do not overlap, individual patients can belong to only one group. For this analysis, we included the nine DSM-IV symptoms for major depression and the four DSM-IV symptoms for generalized anxiety disorder that do not overlap with major depression as latent class indicators. Models with one to five classes were estimated. Each patient was assigned to the latent class to which the largest posterior probability was calculated. The best-fitting model was chosen based on having the lowest values for the following goodness of fit indices: Bayes Information Criterion (BIC), Approximate Weight of Evidence (AWE) (which takes into account classification performance), and the Corrected Akaike Information Criterion (CAIC). The level of contribution of each indicator to the final latent class structure is assessed by the information content statistic (R^2), which can be interpreted similarly to the commonalities in traditional factor analysis. For the clinical interpretation, the mean level and frequency of responses for each psychiatric symptom within each class were examined. After determining the best class solution, we used latent class membership as a between-subject variable in a one-way analysis of variance (ANOVA) followed by post-hoc comparisons using Tukey's HSD, and X^2 analyses to examine demographic and clinical differences among the latent classes. The computer package IBM SPSS Statistics 20 (IBM Corporation, Somers, NY, USA) was used to compare baseline characteristics across the four LCA classes. Data are presented as proportions, mean ± SD, geometric mean (SD range), or, in the case of variables which did not conform to a normal or log-normal distribution, median [inter-quartile range, IQR]. For independent samples, two-way comparisons for proportions were by Fisher's exact test, for normally distributed variables by Student's *t*-test, and for non-normally distributed variables by Mann-Whitney U-test. Multiple comparisons for proportions were by Fisher's exact test or Chi-squared test, for normally distributed variables by one-way ANOVA, and for non-normally distributed variables by Kruskal-Wallis H-test, adjusted using the Bonferroni correction. A two-tailed significance level of $P<0.05$ was used throughout.

Results

Demographic and clinical findings

FDS2 recruited 1,551 participants (90%) with clinically defined type 2 diabetes. Complete data for our study was obtained from 1,337 patients (86%). When compared with the 214 patients with missing data, the latter were more likely to be female (46% vs. 57%, $P=0.005$), and had worse glycaemic control (HbA_{1c} (median [IQR]) 6.8% median [IQR] [6.2%–7.6%] vs. 7.0% [6.4%–8.5%], respectively, $P=0.001$). On the other hand, there were no significant between-group differences in age (mean years

Table 3. Scores for anxiety and depression items for the four LCA classes.

Symptom	No anxious - depression	Subsyndromal anxiety	Minor anxious depression	Major anxious depression	F	*P*
Worrying	0.06 (0.23)	0.65 (0.63)	1.33 (0.87)	2.49 (0.73)	548.6	0.0001
Restlessness	0.01 (0.09)	0.47 (0.53)	1.09 (0.70)	2.17 (0.83)	597.3	0.0001
Tension	0.01 (0.10)	0.57 (0.55)	1.15 (0.72)	2.33 (0.74)	654.6	0.0001
Irritability	0.06 (0.24)	0.52 (0.58)	1.04 (0.69)	2.06 (0.89)	430.5	0.0001
Loss of interest	0.02 (0.17)	0.18 (0.45)	0.96 (0.84)	1.75 (0.91)	398.3	0.0001
Sad mood	0.02 (0.13)	0.12 (0.33)	1.03 (0.74)	2.06 (0.81)	754.3	0.0001
Sleep changes	0.28 (0.66)	0.90 (1.00)	1.35 (1.06)	2.47 (0.85)	162.7	0.0001
Loss of energy	0.20 (0.43)	0.96 (0.83)	1.55 (0.97)	2.55 (0.68)	204.8	0.0001
Appetite changes	0.09 (0.33)	0.44 (0.78)	0.94 (1.03)	1.88 (1.17)	179.0	0.0001
Worthlessness/guilt	0.01 (0.48)	0.09 (0.30)	0.70 (0.77)	1.96 (1.08)	131.1	0.0001
Poor concentration	0.01 (0.08)	0.19 (0.47)	0.72 (0.87)	1.76 (1.04)	104.0	0.0001
Psychomotor changes	0.01 (0.04)	0.08 (0.34)	0.30 (0.59)	1.25 (1.17)	207.7	0.0001
Suicide ideation	0.00 (0.00)	0.01 (0.04)	0.17 (0.50)	0.91 (1.09)	57.7	0.0001

± SD) (65.8±11.1 vs. 64.9±14.4 years, respectively, $P = 0.41$), diabetes duration (8.8 years [2.8–15.6] vs. 10.0 years [3.0–17.8], respectively, $P = 0.12$), or cognition (8.0% vs. 7.1% cognitively impaired (P = 1.00).

Latent class analysis

Items selected for the LCA included all 9 items from the PHQ-9, and the items of worrying/anxiety, feeling restless, feeling tense, and feeling irritable from the GADS (the remaining items were not included due to overlap with PHQ-9 items). The modelling started with probing the presence of conventional latent classes (i.e., cluster modelling), running cluster models of up to 5 latent clusters. Inspection of conditional probabilities showed a reduction in BIC and CAIC values from the 2- to the 5-cluster model, but at the cost of increasing number of parameters (NPar) (Table 2). From the 4-class model onwards, decreased accuracy was unacceptably high (i.e., >10%) and the AWE index has started to ascend. The 4-cluster model showed a pattern of probabilities extending from one extreme (low probabilities for all symptoms) to the other (high probabilities for all symptoms), with the exception of two intermediate classes showing a mixed pattern of probabilities. This finding suggests that a single discrete factor (anxious depression) with 4 ordered levels or classes (e.g., no anxious depression, subclinical anxiety, minor anxious depression and major anxious depression) provides the best explanatory model. Thus, an inter-factorial effect and orderliness of latent classes was obtained, as opposed to random and/or pseudonominal composition of latent classes. Class-specific endorsement profiles for depression and anxiety symptoms are shown in Figure 1.

Latent class 4 included 104 patients (8%) and showed high partial conditional probabilities (>0.60) for all the anxiety and depression symptoms, except for psychomotor changes (>0.40) and suicidal ideation (>0.30). This class was labelled "major anxious depression". Latent class 1 included 439 patients (33%) and showed low partial conditional probabilities (<0.10) for all symptoms of depression and anxiety. This class was labelled "no anxious depression". Latent class 3 included 293 patients (22%) with partial conditional probabilities intermediate between classes 1 and 4, and was labelled "minor anxious depression". Finally, latent class 2 included 501 patients (38%) and showed higher conditional probabilities than class 4 on the anxiety items, sleep changes and loss of energy. This class was labelled "subclinical anxiety". We used final class membership as a between-subject variable to evaluate differences in depressive and anxiety symptoms as a function of latent class membership. The ANOVAs evaluating mean symptom severity differences on each item as a function of latent class membership were all significant at the $P < 0.001$ level. Follow-up pairwise comparisons using Tukey's HSD tests demonstrated the following differences: For GAD worry the ANOVA was significant (Table 3), and all four groups were significantly different to each other (Tukey HSD $P = 0.0001$). Similar results were obtained for GADS restlessness, GADS tension, GADS irritability, loss of interest, sad mood, sleep changes, loss of energy, appetite changes, worthlessness/guilt, and poor concentration. For the items of psychomotor changes and suicide ideation there were significant differences on post-hoc tests between all classes except between classes 1 and 2.

There were significant demographic and clinical differences between classes (Table 4). The *major anxious depression class* was significantly younger than the other classes, whilst the *minor anxious depression class* was significantly younger than the subclinical anxiety class. Depression (major or minor) was significantly more frequent in the *major anxious depression class* as compared to the other classes, and in the *minor anxious depression class* as compared to the remaining two classes. Depression before the onset of diabetes was significantly higher in the *major anxious depression class* as compared to the other classes, and in the *minor anxious depression class* as compared to the remaining two classes. Patients in the *major anxious depression class* had a significantly higher frequency of GAD as compared to the other classes, whilst patients in the *minor anxious depression class* had a significantly higher frequency of GAD than the remaining two classes. Depression (minor or major) and/or GAD were present in 89% of patients in the *major anxious depression class*, 29% in the *minor anxious depression class*, 2% in the *subclinical anxiety class*, and none in the *no anxious depression class*.

Finally, the *major anxious depression class* showed a significantly younger age at onset of diabetes, higher HbA_{1c} levels, higher serum triglycerides levels and a higher frequency of insulin use

Table 4. FDS2 baseline associates of four LCA groups in participants with type-2 diabetes.

	LCA group				
FDS2 baseline variable	**No anxious depression (Cluster 1)**	**Subsyndromal anxiety (Cluster 2)**	**Minor anxious depression (Cluster 3)**	**Major anxious depression (Cluster 4)**	***P*-value**
N (%)	439 (32.8)	501 (37.5)	293 (21.9)	104 (7.8)	
Age (years)	67.4±10.8	66.1±10.8	64.7±11.1††	60.6±12.3***,†††,‡‡	**<0.001**
Any depressive syndrome (%)	0	1.0	26.3***,†††	77.9***,†††,‡‡‡	**<0.001**
Major depressive syndrome (%)	0	0	4.1***,†††	67.3***,†††,‡‡‡	**<0.001**
Taking antidepressant medication (%)	6.6	13.6**	23.5***,†††	35.6***,†††	**<0.001**
No depression/ depression before diabetes/concomitant diagnoses/depression after diabetes (%)	88.2/7.7/1.2/3.0	64.0/19.6/5.4/11.0***	29.8/32.4/10.2/27.6***,†††	2.1/43.3/16.5/38.1***,†††,‡‡‡	**<0.001**
Current GAD (%)	0	0	3.8***,†††	51.0***,†††,‡‡‡	**<0.001**
Lifetime GAD (%):	5.1	14.7***	35.6***,†††	70.3***,†††,‡‡‡	**<0.001**
Any depressive syndrome and/or current GAD (DSMIV) (%)	0	1.6	29.4***,†††	89.4***,†††,‡‡‡	**<0.001**
Male (%)	58.5	52.3	50.2	45.2	**0.030**
Educated beyond primary level (%)	88.2	88.1	88.5	80.4	0.17
Currently married	65.1	65.9	63.1	63.5	0.87
Alcohol consumption (standard drinks/day)	0.1 [0–1.5]	0.1 [0–1.2]	0.1 [0–1.5]	0 [0–0.3]***,†,‡‡	**0.003**
Age at diagnosis of diabetes (years)	57.4±11.7	56.2±11.5	54.7±11.5†	49.9±11.6***,†††,‡‡	**<0.001**
Diabetes duration (years)	8.5 [3.0–15.8]	8.0 [2.3–15.4]	9.0 [2.0–15.5]	10.0 [4.0–15.5]	0.57
Fasting serum glucose (mmol/L)	7.1 [6.2–8.7]	7.1 [6.2–8.5]	7.1 [6.1–8.9]	8.1 [6.2–10.3]*,†	**0.021**
HbA_{1c} (%)	6.8 [6.3–7.5]	6.7 [6.2–7.5]	6.8 [6.2–7.6]	7.5 [6.3–8.9]***,†††,‡‡‡	**0.001**
Diabetes treatment (% diet/OGLMs/insulin/ insulin + OGLMs)	23.9/57.2/3.2/15.7	27.1/52.3/3.4/17.2	24.9/51.2/6.8/17.1	18.3/43.3/9.6/28.8***,††	**0.001**
BMI (kg/m^2)	30.9±5.9	30.9±5.8	32.0±6.6	33.5±7.0**,††	**<0.001**
Central adiposity (% obese by waist circumference)	68.6	70.9	74.4	83.5*,†	**0.013**
Total serum cholesterol (mmol/L)	4.3±1.0	4.4±1.0	4.4±1.2	4.5±1.3	0.09
HDL-cholesterol (mmol/L)	1.26±0.35	1.24±0.34	1.24±0.34	1.15±0.27	**0.033**
Serum triglycerides (mmol/L)	1.4 (0.9–2.4)	1.5 (0.9–2.5)	1.5 (0.9–2.5)	2.0 (1.0–3.8)***,†††,‡‡‡	**<0.001**
eGFR <60 ml/min/ 1.73 m^2 (%)	16.5	18.8	18.2	22.3	0.52
Peripheral sensory neuropathy (%)	57.6	59.7	61.6	56.3	0.67
Any retinopathy (%)	20.6	21.9	22.9	24.5	0.83
Self-reported MI/angina (%)	15.5	14.8	22.5†	25.0	**0.005**
Self-reported stroke (%)	2.5	4.0	6.5	7.7	**0.018**

Table 4. Cont.

FDS2 baseline variable	LCA group No anxious depression (Cluster 1)	Subsyndromal anxiety (Cluster 2)	Minor anxious depression (Cluster 3)	Major anxious depression (Cluster 4)	P-value
Peripheral arterial disease (%)	23.5	20.2	21.8	24.3	0.59

*P<0.05,
**P<0.01,
***P<0.001 vs no depression-anxiety;
†P<0.05,
††P<0.01,
†††P<0.001 vs minor depression-anxiety;
‡P<0.05,
‡‡P<0.01,
‡‡‡P<0.001 vs subsyndromal anxiety after Bonferroni adjustment for multiple comparisons.

than the other three classes. This class also showed a higher BMI than the *subclinical anxiety* and the *no anxious depression classes*. When the class with major anxious-depression was compared with patients meeting DSM-IV criteria for major depression, there were no differences on demographic, diabetes-related or psychiatric variables (Table 5).

Discussion

To our knowledge, this is the first study to examine the validity of diagnostic criteria for depression in diabetes using LCA in a large community sample of patients with type 2 diabetes, and there were several important findings. First, LCA of depressive and anxiety symptoms from our sample produced evidence for a 4-class solution: a *major depression-anxiety class*, a *minor depression-anxiety class*, a *subsyndromal anxiety class*, and a class with *no depression or anxiety*. Second, all nine DSM-IV diagnostic criteria for major depression identified a class of patients with a high frequency of major depression, and further changes to these criteria are not necessary. Third, all symptoms of anxiety had similar high probabilities as symptoms of depression for the *major depression-anxiety class*, suggesting that anxiety symptoms should be added to the DSM-IV/5 diagnostic criteria for major depression to identify a class with more severe psychopathology. Therefore, our findings do not support separating anxiety from depressive symptoms for patients with type 2 diabetes. Fourth, the *major depression-anxiety class* had worse diabetes-related parameters than the class without anxiety or depression, suggesting that anxious depression is a marker of more malignant diabetes. Finally, we also identified a class that included anxiety and depression symptoms of a lesser severity, which we termed *minor depression-anxiety*. About one third of this group had clinically relevant anxiety and/or depression, but there were no demographic or clinical differences when compared to the class without anxiety or depression.

These findings should be considered in the light of some limitations of our study. First, given the large sample of individuals to be assessed and the comprehensive quantity of clinical assessments, we were unable to interview patients with more appropriate structured psychiatric interviews. Nevertheless, we assessed depression using the PHQ-9, a valid and reliable instrument to diagnose depression based on DSM-IV criteria and to measure the severity of depression. Second, anxiety symptoms were assessed with the GADS, a new instrument specifically developed and validated for the present study. As with the PHQ-9, the GADS allows a diagnosis of GAD based on DSM-IV criteria and measures the severity of anxiety. We did not use the Generalized Anxiety Disorder 7-item scale (GAD-7) given that this instrument was not available when our study was designed. However, we believe that the GADS is an improvement over the GAD-7 given that the GADS assesses all the DSM-IV/5 criteria for GAD over the past 6 months, whilst the GAD-7 assesses a partial list of symptoms during the past 2 weeks. This was a cross-sectional study, and the clinical progression of the classes identified in this study will need to be examined in our ongoing biennial follow-up study. Finally, we did not assess for the category of 'diabetes distress' in our study. The syndrome of major depression was criticized for not differentiating an expected emotional reaction to a significant stressor from a pathological reaction, whereas 'diabetes distress' may better capture the worries and fears of a chronic illness [23]. However, the construct of 'diabetes distress' is in need of further validation, and it is not included into the major psychiatric nomenclatures. Our study provides empirical support for a class that includes the symptoms of major depression in diabetes, and demonstrates this class to be significantly related to worse diabetes outcomes.

While depression is recognized as one of the most frequent psychiatric disorders in type 2 diabetes, questions remain regarding the validity of using DSM-IV/5 diagnostic criteria when the symptoms of depression and diabetes can overlap. Given the impact of depression on the management and prognosis of diabetes, it is critical to validate diagnostic criteria for depression for use in clinical practice. Using LCA, we found for the first time that all nine- DSM-IV criteria for major depression identify a class of patients with a high chance of having major depression. Moreover, this group also showed significantly worse clinical parameters, such as higher fasting plasma glucose, higher HbA1c, greater use of insulin, higher BMI, increased central adiposity and increased serum triglycerides than the class without anxious depression, which provides partial validation of the classes obtained.

The classes with high probability of depressive symptoms also included a high probability of anxiety symptoms (worrying, restlessness, tension and irritability) and had a high frequency of GAD. This finding demonstrates the high comorbidity of depression and anxiety in diabetes, and suggests that a new diagnostic category of "major anxious depression" should be used in type 2 diabetes. In the general population, this comorbidity is

Table 5. FDS2 baseline associates of major anxious depression class vs major depression (DSM-IV criteria) in participants with type-2 diabetes.

FDS2 baseline variable	Major depression (DSM-IV)	Major anxious-depression (Cluster 4)
N (%)	82 (6.1)	104 (7.8)
Age (years)	60.6±12.5	60.6±12.3
Any depressive syndrome (%)	100.0	77.9
Major depressive syndrome (%)	100.0	67.3
Taking antidepressant medication (%)	42.7	35.6
No depression/depression before diabetes/concomitant diagnoses/ depression after diabetes (%)	0/38.2/19.7/42.1	2.1/43.3/16.5/38.1
Current GAD (%)	43.9	51.0
Lifetime GAD (%):	67.1	70.3
Any depressive syndrome and/or current GAD (DSMIV) (%)	100.0	89.4
Male (%)	46.3	45.2
Educated beyond primary level (%)	79.0	80.4
Currently married	59.8	63.5
Alcohol consumption (standard drinks/day)	0 [0–0.4]	0 [0–0.3]
Age at diagnosis of diabetes (years)	49.3±11.3	49.9±11.6
Diabetes duration (years)	11.0 [4.0–16.1]	10.0 [4.0–15.5]
HbA_{1c} (%)	7.5 [6.2–9.0]	7.5 [6.3–8.9]
Diabetes treatment (% diet/OGLMs/insulin/insulin + OGLMs)	22.0/41.5/9.8/26.8	18.3/43.3/9.6/28.8
BMI (kg/m^2)	33.5±6.1	33.5±7.0
Central adiposity (% obese by waist circumference)	85.4	83.5
Total serum cholesterol (mmol/L)	4.5±1.4	4.5±1.3
HDL-cholesterol (mmol/L)	1.14±0.29	1.15±0.27
Serum triglycerides (mmol/L)	2.0 (1.0–3.8)	2.0 (1.0–3.8)
eGFR <60 ml/min/1.73 m^2 (%)	18.5	22.3
Peripheral sensory neuropathy (%)	53.7	56.3
Any retinopathy (%)	21.8	24.5
History of ischaemic heart disease (%)	36.6	25.0
History of cerebrovascular disease (%)	12.2	7.7
Peripheral arterial disease (%)	23.2	24.3

associated with a poor prognosis, recurrent depression, worse treatment outcomes of depression, more frequent suicide attempts, greater symptom severity, diminished social supports, and more past-year distressing life events [24]. Starr and Davila [25] proposed a model of depression-anxiety comorbidity in which anxiety symptoms lead to depressive symptoms via maladaptive anxiety response styles.

Another relevant finding from our study was a class with intermediate symptoms of anxiety and depression, which we labelled *minor depression-anxiety*. This class included a relatively large proportion of our sample (22%), and future studies may determine whether this class may evolve into a more severe depression with significant impact upon diabetes variables. Cyranowsky et al [24] recently demonstrated that anxiety commonly emerges alongside subthreshold depressive symptoms. The finding that 29% of this class had depression and/or anxiety suggests that this class is clinically relevant. It has been demonstrated that subclinical depression has a significant negative impact on diabetes control [26] and the relationship between depressive symptoms and poor self-care appears to be linear [1]. A third class, which included 38% of the sample, had minor symptoms of anxiety but no depression. Only 2% of this group had clinical depression and/or anxiety, but had a significantly higher lifetime prevalence of GAD and depression as compared to the class with no anxiety or depression. The clinical relevance of this class should be further examined in longitudinal studies.

In conclusion, we demonstrated that the DSM-IV criteria for major depression may be used unmodified to diagnose depression in diabetes. We also found a high comorbidity between depression and anxiety, suggesting that symptoms of anxiety may be included into a new set of diagnostic criteria for major depression or mixed anxiety-depression in type 2 diabetes. Future longitudinal studies will validate this construct and examine the clinical relevance of minor anxious depression and subclinical anxiety in type 2 diabetes.

Author Contributions

Conceived and designed the experiments: SES WAD MD. Performed the experiments: SES WAD VC. Analyzed the data: MD WAD. Contributed reagents/materials/analysis tools: WAD MD. Wrote the paper: SES DB TMED.

References

1. Blay SL, Fillenbaum GG, Marinho V, Andreoli SB, Gastal FL (2011) Increased health burden associated with comorbid depression in older Brazilians with diabetes. J Affect Disord. 134(1–3): 77–84.
2. Gonzalez JS, Peyrot M, McCarl LA, Collins EM, Serpa L, et al (2008) Depression and diabetes treatment nonadherence: a meta-analysis. Diabetes Care. 31(12): 2398–403.
3. de Groot M, Anderson R, Freedland KE, Clouse RE, Lustman PJ (2001) Association of depression and diabetes complications: a meta-analysis. Psychosom Med. 63(4): 619–30.
4. Bruce DG, Davis WA, Starkstein SE, Davis TM (2005) A prospective study of depression and mortality in patients with type 2 diabetes: the Fremantle Diabetes Study. Diabetologia 48(12): 2532–9.
5. Markowitz SM, Gonzalez JS, Wilkinson JL, Safren SA (2011) A review of treating depression in diabetes: emerging findings. Psychosomatics 1; 52(1): 1–18.
6. Atlantis E, Goldney RD, Eckert KA, Taylor AW, Phillips P (2012) Trends in health-related quality of life and health service use associated with comorbid diabetes and major depression in South Australia, 1998–2008. Social psychiatry and psychiatric epidemiology 47(6): 871–7.
7. Atlantis E, Fahey P, Foster J (2014) Collaborative care for comorbid depression and diabetes: a systematic review and meta-analysis. BMJ open 4(4): e004706.
8. Egede LE, Ellis C (2010) Diabetes and depression: global perspectives. Diabetes research and clinical practice 87(3): 302–12.
9. Campayo A, Gomez-Biel CH, Lobo A (2011) Diabetes and depression. Current psychiatry reports 13(1): 26–30.
10. Atlantis E, Vogelzangs N, Cashman K, Penninx BJ (2012) Common mental disorders associated with 2-year diabetes incidence: the Netherlands Study of Depression and Anxiety (NESDA). J Affect Disord 142 Suppl: S30–5.
11. Kessler RC, Merikangas KR, Wang PS (2007) Prevalence, comorbidity, and service utilization for mood disorders in the United States at the beginning of the twenty-first century. Annual review of clinical psychology 3: 137–58.
12. Collins MM, Corcoran P, Perry IJ (2009) Anxiety and depression symptoms in patients with diabetes. Diabet Med 26(2): 153–61.
13. Edwards LE, Mezuk B (2012) Anxiety and risk of type 2 diabetes: evidence from the Baltimore Epidemiologic Catchment Area Study. J Psychosom Res 73(6): 418–23.
14. Nutt D, Argyropoulos S, Hood S, Potokar J (2006) Generalized anxiety disorder: A comorbid disease. European neuropsychopharmacology: the journal of the European College of Neuropsychopharmacology 16 Suppl 2: S109–18.
15. Davis TM, Bruce DG, Davis WA (2013) Cohort profile: the Fremantle Diabetes Study. Int J Epidemiol 42(2): 412–21.
16. Roy T, Lloyd CE, Pouwer F, Holt RI, Sartorius N (2012) Screening tools used for measuring depression among people with Type 1 and Type 2 diabetes: a systematic review. Diabet Med 29(2): 164–75.
17. Kroenke K, Spitzer RL, Williams JB (2001) The PHQ-9: validity of a brief depression severity measure. J Gen Intern Med 16(9): 606–13.
18. Kroenke K, Strine TW, Spitzer RL, Williams JB, Berry JT (2009) The PHQ-8 as a measure of current depression in the general population. J Affect Disord 114(1–3): 163–73.
19. Kroenke K, Spitzer RL, Williams JB, Lowe B (2010) The Patient Health Questionnaire Somatic, Anxiety, and Depressive Symptom Scales: a systematic review. Gen Hosp Psychiatry 32(4): 345–59.
20. Bruce DG, Davis WA, Cetrullo V, Starkstein SE, Davis TM (2013) Clinical Impact of the Temporal Relationship between Depression and Type 2 Diabetes: The Fremantle Diabetes Study Phase II. PLoS One 8(12): e81254.
21. Vermunt JK, Magidson J (2005) Technical Guide for Latent GOLD Choice 4.0: Basic and Advanced. Belmont, Massachussetts.
22. Ruscio J, Brown TA, Meron Ruscio A (2009) A taxometric investigation of DSM-IV major depression in a large outpatient sample: interpretable structural results depend on the mode of assessment. Assessment 16(2): 127–44.
23. Fisher L, Gonzalez JS, Polonsky WH (2014) The confusing tale of depression and distress in patients with diabetes: a call for greater clarity and precision. Diabet Med 31(7): 764–72.
24. Cyranowski JM, Schott LL, Kravitz HM, Brown C, Thurston RC, et al (2012) Psychosocial features associated with lifetime comorbidity of major depression and anxiety disorders among a community sample of mid-life women: the SWAN mental health study. Depress Anxiety 29(12): 1050–7.
25. Starr LR, Davila J (2012) Responding to Anxiety with Rumination and Hopelessness: Mechanism of Anxiety-Depression Symptom Co-Occurrence? Cognitive therapy and research 36(4): 321–37.
26. Fisher L, Skaff MM, Mullan JT, Arean P, Mohr D, et al. (2007) Clinical depression versus distress among patients with type 2 diabetes: not just a question of semantics. Diabetes Care 30(3): 542–8.

Age-Related Cataract, Cataract Surgery and Subsequent Mortality

E Song[1¶], Hongpeng Sun[2¶], Yong Xu[2], Yana Ma[2], Hong Zhu[2], Chen-Wei Pan[2*]

1 Lixiang Eye Hospital of Soochow University, Suzhou, China, 2 School of Public Health, Medical College of Soochow University, Suzhou, China

Abstract

Purpose: Changes in lens may reflect the status of systemic health of human beings but the supporting evidences are not well summarized yet. We aimed to determine the relationship of age-related cataract, cataract surgery and long-term mortality by pooling the results of published population-based studies.

Methods: We searched PubMed and Embase from their inception till March, 2014 for population-based studies reporting the associations of any subtypes of age-related cataract, cataract surgery with all-cause mortality. We pooled the effect estimates (hazards ratios [HRs]) under a random effects model.

Results: Totally, we identified 10 unique population-based studies including 39,659 individuals at baseline reporting the associations of any subtypes of cataract with all-cause mortality from 6 countries. The presence of any cataract including cataract surgery was significantly associated with a higher risk of death (pooled HR: 1.43, 95% CI, 1.21, 2.02; $P<0.001$; $I^2=64.2\%$). In the meta-analysis of 9 study findings, adults with nuclear cataract were at higher risks of mortality (pooled HR: 1.55, 95% CI, 1.17, 2.05; $P=0.002$; $I^2=89.2\%$). In the meta-analysis of 8 study findings, cortical cataract was associated with higher risks of mortality (pooled HR: 1.26, 95% CI, 1.12, 1.42; $P<0.001$, $I^2=29.7\%$). In the meta-analysis of 6 study findings, PSC cataract was associated with higher risks of mortality (pooled HR: 1.37, 95% CI, 1.04, 1.80; $P=0.03$; $I^2=67.3\%$). The association between cataract surgery and mortality was marginally non-significant by pooling 8 study findings (pooled HR: 1.27, 95% CI, 0.97, 1.66; $P=0.08$; $I^2=76.6\%$).

Conclusions: All subtypes of age-related cataract were associated with an increased mortality with nuclear cataract having the strongest association among the 3 cataract subtypes. However, cataract surgery was not significantly related to mortality. These findings indicated that changes in lens may serve as markers for ageing and systemic health in general population.

Editor: Yingfeng Zheng, Zhongshan Ophthalmic Center, China

Funding: The authors have no support or funding to report.

* Email: pcwonly@gmail.com

¶ These authors also contributed equally to this work.

Introduction

Visual impairment (VI) is a global health burden, associated with increased mortality in different ethnic groups [1–5]. Age-related cataract, including nuclear, cortical and posterior subcapsular (PSC) cataract, is a leading cause of visual impairment worldwide [6–13]. Although age-related cataract seems to increase the risk of death, the relationship of different cataract subtypes and mortality remains unclear. It is important for clinicians and ophthalmologists to understand the associations between different cataract subtypes and mortality as the pathophysiology, treatment and impact on visual functioning of the 3 subtypes are different [14]. A clearer understanding of the relationship between cataract subtypes and mortality may provide further insights into the pathogenesis of these conditions. In addition, if a specific subtype of cataract is associated with increased mortality, lens imaging targeting this subtype may be a useful tool for the assessment of systemic health and ageing of the whole body. This research question is also of great importance from public health perspectives regarding the increasing burden of cataract throughout the world. The question of whether age-related cataracts are associated with an increased risk of death or whether the association between increased mortality and the occurrence of the cataract is caused simply by the relationship with higher age is unclear.

To address this gap, we conducted a systematic review and meta-analysis to examine the association between different subtypes of age-related cataract, cataract surgery and long term mortality from available population-based studies.

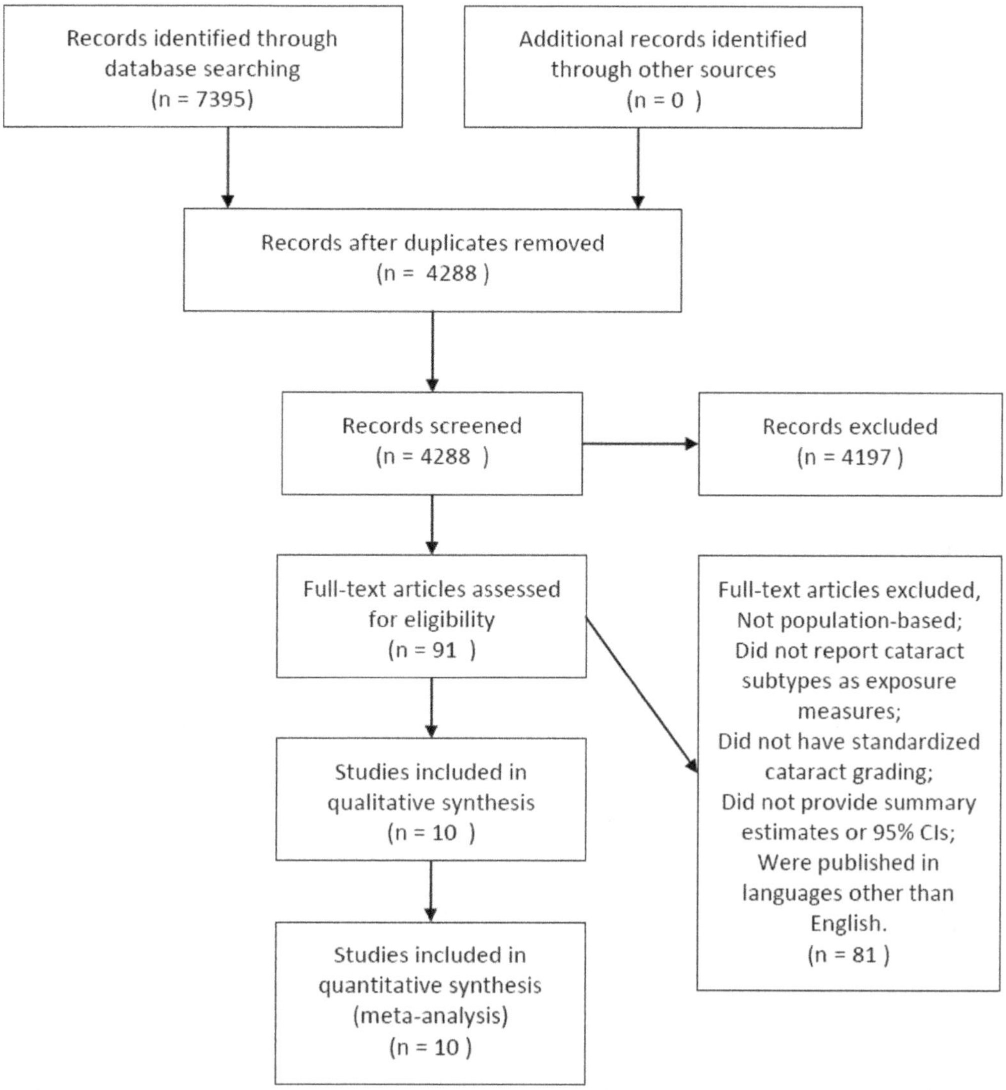

Figure 1. Flow diagram showing the selection process for inclusion of studies.

Methods

Ethnics Statement

The study was approved by the Ethics Committee, Medical College of Soochow University and followed the tenets of the Declaration of Helsinki.

Search Strategy and Inclusion Criteria

The method for performing this meta-analysis is similar with our previously work on overweight/obesity and cataract [15]. We performed this systematic review and meta-analysis to examine the association of different subtypes of age-related cataract, cataract surgery and mortality based on the Meta-analysis of Observational Studies in Epidemiology guidelines [16]. We searched the electronic databases of PubMed and Embase for relevant papers reporting the longitudinal association of age-related cataract, cataract surgery with all-cause mortality published up to March, 2014 with the following search terms (formatted for PubMed search): ((“vision, low”[MeSH Terms] OR (“vision”[All Fields] AND “low”[All Fields]) OR “low vision”[All Fields] OR (“visual”[All Fields] AND “impairment”[All Fields]) OR “visual impairment”[All Fields] OR “vision disorders”[MeSH Terms] OR (“vision”[All Fields] AND “disorders”[All Fields]) OR “vision disorders”[All Fields] OR (“visual”[All Fields] AND “impairment”[All Fields])) OR (“cataract”[MeSH Terms] OR “cataract”[All Fields]) OR (“cataract”[MeSH Terms] OR “cataract”[All Fields] OR (“lens”[All Fields] AND “opacity”[All Fields]) OR “lens opacity”[All Fields]) OR (“cataract extraction”[MeSH Terms] OR (“cataract”[All Fields] AND “extraction”[All Fields]) OR “cataract extraction”[All Fields]) OR (“cataract extraction”[MeSH Terms] OR (“cataract”[All Fields] AND “extraction”[All Fields]) OR “cataract extraction”[All Fields] OR (“cataract”[All Fields] AND “surgery”[All Fields]) OR “cataract surgery”[All Fields])) AND ((“mortality”[Subheading] OR “mortality”[All Fields] OR “mortality”[MeSH Terms]) OR (“mortality”[Subheading] OR “mortality”[All Fields] OR “survival”[All Fields] OR “survival”[MeSH Terms]) OR (“death”[MeSH Terms] OR “death”[All Fields])). Titles and abstracts of the studies were independently reviewed by 2 authors (ES and HPS). All duplicate articles were removed. Inconsistencies during the literature search

Table 1. Characteristics of the included studies.

Author (year)	Study Name	Location	Ethnicity	Sample Size at baseline	Age at baseline (years)	Follow up period (yrs)	Incidence of mortality: N (%)
Knudtson et al (2006)	The Beaver Dam Eye Study	United States	Whites	4926	43–84	14	1576 (32)
Nucci et al (2004)	The Priverno Eye Study	Italy	Italians	860	45–69	7	44 (5.1)
Clemons et al (2004)	The Age-Related Eye Disease Study	United States	Whites	4753	55–81	9	534 (11)
Cugati et al (2007)	The Blue Mountains Eye Study	Australia	Whites	3654	≥49	11	1051 (28.9)
Hennis et al (2000)	The Barbados Eye Study	United States	Blacks	4709	40–84	4	306 (6.8)
Borger et al (2003)	The Rotterdam Study	Netherlands	Whites	6339	≥55	7	1359 (21.4)
West et al (2004)	The Salisbury Eye Project	United States	Whites and Blacks	2520	65–84	2	147 (5.8
Xu et al (2009)	The Beijing Eye Study	China	Chinese	4439	≥40	5	143 (3.2)
McCarty et al (2001)	Melbourne Visual Impairment Project	Australia	White	3271	40–98	5	231 (7.1)
Khanna et al (2013)	The Andhra Pradesh Eye Diseases Study	India	Indians	4188	≥30	11	799 (19.1)

were resolved by consensus and the reference lists of all identified studies were screened.

We included studies if they were population-based, reported any subtypes of age-related cataract or cataract surgery as an independent variable and all-cause mortality as the outcome measure. The Age-Related Eye Disease Study [1] is a multi-center intervention trial rather than a population-based observational study, which has reported the association between major age-related eye diseases and mortality. As the study participants covered a wide geographical areas and the sample size was large, we feel the results should be included in the meta-analysis. We only included studies in which age-related cataract was assessed based on standardized protocols. Furthermore, we included studies only if the summary estimates such as the relative risk (RR) or hazards ratios (HR) with 95% confidence interval (CI) were reported in the paper, or allowed for calculation based on the data presented in the paper. We summarized the measures of association as HR for all the studies. We excluded studies if they were not population-based, did not have standardized cataract grading, or were published in languages other than English. If one study reported two results at different follow-up periods, the result with a longer follow-up period was included in the analysis.

Data Extraction and Assessment of Study Quality

For each study in the analyses, information on first author, publication year, study name, study location, ethnic group, sample size at baseline, age range of the study participants at baseline, follow-up periods, definitions of age-related cataract and mortality, summary estimates and corresponding 95% CI, and confounding factors adjusted for were extracted and recorded in a form designed previously.

The study quality were assessed using the tool described by Sanderson et al [17]. The variables examined included the methods for selecting study participants, methods for measuring exposure (age-related cataract or cataract surgery) and outcome variable (all-cause mortality), design-specific sources of bias, methods for controlling confounding, statistical methods and conflict of interest.

Statistical Methods for the Meta-analysis

The meta-analysis was performed using Stata version 12.0 (StataCorp, College Station, TX). We meta-analyzed the fully-adjusted study-specific risk estimates under random effects model, accounting for both within and between study variability. All-cause mortality was treated as the outcome measure while nuclear, cortical, PSC cataract or cataract surgery were analyzed as the independent variable. Statistical heterogeneity among studies was evaluated using I^2 Statistic [18]. Values of 0 to 24%, 25% to 49%, 50% to 74%, and more than 75% denote no, low, moderate, and high heterogeneity, respectively [19]. Publication bias was assessed using the Egger regression asymmetry test and the Begg's test.

Results

Literature Search and Characteristics of Included Studies

The literature search yielded 4288 unique titles from the two electronic databases. In total, 91 articles were retrieved for full-text review, 12 of which met all the predefined inclusion criteria. However, two studies reported 2 results at different follow-up periods [2,5,20–21] and only the result with a longer follow-up period were included. Finally, 10 unique population-based studies [1–2,21–28] were included in this meta-analysis. (**Figure 1**)

Characteristics of the 10 studies included in the meta-analysis are summarized in **Table 1**. Among the 10 studies, 2 were

Table 2. Assessment of methodological quality of included studies.

Study	Methods for selecting study participants	Methods for measuring exposure (cataract)	Methods for measuring outcome (mortality)	Design-specific sources of bias	Methods for controlling confounding, and statistical methods	Conflict of Interest
Knudtson et al (2006)	4926 persons aged from 43 to 84 years in the period from September 15, 1987, to May 4, 1988, participated in the baseline examination of the population-based Beaver Dam Eye Study and were followed by about 10 years.	Wisconsin Grading System	National Death Index was used for matching against national death data.	Lost to follow up bias; survival bias; chance finding; residual confounding	Adjustments for age, sex, proteinuria, history of cancer, BMI, ratio of total to high-density lipoprotein cholesterol level, smoking, pulse rate,diabetes status, cardiovascular disease history, sedentary lifestyle, education, and systolic blood pressure were made using Cox proportional hazards models	None reported
Nucci et al (2004)	860 legal residents of Priverno represented 70% of a random sample selected to participate in the Di.S.Co. Project—a population-based study on cardiovascular risk factors carried out by the Italian National Institute of Health.	Slit-lamp examination	Review of municipality records	Lack of statistical power; lost to follow up bias; survival bias; chance finding; residual confounding	Adjusting for age, gender, diabetes, serum cholesterol, high-density lipoprotein cholesterol, and cardiovascular diseases using Cox proportional-hazards regression model.	None reported
Clemons et al (2004)	A total of 4757 persons aged 55 to 81 years at enrollment were entered into the study at 11 clinical centers between 1992 and 1998 and were followed up by 9 years	The Age-Related Eye Disease Study (AREDS) system	Hospital records and death certificates.	Lost to follow up bias; chance finding; residual confounding	Cox proportional-hazards regression model adjusting for age, sex, race, education, smoking status, body mass index, diabetes mellitus, angina, cancer, and hypertension	None reported
Cugati et al (2007)	Australian adults aged 49 years and older at baseline in the Blue Mountains area were followed up for about 11 years	Wisconsin Grading System	The Australian National Death Index data	Lost to follow up bias; survival bias; chance finding; residual confounding	Cox regression models assessed associations between cataract and mortality risk during 11 years after adjusting for age, sex, BMI, hypertension, diabetes mellitus, current smoking, and history of stroke, angina, or myocardial infarction	None reported
Hennis et al (2000)	The studies were based on a simple random sample of Barbados African Americans, 40 to 84 years old. 4631 persons completed baseline examinations at the study site. Surviving members of the cohort were invited to return for a 4-year follow-up visit.	Lens Opacities Classification System II	Ministry of Health records	Lost to follow up bias; survival bias; chance finding; residual confounding	Cox proportional-hazards regression. age; gender; self-reported history of diabetes, cardiac disease, and stroke, or combination of these major illnesses; family history of diabetes and hypertension; body mass index; waist-to-hip ratio; alcohol use; and cigarette smoking.	None reported
Borger et al (2003)	A prospective cohort study of all residents aged 55 years and older from a suburb of Rotterdam	Lens Opacities Classification System II	Municipal registry and medical records.	Lost to follow up bias; chance finding; residual confounding	Cox proportional hazard regression analysis, adjusted for appropriate confounders (age, gender, smoking status, body mass index, cholesterol level, atherosclerosis, hypertension, history of cardiovascular disease, and diabetes mellitus)	None reported
West et al (2004)	A random sample of 2520 residents of Salisbury aged 65 to 84 years was recruited for a home interview and an examination at the SEE clinic. Two-year follow-up was conducted.	Wilmer grading scheme.	Hospital records and the National Death Index	Lost to follow up bias; survival bias; chance finding; residual confounding	Logistic regression model adjusting for age, sex, smoking, diabetes, cormorbid conditions and body mass index.	None reported
Xu et al (2009)	At baseline in 2001, the Beijing Eye Study examined 4439 subjects with an age of 40 years or more. In 2006, all study participants were invited for a follow-up examination.	The Age-Related Eye Disease Study (AREDS) system	Death certificate, hospital medical records	Lost to follow up bias; survival bias; chance finding; residual confounding	Logistic regression was used to investigate the associations of the binary dependent variable mortality with the continuous or categorical independent variables.	None reported

Table 2. Cont.

Study	Methods for selecting study participants	Methods for measuring exposure (cataract)	Methods for measuring outcome (mortality)	Design-specific sources of bias	Methods for controlling confounding, and statistical methods	Conflict of Interest
McCarty et al(2001)	Cluster random sampling was employed to identify nine pairs of census collector districts in the Melbourne statistical division from which to recruit eligible residents. Baseline examinations were conducted between 1992 and 1994. In 1997, 5 year follow up examinations of the original cohort commenced.	Wilmer grading scheme.	National Death Index	Lack of statistical power, lost to follow up bias; survival bias; chance finding; residual confounding	Multivariate logistic regression adjusting for age, sex, country of birth, smoking, hypertension, arthritis, best corrected visual acuity, age related maculopathy, glaucoma, uncorrected refractive error,diabetes,gout and cardiovascular disease.	None reported
Khanna et al (2013)	A large-scale prevalence survey of blindness and visual impairment was conducted between 1996–2000 on 10,293 individuals of all ages in three rural and one urban clusters in Andhra Pradesh, Southern India. More than a decade later, participants in rural clusters were traced to determine ocular risk factors for mortality.	Wilmer grading scheme.	Questionnaire	Lack of statistical power, lost to follow up bias; survival bias; chance finding; residual confounding	Cox-proportional hazard model after adjusting for age, gender, diabetes, hypertension, body mass index, smoking and education status	None reported

conducted in Asia [22–23], 2 were in Australia [21,24], 2 were in Europe [25–26] and the remaining 4 were in the United States [1–2,27–28]. The 10 cohort studies comprised a total of 39,659 individuals at baseline. The sample sizes at baseline ranged from 860 to 6,339. The follow-up periods ranged from 2 to 14 years. The range of mortality rates in all identified studies was very wide (from 3.2% to 32%), which may be due to methodological issues including various ages of enrollment at baseline, follow-up periods and ethnic groups.

Quality Assessment of the Included Studies

All studies graded cataract based on standardized protocols such as the Wisconsin grading system, the Wilmer grading system or the Lens Opacity Classification System [29–31]. In most of the included studies, mortality data were reviewed and retrieved from official records or hospital medical records. All studies adjusted for age in the multivariate analysis; however, diabetes, the most important confounding factor was not adjusted for in one study. All studies gave loss to follow-up rates and described sampling methods in the baseline examinations, albeit in varying degrees. However, only 6 studies outlined specific exclusion criteria and provided information on non-responders. Conflicts of interest were not reported in all included studies. The detailed assessment of study quality of the included study is described in **Table 2**.

Age-related cataract and mortality

Adults with any cataract or cataract surgery previously were more like to die (pooled HR: 1.43, 95% CI, 1.21, 2.02; $P<0.001$; $I^2=64.2\%$). In the meta-analysis of 9 study findings, adults with nuclear cataract were at higher risks of mortality (pooled HR: 1.55, 95% CI, 1.17, 2.05; $P=0.002$; $I^2=89.2\%$) (**Figure 2**). In the meta-analysis of 8 study findings, cortical cataract was associated with higher risks of mortality (pooled HR: 1.26, 95% CI, 1.12, 1.42; $P<0.001$, $I^2=29.7\%$) (**Figure 3**). In the meta-analysis of 6 study findings, PSC cataract was associated with higher risks of mortality (pooled HR: 1.37, 95% CI, 1.04, 1.80; $P=0.03$; $I^2=67.3\%$) (**Figure 4**). The association between cataract surgery and mortality was marginally non-significant by pooling 8 study findings (pooled HR: 1.27, 95% CI, 0.97, 1.66; $P=0.08$; $I^2=76.6\%$)(**Figure 5**). After excluding the Salisbury Eye Project with a follow-up period of only 2 years, all cataract subtypes were still associated with mortality (data not shown).

Table 3 shows the association between cataract and mortality by follow-up years of the identified studies and cataract diagnosis. The estimates were more robust in studies with longer follow-up periods or more standardized grading systems (graded by lens photographs).

There was no evidence of publication bias as indicated by a non-significant Egger test (all $P>0.05$) and Begg's test (all $P>0.05$) in all analyses.

Discussion

In this systematic review and meta-analysis of population-based studies, all subtypes of age-related cataract were associated with increased mortality with nuclear cataract having the strongest association among the 3 cataract subtypes. However, cataract surgery was not significantly related to mortality. These findings indicated that changes in lens may serve as markers for ageing and systemic health in the general population.

Our meta-analysis confirmed the longitudinal association between nuclear cataract (nuclear sclerosis of the lens) and increased mortality reported in previous studies. In addition, we found that the association of nuclear cataract with increased

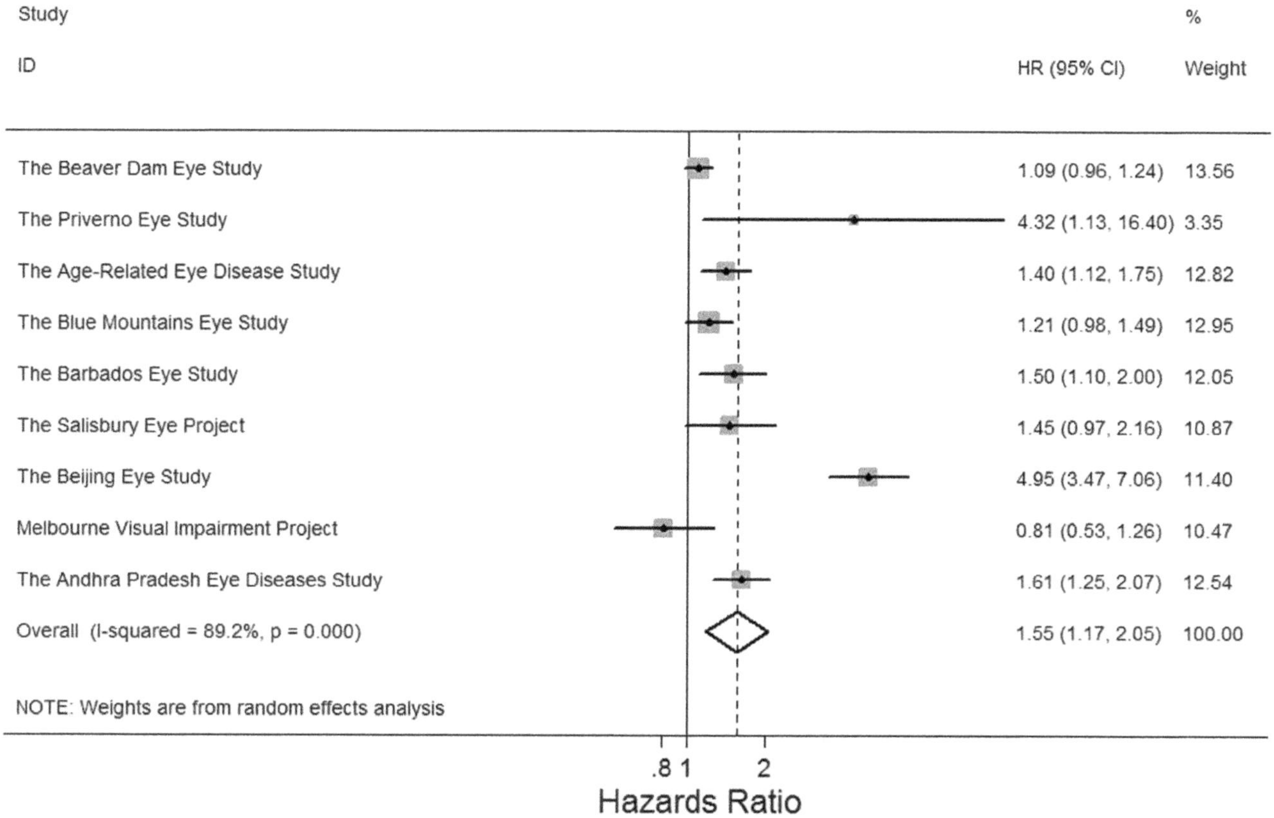

Figure 2. Random effects meta-analysis investigating the association between nuclear cataract and all-cause mortality. HR = hazards ratio; CI = confidence interval.

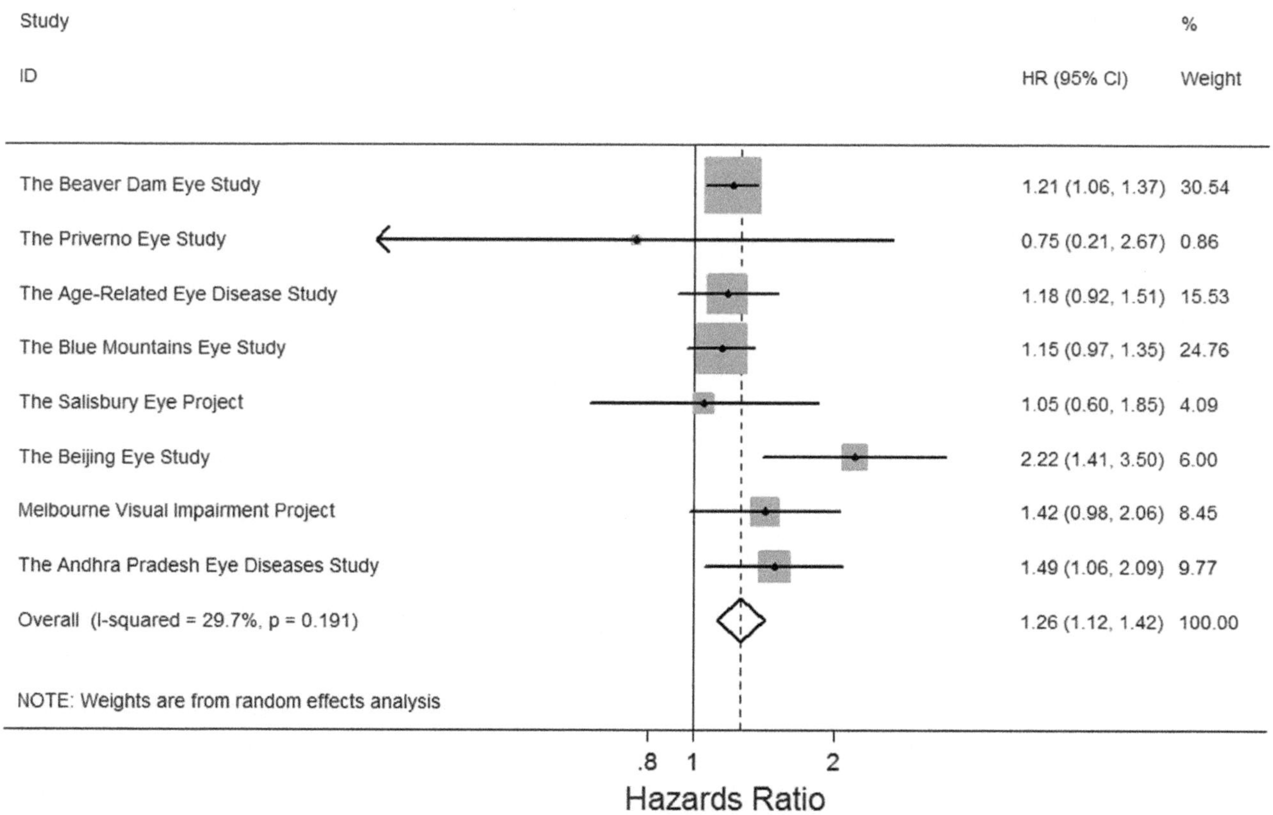

Figure 3. Random effects meta-analysis investigating the association between cortical cataract and all-cause mortality. HR = hazards ratio; CI = confidence interval.

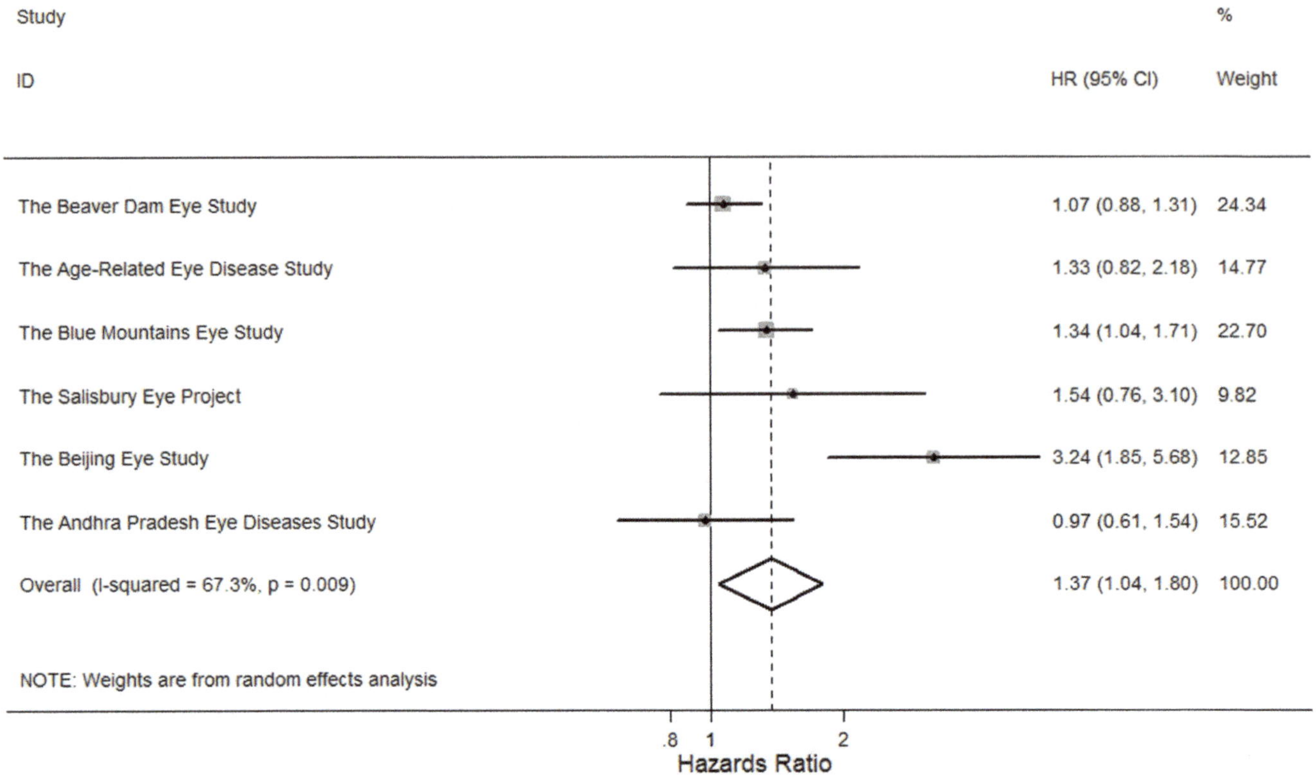

Figure 4. Random effects meta-analysis investigating the association between posterior subcapsular cataract and all-cause mortality. HR = hazards ratio; CI = confidence interval.

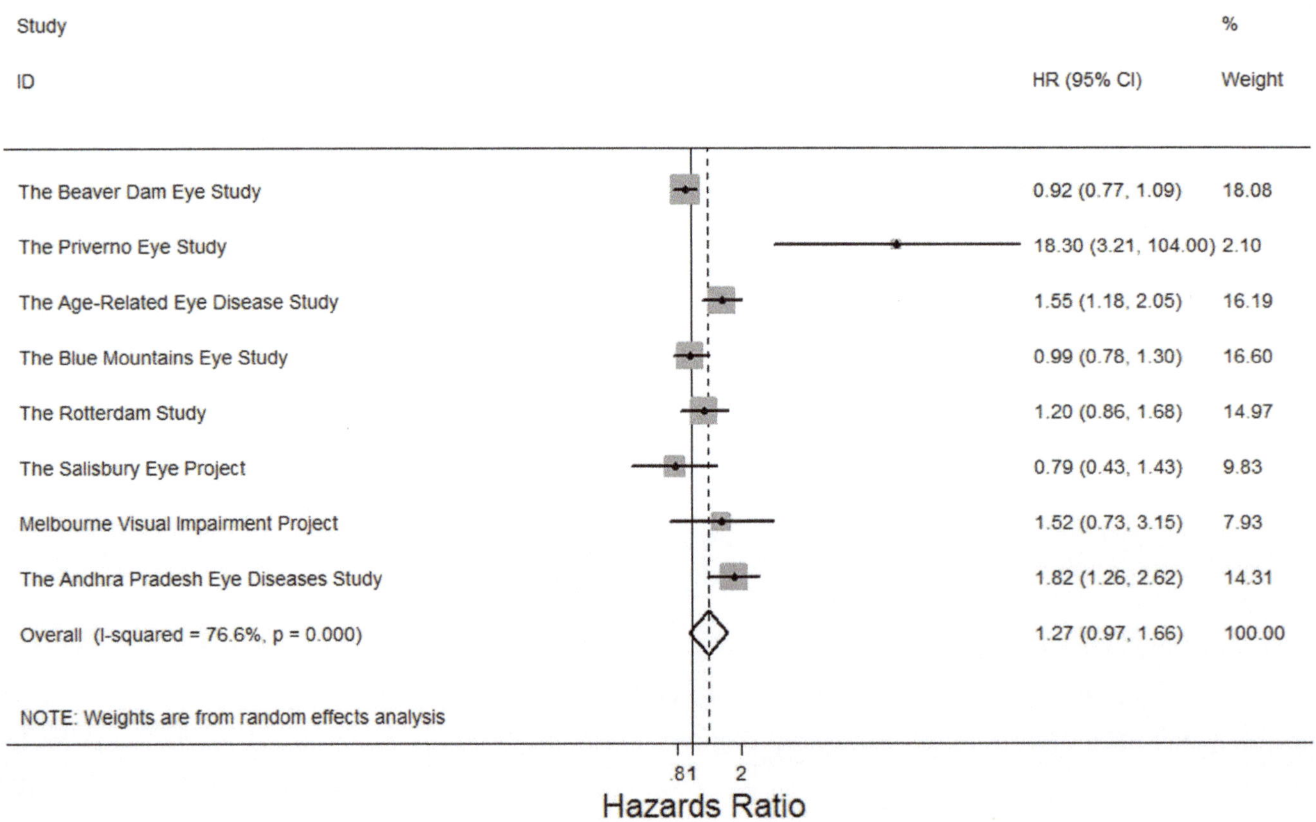

Figure 5. Random effects meta-analysis investigating the association between cataract surgery and all-cause mortality. HR = hazards ratio; CI = confidence interval.

Table 3. Association between cataract and mortality by follow-up years and cataract diagnosis.

	Nuclear cataract				Cortical Cataract				Posterior Subcapsular Cataract				Cataract Surgery			
	N	HR	95% CI	I2 (%)	N	HR	95% CI	I2 (%)	N	HR	95% CI	I2 (%)	N	HR	95% CI	I2 (%)
Follow-up years																
More than 5 years	5	1.32	1.09, 1.60	68.0	5	1.2	1.10, 1.32	0	4	1.16	1.01, 1.33	0	6	1.33	0.98,1.80	82.1
No more than 5 years	4	1.73	0.84, 3.56	93.6	3	1.52	1.03,2.25	55	2	2.31	1.12, 4.77	61.9	2	1.06	0.56,2.00	45.6
Cataract diagnosis																
By photographs	7	1.50	1.09, 2.06	91.5	7	1.27	1.13, 1.44	36	6	1.37	1.04, 1.80	67.3	6	1.2	0.92, 1.56	74.8
By Ophthalmologist clinically	2	2.07	0.80, 5.35	56.3	1	0.75	0.21, 2.67	-	0	-	-	-	2	4.08	0.29, 58.07	89

N = number of studies RR = hazards ratio CI = confidence interval.

mortality was strongest among all of the three cataract subtypes. Nuclear sclerosis of the lens may be a marker for changes in structural proteins of the whole body, mainly resulting from oxidation that cause diminished function [32]. For example, the levels of glutathione (GSH), one of the most important antioxidant agents of the lens, are found to be much higher in the outer cortex fiber cells where GSH is synthesized [33]. Reduced GSH reaches the lens nucleus by diffusion from the surface fiber cells through an abundant network of gap junctions [34]. With increasing age, a greater percentage of GSH is oxidized in the nucleus, making it more susceptible to oxidation [35]. Chronic oxidative stress, especially in brain and immune cells, could accelerate the rate of ageing, leading to an increased mortality in adults with nuclear cataract.

Compared with nuclear cataract, we found a weaker but significant association between cortical cataract and less survival. In the Blue Mountains Eye Study, the association between cortical cataract and increased mortality was no longer significant in persons without diabetes, indicating that the observed association may be confounded by the presence of diabetes [5]. Diabetes is one of the most consistent determinants for cortical cataract [36–38]. In this systematic review, most of the included studies have adjusted for the effect of diabetes in the multivariate analysis (**Table 2**), indicating that the association between cortical cataract and mortality may be, at least partially, independent. UV light exposure could increase the risk of cortical cataract [39]. Exposure to UV light, a known risk factor for cortical cataract, can lead to oxidative stress in the lens, which is a main cause for cortical cataract. This process is similar with other systemic causes of oxidative stress, which may increase the risk of systemic morbidity [40].

The association of PSC cataract and mortality was also positively significant in this meta-analysis although there were fewer studies reporting this association compared with other subtypes. At current stage, we were unable to provide a reasonable biological explanation for this observed association. Animal studies have demonstrated that injection of peroxidative substances into the vitreous resulted in the formation of PSC cataract [41], which may be mediated by peroxidative damage of the whole body.

We found a marginally non-significant association between cataract surgery and mortality, which may be a balanced effect of aged-related cataract and good knowledge of health. Adults who have undergone cataract surgery certainly had cataract previously, which may increase the risk of long term mortality. On the other hand, they tend to have better knowledge of health and healthier lifestyle compared with those who did not. For example, in the Beaver Dam Eye Study, adults with cataract surgery were more likely to take vitamin supplements [2]. Also, adults with previous cataract surgery may have better access to health care services. A clinical trial investigating the effect of cataract surgery on survival in cataract patients may be useful to confirm this finding.

Our meta-analysis may have some important clinical implications. Previous studies have shown that age-related cataract is associated with systemic comorbidities [42] and general functional decline [43] in older adults. We confirmed that these systemic comorbidities and functional decline are sufficient to cause death in the general population. Therefore, we propose that lens imaging may be a necessary clinical examination for normal heath screening of older adults and should not be limited only in eye clinics. Currently, there are various technologies [44–45] for lens imaging and it remains controversial which one is the best to quantify lens opacity in elderly adults.

There are several strengths of the meta-analysis. The qualities of the included studies were relatively high with population-based samples achieving reasonable follow-up rates and the use of standardized grading systems for age-related cataract. Limitations of this meta-analysis should also be acknowledged. First, the potential biases in the original studies, methodological issues and different strategies for adjusting for confounders could affect the results from this meta-analysis. The longitudinal association of age-related cataract and mortality may have been confounded by other unadjusted factors or selection bias. Second, different studies used different cataract grading system, sampling strategies, follow-up period, and ways of mortality measures, which would affect the estimates of mortality. These differences could have also contributed to the observed high heterogeneity across studies. Thirdly, most included studies only reported the association between cataract and all-cause mortality and therefore we were unable to summarize the association between cataract and the cause of mortality. Fourthly, the number of the contributing prospective studies was small and therefore, detailed subgroups analysis may not be feasible. Finally, although there was no evidence of publication bias as indicated by a non-significant Egger test and Begg's test, publication bias could still be of concern because studies that report statistically significant results are more likely to get published than studies that report non-significant results, and this could have distorted the findings of our meta-analyses.

In conclusion, this systematic review and meta-analysis confirmed a longitudinal associations of all age-related cataract subtypes but not cataract surgery with increased mortality. The association was strongest for nuclear cataract. Clinically, ophthalmologists and clinicians should be aware that lens imaging may be a useful tool for the assessment of ageing of the whole body.

Supporting Information

Checklist S1 PRISMA checklist.

Author Contributions

Conceived and designed the experiments: ES HS CWP. Performed the experiments: ES HS. Analyzed the data: HS YX YM. Contributed reagents/materials/analysis tools: CWP. Wrote the paper: ES HS YX YM HZ CWP.

References

1. Clemons TE, Kurinij N, Sperduto RD (2004) Associations of mortality with ocular disorders and an intervention of high-dose antioxidants and zinc in the Age-Related Eye Disease Study: AREDS Report No. 13. Arch Ophthalmol 122: 716–726.
2. Knudtson MD, Klein BE, Klein R (2006) Age-related eye disease, visual impairment, and survival: the Beaver Dam Eye Study. Arch Ophthalmol 124: 243–249.
3. Foong AW, Fong CW, Wong TY, Saw SM, Heng D, et al. (2008) Visual acuity and mortality in a chinese population. The Tanjong Pagar Study. Ophthalmology 115: 802–807.
4. Li Z, Sun D, Liu P, Zhang L, Bai J, et al. (2011) Visual impairment and mortality in a rural adult population (the Southern Harbin eye study). Ophthalmic Epidemiol 18: 54–60.
5. Wang JJ, Mitchell P, Simpson JM, Cumming RG, Smith W (2001) Visual impairment, age-related cataract, and mortality. Arch Ophthalmol 119: 1186–1190.
6. Duerksen R, Limburg H, Carron JE, Foster A (2003) Cataract blindness in Paraguay–results of a national survey. Ophthalmic Epidemiol 10: 349–357.
7. Dunzhu S, Wang FS, Courtright P, Liu L, Tenzing C, et al. (2003) Blindness and eye diseases in Tibet: findings from a randomised, population based survey. Br J Ophthalmol 87: 1443–1448.
8. Zheng Y, Lavanya R, Wu R, Wong WL, Wang JJ, et al. (2011) Prevalence and causes of visual impairment and blindness in an urban Indian population: the singapore Indian eye study. Ophthalmology 118: 1798–1804.
9. Thulasiraj RD, Nirmalan PK, Ramakrishnan R, Krishnadas R, Manimekalai TK, et al. (2003) Blindness and vision impairment in a rural south Indian population: The aravind comprehensive eye survey. Ophthalmology 110: 1491–1498.
10. Murthy GV, Gupta S, Ellwein LB, Munoz SR, Bachani D, et al. (2001) A population-based eye survey of older adults in a rural district of Rajasthan: I. Central vision impairment, blindness, and cataract surgery. Ophthalmology 108: 679–685.
11. Zhao J, Ellwein LB, Cui H, Ge J, Guan H, et al. (2010) Prevalence of vision impairment in older adults in rural China: the China Nine-Province Survey. Ophthalmology 117: 409–416, 416 e401.
12. Hyman L, Wu SY, Connell AM, Schachat A, Nemesure B, et al. (2001) Prevalence and causes of visual impairment in The Barbados Eye Study. Ophthalmology 108: 1751–1756.
13. Varma R, Ying-Lai M, Klein R, Azen SP (2004) Prevalence and risk indicators of visual impairment and blindness in Latinos: the Los Angeles Latino Eye Study. Ophthalmology 111: 1132–1140.
14. Chew M, Chiang PP, Zheng Y, Lavanya R, Wu R, et al. (2012) The impact of cataract, cataract types, and cataract grades on vision-specific functioning using Rasch analysis. Am J Ophthalmol 154: 29–38 e22.
15. Pan CW, Lin Y (2014) Overweight, Obesity, and Age-Related Cataract: A Meta-analysis. Optom Vis Sci 91: 478–483.
16. Stroup DF, Berlin JA, Morton SC, Olkin I, Williamson GD, et al. (2000) Meta-analysis of observational studies in epidemiology: a proposal for reporting. Meta-analysis Of Observational Studies in Epidemiology (MOOSE) group. JAMA 283: 2008–2012.
17. Sanderson S, Tatt ID, Higgins JP (2007) Tools for assessing quality and susceptibility to bias in observational studies in epidemiology: a systematic review and annotated bibliography. Int J Epidemiol 36: 666–676.
18. Higgins JP, Thompson SG, Deeks JJ, Altman DG (2003) Measuring inconsistency in meta-analyses. BMJ 327: 557–560.
19. Higgins JP, Thompson SG (2002) Quantifying heterogeneity in a meta-analysis. Stat Med 21: 1539–1558.
20. Klein R, Klein BE, Moss SE (1995) Age-related eye disease and survival. The Beaver Dam Eye Study. Arch Ophthalmol 113: 333–339.
21. Cugati S, Cumming RG, Smith W, Burlutsky G, Mitchell P, et al. (2007) Visual impairment, age-related macular degeneration, cataract, and long-term mortality: the Blue Mountains Eye Study. Arch Ophthalmol 125: 917–924.
22. Xu L, Wang YX, Wang J, Jonas JJ (2009) Mortality and ocular diseases: the Beijing Eye Study. Ophthalmology 116: 732–738.
23. Khanna RC, Murthy GV, Giridhar P, Krishnaiah S, Pant HB, et al. (2013) Cataract, visual impairment and long-term mortality in a rural cohort in India: the Andhra Pradesh Eye Disease Study. PLoS One 8: e78002.
24. McCarty CA, Nanjan MB, Taylor HR (2001) Vision impairment predicts 5 year mortality. Br J Ophthalmol 85: 322–326.
25. Borger PH, van Leeuwen R, Hulsman CA, Wolfs RC, van der Kuip DA, et al. (2003) Is there a direct association between age-related eye diseases and mortality? The Rotterdam Study. Ophthalmology 110: 1292–1296.
26. Nucci C, Cedrone C, Culasso F, Cesareo M, Regine F, et al. (2004) Association between lens opacities and mortality in the Priverno Eye Study. Graefes Arch Clin Exp Ophthalmol 242: 289–294.
27. West SK, Munoz B, Istre J, Rubin GS, Friedman SM, et al. (2000) Mixed lens opacities and subsequent mortality. Arch Ophthalmol 118: 393–397.
28. Hennis A, Wu SY, Li X, Nemesure B, Leske MC (2001) Lens opacities and mortality: the Barbados Eye Studies. Ophthalmology 108: 498–504.
29. Klein BE, Klein R, Linton KL, Magli YL, Neider MW (1990) Assessment of cataracts from photographs in the Beaver Dam Eye Study. Ophthalmology 97: 1428–1433.
30. Chylack LT, Jr., Wolfe JK, Singer DM, Leske MC, Bullimore MA, et al. (1993) The Lens Opacities Classification System III. The Longitudinal Study of Cataract Study Group. Arch Ophthalmol 111: 831–836.
31. Chylack LT, Jr., Leske MC, McCarthy D, Khu P, Kashiwagi T, et al. (1989) Lens opacities classification system II (LOCS II). Arch Ophthalmol 107: 991–997.
32. Li L, Duker JS, Yoshida Y, Niki E, Rasmussen H, et al. (2009) Oxidative stress and antioxidant status in older adults with early cataract. Eye (Lond) 23: 1464–1468.
33. Giblin FJ (2000) Glutathione: a vital lens antioxidant. J Ocul Pharmacol Ther 16: 121–135.
34. Sweeney MH, Garland DL, Truscott RJ (2003) Movement of cysteine in intact monkey lenses: the major site of entry is the germinative region. Exp Eye Res 77: 245–251.
35. Ye L, Li Q, Cai X, Deng P (2005) Expression of TGF-beta2 mRNA and PCNA, FN protein in lens epithelial cells in age-related nuclear and cortex cataract. J Huazhong Univ Sci Technolog Med Sci 25: 578–581.
36. Machan CM, Hrynchak PK, Irving EL (2012) Age-related cataract is associated with type 2 diabetes and statin use. Optom Vis Sci 89: 1165–1171.
37. Rowe NG, Mitchell PG, Cumming RG, Wans JJ (2000) Diabetes, fasting blood glucose and age-related cataract: the Blue Mountains Eye Study. Ophthalmic Epidemiol 7: 103–114.
38. Klein BE, Klein R, Lee KE (1998) Diabetes, cardiovascular disease, selected cardiovascular disease risk factors, and the 5-year incidence of age-related

cataract and progression of lens opacities: the Beaver Dam Eye Study. Am J Ophthalmol 126: 782–790.
39. Taylor HR, West SK, Rosenthal FS, Munoz B, Newland HS, et al. (1988) Effect of ultraviolet radiation on cataract formation. N Engl J Med 319: 1429–1433.
40. Witztum JL (1994) The oxidation hypothesis of atherosclerosis. Lancet 344: 793–795.
41. Goosey JD, Tuan WM, Garcia CA (1984) A lipid peroxidative mechanism for posterior subcapsular cataract formation in the rabbit: a possible model for cataract formation in tapetoretinal diseases. Invest Ophthalmol Vis Sci 25: 608–612.
42. Nemet AY, Vinker S, Levartovsky S, Kaiserman I (2010) Is cataract associated with cardiovascular morbidity? Eye 24: 1352–1358.
43. Klein BEK, Klein R, Knudtson MD (2006) Frailty and age-related cataract. Ophthalmology 113: 2209–2212.
44. Belikova J, Synek S (2013) Correlation of age-related cataract density graded by the Scheimpflug Imaging System with visual function and phacoemulsification energy. Coll Antropol 37 Suppl 1: 25–30.
45. Grewal DS, Grewal SP (2012) Clinical applications of Scheimpflug imaging in cataract surgery. Saudi J Ophthalmol 26: 25–32.

Identification of Allelic Heterogeneity at Type-2 Diabetes Loci and Impact on Prediction

Yann C. Klimentidis[1]*, Jin Zhou[1], Nathan E. Wineinger[2]

1 Mel and Enid Zuckerman College of Public Health, Division of Epidemiology and Biostatistics, University of Arizona, Tucson, Arizona, United States of America, **2** Scripps Translational Science Institute, La Jolla, California, United States of America

Abstract

Although over 60 single nucleotide polymorphisms (SNPs) have been identified by meta-analysis of genome-wide association studies for type-2 diabetes (T2D) among individuals of European descent, much of the genetic variation remains unexplained. There are likely many more SNPs that contribute to variation in T2D risk, some of which may lie in the regions surrounding established SNPs - a phenomenon often referred to as allelic heterogeneity. Here, we use the summary statistics from the DIAGRAM consortium meta-analysis of T2D genome-wide association studies along with linkage disequilibrium patterns inferred from a large reference sample to identify novel SNPs associated with T2D surrounding each of the previously established risk loci. We then examine the extent to which the use of these additional SNPs improves prediction of T2D risk in an independent validation dataset. Our results suggest that multiple SNPs at each of 3 loci contribute to T2D susceptibility (*TCF7L2, CDKN2A/B*, and *KCNQ1*; $p<5\times10^{-8}$). Using a less stringent threshold ($p<5\times10^{-4}$), we identify 34 additional loci with multiple associated SNPs. The addition of these SNPs slightly improves T2D prediction compared to the use of only the respective lead SNPs, when assessed using an independent validation cohort. Our findings suggest that some currently established T2D risk loci likely harbor multiple polymorphisms which contribute independently and collectively to T2D risk. This opens a promising avenue for improving prediction of T2D, and for a better understanding of the genetic architecture of T2D.

Editor: Shengxu Li, Tulane School of Public Health and Tropical Medicine, United States of America

Funding: YCK was supported by NIH grant K01DK095032. NEW was supported by NIH grant 1UL1TR001114. The funders had no role in study design, data collection and analysis, decision to publish, or preparation of the manuscript.

Competing Interests: The authors have declared that no competing interests exist.

* Email: yann@email.arizona.edu

Introduction

Approximately 65 loci have been shown to be associated with type-2 diabetes (T2D) through genome-wide association studies (GWAS). However, variation at these loci accounts for a small proportion of the expected heritability of T2D [1,2]. Among several potential strategies for identifying additional contributing genetic variation, one approach is to determine whether there are additional genetic markers near established loci that act independently or jointly with the reported marker (lead SNP).

Allelic heterogeneity is a feature of the genetic architecture of many traits, including common traits and diseases such as height, BMI, and T2D [3–6]. In the context of T2D genetics, both Morris et al. [2] and Yang et al. [7] have suggested that additional SNPs in established loci are associated with T2D risk. However, Morris et al. only considered SNPs in weak linkage disequilibrium ($r^2<0.05$) with the lead SNP, and that were not in the same recombination interval. Hence, without formal conditional analysis, they identified two loci as having multiple associations at genome-wide significance (*KCNQ1* and *CDKN2A/B*), and two more at suggestive levels (*DGKB* and *MC4R*). Yang et al. have recently developed a method for identifying additional associated SNPs based on conditional/joint (C/J) analysis using GWAS summary statistics and linkage disequilibrium (LD) information from a reference sample [7]. They applied their method to only a single established T2D locus (*CDKN2A/B*), and identified two novel SNPs at that locus that were significantly associated with T2D when fitted jointly. Finally, on a smaller scale (1,924 cases and 5,380 controls), Ke [8] identified multiple associated loci at the *CDKN2A/B* and *TSPAN8* loci. Although higher power is afforded with the GWAS meta-analysis approach to identify associations with single SNPs, it does not allow for direct C/J analysis since the actual genotype data is not available. The advantage of the method developed by Yang et al. is that it takes advantage of the greater power of GWAS meta-analyses, while also testing for C/J associations, which would otherwise be impossible without individual level data.

Here, we comprehensively examine allelic heterogeneity based on the method developed by Yang et al. at 65 T2D loci discovered by the DIAGRAM consortium, using the summary statistics from their recent meta-analysis of T2D GWAS. We then examine the extent to which these newly identified SNPs increase the accuracy of T2D risk prediction in an independent validation dataset.

Methods

Datasets

We used 6,054 nominally unrelated European-American subjects (genomic relationship coefficient <0.025, based on approximately 2.5 million SNPs) from the Atherosclerosis Risk in Communities (ARIC) study [9] to obtain linkage disequilibrium (LD) estimates. According to Yang et al. [7], this sample size is sufficient for LD estimation with minimal error. In order to maximize the overlap of SNPs between the meta-analysis summary statistics (see below) and the ARIC study, we used IMPUTE2 software [10] along with 1000 Genomes reference data to impute millions of additional SNPs. Prior to imputation, we excluded individuals with a high genotype missing rate (>10%). SNPs were excluded based on extreme minor allele frequency (<0.5%), a high missing rate (>10%), or failed Hardy-Weinberg equilibrium ($p<0.005$). After imputation, we excluded SNPs with 'info' <0.6 (measure of imputation quality), and SNPs with genotype dosage between 0.33 and 0.66, or between 1.33 and 1.66. Intermediate dosages outside of these specified ranges were rounded to the nearest integer. We did not use intermediate genotype dosages since this was not an option with the GCTA software, described below.

The validation dataset consisted of European-American subjects from the Multi-Ethnic Study of Atherosclerosis (MESA) [11], which included 225 T2D cases and 1,985 controls. T2D cases were defined as having a fasting glucose level ≥126 mg/dL, a self-report of taking diabetes medication, or a physician diagnosis of T2D. This dataset can be considered an independent validation dataset since it was not part of the DIAGRAM meta-analysis, whereas ARIC was a part of this meta-analysis, thus precluding it from any validation assessment. We implemented genotype QC and imputation as detailed above. However, we did not round or remove intermediate genotype dosages. The MESA and ARIC dataset were obtained from dbGaP (database of Genotypes and Phenotypes). IRB approval was obtained from the University of Arizona.

Conditional/Joint Analysis

Using the summary statistics from the discovery phase of the latest version (v3) of the DIAbetes Genetics Replication And Meta-analysis (DIAGRAM) consortium, available to the public through an online source [12] and LD estimates from the ARIC dataset as described above, we used GCTA software [13] to perform stepwise model selection. Briefly, SNPs were selected into the model based on p-values in the meta-analysis. An iterative scheme was adopted in which C/J analyses were alternatively performed with the stepwise selection procedure. SNPs with a re-estimated (i.e. through C/J estimation as opposed to marginal estimation) p-value under a certain threshold were selected. For a full description of the method, see Yang et al. [7]. We restricted our analysis to only the genomic regions within 1 Mb of the top SNP at the 65 established T2D loci as reported in Morris et al [2]. This filtering along with the QC filtering described above resulted in 112,329 SNPs being used in this analysis. For each SNP, we recorded the following information as input for the C/J analysis: effect allele, effect size (log of odds ratio), corresponding standard error, p-value, allele frequency of the effect allele (based on ARIC sample described above, as this was not available in the DIAGRAM summary statistic file), and sample size (sum of cases and controls). We used PolyPhen-2 [14] to determine whether any of the newly identified SNPs had any predicted functional effect, and RegulomeDB [15] to determine whether these SNPs may lie in regulatory regions (e.g. transcription factor binding sites) or are associated with specific DNA features (e.g. DNAse sensitivity).

Validation/Prediction

We compared several prediction models. First we constructed a baseline model which only considered demographic information (sex and age). Then we added a weighted genetic risk score [16] based on only the set of lead SNPs with weights corresponding to the log odds ratios according to the DIAGRAM meta-analysis summary statistics. Lead SNPs were defined as those that had the lowest p-value in the respective 2 Mb region according to the DIAGRAM Stage 1 meta-analysis summary statistics. We then considered a weighted genetic risk score based on all SNPs identified by the C/J analysis with weights corresponding to the coefficients estimated from the C/J analysis. We conducted the above analyses at the following p-value thresholds based on the C/J results: 5×10^{-8}, 5×10^{-7}, 5×10^{-6}, 5×10^{-5}, and 5×10^{-4}. We examined the proportion of variance explained by these additional SNPs by calculating the variance explained on the liability scale, estimated through the odds ratios and allele frequencies of the SNPs, and assuming a disease prevalence of 10%, using the Mangrove package [17] in R [18]. We also calculated Nagelkerke's R^2 [19] of the models which include age and sex and each of the GRS, using the fmsb package [20] in R, and report the Akaike information criterion (AIC) [21] for each of these models. Prediction accuracy was estimated using the area under the receiver operating characteristic curve (AUC) as implemented in the pROC package [22] in R. Differences in AUC among models were compared by examining the change in AUC (ΔAUC) and assessed using the DeLong test [23] to determine statistical significance.

Results

Conditional/Joint analysis

We identified novel genome-wide significant ($p<5\times10^{-8}$) SNPs in the C/J analysis at the three following loci: *TCF7L2*, *CDKN2A/B*, and *KCNQ1* (see Table 1). In the *TCF7L2* region, we identified three SNPs (rs7917983, rs17747324, rs12266632) within a 32 kb region. The lead SNP (rs4506565) was not selected in this model, but is positioned in this region and is in moderate LD with each of the novel findings (r^2 between 0.18 and 0.70). For each of these novel findings, the marginal effect sizes and p-values in the meta-analysis are similar to those estimated in the C/J analysis. By relaxing the p-value threshold to $p<5\times10^{-4}$, we discovered an additional SNP in this region (rs10128255). In the *CDKN2A/B* region, the lead SNP (rs2383208) was not selected in the C/J analysis. Instead, two SNPs (rs10757282 and rs10811661) approximately 1.9 kb downstream of the lead SNP were discovered. These SNPs are only 110 bases apart. rs10757282 is in relatively low LD with the lead SNP ($r^2=0.29$). However, rs10811661 is in high LD with the lead SNP ($r^2=0.94$). It should be noted that the correlation between the respective risk alleles is negative ($r=-0.54$), suggesting that estimates obtained through the single marker association were underestimated for both SNPs, as evidenced by the larger effect sizes and lower p-values estimated in the C/J analysis compared to the meta-analysis marginal association results (see Table 1). In the *KCNQ1* region, we identified two SNPs in the C/J analysis ($p<5\times10^{-8}$). One SNP (rs462402) is in moderate LD with the lead SNP, rs231362 ($r^2=0.45$). The other SNP (rs163177) is approximately 121 kb upstream and is not in LD with the lead SNP ($r^2<0.01$). By relaxing the p-value threshold to $p<5\times10^{-6}$, we identified additional novel discoveries in the *DGKB* and *TP53INP1* genes.

Table 1. SNPs identified by conditional/joint analysis with p-value $<5\times10^{-5}$, and corresponding evidence of regulatory function from RegulomeDB.

Gene region	Chr	SNP	bp	refA	freq	b	se	p	n	bJ	bJ_se	pJ	LD (r)	RegulomeDB score
BCL11A	2	rs2192512	59854224	C	0.475	0.058	0.014	6.50E-04	110517	0.060	0.014	2.75E-05	−0.017	
	2	rs243019	60439310	C	0.451	0.086	0.014	2.70E-06	117602	0.087	0.014	3.24E-10	0.000	5
IGF2BP2	3	rs12233623	186712890	C	0.548	0.058	0.014	1.00E-03	111251	0.065	0.014	5.49E-06	−0.074	
	3	rs6767484	187003272	G	0.305	0.122	0.018	3.90E-10	83684.8	0.127	0.018	7.89E-13	0.000	5
ANKRD55	5	rs9686661	55897543	T	0.189	0.095	0.023	9.20E-05	70923.6	0.100	0.023	1.05E-05	−0.063	4
	5	rs1895452	56096152	T	0.635	0.058	0.014	3.10E-03	118858	0.061	0.014	1.69E-05	0.000	
ZBED3	5	rs12522618	75491695	G	0.425	0.058	0.014	3.70E-03	112754	0.058	0.014	4.99E-05	0.009	
	5	rs7708285	76461623	G	0.300	0.122	0.022	1.10E-06	54523.4	0.122	0.022	3.70E-08	0.000	
DGKB	7	rs10282101	13867616	T	0.501	0.077	0.019	7.30E-05	64914.8	0.077	0.019	3.27E-05	−0.011	
	7	rs17168486	14864807	T	0.182	0.122	0.022	6.90E-07	76812	0.126	0.022	1.35E-08	−0.027	3a
	7	rs1974620	15031992	T	0.531	0.068	0.014	1.00E-04	112723	0.069	0.014	1.06E-06	0.000	
TP53INP1	8	rs4735337	96042641	T	0.490	0.077	0.014	6.90E-05	114412	0.078	0.014	2.01E-08	−0.022	5
	8	rs6991742	96533562	T	0.596	0.068	0.014	1.80E-04	116576	0.069	0.014	8.77E-07	0.000	5
CDKN2A/B	9	rs564398	22019547	T	0.579	0.077	0.014	1.70E-05	117268	0.059	0.014	2.48E-05	0.102	
	9	rs10757282	22123984	C	0.430	0.068	0.019	8.80E-04	65000.9	0.163	0.021	1.92E-14	−0.536	5
	9	rs10811661	22124094	T	0.825	0.166	0.021	1.50E-13	86410.9	0.247	0.024	1.08E-24	0.000	
ZMIZ1	10	rs3915932	80611942	G	0.592	0.095	0.018	4.70E-08	69629.2	0.098	0.018	7.10E-08	−0.040	5
	10	rs6480947	80906216	G	0.156	0.113	0.027	2.20E-04	59743.8	0.119	0.027	8.58E-06	0.000	
TCF7L2	10	rs7917983	114722872	C	0.479	0.148	0.013	1.50E-17	131838	0.082	0.014	2.17E-09	0.344	
	10	rs17747324	114742493	C	0.237	0.358	0.021	8.50E-55	70086.8	0.341	0.022	3.07E-54	−0.126	
	10	rs12266632	114754949	G	0.063	0.255	0.042	8.50E-11	53996.4	0.290	0.043	1.12E-11	0.000	5
KCNQ1	11	rs462402	2673869	C	0.507	0.077	0.014	1.10E-05	114391	0.076	0.014	6.49E-08	−0.002	
	11	rs163177	2794989	C	0.506	0.077	0.014	4.80E-05	114382	0.075	0.014	9.55E-08	0.040	5
	11	rs451041	3017301	G	0.496	0.068	0.014	8.20E-05	112303	0.063	0.014	8.89E-06	0.000	5
KCNJ11	11	rs7928810	17329019	C	0.396	0.068	0.014	1.30E-04	117423	0.068	0.014	1.50E-06	−0.004	
	11	rs757984	17576484	T	0.803	0.077	0.019	4.90E-04	102511	0.077	0.019	3.09E-05	0.000	
MTNR1B	11	rs10830962	92338075	G	0.408	0.104	0.014	1.50E-08	124966	0.101	0.014	1.61E-13	0.069	
	11	rs531573	92444531	C	0.182	0.086	0.018	1.70E-04	111150	0.077	0.018	2.75E-05	0.000	
TSPAN8	12	rs11178531	69694957	A	0.449	0.077	0.014	9.20E-06	115565	0.059	0.014	4.73E-05	0.271	
	12	rs1533104	69942814	T	0.338	0.086	0.014	2.80E-06	130115	0.072	0.014	4.26E-07	0.000	
SPRY2	13	rs1616547	78884037	C	0.512	0.058	0.014	3.00E-03	110308	0.058	0.014	4.84E-05	0.006	
	13	rs1327316	79607064	G	0.717	0.095	0.018	9.40E-07	82902.8	0.095	0.018	1.92E-07	0.000	
C2CD4A	15	rs6494307	60181982	C	0.572	0.077	0.014	1.80E-05	116797	0.077	0.014	3.65E-08	−0.001	
	15	rs2456936	60502334	C	0.785	0.077	0.019	1.10E-03	96195.2	0.077	0.019	3.32E-05	0.000	
ZFAND6	15	rs7176681	77714599	C	0.737	0.086	0.018	1.20E-04	85321.9	0.092	0.018	5.42E-07	−0.010	2a

Table 1. Cont.

Gene region	Chr	SNP	bp	refA	freq	b	se	p	n	bJ	bJ_se	pJ	LD (r)	RegulomeDB score
	15	rs1357335	78155918	A	0.684	0.086	0.018	1.60E-05	76497.6	0.086	0.018	2.92E-06	−0.006	5
	15	rs3848174	78531707	T	0.380	0.058	0.014	3.80E-03	117013	0.061	0.014	1.78E-05	0.000	5
HNF4A	20	rs387769	41745269	C	0.881	0.113	0.027	1.40E-05	75082.1	0.113	0.027	2.34E-05	0.008	1f
	20	rs6073708	43386291	A	0.562	0.058	0.014	2.40E-03	111949	0.058	0.014	4.81E-05	0.000	5

Abbreviations: Chr: chromosome, bp: base pair position, refA: reference allele, freq: frequency of the risk allele, b: regression coefficient from meta-analysis summary statistics, se: standard error from meta-analysis summary statistics, p: p-value from meta-analysis summary statistics, n: sample size in meta-analysis, bJ: regression coefficient estimated from conditional/joint analysis, bJ_se: standard error estimated from conditional/joint analysis, pJ: p-value from estimated from conditional/joint analysis, LD (r): linkage disequilibrium between corresponding SNP and the following SNP at the same locus.
(1f: eQTL+transcription factor (TF) binding/DNase peak; 2a: TF binding+matched TF motif+matched DNase Footprint+DNase peak; 3a: TF binding+any motif+DNase peak; 5: TF binding or DNase peak).

Continuing to relax this threshold, we identify 17 ($p<5\times10^{-5}$) (see Table 1) and 34 ($p<5\times10^{-4}$) regions with multiple associated SNPs. According to PolyPhen, none of the SNPs identified through C/J analysis had any predicted functional effect. According to our query in RegulomeDB, rs387769 near *HNF4A* shows evidence of being linked to expression of a gene target, affecting binding of a transcription factor, and shows evidence of a DNase footprint. SNP rs7176681 near *ZFAND6* also displays evidence of being a transcription factor binding site, and evidence of a DNase footprint. SNP rs17168486 in *DGKB* shows evidence of transcription factor binding and a DNase peak. Several other SNPs show evidence of transcription factor binding or a DNase peak (see Table 1).

Validation/Prediction

The AUC of the baseline prediction model which included only sex and age was 0.5702. For each of the three loci with additional SNPs that were significant at the $p<5\times10^{-8}$ threshold (*TCF7L2*, *CDKN2A/B*, and *KCNQ1*), the inclusion of the SNPs identified by the C/J analysis resulted in a higher AUC than a model including only the lead SNP (although not statistically significant) in all regions except for *KCNQ1* (see Figure 1).

Considering all three loci with additional SNPs at the $p<5\times10^{-8}$ threshold collectively, we found that the use of the seven SNPs identified by the C/J analysis resulted in a slightly higher AUC (0.5979) than when using only the three lead SNPs (0.5803). This represents a doubling in ΔAUC over the age+ sex model (see Figure 2), although this difference is not quite statistically significant ($p=0.055$), according to the DeLong test. The inclusion of all SNPs (lead and from C/J analysis) results in a statistically significant ($p=0.049$), yet small, increase in AUC (see Figure 2). At the $p<5\times10^{-6}$ threshold, the use of 11 SNPs at 5 loci (*TCF7L2*, *CDKN2A/B*, *KCNQ1*, *DGKB* and *TP53INP1*), slightly, but not significantly, increased prediction accuracy (AUC = 0.5885) over a model considering only the corresponding 5 lead SNPs (AUC = 0.5779; $p=0.126$). At the $p<5\times10^{-5}$ threshold, we observe a small increase in prediction accuracy when using the 39 SNPs identified by the C/J analysis instead of the corresponding 17 lead SNPs (AUC = 0.5892 vs. 0.5724; $p=0.079$). Finally, at the $p<5\times10^{-4}$ threshold, the use of 120 SNPs identified by the C/J analysis and the lead SNPs results in a slightly higher and nearly statistically significant increase in AUC over that of a model which includes only the 34 lead SNPs at the corresponding loci (AUC = 0.5965 vs. 0.5858; $p=0.067$).

Table 2 shows the proportion of variance explained by the additional SNPs identified by the C/J analysis. For each of the three loci, the SNPs identified by the C/J analysis explained slightly more of the variance in T2D risk than the lead SNP. Similarly, for the collection of SNPs identified by the C/J analysis at various p-value thresholds, we observe an increase in the proportion of T2D variance explained by the SNPs and the GRSs, along with decreasing AIC values.

Discussion

Our analyses confirm previous findings regarding the allelic heterogeneity present at the *CDKN2A/B*, *KCNQ1*, *DGKB*, and *MC4R* loci. We provide novel evidence of allelic heterogeneity at genome-wide significance at the *TCF7L2* locus. We support our finding in *TCF7L2* by showing that the use of the three identified SNPs results in a small increase in AUC (albeit not statistically significant) compared to using the lead *TCF7L2* SNP (rs4506565) alone. We observe similar but much weaker trends at the *CDKN2A/B* and *KCNQ1* loci.

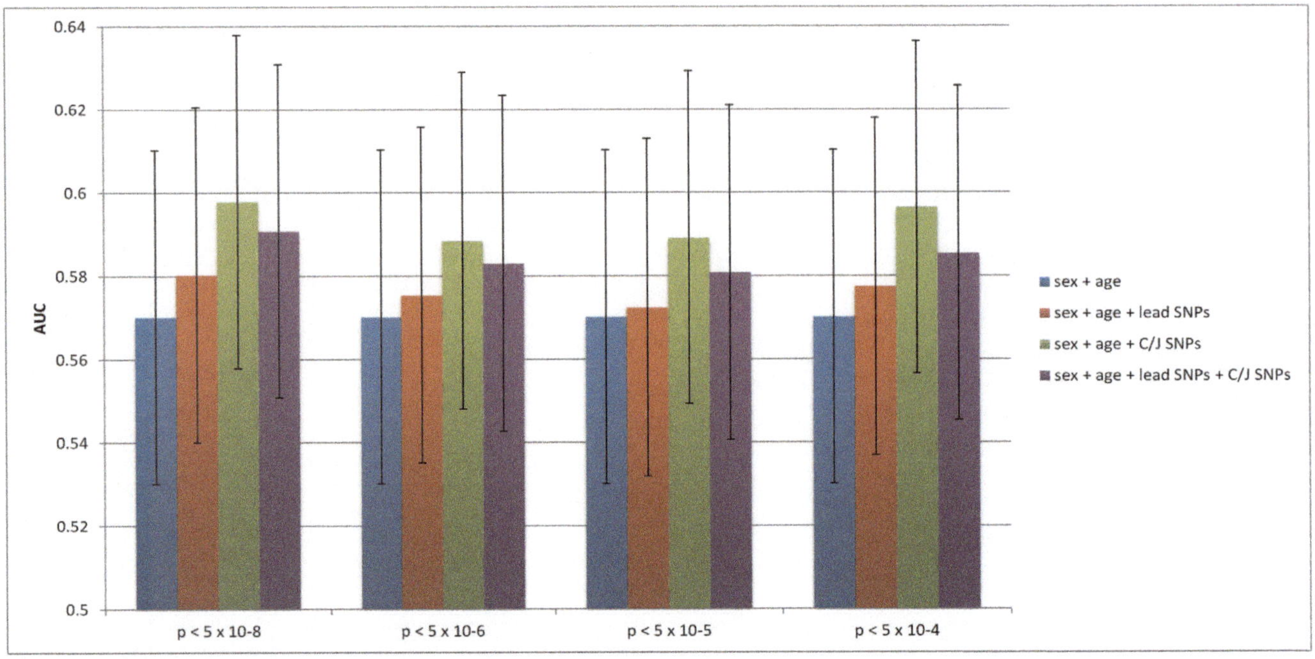

Figure 1. Prediction accuracy in MESA at 3 loci with additional detected SNPs at the 5×10^{-8} threshold.

At less stringent p-value thresholds, we observe additional putatively associated SNPs at up to 34 loci. Considering the collective set of loci in which additional associated SNPs were identified through C/J analysis, prediction accuracy appears to slightly improve with the addition of these additional SNPs in our validation dataset. At all p-value thresholds, the ΔAUC over the sex + age model is at least two-fold greater when using the C/J identified SNPs compared to using the lead SNPs alone.

The strength of the method developed by Yang et al. is well exemplified by the multiple associated SNPs identified at the *TCF7L2* locus, since the use of the three SNPs (which do not include the lead SNP) appears to be more informative than only using the lead SNP, rs4506565. Another example of the strength

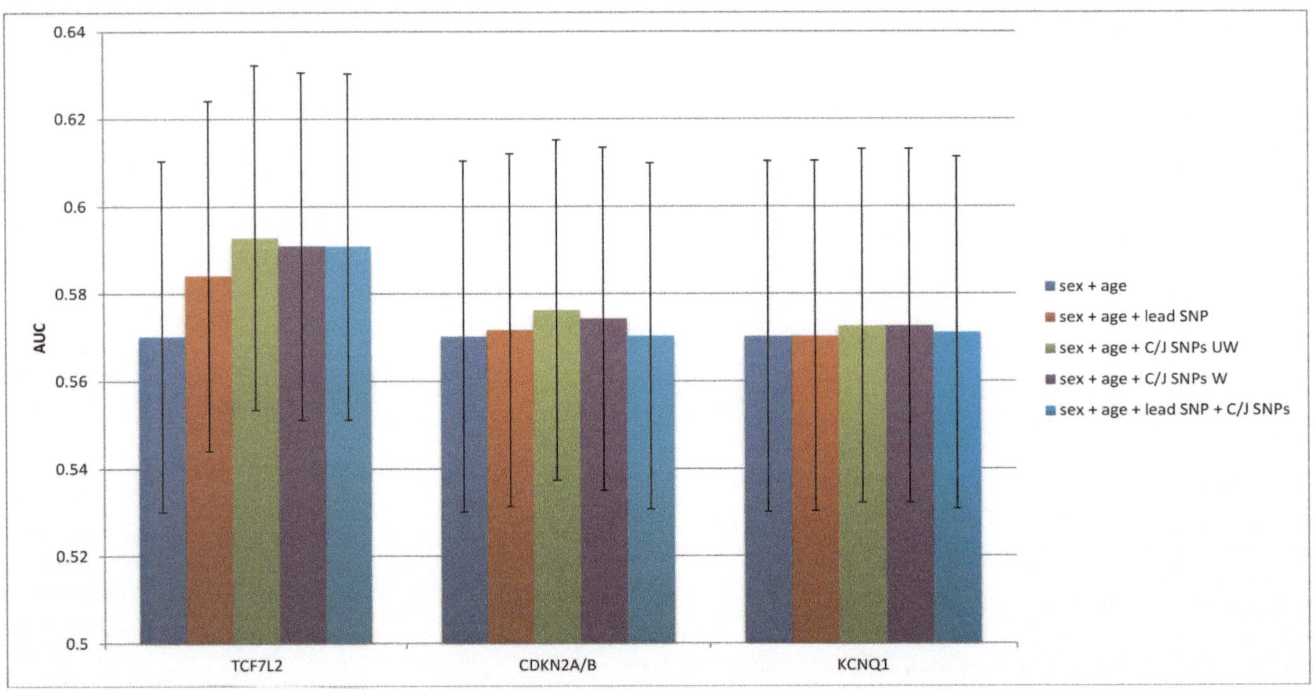

Figure 2. Prediction accuracy in MESA using lead SNPs vs. SNPs identified in C/J analysis at different p-value thresholds.

Table 2. Variance explained at various p-value thresholds in the MESA validation dataset by the collection of individual SNPs on the liability scale, variance explained by, and model fit of, the weighted GRS, using Nagelkerke's R^2, and AIC, respectively.

		Liability-scale variance	Nagelkerke R^2	AIC
age+sex			0.0115	1448.1
TCF7L2	1 Lead SNP	0.0097	0.0178	1443.3
	3 C/J SNPs	0.0189	0.0212	1439.7
	4 Lead+C/J SNPs	0.0282	0.0198	1441.1
CDKN2A/B	1 Lead SNP	0.0004	0.0118	1449.7
	2 C/J SNPs	0.0025	0.0127	1448.8
	2 Lead+C/J SNPs	0.0029	0.0117	1449.8
KCNQ1	1 Lead SNP	3.00E-5	0.0115	1450
	2 C/J SNPs	0.0029	0.0122	1449.3
	3 Lead+C/J SNPs	0.0014	0.0118	1449.8
<5.00E-08	3 Lead SNPs	0.0101	0.0153	1446
	7 GCTA SNPs	0.0225	0.0230	1437.8
	10 Lead+C/J SNPs	0.0322	0.0197	1441.2
<5.00E-06	5 Lead SNPs	0.0130	0.0134	1448.1
	11 GCTA SNPs	0.0258	0.0190	1442.1
	16 Lead+C/J SNPs	0.0381	0.0164	1444.8
<5.00E-05	17 Lead SNPs	0.0277	0.0134	1448
	39 GCTA SNPs	0.0648	0.0209	1440
	55 Lead+C/J SNPs	0.0865	0.0171	1444.1
<5.00E-04	34 Lead SNPs	0.0613	0.0158	1445.5
	91 GCTA SNPs	0.1443	0.0259	1434.6
	119 Lead+C/J SNPs	0.1801	0.0197	1441.2

of this method is the case in which two risk alleles are in negative LD. Without the C/J analysis, the additional SNPs in the *CDKN2A/B* region would not be identified when analyzed on their own.

The main limitation of this method is that associations are not tested directly, but rather through knowledge of marginal associations, and LD patterns in a different dataset (of the same ancestral background). A major limitation of the validation stage of our study is the relatively small sample size which limits the statistical power to detect differences in prediction accuracy between different GRSs. From this perspective, it will be important to continue validating these findings in larger datasets, and to combine actual genotype data across multiple datasets instead of using summary statistics. Furthermore, it will be important to dissect the allelic heterogeneity on a locus-by-locus basis to closely examine the patterns/existence of dependencies and additive or interactive effects. Finally, it will be important to functionally characterize these as well as all GWAS findings to more firmly establish causality and better understand molecular mechanisms leading to T2D.

Nevertheless, this approach is clearly promising for a greater understanding of the molecular basis of type-2 diabetes, and potentially for use in risk prediction scores. As additional loci are identified through GWAS, it will be important to systematically identify instances of allelic heterogeneity and to examine the extent to which additional SNPs can help to shed light on the functional basis of genetic variation.

Acknowledgments

The authors would like to thank the participants and organizers of all studies. Data from these studies was obtained from dbGaP through accession numbers: phs000280.v2.p1, and phs000209.v10.p2. We also thank Akshay Chougule for help with genotype imputation.

Atherosclerosis Risk in Communities

The Atherosclerosis Risk in Communities Study is carried out as a collaborative study supported by National Heart, Lung, and Blood Institute contracts (HHSN268201100005C, HHSN268201100006C, HHSN268201100007C, HHSN268201100008C, HHSN268201100009C, HHSN268201100010C, HHSN268201100011C, and HHSN268201100012C). Funding for GENEVA was provided by National Human Genome Research Institute grant U01HG004402 (E. Boerwinkle). The authors thank the staff and participants of the ARIC study for their important contributions.

Multi-Ethnic Study of Atherosclerosis

MESA and the MESA SHARe project are conducted and supported by the National Heart, Lung, and Blood Institute (NHLBI) in collaboration with MESA investigators. Support for MESA is provided by contracts N01-HC-95159, N01-HC-95160, N01-HC-95161, N01-HC-95162, N01-HC-95163, N01-HC-95164, N01-HC-95165, N01-HC-95166, N01-HC-95167, N01-HC-95168, N01-HC-95169 and CTSA UL1-RR-024156. MESA Family is conducted and supported by the National Heart, Lung, and Blood Institute (NHLBI) in collaboration with MESA investigators. Support is provided by grants and contracts R01HL071051, R01HL071205, R01HL071250, R01HL071251, R01HL071258, R01HL071259, UL1-RR-025005, by the National Center for Research Resources, Grant UL1RR033176, and the National Center for Advancing Translational Sciences, Grant UL1TR000124. This manuscript was not prepared in collaboration with MESA investigators and does not necessarily reflect the opinions or views of MESA, or the NHLBI. Funding for SHARe genotyping was provided by NHLBI Contract N02-HL-64278. Genotyping was performed at Affymetrix (Santa Clara, California, USA) and the Broad Institute of Harvard and MIT (Boston, Massachusetts, USA) using the Affymetric Genome-Wide Human SNP Array 6.0.

Author Contributions

Conceived and designed the experiments: YCK NEW JZ. Performed the experiments: YCK. Analyzed the data: YCK. Wrote the paper: YCK NEW JZ.

References

1. Voight BF, Scott LJ, Steinthorsdottir V, Morris AP, Dina C, et al. (2010) Twelve type 2 diabetes susceptibility loci identified through large-scale association analysis. Nat Genet 42: 579–589.
2. Morris AP, Voight BF, Teslovich TM, Ferreira T, Segrè A V, et al. (2012) Large-scale association analysis provides insights into the genetic architecture and pathophysiology of type 2 diabetes. Nat Genet 44: 981–990.
3. Lango AH, Estrada K, Lettre G, Berndt SI, Weedon MN, et al. (2010) Hundreds of variants clustered in genomic loci and biological pathways affect human height. Nature 467: 832–838.
4. Sim X, Ong RT, Suo C, Tay WT, Liu J, et al. (2011) Transferability of type 2 diabetes implicated Loci in multi-ethnic cohorts from southeast Asia. PLoS Genet 7: e1001363.
5. Williams AL, Jacobs SBR, Moreno-Macías H, Huerta-Chagoya A, Churchhouse C, et al. (2013) Sequence variants in SLC16A11 are a common risk factor for type 2 diabetes in Mexico. Nature.
6. Loos RJ, Lindgren CM, Li S, Wheeler E, Zhao JH, et al. (2008) Common variants near MC4R are associated with fat mass, weight and risk of obesity. Nat Genet 40: 768–775.
7. Yang J, Ferreira T, Morris AP, Medland SE, Madden PAF, et al. (2012) Conditional and joint multiple-SNP analysis of GWAS summary statistics identifies additional variants influencing complex traits. Nat Genet 44: 369–375.
8. Ke X (2012) Presence of multiple independent effects in risk loci of common complex human diseases. Am J Hum Genet 91: 185–192.
9. The Aric Investigators (1989) The Atherosclerosis Risk in Communities (ARIC) Study: design and objectives. The ARIC investigators. Am J Epidemiol 129: 687–702.
10. Howie B, Marchini J, Stephens M, Chakravarti A (2011) Genotype Imputation with Thousands of Genomes. G3 GenesGenomesGenetics 1: 457–470.
11. Bild DE, Bluemke DA, Burke GL, Detrano R, Diez Roux A V, et al. (2002) Multi-ethnic study of atherosclerosis: objectives and design. Am J Epidemiol 156: 871–881.
12. DIAGRAM website. Available: http://diagram-consortium.org/downloads.html. Accessed December 2013.
13. Yang J, Lee SH, Goddard ME, Visscher PM (2011) GCTA: A tool for genome-wide complex trait analysis. Am J Hum Genet 88: 76–82.
14. Adzhubei I, Jordan DM, Sunyaev SR (2013) Predicting functional effect of human missense mutations using PolyPhen-2. Curr Protoc Hum Genet.
15. Boyle AP, Hong EL, Hariharan M, Cheng Y, Schaub MA, et al. (2012) Annotation of functional variation in personal genomes using RegulomeDB. Genome Res 22: 1790–1797.
16. Purcell SM, Wray NR, Stone JL, Visscher PM, O'Donovan MC, et al. (2009) Common polygenic variation contributes to risk of schizophrenia and bipolar disorder. Nature.
17. Package Mangrove website. Available: http://cran.r-project.org/web/packages/Mangrove/index.html. Accessed May 2014.
18. R Development Core Team (2011) R: A language and environment for statistical computing. R Foundation for Statistical Computing.
19. Nagelkerke NJD (1991) A note on a general definition of the coefficient of determination. Biometrika 78: 691–692.
20. Nagelkerke R^2 function (R) website. Available: http://minato.sip21c.org/msb/man/Nagelkerke.html. Accessed June 2014.
21. Akaike H (1974) A new look at the statistical model identification. IEEE Trans Automat Contr 19.
22. Robin X, Turck N, Hainard A, Tiberti N, Lisacek F, et al. (2011) pROC: an open-source package for R and S+ to analyze and compare ROC curves. BMC Bioinformatics 12: 77.
23. DeLong ER, DeLong DM, Clarke-Pearson DL (1988) Comparing the areas under two or more correlated receiver operating characteristic curves: a nonparametric approach. Biometrics 44: 837–845.

22

Hesperidin Produces Cardioprotective Activity via PPAR-γ Pathway in Ischemic Heart Disease Model in Diabetic Rats

Yogeeta O. Agrawal[1,2,3], Pankaj Kumar Sharma[1]*, Birendra Shrivastava[1], Shreesh Ojha[4], Harshita M. Upadhya[5], Dharamvir Singh Arya[2], Sameer N. Goyal[3]*

1 School of Pharmaceutical Sciences, Jaipur National University, Jagatpura, Jaipur, Rajasthan, India, **2** Department of Pharmacology, All India Institute of Medical Sciences, New Delhi, India, **3** Department of Pharmaceutics and Pharmacology, R. C. Patel Institute of Pharmaceutical Education and Research, Shirpur, Maharashtra, India, **4** Department of Pharmacology and Therapeutics, College of Medicine and Health Sciences, United Arab Emirates University, Al-Ain, United Arab Emirates, **5** Sunil's Daibetes and Research Center, Nagpur, Maharashtra, India

Abstract

The present study investigated the effect of hesperidin, a natural flavonoid, in cardiac ischemia and reperfusion (I/R) injury in diabetic rats. Male Wistar rats with diabetes were divided into five groups and were orally administered saline once daily (IR-sham and IR-control), Hesperidin (100 mg/kg/day; IR-Hesperidin), GW9962 (PPAR-γ receptor antagonist), or combination of both for 14 days. On the 15th day, in the IR-control and IR-treatment groups, rats were subjected to left anterior descending (LAD) coronary artery occlusion for 45 minutes followed by a one-hour reperfusion. Haemodynamic parameters were recorded and rats were sacrificed; hearts were isolated for biochemical, histopathological, ultrastructural and immunohistochemistry. In the IR-control group, significant ventricular dysfunctions were observed along with enhanced expression of pro-apoptotic protein Bax. A decline in cardiac injury markers lactate dehydrogenase activity, CK-MB and increased content of thiobarbituric acid reactive substances, a marker of lipid peroxidation, and TNF-α were observed. Hesperidin pretreatment significantly improved mean arterial pressure, reduced left ventricular end-diastolic pressure, and improved both inotropic and lusitropic function of the heart (+LVdP/dt and −LVdP/dt) as compared to IR-control. Furthermore, hesperidin treatment significantly decreased the level of thiobarbituric acid reactive substances and reversed the activity of lactate dehydrogenase towards normal value. Hesperidin showed anti-apoptotic effects by upregulating Bcl-2 protein and decreasing Bax protein expression. Additionally, histopathological and ultrastructural studies reconfirmed the protective action of hesperidin. On the other hand, GW9662, selective PPAR-γ receptor antagonist, produced opposite effects and attenuated the hesperidin induced improvements. The study for the first time evidence the involvement of PPAR-γ pathway in the cardioprotective activity of hesperidin in I/R model in rats.

Editor: Anindita Das, Virginia Commonwealth University, United States of America

Funding: No current funding sources for this study.

Competing Interests: The authors have declared that no competing interests exist.

* Email: jnupharmacyresearch@gmail.com (PKS); goyal.aiims@gmail.com (SG)

Introduction

Ischemic heart disease is the leading cause of morbidity and mortality and is predicted to be the major and most common threat to human life by 2020 [1,2]. Treatments available for myocardial infarction (MI) like ischemic injury targets restoration of blood supply to ischemic tissue and prevent the damage inflicted at the time of injury. While at one hand, imbalance between myocardial blood supply and demand resulting in development of ischemia and induction of necrosis in myocardium results in acute MI [3], oxidative stress produced by generation of free radicals or reactive oxygen species also plays a key role in MI development [4,5]. Therefore, suppressing free radical generation and/or augmentation of endogenous antioxidant enzymes is reported to limit the infarct size and attenuate myocardial dysfunction [6]. Moreover, diabetic like conditions worsen the complications arise due to the ischemic diseases, and also delays the recovery [7].

Hesperidin (30, 5, 9-dihydroxy-40-methoxy-7-Orutinosyl Flavanone) is an abundant and inexpensive byproduct of Citrus cultivation and isolated from the ordinary orange *Citrus aurantium* and other species of the genus Citrus (family: Rutaceae). It is reported to have antiallergic, radio protective, immuno-modulator, anti-hypertensive and anti-oxidant properties. Administered orally, it is hydrolyzed by intestinal micro flora to yield a major active metabolite hesperidin [8]. Previous studies established its bolstering role in oxidative stress, and considered as safe model for protection against free radicals. There is substantial evidence to suggest that hesperidin exerts protective action in cardiac tissue by its antihypertensive and antioxidant properties [9]. A protective effect of hesperidin against oxidative stress in liver and kidney of diabetic rabbits [10] has also been reported. Some reports evidenced that hesperidin targets peroxisome proliferator-activated receptor-gamma (PPAR-γ) to exert biological actions [11]. PPAR-γ being a member of the ligand-dependent nuclear receptor category regulates glucose, lipid and energy homeostasis [12,13]. In addition, PPAR-γ regulates cellular proliferation and differentiation inducing apoptosis in a wide spectrum of human tumor cell lines [12,14]. Various PPAR-γ agonists like pioglitazone have been shown to reduce myocardial injury (infarct size) and inflammation caused by regional myocardial ischemia and reperfusion in rats and rabbits [15]. Therefore, in the present study we attempted to explore the role of hesperidin in cardiac ischemia and reperfusion (I/R) injury in diabetic rats.

Flavonoids like hesperidin are reported to possess satisfactory capability to neutralize free radicals. This antioxidant property may be related to their pharmacological actions and they may be used as protective agents in a number of cardiac diseases. Although the effect of hesperidin on experimentally induced MI by ischemia-reperfusion model has been studied, the mechanisms underlying the effect are yet to be explored. Hence the present study was carried out to investigate the permissive role of PPAR-γ receptors in the cardioprotective activity of hesperidin in diabetic rats using hemodynamic, biochemical, histopathological, ultrastructural and immunohistochemistry in I/R model of MI.

Materials and Methods

Animals

The study protocol was reviewed and approved by the Institutional Animal Ethics Committee, All India Institute of Medical Sciences, New Delhi, India and conformed to the Indian National Science Academy (INSA) Guidelines for the use and care of experimental animals in research. Male Wistar rats weighing 150–250 g were obtained from the Central Animal House Facility of All India Institute of Medical Sciences, New Delhi, India. The rats were maintained under standard laboratory conditions at 25±2°C, relative humidity 60±15% and natural light-dark photo period. Commercial pellet diet (Ashirwad Industries Ltd., Chandigarh, India) and tap water were provided *ad libitum*. The commercial pellet diet contained 24% protein, 5% fat, 4% fibre, 55% carbohydrate, 0.6% calcium, 0.3% phosphorous, 10% moisture, and 9% ash w/w.

Chemicals

Hesperidin was a purchased from Calbiochem, USA. Creatine kinase (CK-MB) isoenzyme detection kit was purchased from Logotech India Pvt. Ltd. (Delhi, India). The ABC staining kit and primary (Bax mouse monoclonal IgG2b and Bcl-2 mouse monoclonal IgGI) and secondary antibodies (anti-mouse IgG) were procured from Santa Cruz Biotechnology, USA. All chemicals were of analytical grade, purchased from Sigma Chemical Co., St. Louis, USA. Double distilled water was used in all biochemical assays and molecular techniques.

Induction of Diabetes

Streptozotocin (50 mg/kg, 0.1 M cold citrate buffer, pH 4.5) was administered by intraperitoneal (i.p.) route to induce diabetes in rats and was confirmed 3 days post injection by glucoseoxidase/ peroxidase method. Briefly, Diabetes was induced by a single intraperitoneal injection of STZ (50 mg/kg body weight) after overnight fasting. Control rats were injected with vehicle buffer only. Blood samples were obtained from the tail vein 72 hr after STZ injection and blood glucose levels were determined. Here in, glucose is oxidized by glucose oxidase (GOD) to produce gluconate and hydrogen peroxide. In the presence of peroxidase (POD), the hydrogen peroxide is then oxidatively coupled with 4 amino- antipyrene (4-AAP) and phenol to yield a red quinoeimine dye that is measured at 505 nm. The absorbance at 505 nm is proportional to concentration of glucose in the sample. Blood glucose level >250 mg/dl was considered as an index of successful induction of diabetes and such rats showing this value were included in the study. Upon confirmation for diabetes, rats were randomly divided into five groups containing 12 rats in each group and used for further experiments (Figure 1).

Experimental protocol

The animals were randomly divided into five main groups as depicted in Figure 1.

Group 1: IR-sham group. Diabetic rats were administered 0.9% saline orally (2 ml/kg) using intra-gastric tubes for 14 days and then sacrificed on the 15th day. The animals were subjected to the entire surgical procedure and thread was passed beneath the coronary artery, but the left anterior descending (LAD) coronary artery was not ligated. The number of animals studied in this group was 12.

Group 2: IR-control group. In this group, 12 diabetic rats were administered 0.9% saline orally (2 ml/kg) using intra-gastric tubes for 14 days; thereafter, on the 15th day, the experimental animals were subjected to a 45-minute LAD coronary artery ligation followed by a one hour reperfusion induced myocardial injury.

Group 3: IR-hesperidin group. Hesperidin (100 mg/kg/ day) was dissolved in saline and was administered orally (50 mg/ ml), using intra-gastric tubes, to additional 12 animals for 14 days. On the 15th day, the rats were subjected to a protocol of a 45-minute LAD coronary artery ligation and a one-hour reperfusion.

Group 4: IR-GW9662 group. In another group of 12 rats, GW9662 (1 mg/kg, ip) was dissolved in saline and was administered to animals for 14 days. On the 15th day, the rats were subjected to a protocol of a 45-minute LAD coronary artery ligation and a one hour reperfusion.

Group 5: IR+GW9662+hesperidin group. In this group, 12 rats were treated with GW9662 (1 mg/kg/day, ip) 15 min prior to the hesperidin (100 mg/kg/day, orally) for 14 days. On the 15thday, the rats were subjected to a 45-minute LAD coronary artery ligation followed by one hour reperfusion.

Experimental procedure for LAD coronary artery occlusion and reperfusion

Following treatments all these groups were subjected to LAD coronary artery occlusion-reperfusion and recording of haemodynamic parameters as described previously [7]. Briefly, rats of all the experimental groups were anaesthetized with pentobarbitone sodium (60 mg/kg, ip) and maintained with 40 mg/kg doses (given at 60 and 120 mins from first dose). Atropine (0.01 mg/kg, ip) was co-administered with the anaesthetic to reduce broncho-tracheal secretions. Body temperature was monitored and maintained at 37°C throughout the experimental protocol. The neck was opened with a ventral midline incision, and a tracheostomy was performed and the rats were ventilated with room air from a positive pressure ventilator (Inco, India) using compressed air at the rate of 70 strokes per minute and a tidal volume of 10 ml/kg. The left jugular vein was cannulated with a polyethylene tube for continuous infusion of 0.9% saline. After that, the right carotid artery was cannulated and the cannula filled with heparinised saline was connected to the cardiac output monitor CARDIOSYS CO-101 (Experimetria, Hungary) via a pressure transducer for measurement of mean arterial pressure (MAP). A left thoracotomy was performed at the fifth intercostal space and the pericardium was opened to expose the heart. The LAD coronary artery was ligated 4–5 mm from its origin using a 5-0 silk suture with an atraumatic needle, and ends of this ligature

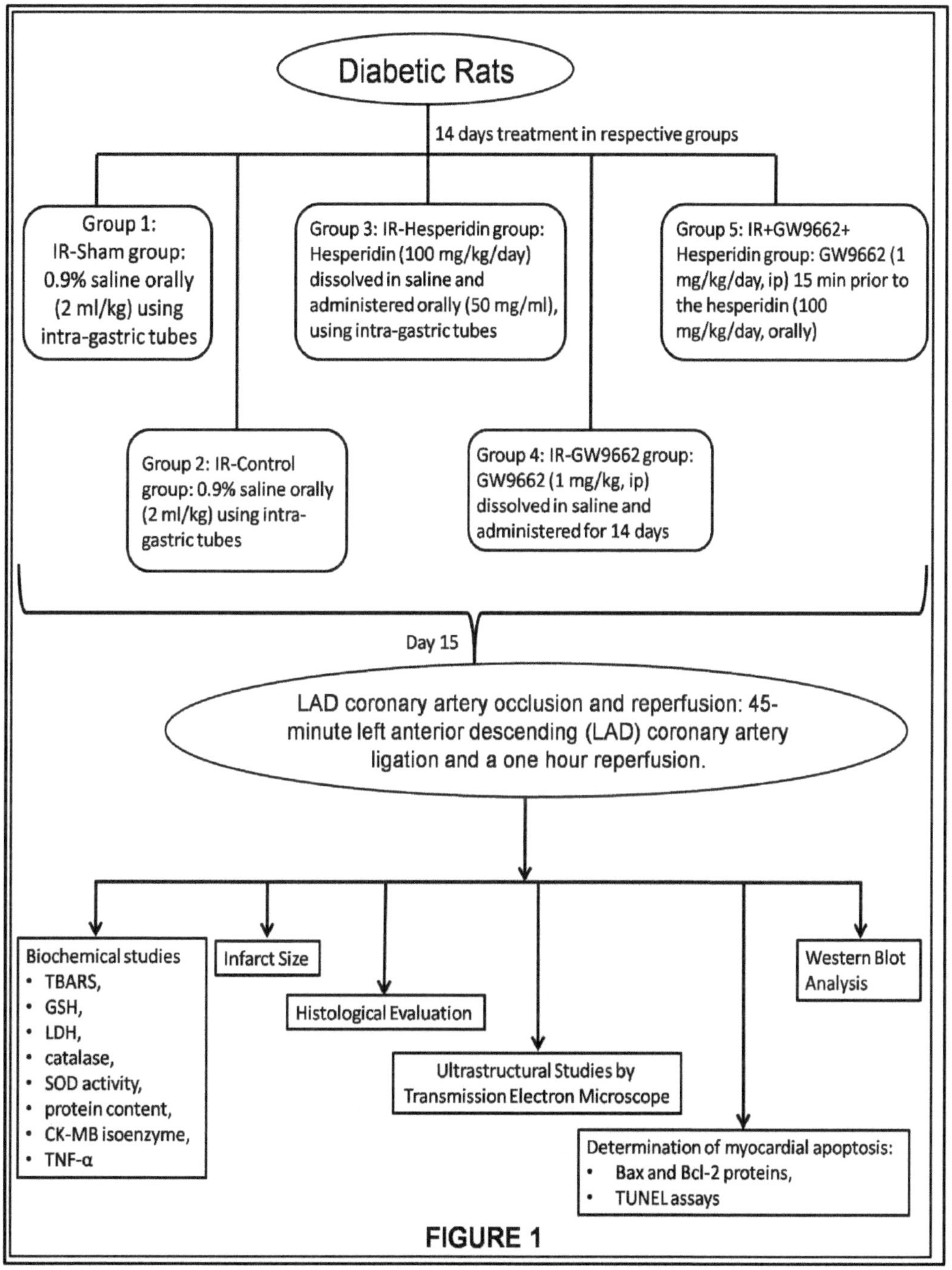

Figure 1. Schematic representation of several groups used in the study showing the treatments received by the diabetic rats for 14 days. On day 15th these rats were subjected to the LAD coronary artery ligation followed by a one hour reperfusion induced myocardial injury. Moreover, these groups were assessed for several biochemical parameters, histological evaluations, ultrastructural studies, myocardial apoptosis markers and western blot analysis.

were passed through a small vinyl tube to form a snare. After completion of the surgical procedure, the heart was returned to its normal position in the thorax. The thoracic cavity was covered with saline-soaked gauze to prevent the heart from drying. The animals were then allowed to stabilize for 15 minutes before LAD coronary artery ligation. Myocardial ischaemia was induced by one stage occlusion of the LAD coronary artery by pressing the polyethylene tubing against the ventricular wall and then fixing it in place by clamping the vinyl tube with a haemostat (except in IR-sham rats). A wide bore (1.5 mm) sterile metal cannula was inserted into the cavity of the left ventricle from the posterior apical region of the heart. The cannula was connected to a pressure transducer (Gold Statham P23ID, USA) and the whole system was filled with heparinised saline (heparin 50 units/ml).

Left ventricular systolic and left ventricular end-diastolic pressure (LVEDP) were measured on a multi channel polygraph (Grass 7D, USA) from the left ventricular pressures curve at lower and higher sensitivity of the preamplifier, respectively. The maximum rates of rise and fall of left ventricular pressure (peak +LVdP/dt and peak −LVdP/dt) were measured by the electronic differentiator from the signal output of the channel recording left ventricular pressure. A bolus of heparin (30 IU) was administered immediately before coronary artery occlusion for prophylaxis against thrombus formation around the snare. The animals then underwent 45 minutes of ischaemia, confirmed visually *in situ* by the appearance of regional epicardial cyanosis. The myocardium was reperfused by releasing the snare gently for a one-hour period. Successful reperfusion was confirmed by visualisation of arterial blood flow through the artery and appearance of hyperaemia over the surface of the previously ischaemic cyanotic segment. The entire surgical process was completed under a terminal anaesthetic during which anaeasthesia was fully maintained with the top-up doses of pentobarbitone sodium (40 mg/kg). At the end of the reperfusion period, animals were sacrificed using an overdose of pentobarbitone sodium (100 mg/kg, i.v.) and the heart was removed for biochemical and immunohistochemical studies. For biochemical estimations, hearts were stored in liquid nitrogen, whereas for immunohistochemistry, hearts were fixed in 10% buffer formalin.

Biochemical studies

The hearts were removed from liquid nitrogen, weighed and a 10% homogenate of myocardial tissue was prepared in ice-chilled phosphate buffer (50 mM, pH 7.4), and an aliquot was used to estimate thiobarbituric acid reactive substance (TBARS) according to the method described by Okhawa [16], and reduced glutathione (GSH) content was measured by the method published by Moron et al. [17]. The homogenate was centrifuged at 5000 rpm for 20 min at 4°C, and the supernatant was assayed for lactate dehydrogenase (LDH), catalase, and superoxide dismutase (SOD) activity, as well as protein content. Creatine kinase-MB (CK-MB) isoenzyme was estimated spectrophotometrically using a kit from Logotech, India whereas, TNF-α was estimated spectrophotometrically using an ELISA kit (Gen-Probe Diaclone SAS, France, UK).

Determination of the Infarct Size

At the end of the reperfusion period, monastral blue (0.5 ml/kg) was injected into the left atrium over 30 s to determine the *in vivo* area at risk as described by Singh et al. (2006) and described in our previous study [7]. Thereafter, animals were sacrificed, and their heart was excised and left ventricle was separated and kept at − 20°C for 30 min for uniform sectioning. In order to visualize the infarction, both masses (unstained and stained with blue dye) of the slices were incubated separately in 1% buffered TTC pH 8.5 for 20 min at 37°C [18].

Histological Evaluation

As described in our previous studies [7,19], tissues fixed in buffered formalin were embedded in paraffin, and serial sections (3 μm thick) were cut using microtome (Labindia Instruments Pvt. Ltd, Chennai, India). Each section was stained with haematoxylin and eosin (H&E). Sections were examined under the light microscope (Nikon, Tokyo, Japan), and photographs were taken. The pathologist performing microscopy was blind to the treatment status of the test subject.

Ultrastructural Studies by Transmission Electron Microscope

As described in [7], tissue fixed with Karnovsky's solution were washed in phosphate buffer (0.1 M, pH 7.4, 6°C) and post fixed for 2 h in 1% osmium tetroxide in the same buffer at 4°C. The specimens were then washed with phosphate buffer, dehydrated with graded acetone and embedded in Araldite CY212 to make tissue blocks. Semithin (1 μm) and ultrathin sections (70–80 nm) were cut with an ultramicrotome (Ultracut E, Reichert, Austria). Sections were stained with uranyl acetate and lead acetate, and examined under a transmission electron microscope (TEM; Morgagni 268D, Fei, the Netherlands) operated at 60 kV by a morphologist blind to the status of the groups studied.

Determination of myocardial apoptosis

Immunostaining for the localization of Bax and Bcl-2 proteins. Indirect immune peroxidase staining was performed as described by Mohanty et al. [20] with some modifications. Briefly, tissue sections (4-μm thickness) mounted on poly-L-lysine-coated glass slides were deparaffinised with xylene. After washing in graded concentrations of ethanol, the specimens were incubated with methanol containing 2% H_2O_2 to inhibit endogenous peroxidase activity. The slides were then washed with PBS for five minutes. The sections were incubated with blocking buffer (10% normal goat serum) for 10 minutes at room temperature. Next, the slides were incubated overnight at 4°C with primary mouse Bax and Bcl-2 monoclonal antibody (1:500). For the negative control, the primary antibody was omitted. After washing with PBS, tissue sections were incubated for one hour with biotinylated goat secondary antibodies (anti-mouse IgG, 1:100). Subsequently, sections were washed and incubated for 30 minutes with peroxidase-conjugated streptavidin-biotin complex. The target protein (Bax/Bcl-2) was visualised by incubation in peroxidase substrate (H_2O_2) using 3,3′-diaminobenzidine as the chromogen and the sections were counterstained with haematoxylin. Myocardial Bax and Bcl-2 proteins were quantitatively analyzed.

TUNEL assays were performed using a cell death detection kit (Roche, Indianapolis, IN, USA) as described by Mohanty et al. [20] and according to the manufacturer's instructions. The percentage of positive apoptotic cells was determined based on the number of positively stained apoptotic myocytes/total number of myocytes ×100.

Western Blot Analysis

Western blot analysis was performed as described in our previous study (Goyal et al., 2011). Briefly, heart tissues (40 μg protein samples) were separated by SDS-PAGE, transferred to nitrocellulose membrane which was blocked for 2 h with 5% bovine serum albumin and incubated for 12 h at 4°C with a rat primary antibody (β-actin and PPAR-γ). The primary antibody was detected with horse radish peroxidase-conjugated secondary antibody. The blots so obtained were scanned and densitometry was performed to quantify the expression of β-actin (primary1: 1000 and secondary goat anti rabbit 1: 2000) and PPAR-γ (primary 1: 1000 and secondary goat anti mouse 1: 5000) using Bio-Rad Quantity One 4.4.0 software (Bio-Rad, Hercules, CA, USA).

Statistical analysis

All numerical data in figures are expressed as the mean±SEM. Two-way analysis of variance (ANOVA) was applied for statistical analysis with *post hoc* Bonferroni's multiple comparison test and one way ANOVA for western blot analysis. Statistical value $p < 0.05$ was considered significant.

Results

Mortality

An overall mortality of 15% was observed during the study period. The animals were lost because of severe diabetes, bleeding or occlusion of the coronary artery during surgery. The groups which were affected with mortality of animals were IR-SHAM (1 animal), IR-Control (3 animals), IR-GW9662 (3 animals) and IR-GW9662-Hesperidin (2 animal). There was a loss of total nine animals due to mortality and these animals were not considered for statistical analysis.

Haemodynamic Parameters

The effects of hesperidin and GW9662 on haemodynamic and LV functions during I/R-induced MI in diabetic rats are depicted in Figure 2 (A–D). While significant decrease ($p<0.001$) was observed in the MAP and ±LVdP/dtmax, increased LVEDP was recorded in the rats subjected to cardiac I/R as compared to diabetic sham group. Fourteen days pretreatment with hesperidin significantly increased MAP, ±LVdP/dtmax and decreased LVEDP throughout I/R period at every time point, as compared to the diabetic I/R group. The dose of hesperidine (100 mg/kg/day for 14 days) was selected depending on the dose dependent study of hesperidine (data not shown). Hesperidine at 100 mg/kg produced significant results as compared to that of 50 and 200 mg/kg. Thus, 100 mg/kg dose was finalized for the entire work and administered to animals to study the effect of cardioprotection in rats. On the other hand pretreatment with GW9662 showed opposite effects as that of hesperidin and worsen the conditions as compared to that in the diabetic I/R group. Interestingly, pretreatment with GW9662 fifteen min prior to hesperidin significantly blocked the reversal effects of hesperidin in the diabetic I/R conditions for MAP, ±LVdP/dtmax and LVEDP throughout I/R period at every time point as compared to respective hesperidin treatment.

Biochemical Parameters

As shown in Table 1, the activities of the CK-MB isoenzyme, LDH, SOD, catalase and GSH content had declined significantly ($p<0.0001$) in the diabetic I/R group, whereas the lipid peroxidation ($p<0.0001$) and TNF-α ($p<0.0001$) levels were markedly increased in the myocardium as compared to diabetic sham group. Hesperidin treatment for 14 days in diabetic I/R rats significantly ($p<0.0001$) reversed the activities of the CK-MB isoenzyme and LDH, and increased the content of these antioxidants in comparison to the diabetic I/R group. In addition, the hesperidin treatment significantly reduced the level of MDA ($p<0.0001$) and prevented the TNF-α increase ($p<0.0001$). In contrast to hesperidin, GW9662 treatment for 14 days produced the opposite effects and when administered 15 min prior to hesperidin in additional group of rats, it significantly attenuated the cardioprotective effects of hesperidin.

Evaluation of the Infarct Size

A major predictor of infarct size in models of regional ischaemia is determination of percent mean area at risk and infarct area. Both the parameters were evaluated in diabetic I/R induced rats in the present study. Chronic hesperidin treatment depicted the significantly decreased infarct area ($p<0.01$) as compared to diabetic I/R group. However, the GW9662 treatment in the diabetic I/R group showed significantly greater infarct area (60.81±5.64, $p<0.001$) as compared to that in the diabetic I/R rats. Furthermore, GW9662 treatment prior to hesperidin also attenuated the cardioprotective effects of hesperidin ($p<0.05$) as compared to that of the hesperidin (Table 2).

Histopathological evaluation

Table 3 and Figure 3 summarizes the histopathological changes following the saline, hesperidin or GW9662 treatments either alone in combination in the diabetic I/R induced rats. While diabetic sham group did not show any inflammation, oedema and necrosis (Figure 3A), myocardial membrane damage with extensive myonecrosis, fibroblastic proliferation, inflammatory cell infiltration and marked oedema were significantly observed in the diabetic I/R induced rats (Figure 3B). On contrary, hesperidin pre treatment in the diabetic I/R rats showed the occasional areas of myofibre loss with necrosis but no oedema and inflammatory cell infiltration (Figure 3C). However, the degree of myocardial damage in the GW9662 pretreated rats was severe as compared to diabetic I/R rats (Figure 3D). Interestingly, the rats pretreated with GW9662 previous to hesperidin showed attenuation in the effects of hesperidin (Figure 3E).

Ultrastructural Results

As shown in Figure 4A, diabetic sham rats showed well preserved mitochondrial structure and glycogen granules throughout the myocardium. Significant disruption of the myofibrils, myonecrosis, depletion of the glycogen reserves, swollen and irregular mitochondria with a loss of cristae and chromatin condensation was observed in the diabetic I/R rats (Figure 4B). On the other hand, hesperidin treatment showed only a mild separation of the mitochondrial cristae without swelling and vacuolation (Figure 4C). More severe ultrastructural complications in conjunction with severe peripheral nuclear condensation were observed in the GW9662-treated group as compared to diabetes I/R rats (Figure 4D). In addition, GW9662 treatment prior to hesperidin blocked the recovery process of hesperidin *per se* (Figure 4E).

Effect of Hesperidin or GW9662 alone or in combination on expression of Bcl-2 and Bax proteins in experimentally induced MI

To confirm the involvement of PPAR-γ receptors in the cardioprotection by Hesperidin, the estimation of apoptosis regulatory proteins (Bax and Bcl-2) using immunohistopathological studies were conducted in the diabetic sham and diabetic I/R rats treated with vehicle, hesperidin and GW9662 either alone or in combination. Photomicrographs in the Figure 5 (A-E), (F-J) and (K-O) shows the effect of hesperidin and GW9662 either alone or in combination on Bcl-2, Bax proteins and TUNEL positive cells, respectively, in the diabetic I/R rats and Figure 5P represents the quantitative analysis of the same. While significant decrease in Bcl-2 was observed (B), Bax proteins and TUNEL positive cells were significantly increased in the diabetic I/R rats (G and L) as compared to diabetic sham control (A, F and K). On the other hand, hesperidin treatment significantly prevented the changes in Bcl-2 and Bax proteins and TUNEL positive cells as observed in the Diabetic I/R group (C, H and M). In contrast to this, GW9662 treatment exaggerated the diabetic I/R induced conditions (D, I and N), and also attenuated the hesperidin induced effects with respect to the Bcl-2 and Bax proteins, and TUNEL positive cells (E, J and O).

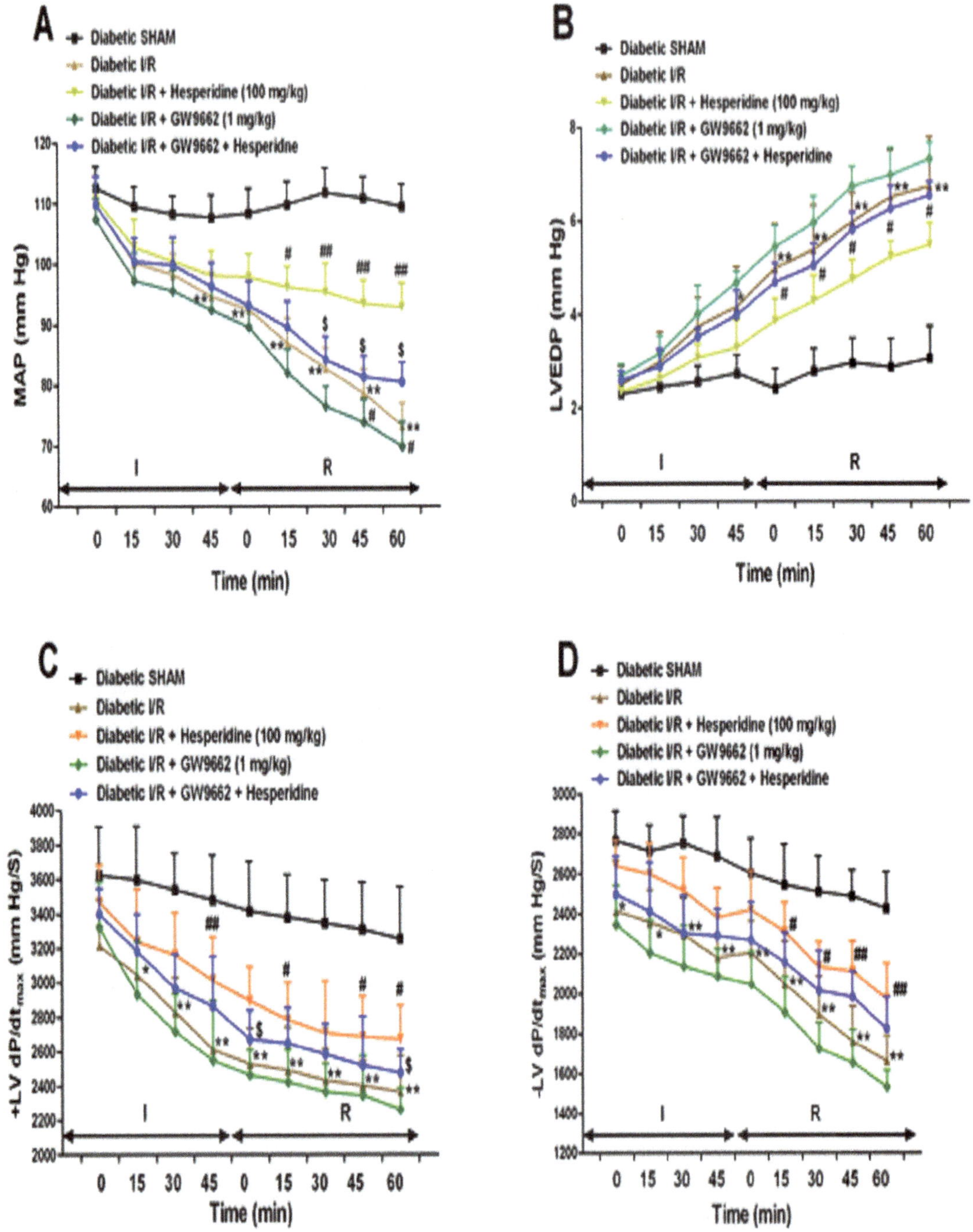

Figure 2. Effect of hesperidin and GW9662 on mean arterial pressure (MAP) and left ventricular (LV) function following ischaemia/reperfusion (I/R) in diabetic rats. (A) MAP, (B) left ventricular end-diastolic pressure (LVEDP), (C) maximal positive rate of left ventricular pressure (+LVdP/dtmax) and (D) maximal negative rate of −LVdP/dtmax. Data are expressed as the mean ± standard error (n = 22/group). Significance was determined by repeated measures analysis of variance followed by the Bonferroni's post hoc test: *$p<0.05$, **$p<0.001$ vs Diabetic SHAM; #$p<0.05$, ##$p<0.001$ vs Diabetic I/R; \$$p<0.01$ vs respective Hesperidin.

Western Blot Analysis

The expression of PPAR-γ was carried out in diabetic sham and I/R rats and those induced diabetic I/R and treated with hesperidin and GW9662 alone or in combination (Figure 6). The expression of PPAR-γ was significantly lower ($p<0.05$) in the diabetic I/R rats as compared to that of the sham rats. Moreover, the hesperidin treated rats showed increased expression of PPAR-γ protein ($p<0.001$) as compared to that of the diabetic I/R group. On the other hand, GW9662 treatment not only significantly decreased ($p<0.05$) the protein expression but also significantly attenuated ($p<0.05$) hesperidin induced increase in the PPAR-γ expression.

Table 1. Effect of hesperidin and GW9662 on cardiac injury marker enzymes, lipid peroxidation, TNF-α and antioxidant parameters.

Parameters	Diabetic sham	Diabetic I/R	Diabetic I/R + Hesperidin	Diabetic I/R + GW9662	Diabetic I/R + GW9662 + Hesperidin
CK-MB (IU/mg protein)	130.19±5.08	89.54±9.16*	126.55±7.89#	93.47±2.98	103.54±7.19@
LDH (IU/mg protein)	82.33±4.89	59.84±3.96*	76.59±6.15#	47.62±5.49	64.29±4.01@
MDA (nmol/g tissue)	34.86±6.21	62.31±6.19*	41.94±4.06#	60.84±5.97	52.37±5.91@
SOD (U/mg protein)	12.64±3.06	7.19±2.06*	10.86±3.19#	4.85±1.21	6.95±1.35@
CAT (U/mg protein)	48.84±6.22	31.97±5.26*	44.61±5.9#	24.41±2.19	39.28±4.64@
GSH (μg/g tissue)	4.28±0.54	1.59±0.81*	3.84±0.67#	1.85±0.41	2.98±0.78@
TNF-α (Pg/mg protein)	58.34±1.96	119.86±6.57*	78.94±6.19#	132.67±7.56	91.48±6.34@

Data are expressed as the mean ± standard error (n = 6/group). CAT, catalase; CK-MB, creatine kinase-MB isoenzyme; GSH, reduced glutathione; I/R, ischaemia/reperfusion; LDH, lactate dehydrogenase; MDA, malondialdehyde; SOD, superoxide dismutase; TNF-α, tumour necrosis factor-alpha. *p<0.001 vs Diabetic Sham; #p<0.001 vs Diabetic I/R; @p<0.01 vs Diabetic I/R + Hesperidin.

Discussion

The present study for the first time evidenced the involvement of PPAR-γ pathway in the cardioprotective activity of hesperidin in the cardiac I/R model in diabetic rats. Herein, streptozotocine was used for the induction of diabetes in rats, since it enters the β-cells in pancreas and alkylates DNA. This depletes NAD+ and ATP and aggravates the diabetogenic effect by activating poly ADP-ribosylation pathway. In addition to this the activation of reactive oxygen species (ROS), superoxide and hydroxy radicals augments cytotoxic action. These results into destruction of β-cells and also cause injury to myocardial tissues leading to ischemia like conditions. Myocardial injury can be experimentally induced in rats using I/R model which mimics the human pathophysiological condition and reduces arterial pressure along with ventricular dysfunction [19,21]. Blockade or occlusion of LAD results in myocardial ischemia which includes complex series of cellular events and lead to myocardial cell death, furthermore, reperfusion (restoration of blood flow) enhances myocardial injury and diminishes cardiac contractile functions and metabolic derangements. Cardiac I/R induced group of rats depicted significantly impaired systolic and diastolic functions (decrease in MAP) and inotropic and lusitropic state (±LVdP/dtmax), and increased ventricular remodeling (preload LVEDP). Further, this impairment was confirmed by pathological assessment as characterized by inflammatory cells, necrosis, edema, and replacement of myofibrils by interfibrillar spaces. While hesperidin treatment improved LVEDP by increasing inotropic (+LVdP/dt_{max}, marker of myocardial contraction) and lusitropic (-LVdP/dt_{max}, marker of myocardial relaxation) states of the heart and decreased systolic, diastolic, and mean arterial pressures, as compared to the diabetic control group, PPAR-γ antagonist GW9662 worsen the conditions. Moreover, prior treatment of GW9662 also prevented the hesperidin induced recovery in rats. PPAR-γ activation is directly correlated to the beneficial effects on all the haemodynamic parameters in spontaneously hypertensive rats [22], salt-sensitive hypertensive rats [23] and in renovascular animal model of hypertension [24]. Geng et al. [25] also found that rosiglitazone (a thiazolidinedione analogue) improves the left ventricular hemodynamic function in rats with MI due to their PPAR-γ agonist activity. Thus, these observations suggest the cardioprotective role of hesperidin in diabetic I/R model of cardiac ischemia via PPAR-γ pathway and that its activation may enhance these effects.

Further to confirm these observations we also studied the biochemical estimations in all the five groups namely sham control, diabetic I/R induced rats treated with saline, hesperidin, GW9662 either alone or in combination. We studied lipid peroxide metabolism and cardiac injury marker enzymes (CK-MB isoenzyme and LDH) and MDA, antioxidant enzymes (SOD, catalase and GSH) and TNF-α. CK-MB isoenzyme and LDH are important hallmarks of I/R injury and plays pivotal role in the pathogenesis of MI. In the present study, while decreased levels of CK-MB and LDH, increased levels of MDA were encountered in the heart of diabetic rats subjected to cardiac I/R injury which denotes oxidative stress. These observations are in accordance with the previous literature where increased lipid peroxidation products and MDA and decreased CK-MB isoenzymes and LDH was observed in hearts exposed to oxidative stress [26]. Myocardial CK-MB isoenzyme and LDH activities were decreased in the diabetic rats [27].Serum LDH activity was found to elevate in the patients with type II diabetes [28]. While, hesperidin treatment increased the levels of CK-MB, LDH and MDA levels in such cardiac I/R injury model, GW9662 treatment worsen the conditions. These observations are in accordance with the

Table 2. Mean area at risk and infarct area in rats in the different experimental groups.

Groups	Mean area at risk (%)	Infarct area (%)
Diabetic I/R	41.68±5.49	51.49±4.65
Diabetic I/R + Hesperidin	37.43±4.91	42.64±6.18*
Diabetic I/R + GW9662	44.29±5.88	60.81±5.64**
Diabetic I/R + GW9662 + Hesperidin	40.05±6.06	46.24±6.98#

Data are expressed as the mean ± standard error (n = 6/group). I/R, ischaemia/reperfusion. *p<0.05, **p<0.01 vs Diabetic I/R; #p<0.01 vs Diabetic I/R + Hesperidin.

Table 3. Histopathological changes in all experimental groups.

	Myonecrosis	Edema	Inflammation
Diabetic Sham	–	–	–
Diabetic I/R	+++	+++	+++
Diabetic I/R + Hesperidin	+	–	–
Diabetic I/R + GW9662	++++	++++	++++
Diabetic I/R + GW9662 + Hesperidin	++	+	+

I/R, ischaemia/reperfusion. Score (–), absence of any myonecrosis, oedema and inflammation; score (+), focal areas of myonecrosis, oedema and inflammation; score (++), patchy areas of myonecrosis, oedema and inflammation; score (+++), confluent areas of myonecrosis, oedema and inflammation; score (++++), massive areas of myonecrosis, oedema and inflammation.

previous literature which also put forward the protective role of hesperidine in similar models [29,30]. Moreover, prior treatment of GW9662 also prevented the hesperidin induced restoration in I/R injury. These results for the first time put forward the involvement of PPAR-γ mechanism in the activity of hesperidin in diabetic I/R injured rats. Further, the antioxidant enzymes like SOD, catalase and GSH were also studied and in addition TNF-α levels were also observed. Dhalla et al. [31] have suggested the

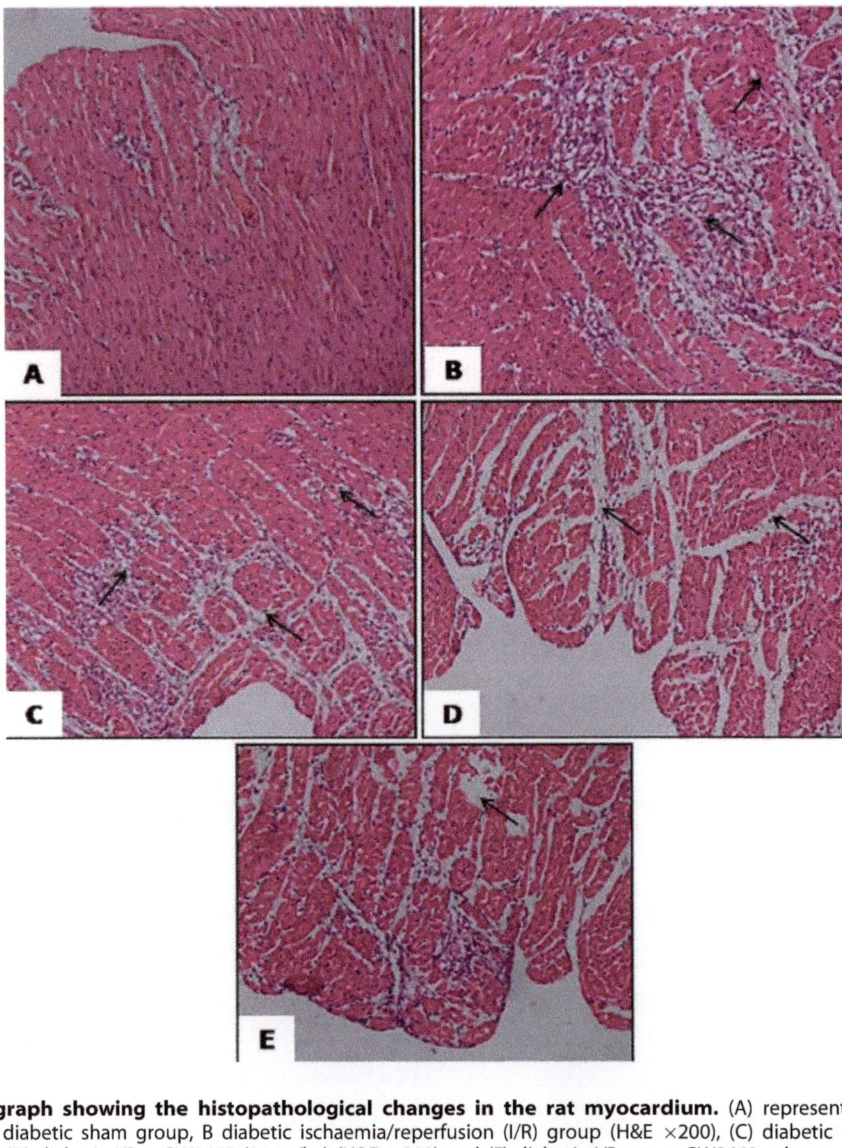

Figure 3. Photomicrograph showing the histopathological changes in the rat myocardium. (A) represents haematoxylin and eosin staining [(H&E) ×200] in diabetic sham group, B diabetic ischaemia/reperfusion (I/R) group (H&E ×200), (C) diabetic I/R + hesperidin treatment (100 mg/kg) (H&E ×200), (D) diabetic I/R + GW9662 (1 mg/kg) (H&E ×200) and (E) diabetic I/R rats + GW9662 + hesperidin (H&E ×200).

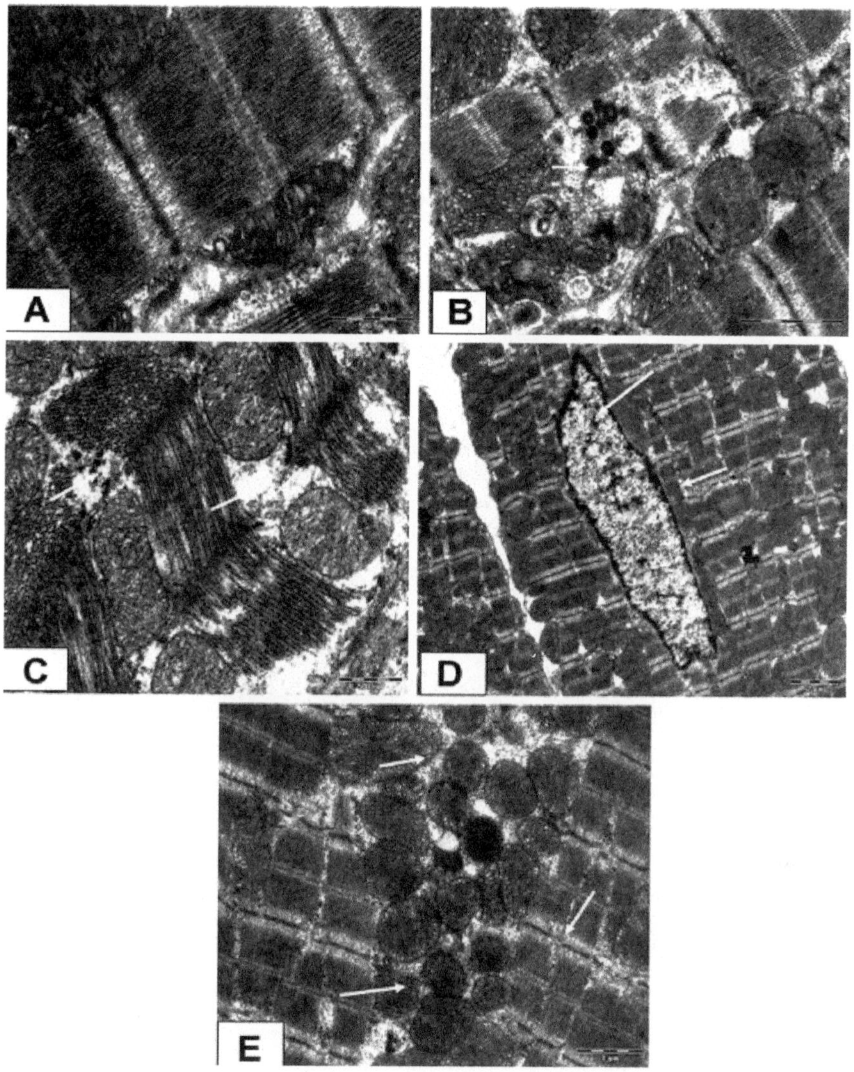

Figure 4. Photomicrograph showing the ultrastructural changes in the rat myocardium. (A) represents transmission electron microscope [(TEM) ×4800] in diabetic sham group, B diabetic ischaemia/reperfusion (I/R) group (TEM ×3500), (C) diabetic I/R + hesperidin treatment (100 mg/kg) (TEM ×3500), (D) diabetic I/R + GW9662 (1 mg/kg) (TEM ×3500) and (E) diabetic I/R rats + GW9662 + hesperidin (TEM ×3500).

importance of these antioxidant enzymes in the protection of myocardial cells against I/R like injury. Significant decrease in the antioxidant enzymes (SOD, catalase and GSH) was observed in the diabetic rats subjected to cardiac I/R injury. The levels were increased significantly in the hesperidin treated group thus categorizing hesperidin as a major antioxidant. In contrast, the GW9662 produced the opposite effects per se and blocked the antioxidant effects of hesperidin which suggests the involvement of PPAR-γ pathway in the hesperidin induced antioxidant effects in the cardiac I/R injury model.

The ability of hesperidin to limit the infarct size in cardiac I/R injured diabetic rats was observed. The percent infarction was significantly decreased in the rats treated with hesperidin, while GW9662 treatment *per se* increased the percent infarct area it also limited the hesperidin induced recovery when given prior to hesperidin. To support this observation TNF-α levels were studied which was found increased in the cardiac I/R injured diabetic rats. The TNF-α levels were decreased in the hesperidin treated rats and the prior treatment of GW9662 prevented this decrease. It seems that, hesperidine treatment may inhibit the TNF-α production, which is known to be one of the major factor in inflammation and infarction [7]. Since, in previous studies PPAR-γ agonists such as rosiglitazone and pioglitazone have been shown to reduce the infarct size following I/R injury [32], and in present study prior treatment of PPAR-γ antagonist attenuated the hesperidin induced recovery, it proves the role of PPAR-γ mechanism in hesperidine induced responses.

In addition to above parameters cardiac apoptosis was also studied, which is suggested to be one of the major pathogenic causes that underlie myocardial I/R injury. Crow et al. [33] suggested that blocking the apoptosis process might help in the prevention of loss of contractile cells, decrease the I/R induced cardiac injury and thus prevent the occurrence of MI. With this information in mind and with a view to explore the underlying mechanisms responsible for the improvement of cardiac functions following hesperidin treatment, the levels of antiapoptotic protein Bcl-2 and the proapoptotic protein Bax were measured and TUNEL staining was performed which is a known marker of DNA

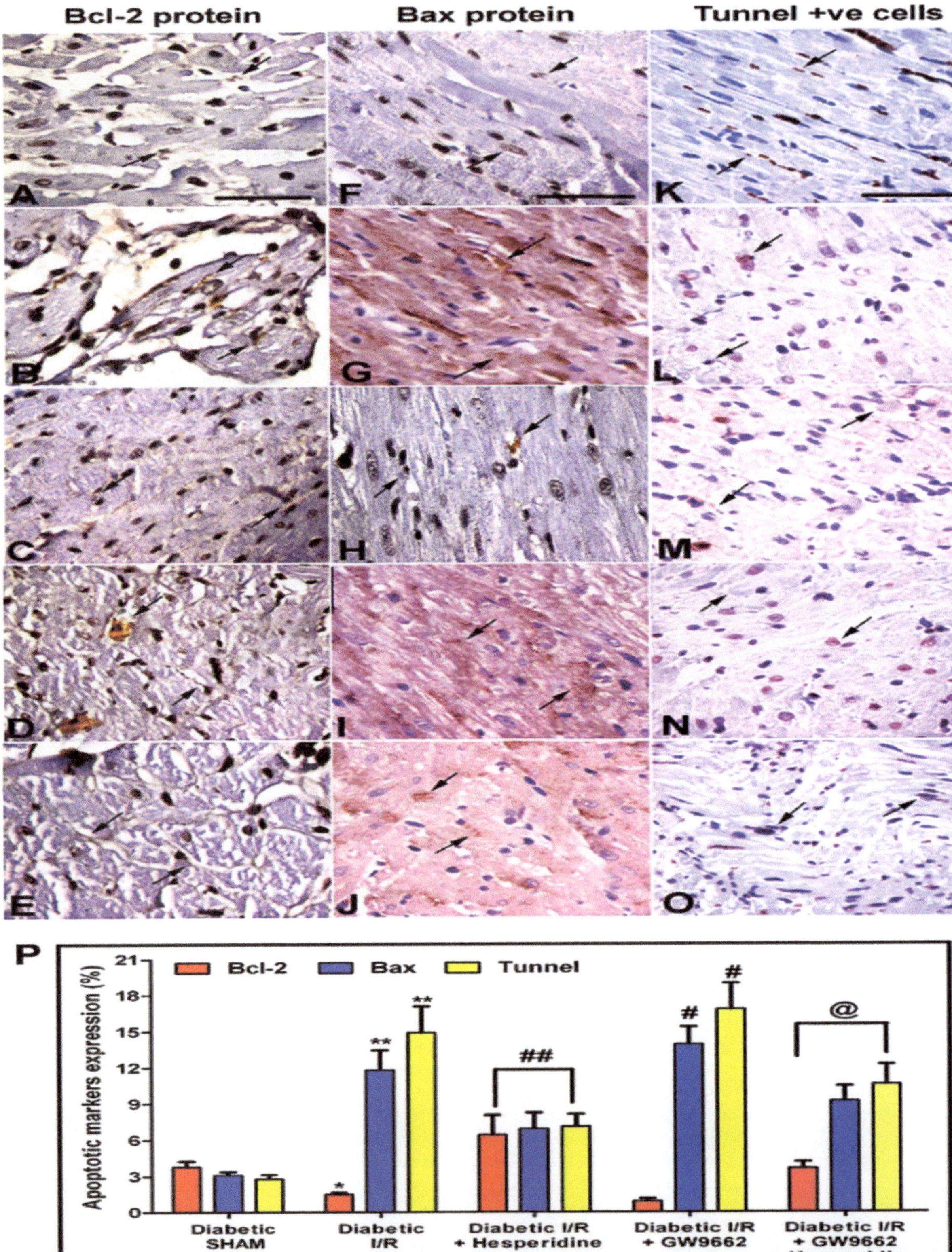

Figure 5. Photomicrograph of myocardial tissue sections showing Bcl-2 (A–E), Bax proteins expression (F–J) and TUNEL-positive cells (K–O). Apoptotic nuclei are indicated by arrows in panels (×400). (A, F and K) represents Diabetic sham rats treated with vehicles, (B, G and L) diabetic ischaemia/reperfusion (I/R) rats treated with vehicles, (C, H and M) diabetic I/R rats treated with hesperidin, (D, I and N) diabetic I/R rats treated with GW9662 and (E, J and O) diabetic I/R rats treated with GW9662 and hesperidin. (P) represents the quantitative analysis of the Bcl-2, Bax proteins and TUNEL-positive cells in the different groups. Data are expressed as the mean ± standard error (n = 6). *$p<0.05$, *$p<0.001$ vs diabetic SHAM; #$p<0.05$, ##$p<0.001$ vs Diabetic I/R group; @$p<0.01$ vs Diabetic I/R + hesperidin.

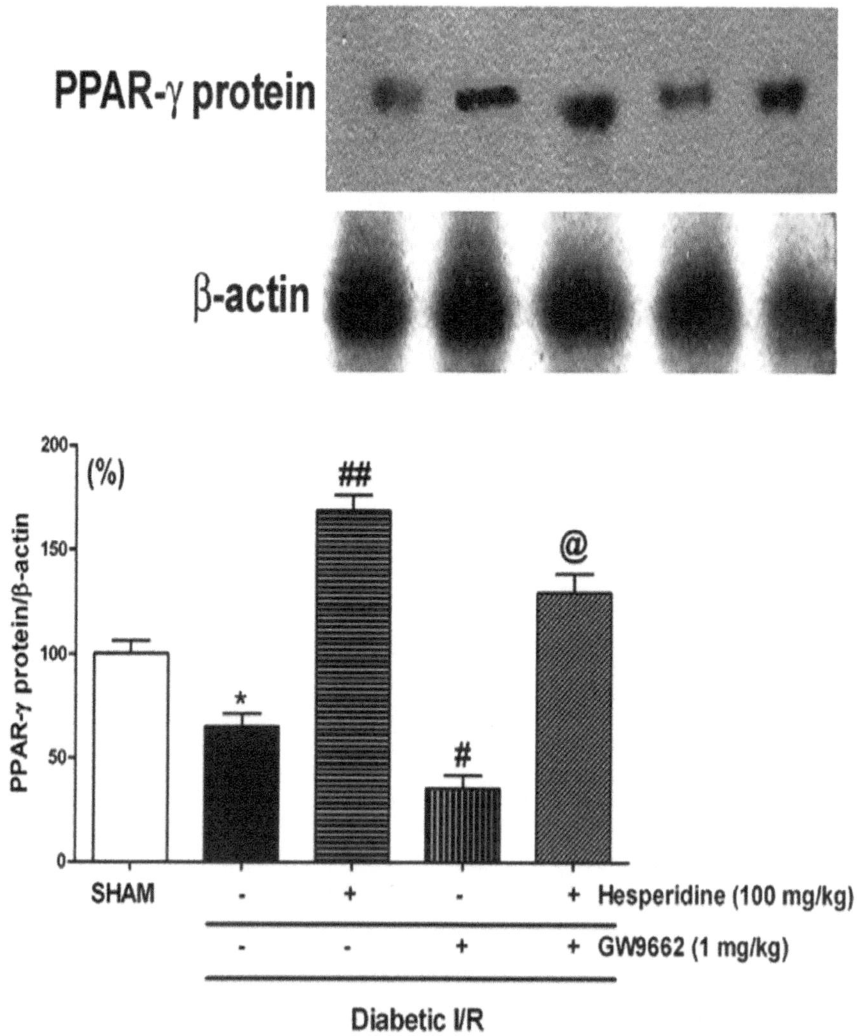

Figure 6. Effect of hesperidin and GW9662 (PPAR-γ antagonist) on PPAR-γ expression (top) in ischaemia/reperfusion (I/R)-induced myocardial infarction in diabetic rats. The bar graphs show PPAR-γ protein expression that has been normalized to β-actin (bottom). Data are expressed as a ration of the value determined for the vehicle (diabetic sham) (set as 100%). Data are expressed as the mean ± standard error. *$p < 0.05$ vs Diabetic SHAM; #$p < 0.01$, #$p < 0.001$ vs Diabetic I/R; @$p < 0.05$ vs Hesperidin.

fragmentation. Cardiac I/R injury in diabetic rats significantly decreased the Bcl-2 and increased BAX proteins and TUNEL-positive cells. Moreover, hesperidin treatment in these diabetic cardiac I/R injured rats showed significant antiapoptotic potential as depicted by augmented Bcl-2 protein expression and decreased Bax protein expression and TUNEL-positive cells. However, GW9662 treatment worsen the conditions in the diabetic I/R injured rats and its prior treatment attenuated the hesperidin induced improvement. The involvement of PPAR-γ mechanism in the antiapoptotic activity is much well known. PPAR-γ agonists, rosiglitazone and pioglitazone, markedly decreased apoptosis in the hearts of rabbits with hypercholesterolaemia and rats subjected to myocardial I/R injury [34,35]. Thus, the attenuation of the hesperidin induced improvement of cardiac functions in the presence of GW9662 (PPAR-γ antagonist) confirms the involvement of PPAR-γ pathway in the hesperidin mediated actions in diabetic cardiac I/R injury.

With a view to confirm the rescuing effects of hesperidin in the diabetic I/R injury model light microscopy and ultrastructural studies were carried out in sham rats, rats subjected to diabetic I/R injury and treated with saline, hesperidin or GW9662 either alone or in combination. Hesperidin treatment in I/R injured diabetic rats showed the protection of normal morphology of myocardium with no infarction, which was impaired in I/R injury control. Similarly, the ultrastructural studies also depicted the cardioprotective effects of hesperidin. On the other hand, GW9662, PPAR-γ antagonist, treatment showed severe infarction of the myocardial fibres, oedema and increased inflammatory cells. Moreover, the prior treatment of GW9662 with hesperidin also attenuated the hesperidin induced improvement. In addition, the western blot analysis depicted the increased expression of PPAR-γ protein, whereas GW9662 significantly decreased the concentration of PPAR-γ expressed *per se* and attenuated hesperidin induced expression. Previous studies also underscore the role PPAR-γ pathway in the different animal models [36,37]. Thus, the observations confirms the involvement of PPAR-γ mediated mechanisms in the I/R injury model in diabetic rats. Several additional confirmative studies may be required for further strengthening of this hypothesis. Limited bioavailability of hesperidin is reported in human volunteers, since low plasma concentration of hesperetin aglycone (<2 μmol/L) was observed after ingesting 0.5–1 L of orange juice [38,39]. Hesperidin is hydrolyzed by β-glucosidase derived from gut microflora into hesperetin when ingested orally, and its conjugated metabolites such as hesperetin glucuronides and sulfoglucuronides are absorbed into the blood in humans and rats [39–41]. However, no free aglycone is detected in the circulating blood. In human plasma the maximum concentrations of hesperetin metabolites following 5–7 h of orange juice ingestion are 1.3–2.2 mM for intake of 130–220 mg [42]. Amongst hesperetin metabolites, hesperetin-7-O-glucuronide and hesperetin-30-Oglucuronide are detected as the predominant metabolites in rat plasma following oral administration of hesperidin (50 mg/kg) [41]. Hesperetin-7-O-glucuronide also exert hypotensive, vasodilatory and anti-inflammatory activities [43]. Thus, the administration of PPAR-γ antagonist may prolong the activity of hesperidin metabolites and produce cardioprotective activity. Taken together, hesperidin treatment reduces oxidative stress and increases blood flow in ischaemic regions of the heart by correcting the I/R induced cardiac dysfunction in diabetic rats. Prior treatment with PPAR-γ antagonist attenuated the effects of hesperidine. Thus, the study for the first time proves the pivotal role of PPAR-γ mechanisms in the hesperidin induced cardioprotective effects in the I/R injury model in diabetic rats. The activation of PPAR-γ pathway along with the hesperidin like agents in the I/R injury like conditions may serve therapeutic importance in diabetic patients.

Author Contributions

Conceived and designed the experiments: YA SG DSA. Performed the experiments: YA SG DSA. Analyzed the data: PS BS SO HU. Contributed reagents/materials/analysis tools: YA SG DSA. Wrote the paper: YA SG DSA PS BS SO HU. Designed, conducted the study, analyzed the data and wrote the first draft YA SG DSA. Analyzed the data, collected references and drafted the manuscript PS BS SO HU.

References

1. Lopez AD, Murrau CC (1998) The global burden disease, 1990–2020. Nat Med 4: 1241–1243.
2. Bibbins-Domingo K, Coxson P, Pletcher MJ, Lightwood J, Goldman L (2007) Adolescent overweight and future adult coronary heart disease. N Engl J Med 6: 2371–2379.
3. De Bono DP, Boon NA (1992) Diseases of the cardiovascular system. In: Edwards CRW, Boucheir IAS, editors. Davidson's Principles and Practice and Medicine. Churchill Livingstone, Hong Kong, pp. 249–340.
4. DeBiase L, Pignatelli P, Lenti L, TocciG, Piccioni F, et al. (2003) Enhanced TNF alpha and oxidative stress in patients with heart failure: effect of TNF alpha on platelet O2- production. Thromb Haemost 90: 317–325.
5. Rajadurai M, Prince PSM (2006) Preventive effect of naringin on lipid peroxides and antioxidants in isoproterenol induced cardiotoxicity in Wistar rats: Biochemical and histopathological evidences. Toxicology 228: 259–268.
6. Nakamura T, Nishi H, Kokusenya Y, Hirota K, Miura Y (2000) Mechanism of antioxidative activity of fluvastatin-determination of the active position. Chem Pharm Bull 48: 235–237.
7. Goyal SN, Bharti S, Bhatia J, Nag TC, Ray R, et al. (2011). Telmisartan, a dual ARB/partial PPAR-γ agonist, protects myocardium from ischaemic reperfusion injury in experimental diabetes. Diabetes Obes Metab 13: 533–541.
8. Park HJ, Kim MJ, Ha E, Chung JH (2008) Apoptotic effect of hesperidin through caspase3 activation in human colon cancer cells, SNU-C4. Phytomedicine 15: 147–151.
9. Wilmsen PK, Spada DS, Salvador M (2005) Antioxidant activity of the flavonoid hesperidin in chemical and biological systems. J Agric Food Chem 53: 4757–4761.
10. Gumieniczek A (2003) Effect of the new thiazolidinedione-pioglitazone on the development of oxidative stress in liver and kidney of diabetic rabbits. Life Sci 74: 553–562.
11. Salam NK, Huang TH, Kota BP, Kim MS, Li Y, et al. (2008) Novel PPAR-gamma agonists identified from a natural product library: a virtual screening, induced-fit docking and biological assay study. ChemBiol Drug Des 71: 57–70.
12. VandenHeuvel JP (1999) Peroxisome proliferator-activated receptors (PPARS) and carcinogenesis. Toxicol Sci 47: 1–8.
13. Hihi AK, Michalik L, Wahli W (2002) PPARs: transcriptional effectors of fatty acids and their derivatives. Cell Mol Life Sci59: 790–798.
14. Ondrey F (2009) Peroxisome proliferator-activated receptor gamma pathway targeting in carcinogenesis: implications for chemoprevention. Clin Cancer Res 15: 2–8.
15. Ito H, Nakano A, Kinoshita M, Matsumori A (2003) Pioglitazone, a peroxisome proliferator-activated receptor-gamma agonist, attenuates myocardial ischemia/reperfusion injury in a rat model. Lab Invest 83: 1715–1721.
16. Okhawa H, Oohishi N, Yagi N (1979) Assay for lipid peroxides in animal tissues by thiobarbituric acid reaction. Anal Biochem 95: 351–358.
17. Moron MS, Depierre JW, Mannervik B (1979) Levels of glutathione, glutathione reductase and glutathione S-transferase activities in rat lung and liver. Biochem Biophys Acta 582: 67–78.
18. Singh AD, Amit S, Kumar OS, Rajan M, Mukesh N, et al. (2006) Cardioprotective effects of bosentan, a mixed endothelin type A and B receptor antagonist, during myocardial ischaemia and reperfusion in rats. Basic Clin Pharmacol Toxicol 98: 604–610.
19. Loh HK, Sahoo KC, Kishore K, Ray R, Nag TC, et al. (2007) Effects of thalidomide on isoprenaline- induced acute myocardial injury: a haemodynamic, histopathological and ultrastructural study. Basic Clin Pharmacol Toxicol 100: 233–239.
20. Mohanty IR, Arya DS, Gupta SK (2008) Withania somnifera provides cardioprotection and attenuates ischemia-reperfusion induced apoptosis. Clin Nutr 27: 635–642.
21. Mohanty I, Gupta SK, Arya DS (2007) Anti-apoptotic and cardioprotective effects of an herbal combination in rats with experimental myocardial infarction. Int J Integr Biol 1: 178–188.
22. Wu L, Wang R, De Champlain J, Wilson TW (2004) Beneficial and deleterious effects of rosiglitazone on hypertension development in spontaneously hypertensive rats. Am J Hypertens 17: 749–756.
23. Bolten CW, Payne MA, McDonald WG, Blanner PM, Chott RC, et al. (2007) Thiazolidinediones inhibit the progression of established hypertension in the Dahl salt-sensitive rat. DiabVasc Dis Res 4: 117–123.
24. de Oliveira Silva-Junior G, da Silva Torres T, de Souza Mendonca L, Alberto Mandarim-de-Lacerda C (2011) Rosiglitazone (peroxisome proliferator-activated receptor-gamma) counters hypertension and adverse cardiac and vascular remodeling in 2K1C hypertensive rats. Exp Toxicol Pathol 63: 1–7.
25. Geng DF, Wu W, Jin DM, Wang JF, Wu YM (2006) Effect of peroxisome proliferator-activated receptor gamma ligand. Rosiglitazone on left ventricular remodeling in rats with myocardial infarction. Int J Cardiol 113: 86–91.
26. CharanSahoo K, Arora S, Goyal S, Kishore K, Ray R, et al. (2009) Cardioprotective effects of benazepril, an angiotensin-converting enzyme inhibitor, in an ischaemia-reperfusion model of myocardial infarction in rats. J Renin Angiotensin Aldosterone Syst 10: 201–209.
27. Hagar HH (2002) Folic acid and vitamin B12 supplementation attenuates isoprenaline-induced myocardial infarction in experimental hyperhomocysteinemic rats. Pharmacol Res 46: 213–219.
28. Huang EJ, Kuo WW, Chen YJ, Chen TH, Chang MH, et al. (2006) Homocysteine and other biochemical parameters in type 2 diabetes mellitus with different diabetic duration or diabetic retinopathy. Clin Chim Acta 366: 293–298.
29. Kakadiya J, Shah M, Shah N (2010) Effect of hesperidin on serum heart marker, myocardial tissues parameter and histopathological of heart in isoproterenol induced myocardial infarction in diabetic rats. Int J Biol Tech 1: 57–62.
30. Kakadiya J, Mulani H, Shah N (2010) Protective effect of hesperidin on cardiovascular complication in experimentally induced myocardial infarction in diabetes in rats. J Basic Clin Pharm 1: 85–91.
31. Dhalla NS, Elmoselhi AB, Hata T, Makino N (2000) Status of myocardial antioxidants in ischemia-reperfusion injury. Cardiovasc Res 47: 446–456.
32. Wayman NS, Hattori Y, McDonald MC, Mota-Filipe H, Cuzzocrea S, et al. (2002) Ligands of the peroxisome proliferator-activated receptors (PPAR-gamma and PPAR-alpha) reduce myocardial infarct size. FASEB J 16: 1027–1040.
33. Crow MT, Mani K, Nam YJ, Kitsis RN (2004) The mitochondrial death pathway and cardiac myocyte apoptosis. Circ Res 95: 957–970.
34. Liu HR, Tao L, Gao E, Lopez BL, Christopher TA, et al. (2004) Anti-apoptotic effects of rosiglitazone in hypercholesterolemic rabbits subjected to myocardial ischemia and reperfusion. Cardiovasc Res 62: 135–144.
35. Cao Z, Ye P, Long C, Chen K, Li X, et al. (2007) Effect of pioglitazone, a peroxisome proliferator-activated receptor gamma agonist, on ischemia-reperfusion injury in rats. Pharmacology 79: 184–192.
36. Ikejima H, Imanishi T, Tsujioka H, Kuroi A, Kobayashi K, et al. (2008) Effects of telmisartan, a unique angiotensin receptor blocker with selective peroxisome proliferator-activated receptor-gamma-modulating activity, on nitric oxide bioavailability and atherosclerotic change. J Hypertens 26: 964–972.
37. Kobayashi N1, Ohno T, Yoshida K, Fukushima H, Mamada Y, et al. (2008) Cardioprotective mechanism of telmisartan via PPAR-gamma-eNOS pathway in dahl salt-sensitive hypertensive rats. Am J Hypertens 21: 576–581.
38. Erlund I, Meririnne E, Alfthan G, Aro A (2001) Plasma kinetics and urinary excretion of the flA (2001) naringenin and hesperetin in humans after ingestion of orange juice and grapefruit juice. J Nutr 131: 235–241.

39. Manach C, Morand C, Gil-Izquierdo A, Bouteloup-Demange C, Remesy C (2003) Bioavailability in humans of the flavanones hesperidin and narirutin after the ingestion of two doses of orange juice. Eur J Clin Nutr 57: 235–242.
40. Ameer B, Weintraub RA, Johnson JV, Yost RA, Rouseff RL (1996) Flavanone absorption after naringin, hesperidin, and citrus administration. Clin Pharmacol Ther 60: 34–40.
41. Matsumoto H, Ikoma Y, Sugiura M, Yano M, Hasegawa Y (2004) Identification and quantification of the conjugated metabolites derived from orally administered hesperidin in rat plasma. Food Chem 52: 6653–6659.
42. Manach C, Scalbert A, Morand C, Rémésy C, Jiménez L (2004) Polyphenols: food sources and bioavailability. Am J Clin Nutr 79: 727–747.
43. Yamamoto M, Jokura H, Hashizume K, Ominami H, Shibuya Y, et al. (2013) Hesperidin metabolite hesperetin-7-O-glucuronide, but not hesperetin-30-O-glucuronide, exerts hypotensive, vasodilatory, and anti-inflammatory activities. Food Funct 4: 1346–1351.

Berberine Improves Kidney Function in Diabetic Mice via AMPK Activation

Long Zhao, Li-Na Sun, Hui-Bin Nie, Xue-Ling Wang, Guang-Ju Guan*

Nephrology Research Institute, the Second Hospital of Shandong University, Jinan, Shandong, China

Abstract

Diabetic nephropathy is a major cause of morbidity and mortality in diabetic patients. Effective therapies to prevent the development of this disease are required. Berberine (BBR) has several preventive effects on diabetes and its complications. However, the molecular mechanism of BBR on kidney function in diabetes is not well defined. Here, we reported that activation of AMP-activated protein kinase (AMPK) is required for BBR-induced improvement of kidney function in vivo. AMPK phosphorylation and activity, productions of reactive oxygen species (ROS), kidney function including serum blood urea nitrogen (BUN), creatinine clearance (Ccr), and urinary protein excretion, morphology of glomerulus were determined in vitro or in vivo. Exposure of cultured human glomerulus mesangial cells (HGMCs) to BBR time- or dose-dependently activates AMPK by increasing the thr172 phosphorylation and its activities. Inhibition of LKB1 by siRNA or mutant abolished BBR-induced AMPK activation. Incubation of cells with high glucose (HG, 30 mM) markedly induced the oxidative stress of HGMCs, which were abolished by 5-aminoimidazole-4-carboxamide ribonucleoside, AMPK gene overexpression or BBR. Importantly, the effects induced by BBR were bypassed by AMPK siRNA transfection in HG-treated HGMCs. In animal studies, streptozotocin-induced hyperglycemia dramatically promoted glomerulosclerosis and impaired kidney function by increasing serum BUN, urinary protein excretion, and decreasing Ccr, as well as increased oxidative stress. Administration of BBR remarkably improved kidney function in wildtype mice but not in AMPKα2-deficient mice. We conclude that AMPK activation is required for BBR to improve kidney function in diabetic mice.

Editor: Shang-Zhong Xu, University of Hull, United Kingdom

Funding: This work was supported by the National Key Technology Research and Development Program of the Ministry of Science and Technology of China 2011BA110B05.

Competing Interests: The authors have declared that no competing interests exist.

* Email: guangj@sdu.edu.cn

Introduction

Diabetes mellitus represents a global threat for premature morbidity and mortality [1]. Diabetic nephropathy (DN) is a major chronic microvascular complication of diabetes and characterized by a progressive increase in albuminuria and a decline in glomerular filtration rate [2]. Mechanisms underlying nephropathy in diabetes include a range of hemodynamic and metabolic factors [3]. A growing number of studies support that the generation of reactive oxygen species (ROS) as a common downstream pathway of most of these mechanisms ultimately leads to inflammation and fibrosis [4]. However, the exact pathogenesis of DN is complex and poorly understood.

Berberine (BBR) is an isoquinolone alkaloid found in plants such as *Phellodendron chinense* and *Coptis chinensis*. In traditional Chinese medicine, BBR from *Coptidis rhizoma* is used as a constituent of the herbal medicine Huanglian [5]. In this form it is reported to exert anti-fungal, anti-bacterial/viral, and anti-oncogenic effects, as well as a beneficial effect on diabetes, and anti-atherogenic properties [6,7]. Several mechanisms are reported to be associated with the beneficial properties of BBR including improvement of sugar and lipid metabolism [8]. BBR has also been reported to reduce the incidence of diabetes through suppression of oxidative stress. Whether BBR exerts its beneficial effects in DN and the molecular targets are undefined.

The AMP-activated protein kinase (AMPK) is a heterotrimeric protein composed of α, β, and γ subunits. The α subunit imparts catalytic activity, while the β subunit contains a glycogen-binding domain that also regulates the activity and the γ subunit forms the broad base of the protein and is required for AMP binding. AMPK is well-conserved among eukaryotic cells and is expressed in endothelial cells of different origins. Activation of AMPK requires phosphorylation of Thr172 in the activation loop of the α subunit and is mediated by at least two kinases, Peutz-Jeghers syndrome kinase LKB1 (LKB1) and Ca^{2+}/calmodulin-dependent protein kinase kinase. AMPK has been shown to mediate angiogenic and anti-inflammatory effects [9]. Indeed, BBR has been reported to activate AMPK in several cell types, such as endothelial cells, smooth muscle cells [10], cardiomyocytes [11,12], cancer cells [13], β-cell [14], liver cells [15], macrophages [16,17], adipocytes [18]. Based on these reports, we hypothesized that the protective effects of BBR on kidney function in diabetes may be due, in part, to the ability of BBR to stimulate AMPK to suppress oxidative stress.

Materials and Methods

Materials

BBR, streptozotocin (STZ) and 5-aminoimidazole-4-carboxamide ribonucleoside (AICAR) were purchased from Sigma (St.

Louis, MO, USA). BBR was dissolved in DMSO to make a 500 mM stock solution (0.1% v/v final concentration) and stored at −80°C. AMPKα1/2 siRNA, LKB1 siRNA, and all primary antibodies were purchased from Cell Signaling Company or Santa Cruz Biotechnology. The siRNA delivery agent Lipofectamine 2000 was purchased from Invitrogen (Carlsbad, CA). Other chemicals were obtained from Sigma-Aldrich (St Louis, MO) unless otherwise indicated.

Animals

C57/BL6 wildtype (WT) mice (6–8 weeks of age, 20–25 g of bodyweight) were purchased from the animal department of Hunan Normal University. AMPKα$2^{-/-}$ mice were generated by Viollet B [19]. They were maintained in a temperature-controlled (22°C) under a 12 h light/dark cycle, pathogen-free environment and fed a standard rodent chow diet and water ad libitum. Male WT mice, 8–12 weeks of age, 20–25 g, were obtained from the Jackson Laboratory (Bar Harbor, ME). A low-dose (50 mg/kg/day for 5 consecutive days) STZ induction regimen was used to induce pancreatic islet cell destruction and persistent hyperglycemia as described by the Animal Models of Diabetic Complications Consortium (http://www.amdcc.org). Hyperglycemia was defined as a random blood glucose level of >300 mg/dL for >2 weeks after injection. The animal protocol was reviewed and approved by the University of Shandong, Animal Care and Use Committee.

Primary cell culture

For isolation of human glomerulus mesangial cells (HGMCs), collected kidney from surgery were washed twice with PBS at 4°C and cut into small pieces. These pieces were purified by 100-mesh sieve to get glomerular. Then the glomerular was incubated in a 0.2% collagenase solution at 37°C for 15–20 minutes. Cell pellets were incubated in 1640 medium with full components. Purity of HGMCs was confirmed through positive staining for collagen and fibronectin. The participants have provided their written informed consent. We recorded the general information and got the permission from the patients to use their kidneys for studying only. The study protocol was approved by the Ethical Committee of the Second Hospital of Shandong University.

Adenovirus infections in cells

Ad-GFP, a replication-defective adenoviral vector expressing green fluorescence protein (GFP), served as control. An adenoviral vector expressing a constitutively active mutant of AMPK (AMPK-CA), was subcloned from a rat cDNA encoding residues 1-312 of AMPK and bearing a Thr172-to-Asp mutation (T172D) into a shuttle vector (pShuttle CMV [cytomegalovirus]). Cells were infected with GFP or AMPK-CA in medium with 2% feta calf serum overnight. The cells were then washed and incubated in fresh growth medium without feta calf serum for an additional 12 h before experimentation. Using these conditions, infection efficiency was typically >80%, as determined by GFP expression.

Transfection of siRNA into cells

Transient transfection of siRNA was carried out according to Santa Cruz's protocol. Briefly, the siRNAs were dissolved in siRNA buffer (20 mM KCl; 6 mM HEPES, pH 7.5; 0.2 mM $MgCl_2$) to prepare a 10 μM stock solution. Cells grown in 6-well plates were transfected with siRNA in transfection medium containing liposomal transfection reagent (Lipofectamine 2000, Invitrogen). For each transfection, 100 μl transfection medium containing 4 μl siRNA stock solution was gently mixed with 100 μl transfection medium containing 4 μl transfection reagent. After 30-min incubation at room temperature, siRNA-lipid complexes were added to the cells in 1.0 ml transfection medium, and cells were incubated with this mixture for 6 h at 37°C. The transfection medium was then replaced with normal medium, and cells were cultured for 48 h.

Western blot analysis

As described previously [20], the protein content in total cell lysates or homogenized tissues was determined using the bicinchoninic acid protein assay reagent (Pierce, USA). Twenty micrograms of protein was separated by SDS-PAGE and then transferred to a membrane. The membrane was incubated with a 1:1,000 dilution of primary antibody and a 1:2,000 dilution of horseradish peroxidase-conjugated secondary antibody. Protein bands were visualized by enhanced chemiluminescence (GE Healthcare). The intensity (area × density) of the individual bands on western blots was measured by densitometry (model GS-700, Imaging Densitometer; Bio-Rad). The background was subtracted from the calculated area. The control was set to 100%.

AMPK activity assay

AMPK activity was assayed using the SAMS peptide. The activity was determined in the presence and absence of AMP (200 μM). AMPK activity was calculated by determining the difference in activity between both conditions.

Determination of kidney morphology

To assess the glomerular sclerotic injury, renal tissues were embedded in paraffin and 4 μm-thick sections were prepared for periodic acid schiff (PAS) staining. Glomerulosclerosis (GS) was evaluated by determining the percentage of glomeruli exhibiting sclerotic lesions (%GS). 200 consecutive glomeruli were examined for each mouse. The data were averaged. Lesion scores related to the glomerular and mesangial area were graded according to the following scale: 0 = preservation of the architecture, 1 = 5-15% glomerular expansion or mesangial expansion and PAS positivity, 2 = 15–30% glomerular expansion or mesangial expansion and PAS positivity, 3 = 30–50% glomerular expansion or mesangial expansion and PAS positivity, and 4 = >50% glomerular expansion or mesangial expansion and PAS positivity, which was described previously [21].

Renal function measurement

Blood samples were centrifuged at 2000 g for 10 min, serum were collected for measuring BUN by using a commercially available kit (ABIN, Cat: 577679). Urine samples were centrifuged in the same way to remove any suspended particles and the supernatant was used to detect 24-hour urine albumin protein by using Albumin Mouse ELISA Kit (abcam, Cat: 108792). The creatinine was measured with a Creatinine Companion kit (Exocell, Cat: 1012). The renal function was assessed by measurement of Cr clearance (Ccr) as urinary Cr X urine volume/serum Cr and expressed as milliliters per minute.

Immunohistochemistry

The expressions of 3-nitrotyrosine (3-NT) and malondialdehyde (MDA) in kidney were measured by immunohistochemistry in paraffin embedded sections following the process as previously described [22]. All morphological analyses and cell counting were performed on blinded slides.

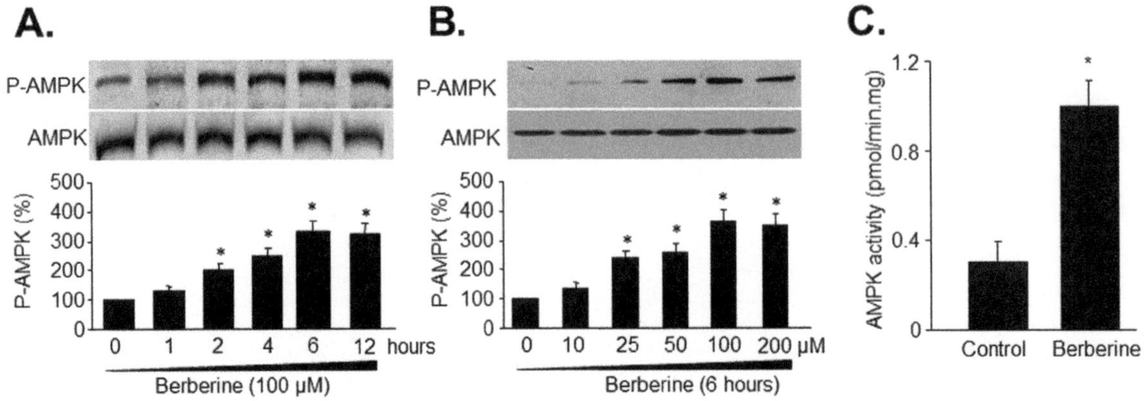

Figure 1. BBR activates AMPK in cultured HGMCs. (**A**) Cultured primary HGMCs were incubated with BBR (100 μM) for indicated time after starvation overnight. AMPK thr172 phosphorylation in total cell lysate was detected by western blot. The blot is a representative of three blots from three independent experiments. *$P<0.05$ VS control. (**B**) Dose-dependent effects of BBR on AMPK-Thr172 phosphorylation in HGMECs. N is 3 in each group. *$P<0.05$ *VS* control. (**C**) Confluent HGMCs were treated with BBR (100 μM) for 2 hours. AMPK activity was assayed using the SAMS peptide as a substrate. N is 5 in each group. *$P<0.05$ VS control.

Detection of ROS

Tissue or cell O_2^- levels were measured using the DHE fluorescence/HPLC assay with minor modifications [23]. Briefly, tissues or cells were incubated with DHE (10 μM) for 30 min, homogenized, and subjected to methanol extraction. HPLC was performed using a C-18 column (mobile phase: gradient of acetonitrile and 0.1% trifluoroacetic acid) to separate and quantify oxyethidium (product of DHE and O_2^-) and ethidium (a product of DHE auto-oxidation). O_2^- production was determined by conversion of DHE into oxyethidine.

Statistical Analysis

Results are expressed as the mean ± SD. Statistical significance for comparison between two groups was calculated using the two-tailed Student's *t* test. To assess comparisons between multiple groups, analysis of variance (ANOVA) followed by the Bonferroni procedure was performed using the Graph-Pad Prism 4 program (GraphPad Software, Inc, San Diego, CA). A *P* value of <0.05 was considered to be statistically significant.

Results

BBR activates AMPK via Thr172 phosphorylation in time- and dose- dependent manner in cultured HGMCs

Earlier studies had established that phosphorylation of AMPK at Thr172 correlates with AMPK activity [24]. BBR is well characterized as a drug to protect diabetes and the vascular complications. To investigate whether BBR activates AMPK in kidney, confluent HGMCs was treated with varying concentrations of BBR from 10 to 200 μM in culture medium for 2 hours. AMPK activation was indirectly assessed by western blot analysis of AMPK phosphorylation at Thr172, which is essential for AMPK activity. As shown in Figure 1A, BBR of 100 μM did not affect phosphorylation of AMPK at 1 hour point. In contrast, BBR began to activate AMPK at 2 hours. Increasing incubating time of BBR (100 μM) further enhanced AMPK phosphorylation. In Figure 1B, the phosphorylation of AMPK gradually increased beginning from 25 μM after incubation with BBR for 2 hours and reached peak levels at 100 μM in HGMCs. BBR treatment did

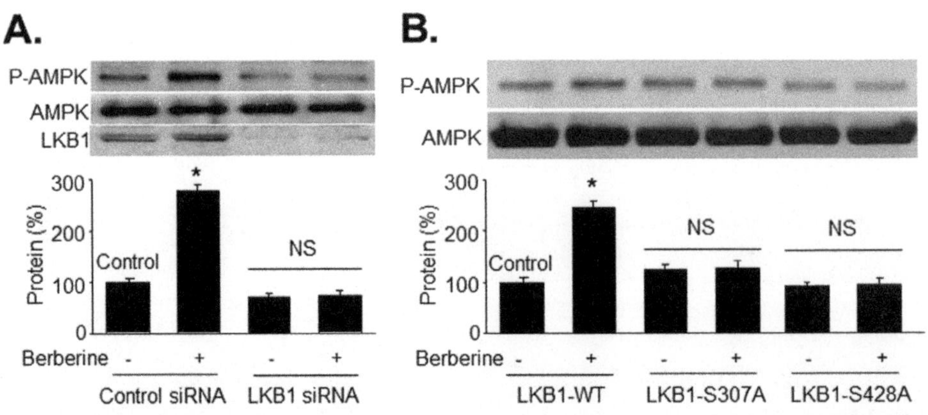

Figure 2. BBR-induced AMPK activation in cultured HGMCs is LKB1-dependent. (**A**) HGMCs were transfected with control siRNA or LKB1 siRNA for 48 h. Then cells were treated with BBR (100 μM) for 2 hours. AMPK thr172 phosphorylation in total cell lysate was detected by western blot. The blot is a representative of three blots from three independent experiments. *$P<0.05$ VS control. NS indicates no significance. (**B**) HGMCs were infected with adenovirus containing LKB1-WT, LKB1-S428A or LKB1-S307A for 48 h. The infected cells were then treated with BBR (100 μM) for 2 hours. AMPK-Thr172 phosphorylation was detected by Western blot. The blot is a representative blot from three independent experiments. *$P<$ 0.05 VS ad-GFP. NS indicates no significance.

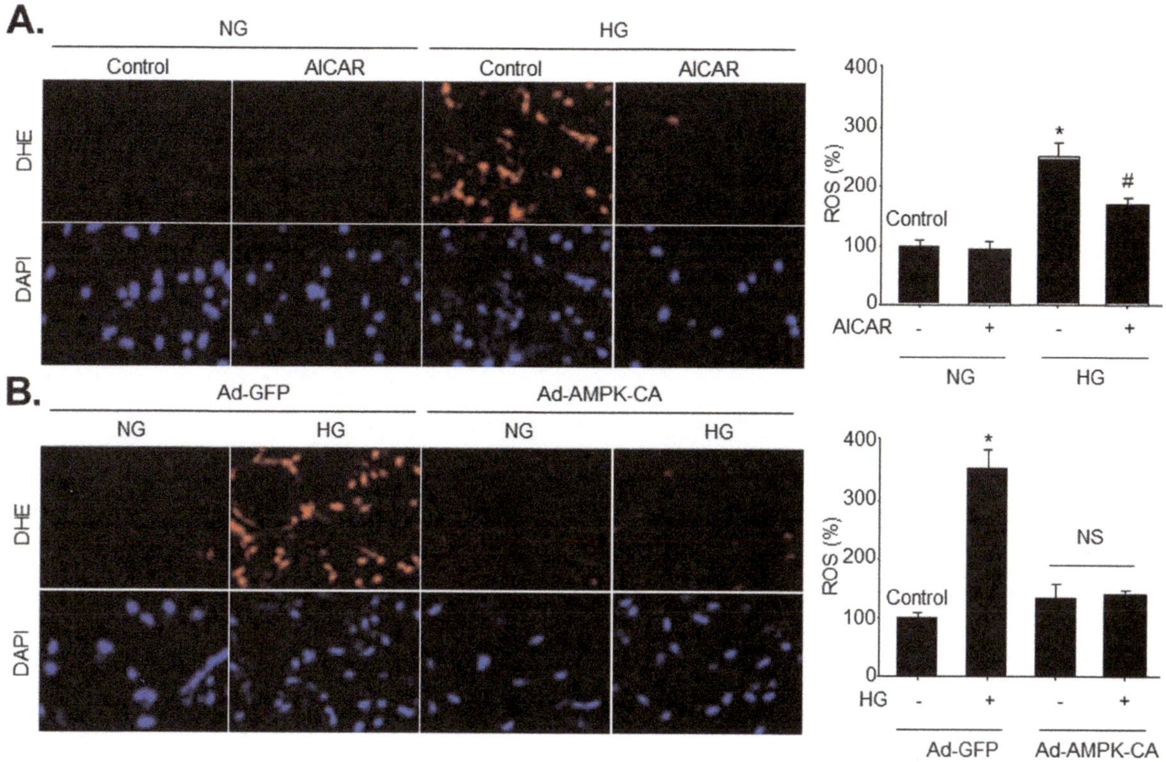

Figure 3. AMPK upregulations by AICAR or gene overexpression attenuate HG-induced oxidative stress in cultured HGMCs. (**A**) HGMCs were incubated with D-glucose (30 mM) in presence or absence of AICAR (2 mM) for 12 hours. ROS productions were detected by DHE fluorescence. N is 5 in each group. $^{*}P<0.05$ vs. control, $^{\#}P<0.05$ vs HG alone. (**B**) HGMCs infected with Ad-GFP or Ad-AMPK-CA for 48 hours were incubated with HG for 12 hours. ROS productions were detected by DHE fluorescence. The picture is a representative from 3 independent experiments. $^{*}P<0.05$ vs. control GFP. NS indicates no significance.

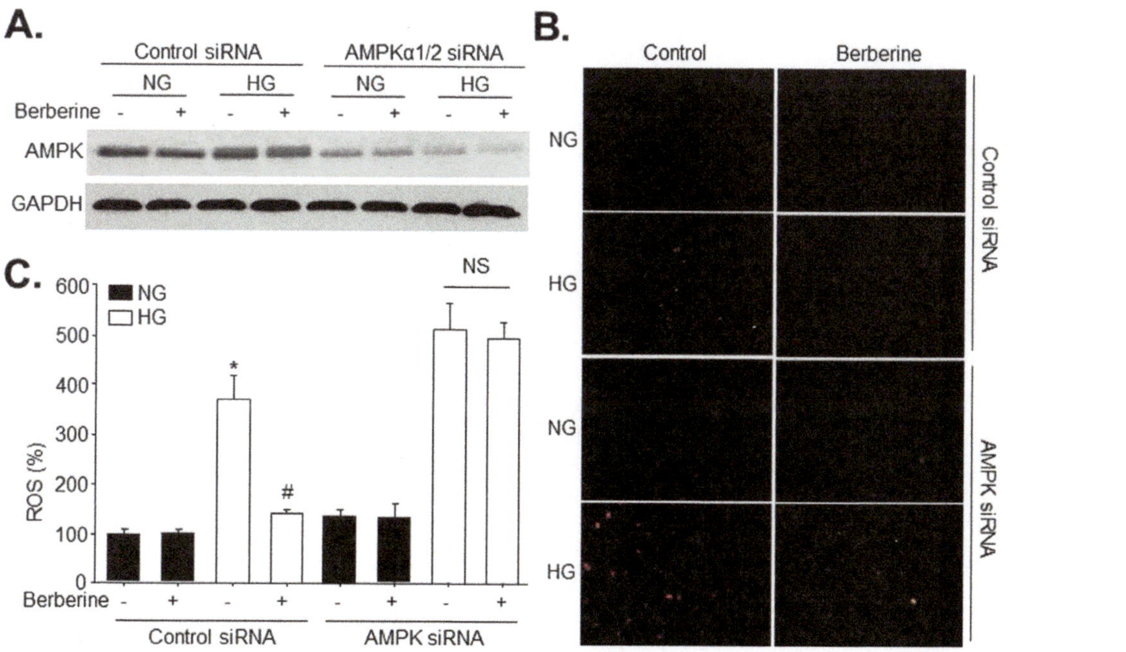

Figure 4. BBR via AMPK activation reverses HG-induced oxidative stress in HGMCs. HGMCs were transfected with AMPKα1/2 siRNA for 48 hours. Then cells were pre-incubated with BBR (100 μM) for 30 minutes followed by treatment with D-glucose (30 mM) for 12 hours. (**A**) AMPKα protein expression in total cell lysates was assayed by Western blot. (**B**) ROS productions were detected by DHE fluorescence. (**C**) Quantitative data of ROS productions. N is 5 in each group. $^{*}P<0.05$ vs. control, $^{\#}P<0.05$ vs HG plus control siRNA. NS indicates no significance.

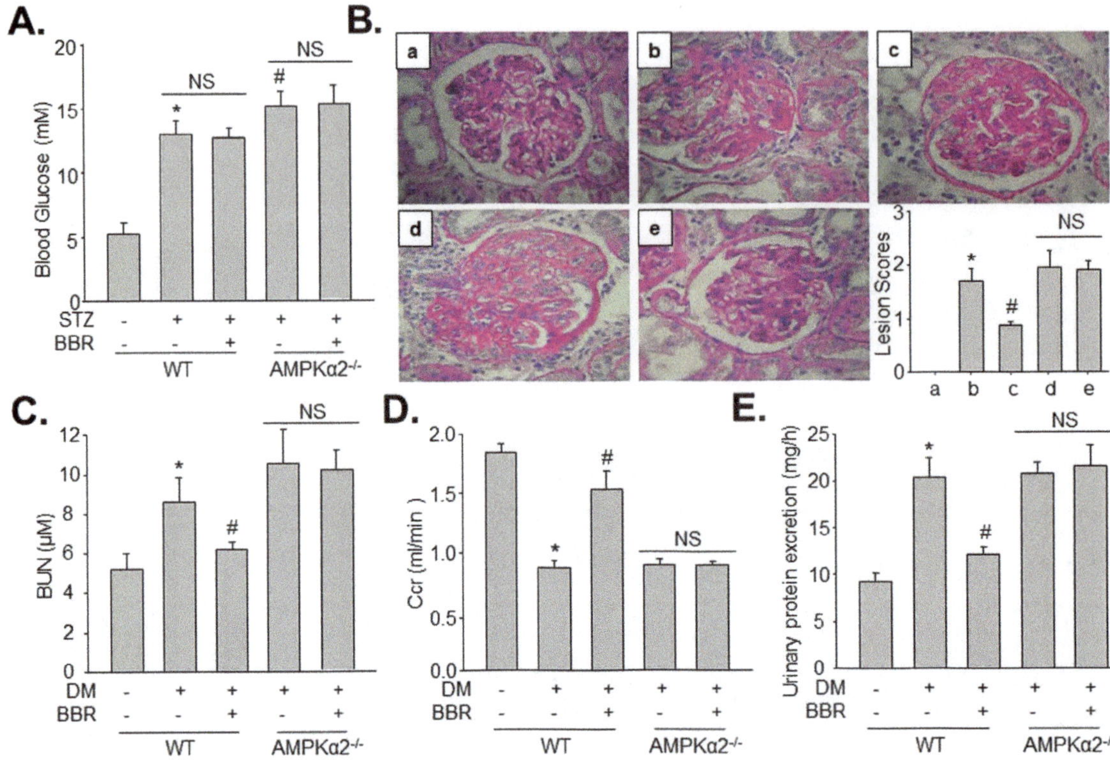

Figure 5. BBR prevents hyperglycemia-induced renal dysfunction in *WT* but not in *AMPKα2*$^{-/-}$ mice. Permanent hyperglycemia in *WT* and *AMPKα2*$^{-/-}$ mice was induced by a low-dose STZ induction. All mice were received with or without BBR administration (200 mg/kg body weight daily) for 8 weeks after the stable diabetic model was established. At the end of experiments, mice were sacrificed. (**A**) Blood glucose in all mice. 5–10 mice in each group. $^{*}P<0.05$ vs. WT alone, $^{\#}P<0.05$ vs STZ plus WT. NS indicates no significance. (**B**) Morphological and quantitative analysis of glomerulus by HE staining. a, WT; b, WT + STZ; c, WT + STZ + BBR; d, *AMPKα2*$^{-/-}$ + STZ; e, *AMPKα2*$^{-/-}$ + STZ + BBR. (**C**) Serum BUN, (**D**) creatine clearance rate (Ccr), and (**E**) urinary protein excretion were assayed. 5–10 mice in each group. $^{*}P<0.05$ vs. control, $^{\#}P<0.05$ vs DM in WT. NS indicates no significance.

not alter total levels of AMPK (Figure 1A and 1B), suggesting that BBR-induced phosphorylation of AMPK was not due to altered expression of the total protein. In addition, increased AMPK phosphorylation was associated with elevated AMPK activity, as measured by the SAMS peptide assay [25] (Figure 1C).

BBR-induced AMPK phosphorylation in HGMCs is LKB1-dependent

To study how BBR activates AMPK, we suppressed LKB1 expression, which is an AMPK upstream kinase by applying siRNA in cells [26]. We found that LKB1 siRNA, but not control siRNA, inhibited BBR-induced phosphorylation of AMPK at Thr172 if LKB1 protein expression was silenced by siRNA (Figure 2A). These experiments offer solid support for the notion that LKB1 is required for BBR-induced AMPK activation in cells.

We next evaluated whether LKB1 phosphorylation at Ser307 or Ser428 was required for BBR-induced AMPK activation [27]. Using site-directed mutagenesis, we developed an LKB1 mutant in which an amino acid essential for LKB1 activation, serine 307 or 428, was mutated to alanine. Since BBR treatment resulted in increased phosphorylation of AMPK in cells infected with adenovirus encoding WT-LKB1, we next investigated whether adenoviral overexpression of the LKB1 mutant would prevent BBR-induced phosphorylation of AMPK. As expected, LKB1-S307A or LKB1-S428A mutant did abolish BBR-enhanced phosphorylation of AMPK-Thr172 (Figure 2B). These data suggest that LKB1 is essential for BBR-induced AMPK activation in cells.

Activation of AMPK attenuates HG-induced oxidative stress

Permanent hyperglycemia is the most common single cause of kidney failure. Oxidative stress and inflammation are proved to be critical for the pathogenesis of diabetes mellitus. In order to induce the injury of kidney cells, we mimicked hyperglycemia by using high glucose (30 mM D-glucose) in culture medium to treat HGMCs. As shown in Figure 3A and 3B, incubation of HGMCs with high glucose (HG) significantly increased the ROS productions. These results are consistent with previous report [25]. Further, activation of AMPK by AICAR (Figure 3A) or gene overexpression (Figure 3B) abolished HG-induced oxidative stress in HGMCs, indicating that HG-induced oxidative stress is AMPK-dependent.

BBR via AMPK activation suppresses HG-induced oxidative stress

We next determined whether BBR suppressed HG-induced oxidative stress through AMPK activation. To test this notion, we performed siRNA transfection to knockdown AMPK α1 and α2 protein levels. As depicted in Figure 4A, the level of AMPK protein was silenced significantly by specific siRNA, but not control siRNA. As expected, BBR treatment dramatically suppressed HG-induced oxidative stress in cultured HGMCs as assayed by DHE fluorescence (Figure 4B and 4C). Collectively, these results demonstrate that AMPK plays a key role in BBR-reduced oxidative stress in HG-treated HGMCs.

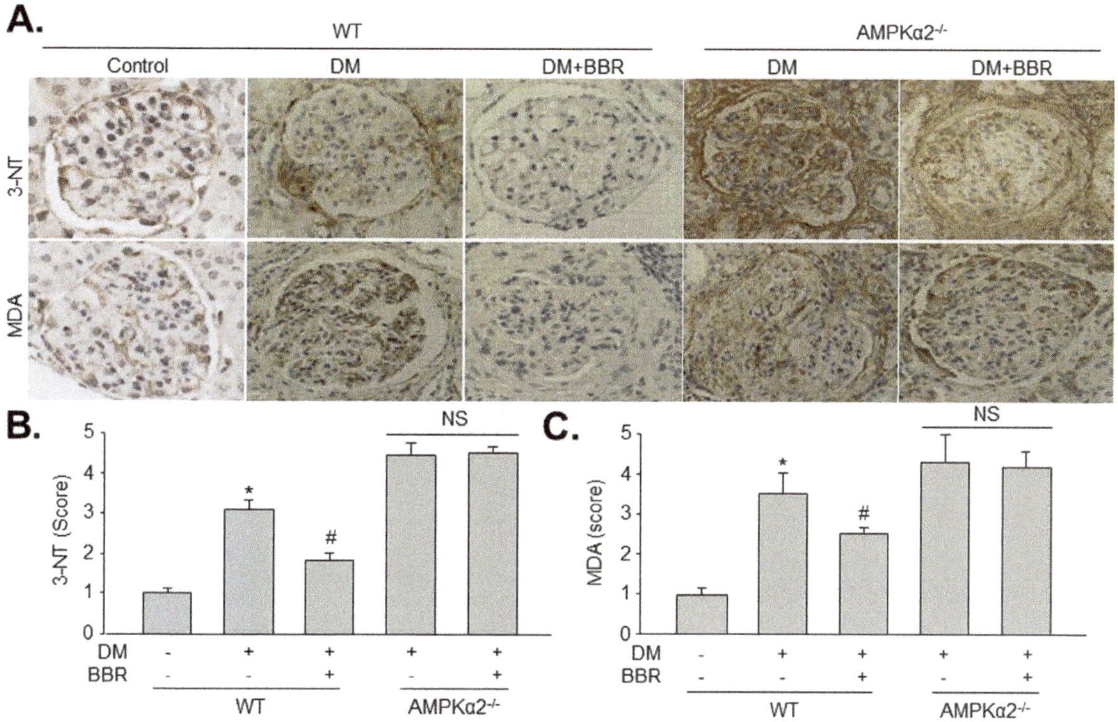

Figure 6. BBR via AMPK prevents hyperglycemia-induced oxidative stress in mice. Permanent hyperglycemia in *WT* and *AMPKα2*$^{-/-}$ mice was induced by a low-dose STZ induction as described in method section. All mice were received with or without BBR administration (200 mg/kg body weight daily) for 8 weeks after the stable diabetic model was established. At the end of experiments, mice were sacrificed to detect MDA and 3-NT by IHC. (**A**) Representative pictures of MDA and 3-NT. (**B**) Quantitative analysis of 3-NT. (**C**) Quantitative analysis of MDA. 5–10 mice in each group. $^{*}P<0.05$ vs. control, $^{\#}P<0.05$ vs DM in WT. NS indicates no significance.

Hyperglycemia induces kidney dysfunction in STZ-injected mice

Then we investigated whether administration of BBR improved kidney function in diabetic mice. After 16-week STZ-induced hyperglycemia duration, morphology of kidneys from all mice was assayed by PAS staining (Figure 5A). Compared to control WT mice, hyperglycemia remarkably caused fibrosis, containing abnormal glomeruli. Similar to formation of glomerulosclerosis, diabetes also induced renal dysfunction as increased serum BUN (Figure 5B), decreased Ccr (Figure 5C), and enhanced urinary albumin excretion (Figure 5D).

Treatment of mice with BBR attenuates diabetes-induced kidney dysfunction in *WT* but not in *AMPKα2*$^{-/-}$ mice

Then we determined the effects of BBR on diabetes-induced renal dysfunction. Injection of STZ dramatically increased blood glucose in WT and *AMPKα2*$^{-/-}$ mice. Interestingly, the increases of blood glucose induced by STZ in *AMPKα2*$^{-/-}$ mice were slightly higher that WT mice. As shown in Figure 5B, BBR significantly inhibited the hyperglycemia-induced the formation of the glomerulosclerosis in WT but not in *AMPKα2*$^{-/-}$ diabetic mice. Quantitative analysis indicated that STZ significantly increased lesion score in WT mice. BBR remarkably reduced the lesion score in WT but not in *AMPKα2*$^{-/-}$ diabetic mice. Similarly, BBR reversed the increased serum BUN (Figure 5C), decreased Ccr (Figure 5D), and enhanced urinary albumin excretion (Figure 5E) induced by hyperglycemia, suggesting that AMPK is a key mediator to perform the protective effects of BBR in diabetic nephropathy.

Diabetes-induced oxidative stress in kidney is reversed by BBR in *WT* but not in *AMPKα2*$^{-/-}$ mice

Pathophysiological processes of diabetes is extreme complex and controversial. A growing number of evidences showed that oxidative stress and inflammation might play important roles in the development of DN. We finally checked the oxidative stress in diabetic mice by assaying 3-NT and MDA, which are makers of peroxidation of protein or lipid [28]. As shown in Figure 6A, 6B, and 6C, our data showed that hyperglycemia increased the levels of 3-NT and MDA in kidney as compared to control group. Treatment of BBR significantly decreased levels of 3-NT and MDA in *WT* diabetic mice but not in *AMPKα2*$^{-/-}$ diabetic mice, suggesting BBR via AMPK activation reduced oxidative stress in diabetic mice.

Discussion

In the present study, we have shown that LKB1-AMPK signaling mediates BBR-protected kidney function in diabetic mice. The underlying mechanism in this process is due to a novel pathway in which kidney dysfunction is inhibited by BBR as a result of AMPK activation. These findings indicate that AMPK pathway is an important mediator for kidney cell function and suggest that BBR therapy that modulates AMPK signaling may be beneficial in treating kidney dysfunction in diabetic nephropathy.

BBR is a natural compound isolated from plants and with multiple pharmacological activities [8]. The emerging role of BBR in modifying sugar and lipid metabolism has been verified in a large amount of experimental and clinical studies. Notably, due to the low toxicity, BBR could be used in diabetic patients with chronic hepatitis. Beneficial effects of BBR were also observed in combating diabetic complications [29]. Diabetes-related endothelial dysfunction, nephropathy, and neuropathy could be relieved after BBR administration. Recently, some groups reported that BBR has some protective effects in different stages of diabetes in rats, such as diabetic nephropathy [30–33]. However, this present study not only demonstrated that BBR improves kidney function and inhibits glomerular fibrosis in diabetic mice, but further uncovered the molecular mechanisms, which BBR activates LKB1-AMPK signaling to suppress oxidative stress in glomerulus mesangial cells. Most importantly, the protective effects of BBR on kidney function in diabetic mice were mediated by AMPK because BBR was unable to protect liver functions in $AMPK\alpha2^{-/-}$ mice, indicating the important role of AMPK in BBR-induced beneficial effects. In fact, BBR has been reported to activate AMPK in vascular endothelial cells and suppressed formation of atherosclerosis [34,35]. Combined with these observations, BBR would be explored to treat kidney and cardiovascular disease, which are related to diabetic complications.

Interestingly, we discovered that STZ-induced type 1 diabetes damaged renal function and induced glomerulosclerosis in mice. This is inconsistent with Qi's report [36]. We reasoned that the discrepancy should be due to the time difference of persistent hyperglycemia. Actually, Zhang M et al. also reported that the kidney function and the morphology of glomerular started to be abnormal at the 6th week and were serve at the 9th week during hyperglycemia [37], as well as the 8th week which we reported. Another issue is that the relationship between AMPK and ROS remains controversial. Recently, Kumar Sharma et al. demonstrated that superoxide is increased by AMPK, which is renal-protective [38]. In fact, AMPK functions as a redox sensor and modulator, in which slight increase of ROS can activate AMPK. However, activation of AMPK reduces ROS production. The disagreement would be due to the different level of ROS productions. Further studies are required to test these possibilities.

In summary, we have demonstrated that BBR attenuates diabetic nephropathy *in vivo* via AMPK activation. In addition, the improvement of kidney function by BBR appears to be mediated by suppression of oxidative stress. The data presented here support the concept that AMPK may be an important therapeutic target for treating diabetic nephropathy and other kidney diseases related to oxidative stress. Therefore, till now, there is no report about the effects of BBR on diabetic nephropathy in clinical patients, indicating the potential application for BBR on treating diabetic kidney disease in patients in future.

Author Contributions

Conceived and designed the experiments: LZ GJG. Performed the experiments: LZ LNS HBN XLW. Analyzed the data: LZ GJG. Contributed to the writing of the manuscript: GJG. Revised the manuscript: LNS HBN XLW.

References

1. Roglic G, Unwin N, Bennett PH, Mathers C, Tuomilehto J, et al. (2005) The burden of mortality attributable to diabetes: realistic estimates for the year 2000. Diabetes Care 28: 2130–2135.
2. Molitch ME, DeFronzo RA, Franz MJ, Keane WF, Mogensen CE, et al. (2004) Nephropathy in diabetes. Diabetes Care 27 Suppl 1: S79–83.
3. Jha JC, Jandeleit-Dahm KA, Cooper ME (2014) New Insights Into the Use of Biomarkers of Diabetic Nephropathy. Adv Chronic Kidney Dis 21: 318–326.
4. Forbes JM, Coughlan MT, Cooper ME (2008) Oxidative stress as a major culprit in kidney disease in diabetes. Diabetes 57: 1446–1454.
5. Yin J, Zhang H, Ye J (2008) Traditional chinese medicine in treatment of metabolic syndrome. Endocr Metab Immune Disord Drug Targets 8: 99–111.
6. Liang KW, Ting CT, Yin SC, Chen YT, Lin SJ, et al. (2006) Berberine suppresses MEK/ERK-dependent Egr-1 signaling pathway and inhibits vascular smooth muscle cell regrowth after in vitro mechanical injury. Biochem Pharmacol 71: 806–817.
7. Cho BJ, Im EK, Kwon JH, Lee KH, Shin HJ, et al. (2005) Berberine inhibits the production of lysophosphatidylcholine-induced reactive oxygen species and the ERK1/2 pathway in vascular smooth muscle cells. Mol Cells 20: 429–434.
8. Li Z, Geng YN, Jiang JD, Kong WJ (2014) Antioxidant and Anti-Inflammatory Activities of Berberine in the Treatment of Diabetes Mellitus. Evid Based Complement Alternat Med 2014: 289264.
9. Wang S, Xu J, Song P, Viollet B, Zou MH (2009) In vivo activation of AMP-activated protein kinase attenuates diabetes-enhanced degradation of GTP cyclohydrolase I. Diabetes 58: 1893–1901.
10. Liang KW, Yin SC, Ting CT, Lin SJ, Hsueh CM, et al. (2008) Berberine inhibits platelet-derived growth factor-induced growth and migration partly through an AMPK-dependent pathway in vascular smooth muscle cells. Eur J Pharmacol 590: 343–354.
11. Chang W, Zhang M, Li J, Meng Z, Wei S, et al. (2013) Berberine improves insulin resistance in cardiomyocytes via activation of 5′-adenosine monophosphate-activated protein kinase. Metabolism 62: 1159–1167.
12. Lv X, Yu X, Wang Y, Wang F, Li H, et al. (2012) Berberine inhibits doxorubicin-triggered cardiomyocyte apoptosis via attenuating mitochondrial dysfunction and increasing Bcl-2 expression. PLoS One 7: e47351.
13. Fan LX, Liu CM, Gao AH, Zhou YB, Li J (2013) Berberine combined with 2-deoxy-d-glucose synergistically enhances cancer cell proliferation inhibition via energy depletion and unfolded protein response disruption. Biochim Biophys Acta 1830: 5175–5183.
14. Shen N, Huan Y, Shen ZF (2012) Berberine inhibits mouse insulin gene promoter through activation of AMP activated protein kinase and may exert beneficial effect on pancreatic beta-cell. Eur J Pharmacol 694: 120–126.
15. Cao S, Zhou Y, Xu P, Wang Y, Yan J, et al. (2013) Berberine metabolites exhibit triglyceride-lowering effects via activation of AMP-activated protein kinase in Hep G2 cells. J Ethnopharmacol 149: 576–582.
16. Mo C, Wang L, Zhang J, Numazawa S, Tang H, et al. (2014) The crosstalk between Nrf2 and AMPK signal pathways is important for the anti-inflammatory effect of berberine in LPS-stimulated macrophages and endotoxin-shocked mice. Antioxid Redox Signal 20: 574–588.
17. Jeong HW, Hsu KC, Lee JW, Ham M, Huh JY, et al. (2009) Berberine suppresses proinflammatory responses through AMPK activation in macrophages. Am J Physiol Endocrinol Metab 296: E955–964.
18. Zhou L, Wang X, Yang Y, Wu L, Li F, et al. (2011) Berberine attenuates cAMP-induced lipolysis via reducing the inhibition of phosphodiesterase in 3T3-L1 adipocytes. Biochim Biophys Acta 1812: 527–535.
19. Viollet B, Andreelli F, Jorgensen SB, Perrin C, Flamez D, et al. (2003) Physiological role of AMP-activated protein kinase (AMPK): insights from knockout mouse models. Biochem Soc Trans 31: 216–219.
20. Wang S, Peng Q, Zhang J, Liu L (2008) Na+/H+ exchanger is required for hyperglycaemia-induced endothelial dysfunction via calcium-dependent calpain. Cardiovasc Res 80: 255–262.
21. Liao J, Soltani Z, Ebenezer P, Isidro-Carrion AA, Zhang R, et al. (2010) Tesaglitazar, a dual peroxisome proliferator-activated receptor agonist (PPAR alpha/gamma), improves metabolic abnormalities and reduces renal injury in obese Zucker rats. Nephron Exp Nephrol 114: e61–68.
22. Wang S, Xu J, Song P, Wu Y, Zhang J, et al. (2008) Acute inhibition of guanosine triphosphate cyclohydrolase 1 uncouples endothelial nitric oxide synthase and elevates blood pressure. Hypertension 52: 484–490.
23. Fernandes DC, Wosniak J Jr., Pescatore LA, Bertoline MA, Liberman M, et al. (2007) Analysis of DHE-derived oxidation products by HPLC in the assessment of superoxide production and NADPH oxidase activity in vascular systems. Am J Physiol Cell Physiol 292: C413–422.
24. Wang S, Liang B, Viollet B, Zou MH (2011) Inhibition of the AMP-activated protein kinase-alpha2 accentuates agonist-induced vascular smooth muscle contraction and high blood pressure in mice. Hypertension 57: 1010–1017.
25. Wang S, Zhang M, Liang B, Xu J, Xie Z, et al. (2010) AMPKalpha2 deletion causes aberrant expression and activation of NAD(P)H oxidase and consequent endothelial dysfunction in vivo: role of 26S proteasomes. Circ Res 106: 1117–1128.
26. Shen Y, Honma N, Kobayashi K, Jia LN, Hosono T, et al. (2014) Cinnamon extract enhances glucose uptake in 3T3-L1 adipocytes and C2C12 myocytes by inducing LKB1-AMP-activated protein kinase signaling. PLoS One 9: e87894.
27. Homolya L, Fu D, Sengupta P, Jarnik M, Gillet JP, et al. (2014) LKB1/AMPK and PKA control ABCB11 trafficking and polarization in hepatocytes. PLoS One 9: e91921.
28. Wang S, Zhang C, Zhang M, Liang B, Zhu H, et al. (2012) Activation of AMP-activated protein kinase alpha2 by nicotine instigates formation of abdominal aortic aneurysms in mice in vivo. Nat Med 18: 902–910.

29. Zhao HL, Sui Y, Qiao CF, Yip KY, Leung RK, et al. (2012) Sustained antidiabetic effects of a berberine-containing Chinese herbal medicine through regulation of hepatic gene expression. Diabetes 61: 933–943.
30. Yang Y, Ni W, Cai M, Tang L, Wei W (2014) The renoprotective effects of berberine via the EP4-Gαs-cAMP signaling pathway in different stages of diabetes in rats. J Recept Signal Transduct Res 22: 1–11.
31. Tang LQ, Liu S, Zhang ST, Zhu LN, Wang FL (2014) Berberine regulates the expression of E-prostanoid receptors in diabetic rats with nephropathy. Mol Biol Rep 41: 3339–3347.
32. Chatuphonprasert W, Lao-Ong T, Jarukamjorn K (2013) Improvement of superoxide dismutase and catalase in streptozotocin-nicotinamide-induced type 2-diabetes in mice by berberine and glibenclamide. Pharm Biol.
33. Wan X, Chen X, Liu L, Zhao Y, Huang WJ, et al. (2013) Berberine ameliorates chronic kidney injury caused by atherosclerotic renovascular disease through the suppression of NFkappaB signaling pathway in rats. PLoS One 8: e59794.
34. Han Y, Wang Q, Song P, Zhu Y, Zou MH (2010) Redox regulation of the AMP-activated protein kinase. PLoS One 5: e15420.
35. Wang Q, Zhang M, Liang B, Shirwany N, Zhu Y, et al. (2011) Activation of AMP-activated protein kinase is required for berberine-induced reduction of atherosclerosis in mice: the role of uncoupling protein 2. PLoS One 6: e25436.
36. Qi Z, Fujita H, Jin J, Davis LS, Wang Y, et al. (2005) Characterization of susceptibility of inbred mouse strains to diabetic nephropathy. Diabetes 54: 2628–2637.
37. Zhang M, Liu M, Xiong M, Gong J, Tan X (2012) Schisandra chinensis fruit extract attenuates albuminuria and protects podocyte integrity in a mouse model of streptozotocin-induced diabetic nephropathy. J Ethnopharmacol 141: 111–118.
38. Dugan LL, You YH, Ali SS, Diamond-Stanic M, Miyamoto S, et al. (2013) AMPK dysregulation promotes diabetes-related reduction of superoxide and mitochondrial function. J Clin Invest 123: 4888–4899.

Permissions

All chapters in this book were first published in PLOS ONE, by The Public Library of Science; hereby published with permission under the Creative Commons Attribution License or equivalent. Every chapter published in this book has been scrutinized by our experts. Their significance has been extensively debated. The topics covered herein carry significant findings which will fuel the growth of the discipline. They may even be implemented as practical applications or may be referred to as a beginning point for another development.

The contributors of this book come from diverse backgrounds, making this book a truly international effort. This book will bring forth new frontiers with its revolutionizing research information and detailed analysis of the nascent developments around the world.

We would like to thank all the contributing authors for lending their expertise to make the book truly unique. They have played a crucial role in the development of this book. Without their invaluable contributions this book wouldn't have been possible. They have made vital efforts to compile up to date information on the varied aspects of this subject to make this book a valuable addition to the collection of many professionals and students.

This book was conceptualized with the vision of imparting up-to-date information and advanced data in this field. To ensure the same, a matchless editorial board was set up. Every individual on the board went through rigorous rounds of assessment to prove their worth. After which they invested a large part of their time researching and compiling the most relevant data for our readers.

The editorial board has been involved in producing this book since its inception. They have spent rigorous hours researching and exploring the diverse topics which have resulted in the successful publishing of this book. They have passed on their knowledge of decades through this book. To expedite this challenging task, the publisher supported the team at every step. A small team of assistant editors was also appointed to further simplify the editing procedure and attain best results for the readers.

Apart from the editorial board, the designing team has also invested a significant amount of their time in understanding the subject and creating the most relevant covers. They scrutinized every image to scout for the most suitable representation of the subject and create an appropriate cover for the book.

The publishing team has been an ardent support to the editorial, designing and production team. Their endless efforts to recruit the best for this project, has resulted in the accomplishment of this book. They are a veteran in the field of academics and their pool of knowledge is as vast as their experience in printing. Their expertise and guidance has proved useful at every step. Their uncompromising quality standards have made this book an exceptional effort. Their encouragement from time to time has been an inspiration for everyone.

The publisher and the editorial board hope that this book will prove to be a valuable piece of knowledge for researchers, students, practitioners and scholars across the globe.

List of Contributors

Song Ding., Longwei Xu, Fan Yang, Lingcong Kong, Yichao Zhao, Lingchen Gao, Wei Wang, Rende Xu, Heng Ge, Meng Jiang, Jun Pu and Ben He
From Department of Cardiology, Ren Ji Hospital, School of Medicine, Shanghai Jiao Tong University, Shanghai, China

Francisco I. Ramirez-Perez
Dalton Cardiovascular Research Center, University of Missouri, Columbia, Missouri, 65211, United States of America
Department of Biological Engineering, University of Missouri, Columbia, Missouri, 65211, United States of America

Angela L. Schenewerk and Rocio M. Rivera
Division of Animal Sciences, University of Missouri, Columbia, Missouri, 65211, United States of America

Katy L. Coffman
Department of Statistics, University of Missouri, Columbia, Missouri, 65211, United States of America

Christopher Foote
Dalton Cardiovascular Research Center, University of Missouri, Columbia, Missouri, 65211, United States of America

Tieming Ji
Department of Statistics, University of Missouri, Columbia, Missouri, 65211, United States of America

Luis A. Martinez-Lemus
Department of Medical Pharmacology and Physiology, University of Missouri, Columbia, Missouri, 65211, United States of America

Hong Yang, Enling Ye, Liangmiao Chen, Lingqiao Cai, Chengfu Ye and Xuemian Lu
Department of Endocrinology, the Third Hospital Affiliate to Wenzhou Medical University, Ruian, Zhejiang, China
Ruian Center of the Chinese-American Research Institute for Diabetic Complications, the Third Affiliated Hospital of the Wenzhou Medical University, Wenzhou, China

Guangxin Si
Department of Endocrinology, Shangdong Jining No. 1 People's Hospital, Jining, Shangdong, China

Chi Zhang
Ruian Center of the Chinese-American Research Institute for Diabetic Complications, the Third Affiliated Hospital of the Wenzhou Medical University, Wenzhou, China

Shanshan Tang, Rong Zhang, Feng Jiang, Jie Wang, Miao Chen, Danfeng Peng, Jing Yan, Yuqian Bao, Cheng Hu and Weiping Jia
Shanghai Diabetes Institute, Department of Endocrinology and Metabolism, Shanghai Key Laboratory of Diabetes Mellitus, Shanghai Clinical Center for Diabetes, Shanghai Jiao Tong University Affiliated Sixth People's Hospital, Shanghai, PR China

Yi-Chun Tsai and Mei-Chuan Kuo
Graduate Institute of Clinical Medicine, Kaohsiung Medical University, Kaohsiung, Taiwan
Division of Nephrology, Kaohsiung Medical University Hospital, Kaohsiung, Taiwan
Faculty of Renal Care, Kaohsiung Medical University, Kaohsiung, Taiwan

Yi-Wen Chiu, Hung-Tien Kuo and Hung-Chun Chen
Division of Nephrology, Kaohsiung Medical University Hospital, Kaohsiung,
Taiwan
Faculty of Renal Care, Kaohsiung Medical University, Kaohsiung, Taiwan

Szu-Chia Chen
Faculty of Renal Care, Kaohsiung Medical University, Kaohsiung, Taiwan Department of Internal Medicine, Kaohsiung Municipal Hsiao-Kang Hospital, Kaohsiung, Taiwan

Shang-Jyh Hwang
Graduate Institute of Clinical Medicine, Kaohsiung Medical University, Kaohsiung, Taiwan
Division of Nephrology, Kaohsiung Medical University Hospital, Kaohsiung, Taiwan

Faculty of Renal Care, Kaohsiung Medical University, Kaohsiung, Taiwan
Institute of Population Sciences, National Health Research Institutes, Miaoli, Taiwan

Tzu- Hui Chen
Department of Nursing, Kaohsiung Medical University Hospital, Kaohsiung, Taiwan

Muralikrishna Gangadharan Komala, Simon Gross, Harshini Mudaliar, Chunling Huang, Katherine Pegg, Amanda Mather, Sylvie Shen, Carol A. Pollock and Usha Panchapakesan
Renal Research Lab, Kolling Institute of Medical Research, Sydney University, Royal North Shore Hospital, St Leonards, Australia

Yinchen Shen, Ning Wang, Zhi Zheng, Kun Liu, Xin Xia, Qing Gu and Xun Xu
Department of Ophthalmology, Shanghai First People's Hospital, Shanghai Jiao Tong University, Shanghai, People's Republic of China, Shanghai Key Laboratory of Fundus Disease, Shanghai, People's Republic of China

Zujia Wen and Yongyong Shi
Bio-X Institutes, Key Laboratory for the Genetics of Developmental and Neuropsychiatric Disorders (Ministry of Education), Shanghai Jiao Tong University, Shanghai, People's Republic of China

Shu-Ching Chen and Pei-Yu Chang
Department of Medical Research, National Taiwan University Hospital, Taipei, Taiwan

Yu-Chia Su
National Laboratory Animal Center, National Applied Research Laboratories, Taipei, Taiwan

Ya-Ting Lu, Hung-Ju Lin and Yo-Ping Lai
Department of Internal Medicine, National Taiwan University Hospital, Taipei, Taiwan

Patrick Chow-In Ko
Department of Emergency Medicine, National Taiwan University Hospital, Taipei, Taiwan

Hong-Nerng Ho
Department of Obstetrics and Gynecology, National Taiwan University, College of Medicine, Taipei, Taiwan

Konstantinos Sombolos
Nephrology Clinic, Papanikolaou Hospital, Thessaloniki, Greece

Demitrios Tsakiris
Nephrology Clinic, Papageorgiou Hospital, Thessaloniki, Greece

John Boletis
Nephrology Clinic, Laiko Hospital, Athens, Greece

Demetrios Vlahakos
Nephrology Clinic, ATTIKON University Hospital, Athens, Greece

Kostas C. Siamopoulos
Nephrology Clinic, Ioannina University Hospital, Ioannina, Greece

Vassilios Vargemezis
Nephrology Clinic, Alexandroupoli University Hospital, Alexandroupoli, Greece

Pavlos Nikolaidis
Nephrology Clinic, AHEPA Hospital, Thessaloniki, Greece

Christos Iatrou
Center for Nephrology, G Papadakis, Nikea Hospital, Athens, Greece

Eugene Dafnis
Nephrology Clinic, PE.PA.G.N.I, Crete University Hospital, Iraklio, Greece

Konstantinos Xynos
AbbVie Pharmaceuticals, Chicago, Illinois, United States of America

Christos Argyropoulos
AbbVie Pharmaceuticals SA, Athens, Greece

Peter Willeit
Department of Neurology, Innsbruck Medical University, Innsbruck, Austria
Department of Public Health and Primary Care, University of Cambridge, Cambridge, United Kingdom

Julia Raschenberger, Margot Haun and Florian Kronenberg
Division of Genetic Epidemiology, Innsbruck Medical University, Innsbruck, Austria

Emma E. Heydon and Adam S. Butterworth
Department of Public Health and Primary Care, University of Cambridge, Cambridge, United Kingdom

Sotirios Tsimikas and Joseph L. Witztum
Department of Medicine, University of California San Diego, La Jolla, United States of America

Agnes Mayr
Department of Laboratory Medicine, Bruneck Hospital, Bruneck, Italy

Siegfried Weger
Department of Internal Medicine, Bruneck Hospital, Bruneck, Italy

Johann Willeit and Stefan Kiechl
Department of Neurology, Innsbruck Medical University, Innsbruck, Austria

Pawel P. Wolkow and Beata Bujak-Gizycka
Centre for Medical Genomics OMICRON, Jagiellonian University Medical College, Krakow, Poland
Department of Pharmacology, Jagiellonian University Medical College, Krakow, Poland

Wladyslaw Kosiniak-Kamysz, Grzegorz Osmenda, Grzegorz Wilk and Adam Ignacak
Department of Internal and Agricultural Medicine, Jagiellonian University Medical College, Krakow, Poland

Mihir Kanitkar and David G. Harrison
Department of Clinical Pharmacology, Vanderbilt University, Nashville, TN, United States of America

Malgorzata Walus-Miarka
Department of Metabolic Diseases, Jagiellonian University Medical College, Krakow, Poland

Ryszard Korbut
Department of Pharmacology, Jagiellonian University Medical College, Krakow, Poland

Maciej T. Malecki
Department of Metabolic Diseases, Jagiellonian University Medical College, Krakow, Poland
University Hospital, Krakow, Poland

Tomasz J. Guzik
Department of Internal and Agricultural Medicine, Jagiellonian University Medical College, Krakow, Poland
Institute of Cardiovascular and Medical Sciences, University of Glasgow, Glasgow, United Kingdom

Shaik M. Fayaz, Valsala S. Suvanish Kumar and Krishnamurthy G. Rajanikant
School of Biotechnology, National Institute of Technology Calicut, Calicut 673601, India

Terri R. Fried
Clinical Epidemiology Research Center, VA Connecticut Healthcare System, West Haven, Connecticut, United States of America
Department of Medicine, Yale School of Medicine, New Haven, Connecticut, United States of America

John O'Leary and Deanna K. Martin
Clinical Epidemiology Research Center, VA Connecticut Healthcare System, West Haven, Connecticut, United States of America
Program on Aging, Yale School of Medicine, New Haven, Connecticut, United States of America

Virginia Towle and Mark Trentelange
Program on Aging, Yale School of Medicine, New Haven, Connecticut, United States of America

Mary K. Goldstein
Palo Alto Geriatrics Research Education and Clinical Center (GRECC), VA Palo Alto Health Care System, Palo Alto, Connecticut, 94304, United States of America
Center for Primary Care and Outcomes Research, Stanford University School of Medicine, Stanford, California, 94305, United States of America

Hyuk Nam Kwon, Yong Jin An, Sunmi Kang and Sunghyouk Park
College of Pharmacy, Natural Product Research Institute, Seoul National University, Sillim-dong, Gwanak-gu, Seoul, Korea, 151-742

Yeon Ji Lee and Ji-ho Choi
Department of Family Medicine, Obesity center, Inha University Hospital, Inha University School of Medicine, Shinheung-dong, Jung-Gu, Incheon, Korea, 400-712

Ju-Hee Kang
Department of Pharmacology and Hypoxia-related disease Research, Inha University Hospital, Inha University School of Medicine, Shinheung-dong, Jung-Gu, Incheon, Korea, 400-712

Dae Hyun Lee
Department of Medicine, Inha University Hospital, Inha University School of Medicine, Shinheung-dong, Jung-Gu, Incheon, Korea, 400-712

Young Ju Suh
Department of Biostatistics, Inha University Hospital, Inha University School of Medicine, Shinheung-dong, Jung-Gu, Incheon, Korea, 400-712

Yoonseok Heo
Department of General Surgery, Inha University Hospital, Inha University School of Medicine, Shinheung-dong, Jung-Gu, Incheon, Korea, 400-712

Ron L. H. Har and David Z. I. Cherney
Division of Nephrology, University Health Network - Toronto General Hospital, Banting and Best Diabetes Centre, University of Toronto, Toronto, Ontario, Canada

Heather N. Reich and James W. Scholey
Division of Nephrology, University Health Network - Toronto General Hospital, Toronto, Ontario, Canada

Denis Daneman, Laura Motran, Yesmino Elia, Livia Deda, Masha Ostrovsky, Etienne B. Sochett and Farid H. Mahmud
Department of Pediatrics, Division of Endocrinology, Hospital for Sick Children, University of Toronto, Toronto, Ontario, Canada

David B. Dunger
Department of Pediatrics, University of Cambridge, Cambridge, United Kingdom

Rahim Moineddin
Family and Community Medicine, University of Toronto Toronto, Ontario, Canada

R. Neil Dalton
WellChild Laboratory, Evelina Children's Hospital, St Thomas' Hospital, London, United Kingdom

Joanna Kern, Robert Drutel, Silvia Leanhart, Marek Bogacz and Rafal Pacholczyk
Center for Biotechnology and Genomic Medicine, Georgia Regents University, Augusta, Georgia, United States of America

Katharina Hellhammer, Tobias Zeus, Jan Balzer, Silke van Hall, Christos Rammos, Rabea Wagstaff, Malte Kelm and Tienush Rassaf
University Hospital Düsseldorf, Medical Faculty, Dept. of Medicine, Division of Cardiology, Pulmonology and Vascular Medicine, Düsseldorf, Germany

Firoz Akhter
Department of Bio-Engineering, Integral University, Lucknow, India
Department of Bio-Sciences, Integral University, Lucknow, India

M. Salman Khan and Saheem Ahmad
Department of Bio-Sciences, Integral University, Lucknow, India

Sarika Singh
Department Toxicology, Central Drug Research Institute (CDRI), Lucknow, India

Sergio E. Starkstein and Milan Dragovic
School of Psychiatry & Clinical Neuroscience, University of Western Australia, Crawley, Western Australia, Australia

Wendy A. Davis, Violetta Cetrullo, Timothy M. E. Davis and David G. Bruce
School of Medicine & Pharmacology, University of Western Australia, Crawley, Western Australia, Australia

E Song
Lixiang Eye Hospital of Soochow University, Suzhou, China

Hongpeng Sun, Yong Xu, Yana Ma, Hong Zhu and Chen-Wei Pan
School of Public Health, Medical College of Soochow University, Suzhou, China

Yann C. Klimentidis and Jin Zhou
Mel and Enid Zuckerman College of Public Health, Division of Epidemiology and Biostatistics, University of Arizona, Tucson, Arizona, United States of America

Nathan E. Wineinger
Scripps Translational Science Institute, La Jolla, California, United States of America

Yogeeta O. Agrawal
School of Pharmaceutical Sciences, Jaipur National University, Jagatpura, Jaipur, Rajasthan, India
Department of Pharmacology, All India Institute of Medical Sciences, New Delhi, India
Department of Pharmaceutics and Pharmacology, R. C. Patel Institute of Pharmaceutical Education and Research, Shirpur, Maharashtra, India

Pankaj Kumar Sharma and Birendra Shrivastava
School of Pharmaceutical Sciences, Jaipur National University, Jagatpura, Jaipur, Rajasthan, India

Shreesh Ojha
Department of Pharmacology and Therapeutics, College of Medicine and Health Sciences, United Arab Emirates University, Al-Ain, United Arab Emirates

Harshita M. Upadhya
Sunil's Daibetes and Research Center, Nagpur, Maharashtra, India

Dharamvir Singh Arya
Department of Pharmacology, All India Institute of Medical Sciences, New Delhi, India

Sameer N. Goyal
Department of Pharmaceutics and Pharmacology, R. C. Patel Institute of Pharmaceutical Education and Research, Shirpur, Maharashtra, India

Long Zhao, Li-Na Sun, Hui-Bin Nie, Xue-Ling Wang and Guang-Ju Guan
Nephrology Research Institute, the Second Hospital of Shandong University, Jinan, Shandong, China

Index